Transcultural
Caring Dynamics
in Nursing and
Health Care
2nd edition

Transcultural Caring Dynamics in Nursing and Health Care

2nd edition

By
Marilyn A. Ray, RN, PhD, CTN-A, FAAN
Col. (Ret.), United States Air Force (USAF), Nurse Corps
Professor Emeritus
Florida Atlantic University
The Christine E. Lynn College of Nursing
Boca Raton, Florida

F.A. Davis Company • Philadelphia

F. A. Davis Company
1915 Arch Street
Philadelphia, PA 19103
www.fadavis.com

Printed in the United States of America

Last digit indicates print number: 10 9 8 7 6 5 4 3 2

Senior Acquisitions Editor: Susan R. Rhyner
Content Project Manager: Julia L. Curcio
Electronic Project Editor: Katherine E. Crowley
Design and Illustration Manager: Carolyn O'Brien

As new scientific information becomes available through basic and clinical research, recommended treatments and drug therapies undergo changes. The author(s) and publisher have done everything possible to make this book accurate, up to date, and in accord with accepted standards at the time of publication. The author(s), editors, and publisher are not responsible for errors or omissions or for consequences from application of the book, and make no warranty, expressed or implied, in regard to the contents of the book. Any practice described in this book should be applied by the reader in accordance with professional standards of care used in regard to the unique circumstances that may apply in each situation. The reader is advised always to check product information (package inserts) for changes and new information regarding dose and contraindications before administering any drug. Caution is especially urged when using new or infrequently ordered drugs.

Library of Congress Cataloging-in-Publication Data

Names: Ray, Marilyn Anne, author.
Title: Transcultural caring dynamics in nursing and health care / by Marilyn A. Ray.
Description: 2nd edition. | Philadelphia, PA : F.A. Davis Company, [2018] | Includes bibliographical references and index.
  | Reprint. Originally published: Philadelphia : F.A. Davis Co., 2016.
Identifiers: LCCN 2018015812 (print) | LCCN 2018019571 (ebook) | ISBN 9780803689763 | ISBN 9780803677548
  (pbk. : alk. paper)
Subjects: | MESH: Transcultural Nursing—methods | Nursing Care | Culturally Competent Care—methods
Classification: LCC RT86.54 (ebook) | LCC RT86.54 (print) | NLM WY 107 | DDC 610.73—dc23
LC record available at https://lccn.loc.gov/2018015812

ISBN: 978-0-8036-7754-8
eISBN: 978-0-8036-8976-3

To the memory of my late husband,
James L. Droesbeke
Loving husband, devoted son, caring person

And
To the memory of my late parents,
Arthur and Elvera Ray
Caring parents, great teachers, spiritual
advisors

And
To all of my family, teachers, colleagues, and
students who have encouraged and supported
me throughout my nursing career

And
Ravil Troncoso, Information Technologist,
for his assistance

The Cover: Sunflower World

Sunflower World

By H. Lea Barbato Gaydos, PhD, RN

Sunflower World is about the interconnectedness of all things. It is in the tradition of a *mandala*, the Sanskrit word for "whole world" or "healing circle." Mandalas are usually very colorful and found in many spiritual traditions. The purpose of a mandala is to provide a focus for meditation and reflection. There are three symbolic elements for reflection in *Sunflower World.*

First, in this work, the earth is encompassed by the sunflower, which is meant to symbolize the beauty and harmony of the world as it exists in nature. Second, the mosaic background represents the multiplicity of peoples and cultures that inhabit our world, different in color, shape, and tradition, but essentially the same in our humanity. Like the sunflower that follows the light, we must look to our intrinsic nature and compassionate caring to transcend our differences and find our wholeness as human beings in relationship with others. Third, the green bars that bisect the image horizontally and vertically represent the four directions; they resemble a ribbon, suggesting a gift, the gift of life.

The aesthetic for this piece was inspired by the work of Lily Yeh, Founder and Director of Barefoot Artists, Inc. and her work with people in Africa who had experienced genocide. With the community of survivors, she created a healing garden memorial to the dead where before they had only had a mass grave of concrete.

Marilyn A. Ray, RN, PhD, CTN-A, FAAN

Colonel, Retired, USAF, Nurse Corps

Marilyn A. (Dee) Ray, RN, PhD, CTN-A, FAAN is a Professor Emeritus at Florida Atlantic University, The Christine E. Lynn College of Nursing, Boca Raton, Florida, where she has served for more than 25 years. Throughout her nursing career, she has worked as a clinical nurse in different roles in various hospitals, held faculty positions at the University of California San Francisco, and the University of San Francisco, the University of Colorado Denver Anschutz Medical Campus, College of Nursing, Denver, Colorado, and McMaster University, Hamilton, Canada, and has served in two Eminent Scholar positions at Florida Atlantic University and Virginia Commonwealth University respectively. She holds a diploma from St. Joseph Hospital, Hamilton, Canada, bachelor of science and master of science degrees in nursing from the University of Colorado, Denver, Colorado, a master of arts degree in cultural anthropology from McMaster University in Hamilton, Canada, and a doctor of philosophy degree in transcultural nursing from the University of Utah. Dr. Ray also participated in the two ethics programs of study at Georgetown University, Kennedy Institute of Ethics. She is a Fellow of the Society for Applied Anthropology, and received the first honorary degree conferred by Nevada State College, Henderson, Nevada. Dr. Ray was inducted as a Fellow of the American Academy of Nursing in 2013. As an officer in the United States Air Force Reserve, Nurse Corps, she retired as a Colonel after more than 30 years of service in flight nursing, clinical practice, administration, education, research, and consultation in aerospace nursing. Dr. Ray was a principal investigator on many federal grants with her colleague and co-principal investigator, Dr. Marian Turkel. Their research using both qualitative and quantitative methods involved the study of nurse and administrative caring in complex organizational cultures with emphasis on technological, political, economic, legal and humanistic and spiritual-ethical caring. The research of Drs. Ray and Turkel earned the Federal Nursing Essay Award for research from the Association of Military Surgeons of the United States (AMSUS), and the coin for excellence in nursing research from the TriService Nursing Research Program of the Uniformed Services University of the Health Sciences (USUHS). As an advanced certified transcultural nurse (CTN-A), and a Transcultural Nursing Scholar, Dr. Ray has published widely on the subjects of caring in organizational cultures, caring theory, and caring inquiry, transcultural caring, transcultural ethics, technological caring, political and economic caring, spiritual caring, complex caring dynamics, complexity sciences, and relational caring theory in the economics of the nurse-patient relationship. She also has published in the qualitative research area, specifically phenomenology and hermeneutics, the grounded theory method, caring inquiry, and critical social theory. Dr. Ray's Bureaucratic Caring Theory has been used in many health-care organizations throughout the world and published in many nursing theory books. The book, *Caring Within an Institutional Culture: The Discovery of the Theory of Bureaucratic Caring,* was published in 2010. Dr. Ray contributed to the core curriculum development for certification of the Transcultural Nursing Society with her model of transcultural caring dynamics, and qualitative research methods. She co-edited a book, *Nursing, Caring, and Complexity Science: For Human-Environment Well-Being,* with Dr. Marian Turkel, in honor of the complexity scientist in nursing, the late Dr. Alice Davidson, which won the 2011 American Journal of Nursing Book of the Year award for professional development. At Florida Atlantic University, Dr. Ray serves as a guest teacher, continues to work with doctoral students, and is a faculty mentor. In addition, she is on the review boards of the *Journal of Transcultural Nursing and Qualitative Health Research* and the on-line journal, *Global Qualitative Nursing Research (GQNR)*. Dr. Ray also presents and keynotes at many national and international conferences, for example, in Switzerland at the World Universities Forum, in Vancouver, Canada, at the Clinical Nurse Society Educators Conference, in Thailand at many universities, in Japan at the 35th International Human Caring Conference, in the Philippines at the Qualitative Health Research Conference, and in Vietnam at the Humanistic Nursing Conference.

Dr. Ray's collection of Caring Science and Bureaucratic Caring Theory, Transcultural Nursing, Complexity Science, and Qualitative Research scholarly works and United States Air Force uniform, insignia, and memoirs are housed in the Museum and Archives of Caring, Florida Atlantic University, The Christine E. Lynn College of Nursing, Boca Raton, Florida. Also, significant information can be found on her website, www.marilynray.com.

With global issues related to health care, economics, hunger, deep poverty, environmental planet changes, rapid growth in technology and innovation, and conflict instead of peace, caring remains the essence of nursing and the core of our humanity. For more than 50 years, nursing scholars have been studying human caring through the lenses of education, practice, and research. The theme for the 35th International Association for Human Caring Conference held in Kyoto, Japan, May 2014, was the Universality of Caring. The conference opened with scholars presenting papers on transcultural nursing and caring. Dr. Marilyn Ray served as a conference cochair. Dr. Ray is a renowned scholar at the national and international levels in the area of caring and an expert in interweaving caring through complexity science and transcultural nursing theory and practices. World-recognized scholars, Dr. Jean Watson and Dr. Ray hosted a special tribute to the late Dr. Madeline Leininger, the founder of transcultural nursing, on the evening of May 24, 2015, to recognize her commitment to transcultural caring and nursing. Dr. Ray is a professional colleague and personal friend of both Dr. Watson and the late Dr. Leininger. Dr. Ray was a doctoral student of Dr. Leininger at the University of Utah and a faculty member at the University of Colorado Denver Anschutz Medical Campus, College of Nursing when Dr. Watson was Dean. The papers at the conference highlighted the universality of human caring, the diversity of our shared humanity, and the scholarship of caring from around the world.

I was privileged to meet Dr. Ray in 1989 when I was a graduate student at Florida Atlantic University and Dr. Ray was the eminent scholar within the College of Nursing. We shared a common research and theoretical interest related to caring within complex systems, caring and economics, and caring leadership. I was co-principal investigator with Dr. Ray on almost $1 million in federally funded research grants focused on caring and economics.

I thank Dr. Ray for her leadership, creative vision for this book, and lifelong commitment and dedication to the advancement of transcultural caring.

Dr. Ray's scholarship and unique contribution to the discipline and profession of nursing are the focus on transcultural caring dynamics within complex systems. Dr. Ray's 1981 doctoral dissertation examined caring within the culture of a hospital. The emerging theory of bureaucratic caring illustrated the integration of humanistic spiritual-ethical caring and organizational foci—the political, legal, technological, and economic systems. The theory reveals that nursing in organizational practice is experiential, contextual, and structural, and caring is influenced by the social structure of the organization, especially the technological, legal, political, and economic. Dr. Ray's ongoing research and scholarship continue to advance the relationship among caring, human care, transcultural nursing, and complexity science. Dr. Ray was inducted as a Fellow in the American Academy of Nursing in 2013 for her seminal and sustaining contribution to the discipline and profession of nursing.

Transcultural Caring Dynamics in Nursing and Health Care shows us the way forward, as the practice of caring in nursing is universal to all cultures. Caring may be expressed differently in various cultures but remains the core of humanity and relationships. Through Dr. Ray's scholarship and the scholarship of the contributors to this book, we recognize and come to know the deeper meaning of caring across cultures. The theoretical and evidence-based exemplars remind us of the need to continue to advance caring across the world as human caring transcends all cultures, and the chapters in this book facilitate the understanding and advancement of culturally congruent care.

This book integrates theory, practice, and evidence of transcultural caring from nurses and healthcare professionals around the world. The structure of this book moves from the theoretical and philosophical tenets of transcultural caring written by

Dr. Ray to narratives of transcultural caring experiences written by a community of scholars including nursing faculty, nursing leaders, and nurses in practice. These exemplars support and extend the need of providing culturally congruent nursing care. This second edition of the book reflects changes in global cultural contexts and includes chapters focusing on Muslim American culture, Ebola and African culture, Japanese culture, the culture of nursing and nursing education, European (Scandinavian) culture and ethics, the role of transcultural nursing and the United Nations within the context of the post 2015 Millennium Development Goals, the Filipino culture with an emphasis on the culture of indigenous people and the culture of poverty, Thai culture from the perspective of Muslim and Buddhist religions, the Haitian culture as a community of caring, and the meaning of the universality of caring.

I am honored and privileged to write the new foreword for this book and endorse this scholarly work as an exemplar of transcultural caring and transcultural nursing. I recommend this book to nursing faculty, nursing students at all levels, nursing leaders, and health-care professionals and nurses in the practice setting. This seminal work keeps alive the legacy of Dr. Leininger and reflects the scholarship and leadership of Dr. Ray to transcultural caring.

As you read this book, I hope you appreciate and value the theoretical tenets, models, and ideas of Dr. Ray and the unique transcultural caring experiences written by a cadre of scholars. I hope that you use the theory and experiences to inform and transform your own practice of nursing as an educator, researcher, or practitioner. I extend an invitation to you, the reader, to reflect on your own practice and look for creative and innovative approaches to make transcultural caring explicit within your own practice and the world. As healers, we have an ethical commitment and obligation to do this work, as transcultural caring is the way to world peace.

Written with intentionality and love, Marian

Marian C. Turkel, PhD, RN, NEA-BC, FAAN
Immediate Past President, International
  Association for Human Caring
Director Professional Practice, Research, Holy
  Cross Hospital, a Magnet® Hospital,
  Fort Lauderdale, Florida
Courtesy Adjunct Associate Professor,
The Christine E. Lynn College of Nursing,
Florida Atlantic University, Boca Raton,
  Florida

©The Magnet Recognition Program is a registered trademark of the American Nurses Credentialing Center.

FOREWORD TO THE 1ST EDITION

Forward to the 1st Edition of this book by the late Dr. Madeleine Leininger, the founder and "mother" of transcultural nursing.

At no time in the history of humankind has there been so many major and subtle changes in the world. Changes and the processes of change are occurring worldwide and influencing the values of human beings, and altering their environments, societies, economics, politics, and spiritual and ethical lifeways. These changes are related to many factors but especially to new technologies, human innovations, rapid transportation, changing economic conditions, new kinds of intercultural relationships, geopolitical challenges, wars, climatic shifts in temperature, and major language and living changes. Granted some of these changes can occur rather quickly and others very slowly over time and geological locations. From an anthropological perspective, many of the major geo-environmental changes have been occurring over millions of years and documented by archaeologists, geologists, climate experts as well as by spiritual leaders and human life specialists. These changes are of major concern to most humans locally and globally, but especially to professional nurses.

In the process of such changes and their consequences, the phenomenon of human caring and its effect on the health and well-being of people is important to study and reflect upon through time and in different geographical environments. Political, economic, social, cultural, spiritual, moral-ethical, and environmental factors play a key role in one's health and well-being. Unquestionably, changes and especially cultural care changes do alter or affect the thinking activities and health status of human beings. In the field of nursing, human life changes have been clearly evident in the care of people in most cultures. Many people struggle to understand and respond to such changes in their daily lives. Amidst these changes the importance of caring for and with humans in order to receive quality health care and/or to survive; grow; be healed; and face death, disabilities, or handicaps are foremost in the minds of professional nurses. Two frequent questions, Who cares for whom, and who cares for health professionals are often heard in the thinking, words, and actions of many nurses.

Over the past 50 years, a cadre of professional nurse scholars have studied and documented human caring. Among these caring scholars has been the author of this book, Dr. Marilyn Ray, who has focused on transcultural caring dynamics in nursing and health care. Dr. Ray has interwoven the essence of caring, transcultural caring ethics, transcultural context and universal sources (spirituality) into a model for awareness, understanding, and choice for patients and families of diverse cultures regarding health, healing, and well-being.

The essence of nursing as human care has been studied in many Western and non-Western societies from holistic, transcultural nursing perspectives, and frequently by using my Theory of Culture Care Diversity and Universality with the Sunrise Enabler and other transcultural care enablers, and the Ethnonursing research method. It was in the late 1950s that I began this movement to study care and caring from transcultural theoretical and research perspectives. At that time, I discovered in nursing and in institutional care settings that cultural factors were woefully missing to understand and help people of diverse cultures. This was, indeed, a major shock to me so I took steps to prepare nurses in transcultural nursing and to incorporate cultural care meanings and research findings into nursing practice. While this was a slow process, my theory gradually became an integral part of many nurses' thinking and nursing practice by the late 1970s. It was during this time period as Dean and Professor at the University of Utah that I had the opportunity and special privilege to know and help prepare Dr. Ray in transcultural care research and theory. As one of the first nurses to pursue graduate study and research in transcultural nursing, Dr. Ray obtained her doctor of philosophy degree focusing on the study of the meaning of caring within institutional contexts. Through her research, she discovered the Theory of Bureaucratic Caring within complex organizations. She is well known and recognized for major research contributions to human caring, organizational caring, and transcultural nursing.

In this book, it was most encouraging to find that Dr. Ray focused on the complex phenomena of human caring dynamics and processes from transcultural nursing viewpoints. This book is truly a breakthrough not only to understand the dynamics of human caring, but to understand how local and global cultural and organizational processes and contexts influence and shape care meanings and expressions that affect choices for health, healing, and well-being. To achieve this goal, Dr. Ray's research and observations provide new and fresh insights about human caring dynamics and the complexities of transcultural relationships within changing local and global cultural contexts.

As I reflect on Dr. Ray's creative work, several factors come to mind in addition to her intellectual astuteness and research abilities. Dr. Ray has had 50 years of professional nursing practice, education, and research, and more than 30 years as an officer culminating with the rank of Colonel in the United States Air Force Reserve. She gained valuable experience in aerospace nursing service and research, which gave her unique insights to explore complex, sometimes invisible, and multifaceted care phenomena. Most importantly, Dr. Ray had the love and compassion of her parents and family, along with many spiritual advisors who instilled in her faith and the love of God's creation and the universe. Moreover, her beloved husband, Jim, and many caring teachers and colleagues over the years were important role models and mentors to discover and know caring.

Today, transcultural nursing with a human care focus has become a major and essential academic area of study and practice. Many transcultural nursing practitioners, faculty, administrators, and other nursing leaders have contributed to the growth of transcultural nursing as a discipline. This positive change is remarkable when contrasted with the fact that specific cultures were often neglected, avoided, or misunderstood. Today, research-based practice using or developing explicit theories and models has facilitated the advancement of transcultural understanding and culturally congruent care. Unquestionably, transcultural care knowledge has become a major national and global trend in the study of human cultures.

Since the purpose of a Foreword is to open the door to all who are interested to explore ideas presented in a book, I believe that the above points should greatly stimulate and encourage readers to read this book, and to discover a true scholar and leader of transcultural nursing. Dr. Ray is to be commended for this milestone contribution and excellent book, *Transcultural Caring Dynamics in Nursing and Health Care*. I recommend it to teachers, beginning students, graduate students, administrators, and practitioners and the many in the health professions who desire to continue to learn about human caring and the multiple factors that influence transcultural nursing care. Dr. Ray has discussed the "rough diamond" and has polished and made it shine as a brilliant gem for nurses and other professionals. I wholeheartedly endorse this scholarly publication that advances human caring and the complexities of transcultural care theory and knowledge to improve the health of and help people of diverse cultures worldwide.

Madeleine M. Leininger, PhD, LHD, DS, RN, CTN-A, FAAN, FRCNA (1925–2012)
Founder and Leader of Transcultural Nursing and Human Care, the Theory of Culture Care Diversity and University, and the Ethnonursing Research Method
Professor Emeritus, Wayne State University, and Clinical Professor, University of Nebraska, Omaha
Distinguished Lecturer and Global Consultant Collection on Human Caring and Transcultural Nursing and Anthropology, Archives of Caring, Christine E. Lynn College of Nursing Museum Archives at Florida Atlantic University, Boca Raton, Florida

PREFACE

In the past few decades, the rapidly changing world around us has produced enormous challenges. Changes in science, technology, transportation, economics, and health care, and expanded knowledge of the meaning of spirituality and religion have affected all cultures at local and global levels. Advancement in the different disciplines of knowledge shows how closely we are interconnected. Science has illuminated new paradigm thinking, the new sciences of complexity that consider the profound relationship between the mind and nature, the mutual human-environment process. New thinking about human values, societies, the environment, cultural diversity, geopolitical communities, health, and our common future is transforming societies. The search for the relationships between nature and consciousness, matter, and mind have helped to illuminate the fertile link among quantum science, art, different worldviews, psychology, language, creativity, theology, and the social-cultural world. Technology has provided the opportunity to learn how we are linked together by information and communication. Technology and transportation are helping us understand the meaning of history, environments, location, space, immigration, affluence, and poverty while seeing the world, people, and cultures in new ways. Economics illustrates the importance of resources and how being stewards of resources worldwide, we can assist with complex human, social, environmental, health, and political problems in every nation and in space. Religions, while often divisive, continue to help us understand the true meaning of spirituality and its illumination of love and compassion and social justice for all people of the world. Health-care research and practice illuminates ways in which we should and can provide improved health care for all. From a nursing perspective, by virtue of our understanding of human caring, awareness of the importance of relationships, holism (i.e., body, mind, and spirit), and integration of the holistic nature of the mutual human-environment process, we show how the scientist and artist in us, engage the *cultural other* and explore new ways of encountering all people in the world. As we begin to recognize the complexity of the universe, we can see culture as transcultural or intercultural and as dynamic and complex. Culture as dynamic complexity mirrors complexity sciences that highlight the meaning of interconnectedness; it shows how we must work together to enact our caring natures, to be ethically responsible for each other and the environment, to find meaning in transcultural contexts—understanding of the person in family, community, organizations, and societies—and to appreciate the spiritual and religious values, beliefs, and creativity of one another. "We are whole and unique. We are diverse but communal. We are in the midst of a remarkable transition to building the global civic culture, to understanding a global civilization that will work for each inhabitant of the universe and for the universe itself."

In nursing, we are fortunate to experience the joy and sorrow of life in our everyday work. Even though we often may feel that our caring efforts are in vain or our good intentions are not appreciated or rewarded, we know that when in an authentic relationship with another person, family, or community who rely upon us for compassion and help, we affect the healing, health, and well-being of those whom we serve. The theory and conceptual model identified in this book, *Transcultural Caring Dynamics in Nursing and Health Care,* with its dimensions: the Essence of Caring, Transcultural Caring Ethics, Transcultural Context for Transcultural Nursing, Universal Sources, and Transcultural Caring Inquiry: Awareness, Understanding, and Choice, enable us to explore and understand nursing as a transcultural caring dynamic process, specifically a transcultural communicative spiritual-ethical caring way of being, knowing, and doing. This theory and conceptual model support the provisions of professional nursing education outlined, for example, in the United States by the American Association of Colleges of Nursing (2006, 2008, 2011) by providing a framework to practice holistically; create a culture of safety and caring; and understand culture, complexity science, and caring science and art. Thus, the central phenomena of the dimensions of this theory and conceptual framework are processes used by each of us when we become aware, seek understanding, and make choices affecting our health, healing, and well-being. Participating in the processes of awareness, understanding, and choice helps us to become more transculturally competent (accountable and responsible) to provide culturally relevant or congruent care to patients, families, communities, and citizens of the globe.

The Essence of Caring highlights the history of caring and its importance in human relationships and various disciplines. Caring in contemporary nursing is illuminated from the commitment of nursing to relationships and the human-environment process beginning first with Florence Nightingale and including Jeanne Mance of Canada through to Martha Rogers and the caring theorists of the past three decades, such as Roach, Watson, and the late Madeleine Leininger. Leininger, the "mother" of transcultural nursing, was instrumental in advancing caring as the essence of nursing and the concept is foundational to her theory in *Culture Care Diversity and Universality: A Worldwide Theory of Nursing* (Leininger, 1991; Leininger & McFarland, 2006, McFarland & Wehbe-Alamah, 2015).

Transcultural Caring Ethics illuminates essentially how we ought to live when we share a common world. Ethics deals with issues and theories of "serving the good" and how cultures have values in common but with contending ideas, theories, and ways of expressing the understanding of morality and what is required of us in professional nursing when examining culture and its diversity and commonality.

Transcultural Context for Transcultural Nursing identifies the centrality of the human-environment process, the unity of persons within their cultural contexts. Transcultural context highlights the human-environment integral relationship, the person (race and identity), and the person in family (kinship system, group, or community), and illuminates ethnicity, panethnicity, societal and organizational systems in local and global communities. As such, the transcultural context also examines multiculturalism, interculturality, and transculturality in the changing world culture and nursing.

Universal Sources outlines the importance of spirituality and/or religion in all choice-making processes in conjunction with the understanding of caring as transcultural ethics and within a transcultural context. Some of the dominant religions or spiritual traditions in the world are presented.

Transcultural Caring Inquiry: Awareness, Understanding, Choice highlights how nurses use the model and its components and the assessment tools for inquiry—knowledge and evidence for awareness, understanding, and the facilitation of choice for the patient, community, and sociocultural healing, health, well-being, or a peaceful death.

The book, *Transcultural Caring Dynamics in Nursing and Health Care,* in the second edition as in the first edition, includes a presentation of transcultural caring experiences (stories/case studies, nursing situations) at the end of each chapter in Section 1 where the conceptual model and dimensions are featured, and in Section 2 where many transcultural caring experiences illuminate the diversity and dynamics of culture and transcultural nursing in a global world. The content of the book helps to reveal information and wisdom that is embedded in each one of us as cultural/multicultural beings. Illuminating information in the conceptual framework presented in this book provides a means to deal with both details and difficulties that nurses as transcultural professionals may encounter each day.

The Online Instructor Resources on DavisPlus available at davisplus.fadavis.com/ feature lesson plans, PowerPoints, and multiple-choice questions for teaching-learning purposes for instructors, including professionals from other healthcare/social science disciplines. Chapters 6 and 7 provide learning tools/models to enhance development of knowledge of patterns and processes of caring, culture, and complexity science in nursing and health-care situations to improve the health and well-being of patients, families, and local and global communities. Becoming culturally competent in transcultural nursing and health-care practice is achieved through the knowledge and skill of transcultural caring ethics or becoming responsible and accountable for the self-in-relation. Transcultural caring competency is a co-creative process of relating formed by awareness, seeking understanding, and facilitating choice making of spiritual-ethical caring knowledge and interaction. Devoting my attention to exploring the complexities of nursing from a transcultural perspective has been a great pleasure for me. I have learned so much from my experiences in nursing practice, education and research, traveling, and from my deep relationships with family, friends, and colleagues. I am pleased to have this opportunity to share with you not only my ideas and experiences but also some ideas and experiences of other people who have contributed to and enriched this book.

The ideas that are discussed in this book are important in an interconnected and global society. They have arisen in the course of exploring nursing through education, research, administration, and practice over time, and observing and studying changes in the contemporary world. They have arisen through teaching and learning opportunities in the classroom and in many countries of our world. They have arisen through my many interactions with people of diverse cultures, including three children I have the privilege to sponsor from Nicaragua, Guatemala, and Honduras. Moreover, the ideas expressed have arisen from the opportunities for service, education, and travel during my career in the United States Air Force Reserve, Nurse Corps. These ideas would not come to life, however, without the participation of each of the readers of this book. For me, the evolution of this book came to fruition only because of love and help from God, the devotion of my late husband and support from my remarkable family, and the many creative students, colleagues, friends, and publishers and editors whom I have had the privilege to know. This book evolved also with my hope in the future despite an often gloomy outlook on the world stage and to the possibilities that may emerge from the readers who are committed to transcultural nursing and caring. The contributions of each one of you will improve the healing, health, well-being, and peaceful deaths of our patients who, although may be different, share a common humanity.

I wish to mention those who have been particularly connected with this work and the activities that have led to its completion. As I mentioned in my dedication, I am deeply grateful to my parents and late husband for their enduring belief in me as a person

and as a transcultural nursing professional, to my family who did not give up on me, to my colleagues and production team at F. A. Davis Company, especially Joanne DaCunha, Susan Rhyner, and Julia Curcio, who always gave me hope and encouragement, and to the many wonderful contributors who made this work a living history and a road map for possibilities, for a truly transcultural caring future in a complex world. I am most grateful to Anne Vitale, and Mary Brigid Martin who assisted me with the Instructor Guide, and to Lea, for her Sunflower World cover painting and narrative that is an inspiration for all transcultural caring nurses.

M. A.R

References

American Association of Colleges of Nursing. (2006). *The essentials of doctoral education for advanced nursing practice*. Washington, DC: American Association of College of Nursing.

American Association of Colleges of Nursing. (2008). *The essentials of baccalaureate education for professional nursing practice*. Washington, DC: American Association of College of Nursing.

American Association of College of Nursing. (2011). *The essentials of master's education in nursing*. Washington, DC: American Association of Colleges of Nursing.

Leininger, M. (1991). *Culture care diversity and universality: A worldwide theory of nursing*. New York, NY: National League for Nursing Press.

Leininger, M., & McFarland, M. (2006). *Culture care diversity and universality: A worldwide theory of nursing* (2nd ed.). Sudbury, MA: Jones & Bartlett.

McFarland, M., & Wehbe-Alamah, H. (2015). *Leininger's culture care diversity and universality: A worldwide nursing theory* (3rd ed.). Burlington, MA: Jones & Bartlett Learning.

CONTRIBUTORS

Charlotte Barry, RN, PhD, NCSN FAAN
Professor and Master Teacher
Florida Atlantic University
The Christine E. Lynn College of Nursing
Boca Raton, Florida
Chapter 17 Haitian Family's Health Experience
and the Public School System
Chapter 32 Coming to Know a Community:
A Community Assessment in Rural Haiti

Anita Beckerman, EdD, ARNP
The Late Associate Professor Emeritus
Florida Atlantic University
The Christine E. Lynn College of Nursing
Boca Raton, Florida
Chapter 20 The Heart of Suffering, Mourning,
and Healing in the Jewish Spiritual Culture:
A Mother's Story

A. Judith Czerenda, RN, DNS, ARNP, LNHA
Nursing Consultant
Fort Lauderdale, Florida
Chapter 11 The Transcultural Social and Health
Experience of an Asian Indian Widow

Charlotte Delmar, RN, PhD
Professor in Clinical Nursing Science
Health Faculty, Institute of Public Health
and Institute of Clinical Medicine
Aarhus University
Aarhus, Denmark
Chapter 29 A Danish/Norwegian Culture
Nursing Care Model: An Ethical Demand

Susana Fortun, PhD
Program Dean—Technology
DeVry University
Miami, Florida
Chapter 14 with Dr. Marilyn Ray: Cuban American
Transcultural Experiences and the Quest for
Freedom in the United States: New Era Beginning

Rhonda Goodman, PhD, ARNP, FNP-BC, NCSN, AHN-BC
Assistant Professor
Christine E. Lynn College of Nursing Florida
Atlantic University
Boca Raton, Florida
Chapter 32 Coming to Know a Community: A
Community Assessment in Rural Haiti

Valarie S. Grumme, MSN, RN, CCRN, PhD(c)
Clinical Manager, MICU/CCU
Memorial Regional Hospital
Hollywood, Florida
Chapter 32 Coming to Know a Community: A
Community Assessment in Rural Haiti

Diane Gullett, PhD Candidate, MSN, MPH, RN
Adjunct Instructor
Christine E. Lynn College of Nursing
Florida Atlantic University
Boca Raton, Florida
Chapter 32 Coming to Know a Community: A
Community Assessment in Rural Haiti

Agnes Hay, RN, MSN
Former Associate Chief Nursing Officer
Boca Raton Community Hospital
Boca Raton, Florida
Chapter 12 with Dr. Marilyn Ray: The Cultural,
Health Care, and Intermigration Experience of
a Filipino Nurse

Mary Enzman Hines, FNP, AHN-BC, RN, PhD

Professor Emeritus
University of Colorado, Colorado Springs
Beth-El College of Nursing and Health Sciences
Colorado Springs, Colorado
Chapter 23 American Nurses and the Native People of Ecuador: The Transcultural Experience of Shamanism

Florence Keane, DNS, MBA, ARNP-NPC

Retired Assistant Professor
Florida International University
College of Nursing and Health Sciences
University Park Campus
Miami, Florida
Chapter 13 Transcultural Diversity Within Unity in Jamaica: Out of Many, One People

Beth M. King, PhD, PMHCNS-BC, RN

Assistant Professor
Christine E. Lynn College of Nursing
Florida Atlantic University
Boca Raton, Florida
Chapter 32 Coming to Know a Community: A Community Assessment in Rural Haiti

Waraporn Kongsuwan, RN, PhD

Professor
Medical Nursing Department
Faculty of Nursing
Prince of Songkla University
Hat Yai, Songkhla, Thailand
Chapter 27 Transcultural Caring for Buddhists and Muslims in Thailand

Rozzano C. Locsin, RN, PhD, FAAN

Professor of Nursing
Institute of Health BioSciences,
Department of Nursing, Faculty of Health Sciences
University of Tokushima
Tokushima Prefecture, Japan.
Professor Emeritus
Florida Atlantic University
Christine E. Lynn College of Nursing
Boca Raton, Florida
Chapter 28 "Like a Moth to a Flame": Ebola and the Culture of Caregiving in Sub-Saharan Africa

Mary Brigid Martin, RN, FNP-BC, CTN-A, PhD

Faculty
Keiser University Graduate Nursing
Nursing Professional Development Specialist
Transcultural Nurse
Ft. Lauderdale, Florida
Chapter 22 Extending Understanding: Transcultural Caring for Muslims in the United States
Chapter 30 Considerations Within the United Nations for Transcultural Nursing: Global Initiatives for Caring, Peace, and Quality of Life

Gerald Amandu Matua, RN, BSN, MNSc, DLitt et Phil

Lecturer of Nursing
College of Nursing, Sultan Qaboos University
Muscat, Sultanate of Oman
Former Head and Senior Lecturer,
School of Nursing, International Health Sciences University
Kampala, Uganda
Chapter 28 "Like a Moth to a Flame": Ebola and the Culture of Caregiving in Sub-Saharan Africa

Tasanee Nasae, RN, PhD

Assistant Professor
Administration of Nursing Education and Nursing Service Department
Faculty of Nursing
Prince of Songkla University
Hat Yai, Songkhla, Thailand
Chapter 27 Transcultural Caring for Buddhists and Muslims in Thailand

Erlinda Castro Palaganas, RN, PhD

Editor-in-Chief, *Philippine Journal of Nursing*
President, Philippine Nursing Research Society, Inc.
Professor, Institute of Management
Head, Graduate Program Office
Member, KASARIAN Gender Studies Program
College of Social Sciences
University of The Philippines
Baguio, The Philippines
Chapter 31 Transcultural Caring Among the Indigenous People of the Cordilleras, The Philippines

Marilyn A. Ray, RN, PhD, CTN-A, FAAN
Professor Emeritus
Florida Atlantic University
The Christine E. Lynn College of Nursing
Boca Raton, Florida
Chapters 2–10, 15, 16, 18, 21, 22, 25, 30

Francelyn Reeder, RN, CNM, PhD
Associate Professor Emeritus
University of Colorado, Anschutz Medical Center
    Campus
Denver, Colorado
Chapter 18 with Dr. Marilyn Ray: The Elderly
    Navajo Native American's Health Experience in
    the Nursing Home Culture

M. Christopher Saslo, ARNP, DNS
Chief Nursing Officer
Veterans Affairs Medical Center
Biloxi, Mississippi
Chapter 24 The Culture of Physical, Mental,
    Spiritual, and Political/Sociocultural Illness:
    Healing Through Education and Love

The 49ers of Booker T. Washington High School
The Late Harold L. Braynon, JD (July 24, 2011)
Sara (Faye) Summons Bullard
Effie R. Fortson
Whittington B. Johnson, PhD
Moses Jones, Jr., Maj. (Ret.), United States Army
Percy L. Oliver
Cortell H. Owens
Chapter 9 with Dr. Marilyn Ray: A Vibrant African
    America Community: The 49ers and the Quest
    for Justice

Mayumi Tsutsui, RN, PhD
Professor
Dean of Graduate School
The Japanese Red Cross College of Nursing
Shibuya-ku, Tokyo, Japan
Chapter 26 Transcultural Nursing and
    Ethnonursing for Japanese Graduate Students at
    Red Cross College of Nursing, Tokyo, Japan

Marian C. Turkel, PhD, RN, NEA-BC, FAAN
Immediate Past President
International Association for Human Caring
Former Director Professional Practice, Research,
    Magnet
Holy-Cross Hospital
Fort Lauderdale, Florida
Associate Professor
The Christine E. Lynn College of Nursing
Florida Atlantic University
Boca Raton, Florida
Chapter 33 Reflections on The Universality of
    Caring

Josie A. Weiss, ARNP, PhD
Professor
University of Central Florida
Orlando, Florida
Retired Associate Professor
Florida Atlantic University
The Christine E. Lynn College of Nursing
Boca Raton, Florida
Chapter 19 The Transcultural Caring Experience
    of a Haitian Girl and a Nurse Practitioner in an
    Adolescent Correctional Facility

Sara Fuller, PhD, APRN, CPNP
Associate Professor
University of South Carolina
College of Nursing
Columbia, South Carolina

Nelma B. Shearer, PhD, RN
Associate Professor
Arizona State University
College of Nursing and Healthcare Innovation
Phoenix, Arizona

Joyce M. Varner,
RN, MSN, GNP-BC, GCNS, DNPc
Clinical Assistant Professor
University of South Alabama
College of Nursing
Springhill Campus
Mobile, Alabama

ACKNOWLEDGMENTS

I wish to acknowledge and thank my teacher, mentor, colleague, and friend, the late Dr. Madeleine Leininger, the first nurse anthropologist, "mother" of transcultural nursing, and inspiration for the development of nursing as a human science, and caring as the essence of nursing. Dr. Leininger guided me through my bachelor and master of science in nursing, supported me through my master of arts in anthropology, and directed my efforts to achieve the doctor of philosophy in transcultural nursing.

I wish to acknowledge all of the people who helped me begin to understand myself as a cultural, multicultural, caring, and spiritual being, beginning first with my family; the aboriginal, French Canadian and immigrant people of my native land, Canada; and, after coming to the United States as an immigrant myself, the many people of diverse cultures who also have made their home in the United States. All have enriched my life with their fascinating histories, stories of the Diaspora, immigration, and the struggle and joy in finding meaning in new diverse and exciting communities. I am also grateful to all the people I met through my commission as an officer and affiliation with the United States Air Force, Nurse Corps. With nurturing from my loving husband and family, and many wonderful friends—in particular Drs. Francelyn Reeder, Carolyn Brown, and Marian Turkel, my Deans, students, and colleagues—I was able to achieve the goals in my life: the ability to explore the interrelationship among science, art, and the sacred and how nursing as a science and art embraces holism, human caring, ethical responsibility, transcultural awareness, and spirituality. I wish to acknowledge all of those who have encouraged me not only to reach for the stars in my personal life but also to find deep meaning in a career dedicated to the study and practice of human caring, human science, and transcultural nursing.

I wish to thank all the contributors to this book. I thank Dr. H. Lea Barbato Gaydos for her cover painting. I am grateful to all of the nurses who have shared their stories of transcultural caring at home and around the world in the second section of this book. I wish to thank Joanne DaCunha, retired Publisher and Editor, F. A. Davis Company, for her belief in me and transcultural caring, and her constant encouragement and patience to complete this work. I wish to thank Editors Susan Rhyner and Julia Curcio for their support with the 2nd edition of my book. I would not have been able to accomplish this book without the commitment, perseverance, and assistance of my Developmental Editor, Caryn Abramowitz. I am so appreciative of the talent and skill my co-authors of the Instructor Guide, Dr. Anne Vitale and Dr. Mary Brigid Martin who, with their knowledge of both in-class and online education will help to make this work accessible to many faculty and students around the world. Lastly, I am indeed grateful to my first edition copy editor, Julie Vitale, Lisa Thompson, my 2nd edition content project manager, Julia Curcio, and the whole production team at F. A. Davis Company.

May this book inspire students as the late Dr. Leininger inspired me. May this book help professionals seek understanding of the transcultural theory/model and meaning of professional nursing as a transcultural caring discipline and practice.

TABLE OF CONTENTS

SECTION 1
Theory and Conceptual Model and Applications   *1*

CHAPTER 1 Theoretical and Transcultural Caring Dynamics in Nursing and Health Care   3
By Marilyn A. Ray

CHAPTER 2 The Essence of Caring   35
By Marilyn A. Ray

CHAPTER 3 Transcultural Caring Ethics   67
By Marilyn A. Ray

CHAPTER 4 Transcultural Context for Transcultural Nursing   100
By Marilyn A. Ray

CHAPTER 5 Universal Sources   131
By Marilyn A. Ray

CHAPTER 6 Transcultural Caring Inquiry: Awareness, Understanding, and Choice   166
By Marilyn A. Ray

SECTION 2
Transcultural Caring Experiences   *199*

CHAPTER 7 Transcultural Caring Competency in Transculturally Dynamic Communities   201
By Marilyn A. Ray

CHAPTER 8 The Border and Pueblo: An American Mexican Cultural Experience   216
By Marilyn A. Ray

CHAPTER 9 A Vibrant African American Community: The 49ers and the Quest for Justice   223
By The Community of 49ers with Marilyn A. Ray

CHAPTER 10 The Story of a Guatemalan Mayan Farmworker   230
By Marilyn A. Ray

CHAPTER 11 The Transcultural Social and Health Experience of an Asian Indian Widow   235
By A. Judith Czerenda

CHAPTER 12 The Cultural, Health-Care, and Intermigration Experience of a Filipino Nurse   239
By Marilyn A. Ray with Agnes Hay

CHAPTER 13 Transcultural Diversity Within Unity in Jamaica: Out of Many, One People   244
By Florence Keane

CHAPTER 14 Cuban American Transcultural Experiences and the Quest for Freedom in the United States: A New Era Beginning   250
By Susana Fortun and Marilyn A. Ray

CHAPTER 15 Puerto Rican Transcultural
and Health Beliefs in a
Western New York
Community   256
By Marilyn A. Ray in memory of
Barbara Higgins

CHAPTER 16 The Nurse Manager in a
Cardiovascular Intensive
Care Unit and the
Organizational Complexity
of a Hospital Culture   260
By Marilyn A. Ray

CHAPTER 17 Haitian Family's Health
Experience and the Public
School System   267
By Charlotte Barry

CHAPTER 18 Elderly Native American
Navajo's Health Experience
in the Nursing Home
Culture   271
By Marilyn A. Ray with Francelyn
Reeder

CHAPTER 19 The Transcultural Caring
Experience of a Haitian Girl
and a Nurse Practitioner
in an Adolescent
Correctional Facility   277
By Josie A. Weiss

CHAPTER 20 The Heart of Suffering,
Mourning, and Healing in
the Jewish Spiritual
Culture: A Mother's
Story   282
By Anita Beckerman

CHAPTER 21 The American Chinese
Transcultural Maternal-
Child and Family
Experience in China   290
By Marilyn A. Ray

CHAPTER 22 Extending Understanding:
Transcultural Caring for
Muslims in the United
States   296
By Mary Brigid Martin

CHAPTER 23 American Nurses and the
Native People of Ecuador:
The Transcultural
Experience of
Shamanism   307
By Mary Enzman Hines

CHAPTER 24 The Culture of Physical,
Mental, Spiritual, and
Political/Sociocultural
Illness: Healing Through
Education and Love   313
By M. Christopher Saslo

CHAPTER 25 The Political-Legal Culture
of Multiculturalism and
Interculturality: The Story
of Canada   320
By Marilyn A. Ray

CHAPTER 26 Transcultural Nursing
and Ethnonursing for
Japanese Graduate
Students at Red Cross
College of Nursing,
Toyko, Japan   328
By Maymi Tsutsui

CHAPTER 27 Transcultural Caring
for Buddhists and
Muslims in Thailand   342
By Waraporn Kongsuwan and
Tasanee Nasae

CHAPTER 28 "Like a Moth to a Flame:"
Ebola and the Culture
of Caregiving in
Sub-Saharan Africa   352
By Gerald Amandu Matua, and
R. Locsin

CHAPTER 29 A Danish/Norwegian
Culture Nursing Care
Model: An Ethical
Demand   374
By Charlotte Delmar

CHAPTER 30 Considerations Within the United Nations for Transcultural Nursing: Global Initiatives for Caring, Peace, and Quality of Life 388
By Mary Brigid Martin and Marilyn A. Ray

CHAPTER 31 Transcultural Caring Among the Indigenous People of the Cordilleras, The Philippines 401
By Erlinda Castro Palaganas

CHAPTER 32 Coming to Know a Community: A Community Assessment in Rural Haiti 420
By Charlotte D. Barry, Beth M. King, Rhonda Goodman, Valarie Grumme, and Diane Gullett

CHAPTER 33 Reflections on the Universality of Caring 431
By Marian C. Turkel

INDEX 440

Section 1

Theory and Conceptual Model and Applications

Objectives

1. To present an introduction to the *Transcultural Caring Dynamics in Nursing and Health Care* book, theory, and model, and each dimension of the model (i.e., the essence of caring, transcultural caring ethics, transcultural context for transcultural nursing, and universal sources) to develop an awareness of, assess, guide, and evaluate nursing from transcultural, multicultural, and global perspectives. (See Section 2 for application of the dimensions of this book in diverse transcultural caring experiences [i.e., case studies/stories] to facilitate health, healing, well-being, or a peaceful death.)

2. To illuminate the processes of globalization and its effect on nursing and the meaning of nursing as transcultural caring.

3. To understand the meaning of culture as dynamic complexity that incorporates traditional views of culture and the new sciences of complexity.

4. To appreciate the notions of cultural diversity and cultural universality in co-creating a common humanity.

5. To present the history and emergence of caring in human culture.

6. To appreciate the emergence of caring in the discipline and profession of transcultural nursing.

7. To identify transcultural caring ethics in relation to the history of ethical theories (primarily Western) that has influenced the discipline and profession of transcultural nursing.

8. To appreciate the person, family, community, and organizations within a transcultural context for transcultural nursing.

9. To understand concepts such as identity, ethnicity, panethnicity, and interculturality/transculturality.

10. To appreciate the concept of universal sources—the roles of religion and spirituality in the choice-making process in transcultural nursing.

11. To identify major dimensions of the major religions and beliefs in world culture.

12. To present a transcultural caring inquiry that integrates the dimensions of the theory and conceptual model for awareness, understanding, and choice in transcultural nursing practice.

13. To identify for purposes of application a variety of tools for inquiry and culturological assessment, planning, and evaluation to enhance the Transcultural Caring Dynamics for Nursing and Health-Care model. The tools include: Transcultural Caring Dynamics Assessment Tool, Ray's Transcultural Spiritual-Ethical Communicative Caring (CARING) Tool, Transcultural Caring Culture Value Conflict Assessment Tool, and Negotiation Tools for Choice—the Dynamics of Transcultural Caring Tool for Choice and the Transcultural Caring Negotiation Tool.

14. To present transcultural caring experiences (i.e., case studies/stories) at the end of each chapter in Section 1 to highlight the discussions of each chapter dimensions (i.e., essence of caring, transcultural caring ethics, transcultural context for transcultural nursing, and universal sources) for teaching-learning and reflection.

CHAPTER 1

Transcultural Caring Dynamics in Nursing and Health Care

Our era lures us to create the first global civilization on earth.
We are the generation that begins the creative transformation of
the whole world into a single community out of the diverse
peoples of the planet. (Fox & Swimme, 1982, p. 6)

Chapter Objectives

1. Develop awareness of nursing from transcultural, multicultural, and global worldviews.
2. Examine the concepts of caring, transcultural caring, caring for self and self-reflection, ways of knowing, and culture as dynamic complexity.
3. Identify issues in globalization—diversity, cultural identity, economics, technology, multiculturalism, and immigration.
4. Apply the concepts of the multicultural self and transcultural consciousness.
5. Conceptualize the theory and conceptual model of Transcultural Caring Dynamics in Nursing and Health Care.
6. Analyze the transcultural caring experiences of Monique, Kathleen, and Lian to appreciate the concepts in transcultural caring in nursing practice and enhance awareness and understanding of transcultural caring dynamics in nursing and health care.

KEY WORDS

Globalization • culture • technological culture (internet and social media) • multiculturalism • culture as dynamic complexity • cultural sensitivity • health-care issues • alternative therapies • caring • holistic nursing • transcultural worldview • transcultural nursing • transcultural caring • ways of knowing in nursing • Transcultural Caring Dynamics in Nursing and Health-Care Model • Theory and Model

*T*he purpose of this book is to teach nurses transcultural caring dynamics, to understand and care for people of different cultures as they interact with each other locally, nationally, and transglobally. Readers will explore each dimension of the Transcultural Caring Dynamics in Nursing and Health-Care Theory and Model (Fig. 1-1)—the essence of caring, transcultural caring ethics, transcultural context, and universal sources—as the foundation for awareness, understanding, and choice. The chapters outlining each dimension of the model will be followed by case studies that illustrate the dimension being explored. The book will then delve into use and application of a variety of tools for inquiry, culturological assessment, planning, and evaluation; the Transcultural Caring Dynamics Assessment Tool; Ray's Transcultural Spiritual-Ethical Communicative Caring (CARING) Tool; Transcultural Caring Culture Value Conflict Assessment Tool; and Negotiation Tools for Choice—the Dynamics of Transcultural Caring Tool for Choice and the Transcultural Caring Negotiation Tool. The final part of the book will present a variety of transcultural caring experiences to discuss and analyze using the Transcultural Caring Based Learning (TCCBL) model, the Transcultural Caring Dynamics in Nursing and Health-Care Model, and the assessment tools. These practical applications will guide students and professionals in developing culturally sensitive, creative transcultural caring practice

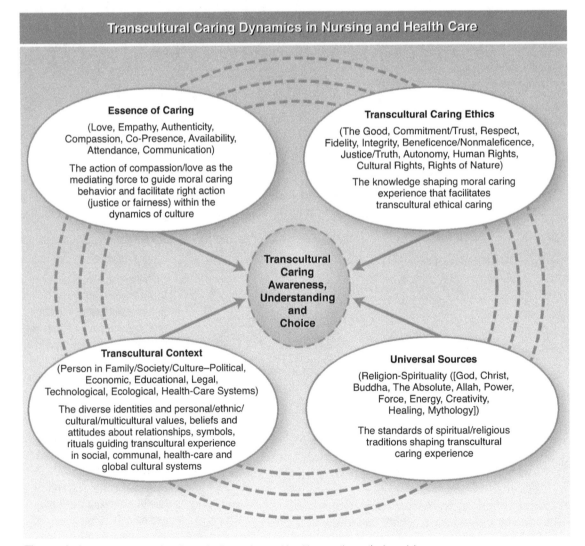

Figure 1–1: Transcultural caring dynamics in nursing and health-care theoretical model.

skills when working with individuals and families from diverse cultures, communities, and nations.

Before going into details, we must first grasp the basics, which is the purpose of this chapter. Transcultural caring dynamics is a theory with four dimensions (the essence of caring, transcultural caring ethics, transcultural context, and universal sources (spirituality/religions). This theory is an interrelational, transcultural human-environmental process (a conceptual system organized for a co-created purpose or intention of communicative-spiritual ethical caring) that features the dominant constructs of the sciences of complexity (human-environment interconnectedness, dynamism, holography, chaos), the discipline of nursing (humanism, caring science, relationship, love, compassion, health), transcultural ethics (values, honoring the good and respect for persons, human and cultural rights), the social sciences (the sociocultural, political, economic, technological, legal, and educational contexts—weaving of the themes of human-environment relationship), and spirituality or religions (universal sources of beliefs and values across all cultures). Each of these theoretical constructs or phenomena interacts to facilitate awareness, understanding, and choice making for health, healing, well-being, or a peaceful death (the center of the model). The fundamental assumptions of the theory (illumination of the meaning of transcultural caring) are the following:

- caring is holistic—mind, body, spirit;
- caring is transcendent;
- caring is the unfolding of the sacred art of divine love;
- caring is the human mode of being
- caring is the process of relationship and interconnectedness;
- caring is love and co-presence as the essential nature of nursing;
- caring involves understanding of compassion as love and right action and as justice (fairness) in culturally dynamic nursing and health care situations;
- caring is dynamic, relational, transcultural, complex, and emergent, grounded in the sciences of complexity, communication, and transculturality (collaboration);
- caring involves ways of knowing, personal, empirical (scientific knowledge), ethical (moral knowledge), and aesthetic (artistic knowledge and the art of nursing), and is recognized as transcultural and knowledge-in-process (culturally sensitive, dynamic, and emergent);

- caring includes the cultural context of nursing and health-care situations and society and organizations (weaving or integration of the economic, political, technological, legal, and sociocultural);
- caring involves forgiveness and reconciliation;
- caring fosters spiritual-ethical communication that illuminates transcultural and multicultural competency (accountability and responsibility for self and others within a process of negotiation for choice making);
- caring enhances awareness, understanding, and choice making for health, healing, well-being, and peaceful dying and death.

Transcultural caring in nursing is a culmination of a number of forces, each of which we will review and define in this chapter: globalization, caring, holistic nursing, nursing paradigms and ways of knowing, culture, transcultural consciousness, transcultural caring, health, and multiculturalism and transculturality. After examining these basic components, we will turn to a discussion of the Transcultural Caring Dynamics in Nursing and Health-Care as a Theory and Model and its application to transcultural nursing practice.

Globalization

Globalization is causing a worldwide reformation, transformation, and integration of cultures, and it is here to stay. Science is manifesting that "this universe is a single, multiform energetic unfolding of matter, mind, intelligence and life" (Swimme, 1996). New technologies, including transportation, space, and communication infrastructures, and changing ideological, economic, environmental, and social forces have thrust countries around the world toward globalization, causing shifts in every sector from economics to technology, politics to military, and entertainment to health (Breda, 2009; Friedman, 2006; Gutierrez & Kendall, 2000; Pensky, 2005; Rogers, 2003; Sachs, 2005; Zwingle, 1999). This worldwide shift toward globalization intimately affects our encounters with, and our perception of, culture, cultural diversity, and cultural universality. Migration is also a critical factor (Leininger, 1991; Leininger & McFarland, 2006; McFarland & Wehbe-Alamah, 2015). East is meeting west and south is meeting north, so it is our responsibility to be mindful of the differences and not take for granted the similarities.

As the world is becoming more dynamic and complex, new patterns of relationships are emerging. Each nation and culture, with its unique values

Learn More

The racial and ethnic populations of North American countries are growing differently than they have in the past. Immigration is having a greater impact on population growth. According to the U.S. Census Bureau (2008), the population is expected to grow from 320 million in 2014 to 438 million in 2020 to 500 million in 2050 (https://www.census.gov/population/projections/data/national/2008.html). A good portion of the increase will be attributable to immigrants of non-English speaking countries. The Pew Research Report (Passel & Cohn, 2008) projected that 82% of the increase will be due to immigrants arriving (67 million), and their U.S.-born descendants (50 million) during this period. By 2042, the minority population will be the majority (Winslow, 2008). One in five Americans (19%) will be an immigrant in 2050. The Latino/Hispanic population is the nation's largest minority (15% in 2008 and projected to be 30% by the year 2050). Population growth of the black population in 2050 is projected to rise to 15% at 65.7 million from 14% in 2008. Asian American population growth is expected to rise in 2050 to 9% from 5 % in 2008. Population growth of American Indians/Alaska Natives is expected to rise from 1.6% to 2% (4.9 million to 8.6 million). Native Hawaiians and Pacific Islanders are projected to double from 1.1 million to 2.6 million. The white population is expected to decrease from 67% to 47% in 2050. (https://www.census.gov/population/projections/data/national/2008/downloadablefiles.html).

and perspectives, must rise to the challenges presented by globalization by reflecting upon creative ways to handle complex problems, and cultural differences while sharing worldwide resources (Bar-Yam, 2004; Boulding, 2000; Eisler, 2007; Lindberg, Nash, & Lindberg, 2008; McFarland & Wehbe-Alamah, 2015; Sachs, 2005). Individual cultures need to be aware of how they will change and grow as cultures interact. Technology, communication technology, travel, and immigration especially have joined people together. We are all aware of the impact of the social media culture (Behar, 2013; Floridi, 2013) and how porous borders for potential migration are between and among nations (Chomsky, 2014). Such challenges present extraordinary opportunities for health-care professionals, such as nurses. Different cultures perceive wealth and health, disease and illness, caring and death in very different ways. But there is a force toward understanding the universality of what it means to be human in the world, and the practice of securing competency and human rights in health and cultural care (Breda, 2009; Douglas & Pacquiao, 2010; Giger, Davidhizar, Purnell, Harden, Phillips, & Strickland, 2007; *Journal of Transcultural Nursing*, 2007, Special Issue, Vol. 18, No. 1; Martin, 2015; Miller, Leininger, Leuning, Pacquiao, Andrews, Ludwig-Beymer, & Papadopoulous, 2008; Ray & Turkel, 2014; Sager, 2012). As more cultures seek access to health resources, nurses will be the ones responsible for understanding, facilitating, and integrating traditional culture into modern approaches to health and

nursing care. Transcultural caring-based nursing practice can improve the quality of care and health for diverse and vulnerable populations.

In 21st century North America, individuals are challenged with globalization and identity (Brush, 2008). Different cultures are assimilating less and blending more despite struggles in some parts of the world. More frequently, individuals of different

Learn More

The population of Canada is more than 34 million people. Seventy percent of ethnic groups are visible minorities (a term used in Canada) and were born outside the country. One hundred languages are represented. In 2017, one in five Canadians is projected to be a visible minority or between 19% to 25% of the population (2006 Canadian Census, Statistics Canada, 2006). *The Daily* (Statistics Canada, March 22, 2005) reported that currently, most minorities, about 58%, are from China, South Asia, Korea and Japan, and the Middle East (West Asia). The remaining immigrants are from the United States, Latin America, and Europe. In 2017, Canada's First Nations' and Inuit peoples (aboriginals) will represent 4.1% of the population, up from 3.4% in 2001, a rise from 1.39 million to 1.43 million (2014 Canadian Census, Statistics Canada. www.statcan.ca).

cultures are preserving their cultural diversity by choice and in symbol and rituals, and adding their diversity to the ever-changing mix of values, customs, lifeways, norms, and artifacts already in place. Out of this mix emerges a new understanding and an interconnectedness that will open humans to emotional and intellectual cultural innovation. One common feature to all cultures and people is the human capacity to care deeply for people and, now, the environment, regardless of origins.

GLOBALIZATION IN NURSING

And this brings us to the heart of nursing—caring for others. Nursing is becoming increasingly dedicated to holism, healing the split among body, mind, and spirit, and renewing a commitment to the focus of nursing as global health, and caring in the human health experience (Gennaro, 2008; Leininger & McFarland, 2006; Newman, 2003; Newman, Smith, Dexheimer-Pharris & Jones, 2008; Ray & Turkel, 2014; Watson, 1999, 2005, 2008a, 2008b). In these times of cultural intermixing, this central phenomenon of caring, although a universal value, becomes more complex. Different cultures express care and caring in different ways and it is incumbent upon nurses in North America and around the world to understand, acknowledge, and incorporate innovative and varied transcultural caring expressions into their practice.

Ironically, for a profession charged with the obligation to learn about and effectively care for many different cultures, nursing is not very representative of the country's cultural diversity, representing only 19% of the population (www.allnursingschools.com, 2014). Despite the fact that by the year 2042, the U.S. Census Bureau projects that the nation will become much more diverse and minorities will become the majority (Winslow, 2008), the majority of registered nurses are Caucasian (The Registered Nurse Population, 2004; National Coalition of Ethnic Minority Nurse Associations [NCEMNA], 2014). In American baccalaureate nursing education, the dominant racial group continues to be white, followed distantly by blacks/African Americans, Hispanics/Latinos, Asian Americans, and American Indians (Fang, Wilsey, & Bednash, 2007).

The registered nurse *minority* population in the United States, Canada, and other countries has increased in the past few decades largely due to the scope and magnitude of global migration to fulfill staff nurse shortages in hospitals and elsewhere (Brush, 2008). In the United States, there are more than 350,000 minority

❖ *Nursing Reflection*

Why Must Nurses Become More Transculturally Caring?
Technology, economics, class structure, immigration, increasing needs of vulnerable populations, and changing views of the *meaning* of race, ethnicity, and gender are altering the face of North America, the world, and the delivery of health and nursing care.

nurses (NCEMNA, 2014). Organizations, such as the American Association of Colleges of Nursing (AACN), the Canadian Association of University Schools of Nursing (CAUSN), and the American Academy of Nursing (Giger et al, 2007) have recognized that respect for cultural diversity must be a core value of the nursing profession and of institutions that hire nurses. Moreover, nursing education and research recognize the importance of teaching and learning about cultural diversity and initiating culturally competent care (*Journal of Transcultural Nursing*, 2007, Special Issue, Vol. 18, No. 1; Pacquiao, 2007).

The late Madeleine Leininger, the first nurse-anthropologist and mother of transcultural nursing (Leininger, 1970, 1991; Leininger & McFarland, 2006) advocated for the incorporation of transcultural nursing content in education and has promoted research for culturally focused practice for more than 50 years.

In 1970, the late Leininger stated the following:

> *The cultural context approach [for nursing] strives for specificity in the consideration of patient problems and for reducing ambiguity in nursing goals. . . . Each cultural group in various places in the world has its own life style, patterns of living, and its own special way of viewing the world about it. Its special world view is the essential basis of a people's modes of acting and thinking, and its world view serves as the basic framework for their unique cultural context of behavior.*
> Leininger (1970, p. 111)

More and more, schools and clinical agencies are responding to the demand and are incorporating content and teaching-learning processes related to culture and transcultural nursing (Dougherty & Tripp-Reimer, 1991; Giddens, 2008; McFarland & Wehbe-Alamah, 2015; Pacquiao, 2007; Ryan,

Learn More

One example of the way that ethnic and professional cultures can change and merge is illustrated by the recent surge in the use of complementary or alternative therapies. Such therapies—acupuncture, meditation, therapeutic touch, Reiki, massage, Ayurvedic, Chinese, and other herbal remedies—generally come from non-Western cultures and are gaining in not only popularity, but also acceptance in some nursing and medical circles (Dossey & Keegan, 2012; National Center for Complementary and Alternative Medicine [www.nccam.nih.gov]). What was once shunned as "quack medicine" is now viewed by some Western health-care practitioners as viable and meaningful. Western healing is beginning to take on a new holistic light, as a combination of traditional and modern practices.

Carlton, & Ali; 2000; Simpson, 1989). Building on the educational organizations in nursing, and the Transcultural Nursing Society (TCNS), there is a call for *more* action on the part of the nurse accrediting agencies to require transcultural education as part of curricula and the accreditation criteria. By acknowledging the importance of transcultural knowledge development in nursing education, administration, and research, nursing practice gradually will become more culturally aware, caring, sensitive, and competent.

GLOBALIZATION YIELDS HEALTH ISSUES

With the benefits of globalization come the shortcomings. Health issues emerging from diverse viewpoints about health and illness; geopolitical strife; war, communicable and infectious diseases; poverty; nutrition deficiencies; global spread due to travel; or characteristics of genetic engineering, biotechnology, and environmental pollution all pose serious health concerns that are exacerbated by globalization. ". . . [T]he health of one affects the health of all" (Simpson, 1989, p. 196). The extent to which scientists should interfere with nature to develop new products or inventions creates ethical dilemmas for health-care practitioners and governments. A greater divide exists now between the world's affluent and the world's poor, creating responsibility on the part of the affluent to care for the disenfranchised

(Chamberlin, 1999; Chomsky, 2014; Eisler, 2007; Pope Francis, 2013; Sachs, 2005). Global changes and monetary regulation issues have led to insecurities and uncertainty about the world's financial markets. Moreover, political instability in many regions of the world affects all nations, and presses many to seek asylum in North America and Western Europe. This influx of immigrants often leads to additional poverty and substandard access to health care. Often, immigrants, both documented and undocumented, and others such as the working poor with different ethnic and racial identities are prevented from availing themselves of quality health care. Globalization also has led to local job losses in varied industries. The general accelerated costs in health care, not only in North America but also in the world community over the past decades, have made health-care costs and access prohibitive in many nations (Hannerz, 1993, 1999; Mander & Goldsmith, 1996; Ray & Turkel, 2014; Ray, Turkel & Marino, 2002; Sorbello, 2008a, 2008b).

Globalization has affected society and nurses feel its effects when they provide health care. Understanding oneself in the context of diverse cultures helps the nurse to evaluate the affect of globalization on culture and health. Self-reflection and awareness propels nurses to engage in transcultural caring practices that demonstrate moral responsibility, cultural relevancy, and innovation in the care to people within complex organizational systems and nation-states. Consider the case study of Monique and its accompanying questions at the end of the chapter to further your understanding of issues presented by globalization.

The Concept of Caring

Caring, for many nurse theorists, is considered to be the foundation of the discipline and practice of nursing, and thus nursing is now considered the science of caring (Bishop & Scudder, 1991; Boykin & Schoenhofer, 2001; Coffman, 2006; *International Journal for Human Caring* Volumes, 1997-present; Leininger, 1991; Leininger & McFarland, 2006; Newman, Sime, & Corcoran-Perry, 1991; Newman et al, 2008; Ray, 2006, 2010a, 2010b, 2010c; Ray & Turkel, 2014, 2015; Roach, 2002; Watson, 1985; 2005). However, it is not a simple concept. (See significant articles in ongoing quarterly volumes of the *International Journal for Human Caring*, first launched in 1997.) Disparaged as too illusive, vague, and ambiguous (Paley, 2001), caring remains the most important concept for illuminating *what*

❖ *Nursing Reflection*

Understanding oneself as a cultural or multicultural being in relationship to other diverse culture groups helps the nurse to evaluate the effect of globalization—potential poverty, inequality, commercialism, conflict or war, and environmental degradation—on culture and health. Subsequently, there is a call to action in developing a more caring and just global society.

happens in the nurse-patient relationship and the mutual human-environment nursing process. Caring is a complex, relational concept that relies on the intricate interactions between individuals and others in their life world (Davidson, Ray, & Turkel, 2011; Ray, 1994b; Ray & Turkel, 2014; Turkel & Ray, 2000, 2001; Watson, 1999, 2005, 2008a, 2008b). Newman et al (1991) viewed caring in the human health experience as the central phenomenon of nursing that facilitates health and healing. Roach (1987, 2002) defined caring as compassion, commitment, conscience, confidence, competence, and comportment. Mayeroff (1971) focused on caring as helping others grow. Watson (1985, 1999, 2005) (1) advanced the idea of nursing as a sacred science, and knowledgeable caring intended to protect and enhance human dignity. Ray (1981a, 1981b, 1989a, 1989b, 1997a, 1997b, 2010a, 2010b, 2010c) (2) explicated the meaning of caring as love and co-presence, and (3) in practice illuminated spiritual-ethical caring as interrelated with political, economic, legal, and technological dimensions of the organizational environment.

Over the course of 40 years of scholarship in caring, new ideas and multiple meanings of caring have been advanced. Although there are many different ways of caring and definitions of caring, there are several common threads. Every human being is in need of and capable of caring (Boykin & Schoenhofer, 2001). Furthermore, "the human expression of caring may be shown through love or compassion, sorrow or joy, sadness or despair. . . ." (Roach, 1987, p. 2). Caring is an art, a science, and a philosophy. Thus, caring is an ontology (a way of being), an epistemology (a body of knowledge and way of knowing), an ethic (a moral ideal), an aesthetic (an artful practice), and a sociocultural phenomenon. Caring is central to the notion of well-being; self-care (Brown, 2009);

growing into wholeness, body, mind, and spirit (Nouwen, 1979); cultural competence (Pacquiao, 2007); and quality nursing care practices (Leininger, 1991; Leininger & McFarland, 2006; McFarland & Wehbe-Alamah, 2015; Ray, 1989a, 1989b, 1997b; 2006; Turkel & Ray, 2000, 2001, 2004a, 2004b, 2009; Turkel, 2007; Watson, 1985, 2005). Through the efforts of more than 30 years of scholarship, the International Association for Human Caring (www.humancaring.org), and the *International Journal for Human Caring* have disseminated knowledge, held conferences, and published articles on caring that have reached countless numbers of nurses and others interested in human caring, including caring in educational, political, economic, legal, and technological spheres (Barnard & Locsin, 2007; Boykin, Schoenhofer & Valentine, 2014; Eggenberger & Keller, 2008; Ray, 2006; Ray & Turkel, 2014; Smith, Turkel, & Wolf, 2013; Touhy & Boykin, 2008; Turkel & Ray, 2000, 2001, 2004a; Watson, 2005, 2008a, 2008b).

CARING THROUGH SELF-REFLECTION

Because every individual is unique, caring also is unique in terms of how to care for self and each individual (Boykin & Schoenhofer, 2001; Boykin, Schoenhofer, & Valentine, 2014). Caring is a learned art and science (see *International Journal for Human Caring*, Vol. 12, 2008 and volumes 1997 to the present). Self-reflection is one way to learn this art (Brown, 2009; Johns, 2007; Johns & Freshwater, 1998). Not only does caring for self through reflection offer solitude, inspiration, and lessons for self-growth, caring also enhances human understanding and human awareness in general (Johns, 2007; Lauterbach & Becker, 1996). Self-reflection focuses on the meaning and interpretation of one's living as a person with multiple worlds—personal, social, cultural, spiritual, and professional. Strategies for nurses to reflect inwardly include meditating, journaling, and dialoguing about values, beliefs, attitudes, and human experiences. This type of multifaceted internal exploration can help prepare nurses to understand themselves as cultural beings or even multicultural beings, and the complex meanings in the human health and sociocultural experience ultimately to care effectively across cultures.

TRANSCULTURAL CARING

Caring, for purposes of this text, means transcultural caring. Transcultural caring is defined as "the relationship between charity and right action—between love as compassion and response to suffering and need, and justice or fairness of doing what ought to be done within the [dynamics] of culture [nursing situations, organizations], or society" (Ray, 1989a, p. 19). This definition contains several components of caring and culture:

- Love
- Compassion
- Empathy
- Justice or fairness
- Dynamics of culture
- Nursing situations/organizational cultures/ society

Caring integrates love and compassion because of its unity of purpose, agape love, that is expressing limitless or unconditional altruism for its own sake and for the benefit of others without expecting anything in return (Templeton, 1999). In essence, agape love is working for the good of others and society (Eriksson, 1997, 2006; Ray, 1981a, 1981b, 1997b; Templeton, 1999). The good in nursing is holistic, facilitating the integration of body, mind, spirit, and choice in the mutual human-environment process (Davidson & Ray, 1991; Rogers, 1970). Love should transcend religious, cultural, or ethnic differences. Caring requires compassion because it embodies a loving, empathic response, a deeply felt awareness of the human race with recognition that we are all bound together by the human condition (Nouwen, 1977). Caring involves empathy because empathy entails seeing the other as our self and treating the other as we would want to be treated (*The New American Bible*, 1970). Justice and fairness are implicit in caring because they speak to the societal need for everyone to be treated equitably and with respect (Rachels, 2003; Ray & Turkel, 2014). Cultural dynamics involves relating to the complexity and ever-changing process of complex human interactions in nursing situations, and moral responsibility; and facilitation of choice for wholeness, well-being, health, healing, and a peaceful death (Barry, Gordon, & King, 2015; Ray, 1994a, 1994b; 1997a, 1997b).

Transcultural caring as compassion and justice for people of diverse cultures is a worldview and a philosophy, and theory but it also is a practical approach. Transcultural caring as a way of practicing encourages nurses to be mindful of themselves as cultural/multicultural beings, and work carefully and ethically to communicate and interpret the multiple meanings of cultural expressions, and of diverse health and illness practices. Nurses practicing transcultural caring recognize the influence of diverse cultural aspects like spirituality and/or religion on choice-making. Transcultural nurses consider values, beliefs, and attitudes of others within cultural, environmental, political, technological, and economic contexts (Ray, 1989b, 2010a, 2010b; Ray & Turkel, 2014, 2015). By concentrating on the changing nature and meaning of population groups, cultural diversity, panethnic identities, and multiculturalism, nurses can care more competently for culturally complex patients.

Panethnicity

Panethnicity refers to the *dynamic* interrelationship between culture and identity that reflects the notion of many intersecting "coethnics" and evolving intercultural patterns or multicultural/postmulticultural frames of reference of people who share complex transcultural and sociopolitical experiences in the emerging global community, especially the dynamic community in postmulticultural North and South America, and Europe (Postero, 2007; Tuan, 1998).

[Panethnicity, multiculturalism, or the newer terms postmulticulturalism, interculturality or transculturality supercede the concepts of ethnicity and even race. Race, in the sense of classification, in the anthropological literature is considered controversial and difficult to define and, in the United States, to a large extent it has been rejected academically and viewed as negative in the study of human variation (Kaszycka, Strkalj, & Strzalko, 2009)].

The Concept of Culture

Culture, like caring, is a term and concept with multiple definitions and meanings (Andrews & Boyle, 2007, 2015; Frelich, 1989; Smircich, 1985). Historical conceptions of culture ground contemporary ones. Different culture groups view the concept of culture in different ways. Yet, there is a growing commitment to recognition of our common humanity, a sense of interconnectedness and belongingness in a complex universe (Bar-Yam, 2004; Capra, Steindl-Rast, & Matus, 1991). Through this knowledge of interconnectedness and the living history behind the concept of culture, we can begin to appreciate the process of the complexity and dynamics of an emerging world culture in the 21st century that incorporates global change and transcultural caring.

HISTORICAL MEANINGS

Culture generally has been part of the parlance of anthropology, a human science discipline dedicated to the study of the meaning of culture. In its simplest form, culture refers to humankind, tribes of humanity from a common ancestry of races, and a family of languages from one ancestral tongue (Tylor, 1930, pp. 4–5). Culture equals race, ethnicity, or panethnicity (integrating multiple identities and practices as people interact with one another) (Tuan, 1998). The concept of culture, emerging from the Latin, *cultura*, was originally associated with cultivation or agriculture—cultivation of the soil. Over time, however, culture became associated with *humanitas* (humanity), society, and civilization. The first professional anthropologist, Sir Edward Tylor (1871), stated the following:

> *Culture, or civilization, taken in its wide ethnographic [descriptive] sense, is that complex whole which includes knowledge, belief, art, moral, law, custom, and any other capabilities and habits acquired by man as a member of society* (p. 1).

Tylor presented culture in a number of ways: as *creative* because people create culture and it is progressive; as *information* because culture is communicated and transmitted through acquired languages; as *problem-solving* because people develop systems to deal with human and environmental challenges; and as *everywhere* because culture is the complex whole (Tylor, 1871). Culture has been defined in various ways since Tylor. Although controversies exist in its meaning from the superorganic to the material, from the empirical to the interpretive, and from the diverse to the universal (Freilich, 1989; Kroeber, 1917), some dominant ways that culture has been defined include: social habits of people (Boas, 1928); designs for living (Kluckhohn & Kelly, 1945); the way of life of a people (Leininger, 1970); ideas and perception or cognitive and behavioral elements like values, beliefs and attitudes that are transmitted from one group to another (Leininger, 1995); and shared systems of meaning that are socially constructed, interpreted, and reproduced through interaction (Geertz, 1973).

Helman (1994) defined culture as a set of guidelines that individuals inherit as members of a group. These guidelines are a moral compass and direct individuals how to view and experience the world, and how to behave in relation to others, supernatural forces, and the environment. Culture includes most social structural elements in society, such as kinship, religion, politics, law, economics, technology, ecology, and health care (Leininger, 1991; Leininger & McFarland, 2006; Ray, 1989b, 2010a, 2010b). Moreover, culture today includes complex adaptive systems, social norms, creative ideas, complex problem-solving processes, explanatory models, and action (Bar-Yam, 2004; Brown, 1998, Davidson, Ray, & Turkel, 2011). With the continuation of exploration and the advent of computers, culture includes the exploration of *outer* space, including the moon, Mars, and NASA's New Horizons spacecraft exploration of the "planet" Pluto (Aldrin, 2015; www.NASA.gov/newhorizons (July 2015), and the cultures interfacing in the international space station (Aldrin, 2015; Duggins, 2007; Furniss, 2006); the *MySpace* culture (Platt & Platt, 2007), *thumb culture* (cell phones and text messaging, etc.) (Glotz & Bertsch, 2005), and the culture of the *F generation*— Facebook, Twitter, Instagram, YouTube, video, etc. (Behar, 2014) (moreover, this culture is referred to as the fourth revolution of the infosphere because of how it is reshaping reality (Floridi, 2014); the culture of place making (Zúñiga & Pellow, 2008) and *biltechnology* (sociocultural behavior and the built environment), simulation, and robotics (Barnard & Locsin, 2007; Locsin, Purnell, Tanioka, & Osaka, 2011); and, more recently, the culture of terrorism, cyberterrorism, and extremist tyranny (Jarvis & Macdonald, 2014; Libicki, 2007). In his book, *The Predicament of Culture*, Clifford (1988) wrote that in many ways, "culture is a deeply compromised idea . . . it comprises local and global perspectives"

❖ *Nursing Reflection*

Nurses practicing transcultural caring recognize not only the personal and social aspects of culture or multiculturalism but also the ethical, spiritual, or religious aspects of culture when facilitating choices for health and healing with patients.

(p. 10), and permeates every aspect of life. Culture is in a constant state of unfolding and transformation. Thus, culture is the preservation through ethnography (narrative description or stories) and history of diverse processes and patterns, including social media patterning of reality, of the interaction of individuals within groups, and, at the same time, culture captures the collective identity of humankind, the universal or the unified whole within the universe.

A NEW VIEW OF CULTURE

Transglobalization and the global exchange of information, has enhanced our view of culture (Zwingle, 1999). As we have learned, all cultures as we knew them are changing. Cultures are being redefined as outside influences are incorporated. Some cultures have become more insular in the wake of global pressures; some cultures have become what is known as terroristic; many cultures have conformed to a more technologically material or economic worldview; most cultures have blended traditional ideas and ways of life with modern material or technological culture. Cultures thus are dynamic and complex. Old cultural conflicts may continue to threaten the positive growth and development of different cultures or nations, but on the whole there is a growing desire *to choose* to belong to a world community that is committed to preservation of humanity and the rich cultures that have evolved through the centuries. There is a desire on the part of peoples of the world to develop relationships that honor traditional and diverse ways of life while, at the same time, cocreate a shared vision for living in an interconnected universe. In the complex world of today, individuals must transcend their own culture-bound assumptions. "The human person is a centre of consciousness, which is capable of infinite extension and as it grows it becomes more and more integrated with the whole complex of persons who make up humanity" (Griffiths, 1989). We must all move toward growth–producing intercultural/transcultural relationships. For the most part, respect for ways of life that serve the *good* of people in a complex and dynamic world have become a goal (Harman, 1998; Leininger & McFarland, 2006; McFarland & Wehbe-Alamah, 2015). In essence, a transglobal culture has become more purposeful, more open, and more universal. People are beginning to participate in transcultural dialogue to share visions for the future, and to engage in moral actions to benefit all in a universe that cares (Eisler,

2007; Harman, 1998; Henderson, 2006; Ray, 1994a; Turkel & Ray, 2000, 2001, 2010a, 2010b; Ray & Turkel, 2014). The idea of dynamic complexity becomes a new metaphor for culture.

Dynamic Complexity

Dynamic Complexity, as a new metaphor for a transglobalizing culture and transculturality, draws its meaning from the new sciences of complexity (Arntz, Chasse, & Vicente, 2005; Briggs & Peat, 1989, 1999; Wheatley, 1999), and complex caring dynamics (Davidson, Ray, & Turkel, 2011; Ray, 1989a, 1994b, 1998, 2010a, 2011). Complexity refers to a new way of perceiving the universe by discovering through science, art, and theology the dynamics of the mutual human-environment process as creative, good, irreversible, pandimensional, and moving toward increasing complexity and diversity with continuously changing patterning affected by choice (Davidson & Ray, 1991; Davidson, Ray, & Turkel, 2011; Goodwin, 1994; Newman et al, 2008; Rogers, 1970). Complexity sciences emerged first from Einstein's discovery of relativity as the way to describe the relationships between different observers in a world where communication was not instantaneous but limited by the speed of light. Second, complexity sciences emerged from the development of quantum mechanics where the physical world was revealed as holistic rather than independent particles. Third, complexity science emerged with the realization that the laws governing the motion of the planets and weather were chaotic and unpredictable. The final phase of development in complexity sciences was the dynamic view of nature, the revelation that the earth is like a living organism with unpredictable qualities known as emergent properties whereby through direct participation and knowing, scientists and others have insight into the qualities of organisms, systems, families, communities, and organizations allowing people to recognize their health or fragmentation (Goodwin, 2003, pp. 13–14). Complexity sciences emphasize wholeness, interconnectedness, and quality of life. Wholeness or holography (i.e., the description of the holon) as a subset of complexity illustrates that all reality, including the reality of human beings and social systems, reveal holons, wholes and parts that emerge into more complex forms from the connection and nesting of parts into greater complexity. In the physical world, atoms, molecules, cells, and organs nest together. Each is dependent on the other for existence. "All wholes are part of something more complex [the earth, solar system, families, organizations, communities, nations], and all are contained in the one Universe that is home to all" (Cannato, 2006, p. 98). For example, when the metaphor is extended to the global community, each member of the society is interconnected and brings forth consciousness that is essential to understanding the whole (Newman et al, 2008). Thus, the whole global society with diverse co-existing cultures as an illumination of our social interrelatedness is to understand any one culture in relationship to the whole (Capra et al, 1991). This epistemology (way of knowing) of interrelatedness and wholeness is brought forth as knowledge-in-process, a dynamic informational/communication process that is formed in and by relationships (Bar-Yam, 2004; Davidson, Ray, & Turkel, 2011; Harman, 1998; Ray, 1994b; Ray & Turkel, 2014). This unfolding of knowledge is *intrinsically* grasped in consciousness and conscience through "informational patterns of relationship"—a compassionate relationship that calls forth the spiritual (creativity) within—and *extrinsically* understood through shared and ethically responsible communication with persons who are integral with their environment and who share beliefs, values, attitudes, feelings, and memories (Arntz et al, 2005; Cannato, 2006; Davidson, Ray, & Turkel, 2011; Newman et al, 2008; Ray, 1994b, 1997b).

Complexity theory in science is important because it provides a mechanism for understanding multivariate evolving patterns of order. At the root of all complex systems, from the behavior of molecules to the operation of nation-states to the balance of nature, is a set of rules that, when identified, will yield transformation and "unification." Chaos theory, another subset of complexity, helps us to understand this transformative process in nature, human, social, and economic systems, including health-care systems, and the concept of culture as dynamic complexity. Chaos theory advanced from researching movements and changes in *patterns of nature,* such as hurricanes, powerful rivers, and even insects, such as butterflies flapping wings, and making a difference in weather patterns far away from the source. Over time, these patterns exhibit no rational predictable behavior but produce new, more complex structures known as nonlinear emergent properties (Briggs & Peat, 1999; Davidson, Ray, & Turkel, 2011; Lindberg et al, 2008; Ray, 1994b; Ray & Turkel, 2014; Turkel & Ray,

2000, 2001). Chaos theory thus represents a nonlinear dynamic, where chaotic, disorderly, or turbulent systems in nature or society appear to behave in a random or unpredictable manner at the *edge of chaos* (disorder and order). On closer inspection, the patterning demonstrates an underlying order at a bifurcation point from fluctuations or turbulence that becomes dominant and a new pattern forms with greater order (Ray, 1994b, 1998, 2011; Davidson, Ray & Turkel, 2011). In this information process, observations ". . . include the way patterns are established in living and nonliving systems, how these patterns interconnect, and how they are linked to corresponding principles of order" (Ray, 1994b, p. 23). In the social system, as we interact with people who are diverse and complex cultural beings, we learn through interaction, that the essential picture of complexity or dynamic relational activity is seen at the boundary between evolving human-environment systems. The edge of chaos is a communication and information process that feeds back on itself and coordinates system behavior through continual, mutual interaction. "Opposing things can happen at the same time, in the same space, without contradicting each other" (Thoma, 2003, p. 17). Thus, there are forces of reciprocity between order and disorder (unpredictability) at what is termed the edge of chaos, where transformation or disintegration take place (Ray, 1994b). This creative and informational process is brought forth in relationship in, what is termed a phase space at the edge of chaos. (The edge of chaos can represent all forms of diversity, conflict, disagreement, linguistic challenges, etc.). At this edge, interacting systems in the *phase space* are pulled in a trajectory, a certain direction by a magnetic attractor toward self-organization (change). The chaotic state thus contains the possibilities for order (self-organization) at a bifurcation point allowing the structure, pattern, and process freedom to seek out its own solution. Solutions in the social, economic, and health-care world are resolved in relationships through rational thought, dialogue, negotiation, and choice. The seemingly unpredictable emergent natural, human, or social system "chooses" a possible future while leaving others behind (Briggs & Peat, 1989). In the *Tree of Knowledge,* Maturana and Varela state the following: "We have only the world we can bring forth with others, and only love helps bring it forth . . . This is the biological foundation of social phenomena: without love, there is no social process and, therefore, no humanness" (in Goodwin, 2003, p. 14). Thus, as Goodwin (2003) points out, "This is the way of 'science with love,' which is the essence of the holistic approach to understanding and action" (p. 14).

Concepts in complexity sciences are well represented in the nursing literature. They include the shared concepts of human-environment integrality (Davidson, Ray, & Turkel, 2011; Rogers, 1970), interconnectedness, belongingness, complexity, holism, value, purpose, love, caring, information, energy patterns, choice, and quality of transcultural relationships for transformation to health, well-being, healing, or a peaceful death (Davidson & Ray, 1991; Newman et al, 2008; Ray, 1994b, 2011; Watson, 2005). When nursing addresses the use of chaos theory to increase understanding of relational and communicative patterns of behavior, it is cognizant of the magnetic appeal of the nurse, the quality of caring in the nurse-patient relationship, whether formed through direct interaction or computer-assisted interaction (e.g., telephone, video, etc.) to communicate about human need and suffering in terms of the lack of well-being or disease (Ray, 1994b, 1998, 2011) at the edge of chaos. Caring is the force; it is a spiritual-ethical knowing—a communicative process understood as compassion within the virtues of faith, hope, love, and social and technical competency (Ray, 1981b, 1989a, 1994b, 1997b, 2011). The action of compassion and social-cultural justice at the edge of chaos pulls the other, the patient or community, in such a way that the power of the caring relationship brings forth trust, a courageous trust in the authenticity of the caring relationship itself to initiate change or relational self-organization. In this emergent process, reasoned moral choice-making occurs simultaneously within the will to act or choose for the best possible future. Both the nurse and the patient (also family or community) are transformed (relational self-organization). New insights for health and healing are attained.

Using complexity science as a foundation for understanding culture as dynamic complexity, and complex caring dynamics provides a way of understanding how complexity in the nurse-patient relationship nursing is addressed in this book. The Transcultural Caring Dynamics in Nursing and Health-Care Theoretical Model (see Fig. 1-1) is holographic (showing the integrated whole and the parts); and it is knowledge-in-process (illustrating interaction of whole and

parts). Thus the theoretical model illuminates how the knowledge of caring, transcultural caring ethics, transcultural context, and universal sources (spirituality) can be integrated when one or more interact together (the multicultural self and other) to facilitate awareness, understanding, and choice in the provision of culturally competentand relevant care. In transcultural nursing, the nurse-patient *caring* relationship as a magnetic attractor demands cocreative participation in the *choice* for change or transformation to health, well-being, healing, or a peaceful death.

The metaphor of culture as dynamic complexity reveals "timeless wisdom" for change (Briggs & Peat, 1999). In transcultural caring, patterns of meaning are cocreated by nurses and patients interacting in complex systems, to make choices for relational self-organization for the best possible culturally relevant future. Caring as an intellectual and emotional process is transcultural, spiritual, and ethical communicative action (Ray, 1994b, 2011). Personal and cultural change takes place in the context of recognizing human and spiritual interconnectedness. Human interactions shape and are shaped in a dynamic way by transcultural spiritual-ethical caring communication, moral commitment, and responsibility.

Overall, culture as dynamic complexity is a foundation for cocreating cultural unity within diversity. In our transglobal world, manifestations of intercultural brutality exist; however, thoughtful leaders,

Learn More

"As a global community, we are in the middle of a transition from the industrial age to the information age, and this transformation is reflected and re-reflected in everything around us. The amount of information that is flowing and the rate of change of society are both aspects of the growing complexity of our existence. . . . Professional activities, from corporate management to systems engineering [including nursing], require new approaches, insights and skills" (Bar-Yam, 2004, p. 13). Transcultural caring, incorporating knowledge of the complexity of relationships and diverse cultures, is an important way of making progress in the profession of nursing to deal with the changing multicultural/intercultural population and the provision of authentic and compassionate caring in nursing and health care.

including nurses, must examine both good and harmful patterns of behavior and choose to seek understanding of the meaning of differences in cultures and negotiate change toward a new order (relational self-organization/transformation). Choosing to cocreate a better world comes by understanding our common humanity within diversity, and the conditions that have contributed to the bitter historical struggles between and among cultures. Culture as dynamic complexity helps to explain the process of transglobalization of life and living; transcultural caring is the magnetic attractor and choice point to facilitate the potential for healing and health to ultimately enhance well-being and build the global civic culture (Briggs & Peat, 1989, 1999; Davidson, Ray, & Turkel, 2011; Leininger, 1991; Ray, 1989a, 1994b, 1997a, 1997b; Teilhard de Chardin, 1965; Watson, 2005; Wheatley, 1999).

MULTICULTURALISM

From a practical perspective, diversity in American culture and around the world, especially in the industrialized nations, is increasing. At the same time, there is a vision of a common humanity (Harman, 1998; Leininger, 1991; Leininger & McFarland, 2006). As stated earlier, the recent trend is to try to preserve these cultures, rather than to assimilate them completely. The term *multiculturalism* refers to people of diverse origins and communities who are free to preserve and enhance their own cultural heritage. From reports, the term was coined in Canada (Davidhizar & Giger, 1998; Taylor, 1994), where multicultural values and cultural pluralism are respected. In Canada, biculturalism (bilateral French and English legal/parliamentary agreements from two of the founding European cultures) was first institutionalized, and then later the concept of multiculturalism with rights and privileges for aboriginal (First Nations' and Inuit people) and other ethnic cultures, especially Ukrainians (Lupul, 2005), was institutionalized. In 1982, there was the creation of federal and provincial Ministries of Multiculturalism (*The New Canadian Constitution*, Milne, 1982; Canadian Multiculturalism, Library of Parliament, Revised 16 March, 2006). The country has been successful in preserving cultural diversity in most environments, especially urban environments, and the northern Arctic Inuit community of Nunavut. Still, conflicts between and among cultures continue and questions arise about the meaning of the "politics of recognition" of

diverse and aboriginal cultures in Canada (Taylor, 1994). In Quebec, there is a desire for increased political autonomy among French Canadians (Canadian Election Results, CSPAN, October 14, 2008).

Maintaining one's cultural identity in the United States is evolving with the seeking of a stronger voice among Native Americans (Jennings & Lowe, 2013; Lowe & Nichols, 2014), and the increase in immigration, especially from Mexico, Central American countries, the Caribbean, and Latin American countries. Until more recently, the government focused more on assimilation into the dominant Anglo-American culture rather than on promoting and maintaining diversity of cultures. Some leaders say that this tradition of assimilation of a variety of cultures has led to "imprisonment of the spirit rather than that of the flesh" (Okinaka, in Tuan, 1998, p. 140). Despite a growing interest in multiculturalism because of increasing educational and human rights' laws and policies, more vocalization, and interracial and interethnic marriage, even exposure to ethnic food choices and shops that feature ethnic artifacts, the demands and influence of Anglo-American culture on all citizens are still far-reaching. Anglo or Caucasian cultural groups from European heritages have more opportunities for "ethnic options" or the ability to choose whether or to what extent ethnicity will matter in their lives. Asian Americans, for instance, do not necessarily have this option. Ethnicity will be a part of their lives whether they choose it or not, because of the obviousness of physical appearance and the historical American stigma of racial distinctiveness and foreignness (Tuan, 1998). African Americans likewise do not have ethnic options. Ethnicity in the form of race, although changing (especially with the historic election in 2009 and reelection in 2013 of Barack Obama as the 44th President of the United States in 2009), factors heavily into black and Asian American lives whether they or others would like it to or not (Tuan, 1998).

Even as multiculturalism gains support politically in the United States, many people from different cultures continue to experience marginalization, including health disparities (Osajima in Tuan, 1998, p. 3). Many citizens in the dominant Caucasian or Anglo cultures in the United States and Canada are exhibiting "diversity fatigue" (DeSantis, 1997, p. 28; Taylor, 1994); there is growing intolerance to the increasing preservation of diverse ethnic identities. For example, some Californians are complaining about how Asians are taking over many areas in the state (Tuan, 1998). Similarly, at the United States–Mexico border, many Mexicans encounter suspicion and are denied opportunities to emigrate due to profiling, cultural prejudice, and what is known as "compassion fatigue" (Chomsky, 2014; Heyman, 1999). The tension is clear. The demand for the preservation of cultural identities is increasing. Simultaneously, there is a push to homogenize diverse cultural groups into one dominant metaculture (Chomsky, 2014; DeSantis, 1997; Tuan, 1998).

Despite multiple interpretations and critiques, multiculturalism is moving toward what the Latin Americans call interculturality (transculturality) (Postero, 2007), a transcultural caring relationship where the voice-lacking minorities can achieve a more equal voice in political and economic spheres. Thus, multiculturalism will find success only in transcultural compassion, innovation, political and economic mutuality in choice-enhancing processes. Although the dominant culture continues to be pervasive in many nations, new ideas, insights, and increased compassion will help discover the best ways to seek understanding of differences and create the best possible future for *all* people (Ray, 1989a, 1994a, 2010a, 2010b; Semotiuk, 2014).

The Multicultural Self

Not only are we becoming multicultural from a community perspective; we are also recognizing multiculturality from a personal perspective. Changing demographics, the media, the Internet, social media, immigration, travel, knowledge and internal integration of other cultures lead us to establish multiple intersecting identities. In other words, the diversity of our interactions and affiliations create within us multicultural selves. In the past, cultures usually were bound by family, kin, the culture group, geography, climate, and socioeconomic structures. Today, this is not the case; everything overlaps. So many individuals have incorporated aspects of other cultures into their own ways of thinking and feeling. Native Americans are fascinated, for instance, by what is happening on Music Television (MTV) and the Caucasian community, non-Native Americans, are fascinated by the Native American way of life, art, storytelling, and culture (Peat, 2002, 2003). Similarly, Japanese young people, for example, have taken on lifestyle patterns from the West, which have altered the traditional patterns and practices that focus on family, kinship, and the social structures of Eastern culture (Tuan, 1998). The average white North American no longer thinks of herself or himself primarily in ethnic terms, such as Irish, French, German, and so forth. Rather, ethnic culture takes a backseat to other cultural communities of which individuals find themselves a part—professional, social, social media, religious, or familial. Knowledge of the different components of our multicultural self helps us to understand how we function and communicate. Consider the concept of multicultural self when you read and evaluate the case study on Kathleen at the end of the chapter.

Paradigms and Ways of Knowing in a Transcultural Worldview

A paradigm is a set of basic assumptions about the world, and in science a paradigm refers to a *matrix* of information that embodies elements of a discipline of knowledge (Omery, Kasper, & Page, 1995, p. 44).

Learn More

Despite reports that our world is becoming homogenous and that native cultures are perishing, about 5,000 indigenous cultures have survived for thousands of years (Davis, 1999). Groups, such as the Inuit of Canada and the Aborigine of Australia are preserving their cultural identities and asserting their rights to control their future and ancestral land (e.g., consider the new territory of the Inuit in Arctic Canada, called Nunavut). The new global culture is, in fact, a blend of experimentation and innovation, in which developed countries and less developed societies learn and benefit from one another (Lowe & Nichols, 2014; Zwingle, 1999).

❖ *Nursing Reflection*

The Multicultural Self

To understand more fully the concept of the multicultural self, look at gender, race, ethnicity, panethnicity, culture, religion, generation, sexual orientation, socioeconomic class, disability, and professional roles (Tuan, 1998, p. 25).

Thus, "a scientific discipline is a body of knowledge that encompasses more than one paradigm to guide inquiry toward an understanding of phenomena" (Parse, 1987, p. 2). Although in a multicultural or transcultural world, we are trying to assist people to transcend their fundamental assumptions, individuals do filter knowledge and experiences through their own ways of seeing the world, or through their paradigm(s) (Smircich, 1985). Nursing has its own different paradigms to guide its practice. Viewed in conjunction with the conception of culture as a dynamic complexity, reviewing nursing paradigms can help to create a basic structure for transcultural nursing practice.

NURSING PARADIGMS

The nursing profession claims three main paradigms that encompass basic nursing assumptions about human beings and health: totality, simultaneity, and unitary-transformative (Fawcett, 1993; Newman, 1992; Newman et al, 2008). In the past two decades, debate has ensued about which paradigm of nursing should prevail.

The human-environment totality paradigm is the most common view. It states that people are biological, psychological, social, and spiritual organisms and thus are systems. The environment includes the internal and external stimuli surrounding human beings. We relate to the environment linearly; and the environment can be manipulated to suit our health and well-being (Parse, 1987).

The simultaneity paradigm, advanced by Parse (1987, 1996), views human beings and health in a different way. Under this perspective, humans are more than a mere sum of their parts; they are whole in themselves. Human beings are in a process of becoming, and thus live in relationship—a mutual, rhythmical, and cocreative interchange with the environment. Human beings freely choose, and thus freely choose health based upon a set of value priorities that is often paradoxical yet always open to possibilities.

The unitary-transformative (UT) paradigm espoused by Newman (1992; Newman et al, 2008) takes the position that human beings evolve holistically as self-organizing energy fields. Human energy fields are identified by pattern and interaction with the larger whole. These energy fields, or holistic systems, organize and reorganize to become more complex patterns (Fawcett, 1993; Newman, 1992; Newman et al, 1991; 2008). Human beings are characterized by wholeness (i.e., body, mind, and spirit), complexity, and consciousness. A person is identified by a pattern or consciousness, which includes awareness of self within a larger system of consciousness (the totality of information). Health in this view is expanded consciousness—all forms of information, sensations, physiology and intellect, emotion, and intention (Newman et al, 2008). The essence of nursing is the nurse-patient caring relationship and health is the focus of nursing.

The dynamic complexity view of culture mirrors phenomena in all these paradigms but is represented most in the UT paradigm because of its illumination of complexity, holism, the concepts of unitary and universal, patterning, consciousness, and caring. In this presentation, health (i.e., values and beliefs of diverse culture groups that include well-being, healing, or a peaceful death) is highlighted (as with Newman and Leininger). The focus of nursing from the perspective of culture as dynamic complexity, including multiculturalism and interculturality/transculturality (giving equal voice to the voiceless), underscores transcultural caring as the essence of nursing.

WAYS OF KNOWING

Carper (1978), widely known for advancing the nursing profession's philosophy, stated that "the body of knowledge that functions as the rationale for nursing practice has patterns, forms and structures that serve as horizons of expectations and exemplify characteristic ways of thinking about phenomena" (p. 13). In other words, each paradigm communicates an epistemology, philosophical orientation, or "way of knowing."

In the totality paradigm, the way of knowing is considered to be objective and linear. In the simultaneity paradigm, the way of knowing is subjective and mutual. The way of knowing in the UT paradigm is holistic and self-organizing. Carper identified four fundamental ways of knowing that are applicable in all paradigms. The ways of knowing are:

1. Personal (personal knowledge)
2. Empirical (scientific knowledge)
3. Ethical (moral knowledge)
4. Aesthetic (artistic knowledge or the art of nursing)

The sociocultural including sociopolitical, caring, and complex caring dynamics emerged as ways of knowing, and were articulated and advanced by many scholars, including Leininger (1970, 1991;

Leininger & McFarland, 2006), McFarland and Wehbe-Almah (2015); Roach (1987, 2002); Ray (1981, 1989a, 1989b, 1994a, 1994b, 1997a, 1997b, 1998, 2010a, 2010b; Davidson & Ray, 1991; Davidson, Ray, & Turkel, 2011; Ray & Turkel, 2014); White (1995); and Watson (1979; 1985, 1988, 2005, 2008a,b). The concepts are listed as follows:

1. Sociocultural (cultural knowledge as the foundation to ways of knowing/transcultural nursing)
2. Caring (caring knowledge as the essence of nursing, and integral with the UT paradigm)
3. Complex caring dynamics (transcultural caring as integral with the new sciences of complexity (relational complexity), transcultural nursing, and the Totality, Simultaneity, and UT paradigms in nursing)

To be competent and successful professionals, nurses must employ each way of knowing in conjunction with the others; none of the ways of knowing by themselves prepares nurses sufficiently.

The dimensions of this text's *Transcultural Caring Dynamics in Nursing and Health Care* theory and conceptual model (Fig. 1-1) mirror the ways of knowing, and will be discussed later in this chapter, and throughout this book.

- The first dimension, *the essence of caring*, models the aesthetic and complex caring dynamical ways of knowing.

Learn More

The Transcultural Caring Dynamics in Nursing and Health-Care (theoretical and conceptual) Model augments Carper's *Ways of Knowing* by adding several components to all the ways of knowing. The conceptual model recognizes the *quality* of the human-environment caring relationship and therefore adds to the ways of knowing, culture as dynamic complexity, and transcultural caring as complex caring dynamics. Within these views, the model as a way of knowing illuminates knowledge-in-process as people of diverse cultures interrelate and make choices for health and healing. The model thus illuminates the importance of the political, legal, economic, and technological aspects, and the humanistic, ethical and universal (spiritual) sources.

- The second dimension, *transcultural ethics,* clearly mirrors the ethical way of knowing.
- The third dimension, *transcultural context,* resembles the empirical, sociocultural, and complex transcultural caring dynamical ways of knowing.
- And the fourth dimension, *universal or spiritual sources*, can be likened to the personal, ethical and complex caring dynamical ways of knowing.

The Meaning of Health in the Dynamics of Complex Culture

Health is a universal phenomenon. It is harmony of body, mind, and spirit (Watson, 1985, 2005) and is espoused and desired by people of all cultures, although expressed differently depending upon the transmission of values, beliefs, attitudes, and behaviors, and the ability to meet basic needs. Newman (Newman et al, 2008) stated that health is expanded consciousness, which is the total informational field (i.e., sensation, awareness, physiology and intellect, emotion, and intention)—the informational pattern of the relationship that is constantly receiving and sending information. In Western culture, health has been characterized by Maslow as a hierarchy of needs (i.e., physiological needs, safety, belongingness, esteem, and self-actualization) (Hoffman, 2008). Physiological needs must be met first followed by personal growth and esteem needs. "When a lower-level need is satisfied, the next-higher need occupies our main attention until it, too, is satisfied. The highest need, self-actualization [self-organization using complex caring dynamics' information], is to become all that one is capable of becoming in terms of talents, skills, and abilities" (Hoffman, 2008, p. 26). This *human becoming* is the essence of health and one of the foci of the discipline of nursing (Parse, 1981, 1996).

The meaning of health in different cultures is defined by the health-belief model, patterns of coping, help-seeking behaviors, and social and spiritual parameters (Kleinman, 1998). Some diseases are culture-bound, for example, in terms of the sense of shame with psychiatric disorders, or the integration of the evil-eye syndrome and its alleviation through cultural rituals. Some diseases may bear a family resemblance (Kleinman, 1998), and in the modern era could be associated with genetic inheritance. Some diseases are stress-related and, thus, social. In essence, values, beliefs, attitudes, and behaviors of culture groups that illuminate diverse physical, psychological, spiritual, political, economic, health policy, and health-care delivery factors, including transcultural nursing (Leininger, 1991; Leininger & McFarland, 2006; McFarland & Wehbe-Alamah, 2015), contribute to the meaning of health.

The success—or lack thereof—of a health-care system is determined by morbidity (illness) and mortality (death) rates in a given population. And morbidity and mortality rates often fluctuate according to governmental policies, health-care access, and the provision of culturally relevant and competent care (Andrews & Boyle, 2007, 2015; Leininger & McFarland, 2006; McFarland & Wehbe-Alamah, 2015); Lipson & Dibble, 2005). Decisions at all levels of government come into play with regard to health-care provision, reimbursement, access, privacy, and research.

As we can see, health is not simply an individual's physical state. It is intimately intertwined with societal culture and perception. The concept of health, therefore, contains beliefs and values about a person's own social and psychological significance, and is affected by the political, economic, legal, spiritual, and ethical social structures in place in communities, nations, and the world.

Transglobal health-care systems reveal struggles facing nations, immigrants, and minorities (Albrecht, Fitzpatrick, & Scrimshaw, 2000). Globalization, the changing patterns of global politics and economies, diffusion of innovations, ethical issues, political theologies, wars, immigration or migration, the nursing shortage, and global nurse migration are some of the factors that have affected the causes and prevention of disease and death (Brush, 2008; Burkhardt & Nathaniel, 2008; Chomsky, 2014; de Vries & Sullivan, 2006; Eisler, 2007; Gennaro, 2008; Henderson, 2006; Pensky, 2005; Rogers, 2003; Slatterly, 2004). Some systems, like that in the United States, demonstrate how economics and politics can influence health-care policies. A new program, the Patient Protection and Affordable Care Act (PPACA), was initiated in 2010 to improve health-care quality and access to care in the United States. Other developed countries are committed to providing health care for all citizens, despite countervailing forces such as economics. Health-care professionals, along with health organizations, such as the American and Canadian Nurses Associations, the World Health Organization, and the International Council of Nurses, have considerable influence on the health of the population (Chinn, 2013; Ray & Turkel, 2014).

Traditional and contemporary health and healing practices form out of a combination of evolving human and organizational systems, and professional values (Leininger, 1991; Leininger & McFarland, 2006; Ray, 1994b, 2010a, 2010b). As discussed, health status varies by culture and it varies according to the values and beliefs of a health-care organization. It also varies by the social, political, and economic structure of a nation. In any event, the meaning of health in any culture or society determines the type of care that is most appropriate and effective (Lipson & Dibble, 2005; Spector, 2004).

Transcultural Nursing in Practice

With all of these components in mind, then, what does it mean to practice transcultural caring? Nurses care for patients in a very complex environment with multifarious cultures. They must care in the context of their own cultural backgrounds, their education about diversity, and their own abilities to relate to others of different cultures. Furthermore, health status varies according to cultural perception, the nurse's perception, cultural competence, the organization's (hospital or health-care clinic) mission and perception, and the nation's social structure, including human and cultural rights, the rights of nature, and political and economic perceptions. These various perceptions often are not in line with each other (i.e., the edge of chaos from a complexity science perspective), prompting turbulence, tensions, and competing interests for patients and for health-care providers, such as nurses. For example, Medicare and Medicaid government systems of health insurance in the United States, including insurance provisions from the Patient Protection and Affordable Care Act (2010) legislation, may not perceive an individual's health status as requiring comprehensive health-care coverage even though the patient and the nurse caring for that patient perceive the individual as requiring extensive care or treatment. Culture finds its way into everything that we do, from our reactions to illness to the way that we seek care (Leininger & McFarland, 2006; Ray, 2010a, 2010b; Spector, 2004). If nurses understand the meaning of caring and the dynamic complexity of culture, and acknowledge its critical role, they can facilitate effective choices with patients and significant others to provide high-quality transcultural care, and the best possible future. Nurses have to be committed to caring and healing, to advocating for patients, securing the welfare of their organizations, participating in political arenas, and bridging the cultural chasms among all of them.

THE GROWTH OF TRANSCULTURAL NURSING

The late Dr. Madeleine Leininger led the way to building the knowledge base and understanding of the discipline and practice of transcultural nursing (Leininger, 1970, 1978, 1991, 1995; Leininger & McFarland, 2002, 2006; McFarland & Wehbe-Alamah, 2015). Since the 1960s, many nurse scholars have followed in Leininger's path and advanced transcultural nursing in unique ways (Andrews & Boyle, 2015; Coffman, 2006; Giger & Davidhizar, 2004; Purnell & Paulanka, 2008; Ray, 1989a, 1989b, 1994a, 1994b, 2005, 2010a, 2010b; Spector, 2004; Turkel, 2007). Leininger (1981) emphasized caring as the critical factor for human growth, self and group actualization, human development, and survival for human cultures. In the past 40 years, transcultural nursing has become a dominant force in nursing and the knowledge application is beginning to yield significant results in nursing administration, education, practice, and research (Andrews & Boyle, 2007, 2015; Giddens, 2008; Giger & Davidhizar, 2004; Leininger & McFarland, 2002, 2006; McFarland & Wehbe-Alamah, 2015).

TRANSCULTURAL CONSCIOUSNESS

To practice transcultural nursing, nurses must first develop transcultural consciousness. Transcultural consciousness is a combination of (1) self-reflective awareness (Davidson, Ray & Turkel, 2011; Johns, 2007; Ray, 1994a); (2) transcultural caring (Leininger & McFarland, 2006; Ray, 1989a, 2010a, 2010b); (3) influence by people who share diverse cultural human experiences (Andrews & Boyle, 2007, 2015; Newman et al, 2008; Spector, 2004); and (4) a knowledge of complexity science (Davidson, Ray, & Turkel, 2011; Newman et al,

2008; Ray, 1998; Ray & Turkel, 2014). Transcultural consciousness engenders an appreciation of both diversity, and the reality of sharing a common humanity. Through self-reflecting, nurses can set aside preconceptions about life and people and view life and health and make choices in a different way, in essence become compassionate. Nurses also have a unique opportunity to share human experiences with those of different cultures and, as a result, to enhance their transcultural consciousness. Through everyday life encounters, nurses work with people of different cultures, experience their obstacles, and explore culturally viable and dynamic solutions. For nurses, self-reflection and shared transcultural experiences are the two components to building transcultural consciousness, relatedness, trust, and competency (Meleis, 1996) and developing cultural competencies (DeSantis & Lipson, 2007; Lipson & DeSantis, 2007; Ray, 2010a). To understand transcultural consciousness better, read and respond to the questions in the transcultural caring experience/case study on Lian at the end of the chapter.

Transcultural Caring Dynamics in Nursing and Health-Care Theoretical Model

The Transcultural Caring Dynamics in Nursing and Health-Care Theoretical Model was developed to help answer the following questions about caring for patients of diverse cultures.

- What is the meaning of caring to you?
- Do you have a perspective about transcultural caring?
- How do the beliefs, values, attitudes, and behaviors that make up your experience affect how you give care?
- Does nursing have a culture? If so, what are the dominant characteristics?
- Do other disciplines/professions, such as medicine and social work, have specific cultures? What are the dominant characteristics?
- How does a person's culture, including your own, affect health, illness, healing, and caring?
- How does the health-care organization (as a transcultural context) in which you practice or that supports your student experiences convey its values, and what are they?
- How does the organization in which you work, or that supports your student experiences,

understand cultural diversity and encourage culturally competent caregiving?

- What does transcultural ethics mean to you?
- What do human rights and cultural rights mean to you?
- How do political, legal, economic, and technologic factors influence health, illness, and healing?
- How can you communicate better with someone of a different culture? What does it mean to understand another's language, symbols, and rituals?
- What is the language of caring? Do you try to convey understanding by knowing the language of caring—the nurse-patient/family/community relationship—in nursing?
- How can you help patients find the cultural and material resources necessary to improve their health?
- How do the economics of health play a role in the provision of health care to culturally diverse patients?
- How do your beliefs about spirituality contribute to your values and beliefs, and interactions toward people of diverse cultural beliefs?
- What does spirituality have to contribute to being culturally relevant in patient care?
- What culturally relevant spiritual practices are supported by the organization within which you work or that supports your educational pursuits?
- How can you assess your progress toward transcultural caring competence?
- What is meant by the term *multicultural self*?
- How can you help to create a transcultural caring environment in the workplace or in school?
- What does patient choice mean to you in terms of the practice of transcultural nursing?
- How do you as a cultural/multicultural being negotiate for self in the context of daily life?
- How do you perceive vulnerable people negotiating for their health and well-being in multicontextual environments?
- What does transformation or change mean to you in the lifeworld?
- What does health, well-being, healing, and peaceful death mean to you?

THEORETICAL MODEL OVERVIEW

Transcultural Caring Dynamics in Nursing and Health Care uses a theoretical and conceptual model, which is derived from the notion of culture as dynamic complexity. Theoretical and conceptual models are explanatory, representational, and operational and guide for the most part transcultural behavior in a given situation (Holland & Quinn, 1987). Theoretical and conceptual models in nursing focus on nursing's purpose and communicate what is most influential in shaping nursing knowledge and guiding practice (Fitzpatrick & Whall, 1996). This model points to the processes that shape transcultural caring in nursing. The theoretical model points to culture as dynamic complexity; it points to understanding of the paradigms of nursing, and the ways of knowing, and caring as the essence of nursing; and it points to transcultural ethics, transcultural context, and universal sources (spirituality) as the foundation for awareness, understanding, and choice. In essence, given these dimensions, including the center of the theoretical model, the Transcultural Caring Dynamics in Nursing and Health Care Theoretical Model can be viewed as a human rights theory in terms of empowering lives and helping "to develop resilient nations" (www.undp.org). For example, see the United Nations Millennium Development Goals (MDGs) 2015 and Healthy People 2020 (www.healthypeople.gov). We all should be prepared to improve the goals of the MDG post 2015 (www.undp.org). Thus, culture as dynamic complexity represents the values, beliefs, and meaningful systems that are cocreated as people interact with one another and the environment, and facilitate or make choices for health and well-being in mutual caring relationships.

Although the theoretical model is depicted as two dimensional, it is holographic; the separate parts depicted are considered integral to the whole; in each part, the whole structure of the model exists (Briggs & Peat, 1989). The theoretical model applies to professionals and patients, families, and communities in a reciprocal relationship and engaged in choice making regarding caring, health, illness, death, healing, and well-being (see Fig. 1-1).

The theoretical model considers transcultural caring to be an integrated mode of being, thinking, and doing, in the context of caring, ethics, sociocultural phenomena, and religion or spirituality. These are the creative transcultural forces that constitute the foundations for personal awareness, understanding, and choice-making. Overall, the theoretical model reveals nursing or any discipline as the practice of relatedness, complex communicative spiritual-ethical caring, and knowledge-in-process, the process of facilitating choice through awareness and seeking understanding of self and others. Cultural dynamics unites and facilitates the interplay among compassion and justice, transcultural ethical principles, the transcultural context, and the universal sources (spiritual traditions). Through this process, one is authentic and sees beyond the self toward the other and the community in an I-Thou way of relating, that is, seeing or "... regarding the other as the very person he or she is" (Buber in Ray, 2010c, p. 45). The four dimensions have the capacity to guide and shape moral caring experiences to form the foundation for awareness, understanding, and choice for health, well-being, healing, and a peaceful death.

The theoretical model explains the impact of culture and transcultural caring phenomena in health and nursing care as well as the environment. In transcultural interactions, we shape and are shaped by aesthetic, moral, empirical, environmental, and personal and ethical interactions. Interacting structures are the foundation for co-creating culturally relevant choice making, facilitating patient choices, and building transcultural competency. The transcultural structure clarifies the complexity of the interactive and communicative processes in professional transcultural nursing practice (Ray, 2010c).

A fundamental assumption for transcultural caring is that caring itself is the human mode of being (Roach, 2002; Solecki, 1971; Spikins, 2015), and caring is the most unifying, dominant and central intellectual and practice focus in nursing

around the world (Leininger, 1981, 1996; Leininger & McFarland, 2006; Ray, 1981a, 1981b, 1989a, 2010a, 2010b, 2010c). Moreover, caring is thought of as a moral enterprise because it is universal in terms of seeking meaning and ultimately seeking the good of the self, other, and the environment (Davidson, Ray, & Turkel, 2011; Gadow, 1988; Ray, 1989a; 1994a; Ray & Turkel, 2014; Watson, 1988). Reality changes and shapes meaning and meaning shapes reality because of our moral activity, transcultural communicative spiritual-ethical caring action. Transcultural caring is transcultural compassion and empathy and thus incorporates the "compassionate we" by declaring that entering into the life of, and aspiring to understand, the self and other inspires culturally relevant choices (Davidson & Ray, 1991; Davidson, Ray, & Turkel, 2011; Ray, 1989a, 1989b, 1994a, 1994b, 2010a, 2010b, 2010c).

Summary

This chapter addressed the following:

* Appreciation of the concept of globalization, diversity, multiculturalism, cultural innovation, transglobal, and transculturality/interculturality.
* Identification of and definitions of concepts of caring, transcultural caring, caring for self, transcultural nursing, transcultural consciousness, and spiritual-ethical communicative caring.
* Presentation of the historical and contemporary concepts of culture, including culture as dynamic complexity.
* Presentation of the sciences of complexity, holography, and chaos theory.
* Examination of ways of knowing in nursing, nursing paradigms, and ways of knowing in nursing and transcultural caring.
* Presentation of the evolution of transcultural nursing.
* Presentation of the Transcultural Caring Dynamics in Nursing and Health-Care Theoretical Model.
  * Cultural models are explanatory, representational, and operational (Holland & Quinn, 1987).
  * The *explanatory* aspect of the Transcultural Caring Dynamics in Nursing and Health-Care

BOX 1–1 ❖ Ensuring Transcultural Caring

COMPASSION through LOVE
In response to suffering/need with
RIGHT ACTION or JUSTICE/FAIRNESS
within an understanding of cultural dynamics

Theoretical Model helps professionals gain the knowledge needed to understand personal and relational culture and multiculturalism and their effects on choices and choice-making.

- The *representational (illustrative)* aspect contains material that all cultures can appreciate because each culture can respond to the significance of the structural information, the essence of caring, transcultural ethics, transcultural context, and universal sources.
- The *operational (applicability)* aspect guides understanding, meaning, and behavior to cocreate choices and the best possible future in the nurse-patient/family/community relationship in given transcultural situations.
- Overall, the theoretical model presents a holistic, complex, and dynamic approach to understanding personal and professional culture and facilitating transcultural choice-making in nursing and health care.

Review Questions to Integrate the Transcultural Caring Dynamics in Nursing and Health-Care Theoretical Model into Nursing Education and Practice

Review the following questions to evaluate the meaning of the ideas presented in this chapter, and the meaning the theoretical model has for you as a nurse or nursing student or a professional from another discipline.

- How does the Transcultural Caring Dynamics in Nursing and Health-Care Theoretical Model speak to you?
- What does the concept of transglobal mean to you?
- How can meaning be established and shared in the lives of nurses, other health professionals, and clients interacting in diverse communities?
- How can people of different cultures, including health-care professionals, relate to each other from a caring perspective?
- How does communication, language, or linguistic patterns make a difference in the meaning structure of transcultural caring?

- What is the meaning of adding to the perspective of homo sapiens, the concept of homo socialus (Behar, 2014)? In view of the history of caring, human beings are social and relational. What does it mean to contemplate the idea of virtual presence or the human dimension in virtual reality (Grumme et al., 2015)?
- How do gaps in communication arise?
- What is the meaning of transcultural communication, transcultural spiritual-ethical caring communication?
- What does spiritual-ethical caring mean to you? (Discover the meaning expressed in this book in other chapters in the book.)
- What are the cultural meanings of health and illness in contemporary Western culture or other cultures? How do they present themselves from a multicultural perspective?
- How do social, legal, political, economic, and technological forces in the society in which you live affect ways of being and the meaning of health?
- How does transcultural caring cocreate relationships? (Refer to Chapter 2, The Essence of Caring.)
- What are the transcultural ethical principles that connect people to one another? (Refer to the chapter on Transcultural Caring Ethics in this book.)
- How can culture-value conflict be reduced by transcultural awareness and understanding? (Refer to the chapters on Transcultural Context, and Awareness, Understanding, and Choice.)
- What are some of the factors that contribute to culture-value conflict? (Refer to your own views and others presented in this book.)
- How do culturally oriented spiritual and religious practices influence health-care choices? (Refer to the chapter on Universal Sources.)
- How should nurses and other health-care professionals provide culturally relevant, competent, and innovative care?

Transcultural Caring Experiences

Monique

Monique's story is about the global effect of poverty, seeking freedom, immigration, and the emotional impact that these facts have on a person's health and well-being, and on the nurse(s) who care for her.

Transcultural Facts

You have just had a female patient come into the Emergency Department Fast Track Clinic. The patient is fragile, malnourished, and weary and has a persistent cough with green sputum. She speaks Creole (Haitian traditional language), but she has an English-speaking friend with her. Monique's friend weeps and appears fearful when sharing Monique's story. She states that Monique hopes someone will understand her and help her. She tells Monique's story of fleeing from Haiti to the Bahamas and from the Bahamas, on a boat across the Atlantic, to Florida. She cries as she describes the images of the trip, fleeing from her homeland, poverty, political unrest, and the pain of leaving her family. Monique has had a severe cough for several months. It got worse after landing in Florida and going into hiding. The herbal remedies she was using stopped working and she has pain in her chest. Monique's friend decided they had to seek assistance in the Emergency Department.

Transcultural Nursing Issues

You wonder about your ability to assist this patient. You know that you can handle the physical symptoms of the cough but are more concerned with the transcultural challenges. You are worried about communicating with Monique, her potential undocumented status, and your responsibilities as a nurse with legal sovereign immunity status. You are concerned about Monique's mental state and about your ability to empathize with her over what it is like to leave your homeland and family and come to a strange country to go into hiding. At the same time, you feel compassion for a woman so alone and so sick. You know that an interpreter is necessary and you want to find a way to find an interpreter of the Creole language to help you be a more culturally competent nurse.

Nursing in the hospital and in such a situation is complex. There is little time, money, or incentive to sit down and understand and listen to people from other cultures. It takes effort to provide both physical and culturally relevant care. However, as a nurse, you know that there is an ethical obligation to respect and care for all people of different cultures, races, and behaviors.

Self-Reflection

Answer these questions in the best way possible to test your own cultural knowledge of self and other.

1. What does culture mean to me? What are *my own* beliefs, attitudes, and behaviors that make up my experience about people of different cultures?

2. What are my nursing (student or professional) beliefs, attitudes, and behaviors? How do they affect my professional relationship with this patient and friend? How much education in this area of transcultural nursing did I have in college? What content was emphasized?

3. How do political (including health-care policies), legal (including immigration and homeland security laws), and economic factors affect living, health, illness, and healing, specifically in the case of Monique?

4. How can I communicate better with someone of a different culture? For instance, how could I communicate better with Monique?

5. What language services should be available in hospitals and, in particular, in communities that have diverse yet specific culture groups?

6. How can I help Monique and other patients find the cultural and material resources necessary to improve their health (even in an Emergency Department)?

7. How can I help to create a transcultural caring environment in the workplace?

Kathleen

Kathleen's story is an illustration of our multicultural self.

Transcultural Facts

Kathleen is a nurse from Montreal, Quebec. She comes from a large Irish, Catholic family with roots in Dublin, Ireland. Kathleen loved living in the French Canadian city throughout her childhood. She went to a French-speaking elementary school where she met not only French Canadians but also other Euro-Canadians. She has a slight accent when she speaks French, denoting that French was not her first, or native, language. Kathleen studied nursing in a midsized city in the province of Ontario, which has Scottish roots. There were many activities and festivals that harkened back to the ancestry of the United Kingdom. Kathleen enjoyed being a professional nurse and was challenged by the symbols and rituals of the nursing culture. She loved patients and wanted to meet their needs. After completing her nursing program, she decided to move to California where she worked in a large medical center in Los Angeles, in an upper-class neighborhood. She and some friends found an attractive apartment near the medical center. Kathleen's work life brought her in contact with different culture groups, different from those she had been used to when she grew up. She worked with many multicultural health-care personnel. Many diverse cultures immigrated to southern California. Kathleen even cared for patients who were "big names" in the entertainment industry. Kathleen liked all the transcultural experiences but longed for a family and to create a home of her own. She soon fell in love and married a lawyer, originally from Lebanon with Islamic roots, who was contemplating a new job with a law firm in Houston, Texas.

Transcultural Nursing Issues

Consider the complexity of Kathleen's national and bicultural heritage and about the new cultural groups she encountered and joined after moving from Canada. Explore the meaning of the multicultural self, using Kathleen as an example.

Think about nursing and about how the rituals and symbols of nursing practice affect and ground transcultural nursing practice. Consider how the culture of nursing practice differs among different countries and different American states.

You ponder the impact on Kathleen's marriage. Consider the complexity of Kathleen's new marriage and the cultural challenges that she will encounter—marrying a man originally from the Middle East with a culture and religion different from her own. Now think about how she will adapt to living with and supporting the profession of an attorney in the Texas city of Houston, which is culturally different from Los Angeles.

Self-Reflection

1. Compare and contrast the identities outlined in Kathleen's story.

2. What are the familial, linguistic, community, geographical or nation-state, professional, work, and social parameters? Are there fixed boundaries?

3. How would you analyze Kathleen's multicultural self in terms of gender, kinship, ethnicity, culture, generation, and socioeconomic?

4. What are the potential conflicts or tensions that may arise in a multicultural self? Give some examples using Kathleen's or your own experiences.

5. How does choice enter in the picture? What is meant by defining culture as Dynamic Complexity and choice in the contemporary North American culture?

6. What is your own multicultural self? What makes up your identity? How does social media affect identity and understanding of the self? What choices have you made in your personal and professional lives that contribute to your understanding or misunderstanding of the culture of self and other?

7. How does this notion of the multicultural self affect your role as a student, a professional nurse, and how does it affect relationships with patients?

Lian

Lian's story will assist you in learning about building a transcultural consciousness and understanding issues of marginalization, discrimination, and bullying.

Transcultural Facts

Lian is a senior in high school and is considering a career in nursing. He came to the United States from Cambodia with his parents when he was 10 years old. His parents disapprove of nursing and would prefer that he be a physician or a computer technology professional so that he will receive more money and respect. Nonetheless, Lian is drawn to nursing because of his experience with the school nurse, Ms. Blanchard. Ms. Blanchard had defended and cared for him when he experienced discrimination, marginalization, and bullying by his fellow students. Ms. Blanchard talked to Lian and other students and helped them address and cope with their problems, specifically those related to discrimination and feelings of isolation, marginalization, and bullying, especially now with the use of the Internet, Facebook and Twitter.

Although at first Lian was enticed by the idea of money and prestige offered by other career options, such as the computer industry, which features opportunities for positions in social media—areas to which Lian is attracted. He, however, was more inspired by Ms. Blanchard and intrigued by the challenges of helping others and caring for people with needs. He wanted to understand more about racial identity, marginalization, and cultural diversity, and more about caring for others. He did some research and found that the local nursing school offered a course in transcultural nursing in addition to the required courses. He decided to enroll in the local nursing program.

Self-Reflection

Here are some relevant questions you may ask yourself related to building a transcultural consciousness. Try to answer these questions in light of what you have learned in this chapter about transcultural consciousness and nursing.

1. As a person and nurse, how do you see Lian's situation? Why is nursing not recognized strongly as a profession in the dominant culture?

2. What is the role of example in human experience and in developing a transcultural consciousness? Is caring learned only by example, or can it be learned in other ways?

3. Talk about the caring and empathy that the nurse showed to the culturally diverse students. Reflect on and illuminate the meaning of transcultural caring empathy/compassion. What is the meaning of marginalization, discrimination, and bullying?

4. Why is it that nurses exhibit an emotional intimacy and compassion and a sense of justice?

5. What is the meaning of caring for others who are not family?

6. What examples from the social world (i.e., family, teachers, friends, counselors and school, television, YouTube and other social media) make nursing an attractive career and facilitate understanding of why a person would choose nursing?

7. What is self-reflective consciousness and how does it underlie transcultural awareness?

8. What strategies can be used to develop a self-reflective and transcultural consciousness?

9. Reflect on and illuminate the meaning of transcultural empathy/compassion.

References

Albrecht, G., Fitzpatrick, R., & Scrimshaw, S. (Eds.). (2000). *Handbook of social studies in health and medicine*. London: Sage Publications.

Aldrin B. (2015). *Mission to Mars*. New York: National Geographic.

American Nurses Association. http://www.nursingworld.org, Retrieved December, 14, 2014.

Andrews, M., & Boyle, J. (2007). *Transcultural concepts in nursing care* (5th ed.). Philadelphia: Lippincott.

Andrews, M., & Boyle, J. (2015). *Transcultural concepts in nursing care* (7th ed.). Philadelphia: Lippincott.

Arntz, W., Chasse, B., & Vicente, M. (2005). *What the bleep do we know!?* Deerfield Beach, FL: Health Communications, Inc.

Bar-Yam, Y. (2004). *Making things work: Solving complex problems in a complex world*. Boston, MA: Knowledge Press.

Barnard, A., & Locsin, R. (Eds.). (2007). *Technology and nursing: Practice, concepts and issues*. Hampshire, United Kingdom: Palgrave MacMillan.

Barry, C., Gordon, S., & King, B. (2015). *Caring in nursing situations*. New York: Springer Publishing Company.

Behar, M. (2013). *Generation F.* Bulgaria: Alto Communications Publishing Ltd.

Berman, P. (2003). *Terror and liberalism*. New York: W. W. Norton.

Bishop, A., & Scudder, J. (1991). *The practice of caring*. New York: National League for Nursing Press.

Boas, F. (1928). *Anthropology and modern life*. New York: Norton.

Boulding, E. (2000). Peace culture: The vision and the journey. *Friends Journal, 9*, 6–8.

Boykin, A., & Schoenhofer, S. (2001). *Nursing as caring* (2nd ed.). New York: Jones and Bartlett. (Original work published 1993)

Boykin, A., Schoenhofer, S., & Valentine, K. (2014). *Health care system transformation for nursing and health care leaders: Implementing a culture of caring*. New York: Springer Publishing Company.

Breda, K. (Ed.) (2009). *Nursing and globalization in the Americas*. Amityville, NY: Baywood Publishing Company, Inc.

Briggs, J., & Peat, F. (1989). *Turbulent mirror*. New York: Harper & Row.

Briggs, J., & Peat, F. (1999). *Seven lessons of chaos*. New York: HarperCollins Publishers.

Brown, C. (2009). Self-renewal in nursing leadership: The lived experience of caring for self. *Journal of Holistic Nursing, 27*(2), 75–84.

Brown, P. (1998). *Understanding and applying medical anthropology*. Mountain View, CA: Mayfield Publishing Company.

Brush, B. (2008). Global nurse migration today. *Journal of Nursing Scholarship 40*(1), 20–25.

Burkhardt, M., & Nathaniel, A. (2008). *Ethics & issues in contemporary nursing* (3rd ed.). New York: Thomson Delmar Learning.

Cannato, J. (2006). *Radical amazement*. Notre Dame, IN: Sorin Books.

Capra, F., Steindl-Rast, D. with Matus, T. (1991). *Belonging to the universe*. San Franscisco: HarperSanFrancisco.

Carper, B. (1978). Fundamental patterns of knowing in nursing. *Advances in Nursing Science, 1*(1), 13–23.

Chamberlin, J. (1999). *Upon whom we depend: The American poverty system*. New York: Peter Lang.

Chinn, P. (2013). *Peace and power: New directions for building community* (8th ed.). Burlington, MA: Jones & Bartlett Learning.

Chomsky, A. (2014). *Undocumented: How immigration became illegal*. Boston, MA: Beacon Press.

Clifford, J. (1988). *The predicament of culture*. Boston, MA: Harvard University Press.

Coffman, S. (2006). Marilyn Anne Ray: Theory of bureaucratic caring. In A. Marriner Tomey & M. Alligood (Eds.), *Nursing theorists and their work* (6th ed., pp. 116–139). St. Louis: Mosby Elsevier.

Coffman, S. (2014). Marilyn Anne Ray: Theory of bureaucratic caring. In M. Alligood (Ed.), *Nursing theorists and their work* (8th ed.) (pp. 98–119). St. Louis: Elsevier.

Davidhizar, R., & Giger, J. (1998). *Canadian transcultural nursing*. St. Louis: Mosby.

Davidson, A., & Ray, M. (1991). Studying the human-environment phenomena using the science of complexity. *Advances in Nursing Science, 14*(2), 73–87.

Davidson, A., Ray, M., & Turkel, M. (Eds.) (2011). *Nursing, caring, and complexity science: For human-environment well-being*. New York: Springer Publishing Company. [AJN Book of the Year, 2011]

Davis, W. (1999). Vanishing cultures. *National Geographic, 196*(2), 64–89.

DeSantis, L. (1997). Building healthy communities with immigrants and refugees. *Journal of Transcultural Nursing, 9*(1), 20–31.

DeSantis, L., & Lipson, J. (2007). Brief history of inclusion of content on culture in nursing education. *Journal of Transcultural Nursing, 18*(1), 7S–9S.

De Vries, H., & Sullivan, L. (2006). *Political theologies: Public religion in a post-secular world.* New York: Fordham University Press.

Dewing, M., & Leman, M. (2006). *Canadian multiculturalism.* Library of Parliament: Parliamentary Information and Research Services, Political and Social Affairs Division. (Original Publication 1994, Revised Publication 16 March, 2006). Ottawa, ON: Parliamentary Research Branch. Retrieved May 24, 2009, from www://par..gc.ca/information/library/PRBpubs/936-e.htm-65k

Dossey, B., & Keegan, L. (2008). *Holistic nursing: A handbook for practice.* Sudbury, MA: Jones & Bartlett Publishers.

Dossey, B., & Keegan, L. (2012). *Holistic nursing: A handbook for practice* (6th ed,). Burlington, MA: Jones & Bartlett Learning.

Dougherty, M., & Tripp-Reimer, T. (1991). Nursing and anthropology. In T. M. Johnson & C. Sargent (Eds.), *Medical anthropology: A handbook of theory and research.* Westport, CT: Greenwood Press.

Duggins, P. (2007). *Final countdown: NASA and the end of the space shuttle program.* Gainesville, FL: University Press of Florida.

Eggenberger, T., & Keller, K. (2008). Grounding nursing simulations in caring: An Innovative approach. *International Journal for Human Caring, 12*(2), 42–46.

Eisler, R. (2007). *The real wealth of nations: Creating a caring economics.* San Francisco: Berrett-Koehler Publishers, Inc.

Eriksson, K. (1997). Caring, spirituality and suffering. In M. Roach (Ed.), *Caring from the heart: The convergence of caring and spirituality.* New York: Paulist Press.

Eriksson, L. (2006). *The suffering human being.* Chicago: Nordic Studies Press.

Ess, C. (2014). *Digital media ethics.* United Kingdom, Palgrave McMillan: Polity.

Fang, D., Wilsey, S., & Bednash, G. (2007*). 2006–2007 Enrollment and graduations in baccalaureate and graduate programs in nursing.* Washington, DC: American Association of Colleges of Nursing (AACN).

Fawcett, J. (1993). From a plethora of paradigms to parsimony in worldviews. *Nursing Science Quarterly, 6*(2), 56–58.

Fitzpatrick, J., & Whall, A. (Eds.). (1996). *Conceptual models in nursing* (3rd ed.). Stamford, CT: Appleton & Lange.

Floridi, L. (2014). *The fourth revolution: How the infosphere is reshaping human reality.* Oxford: Oxford University Press.

Fox, M., & Swimme, B. (1982). *Manifesto! For a global civilization.* Santa Fe, NM: Bear and Company.

Frelich, M. (Ed.). (1989). *The relevance of culture.* New York: Bergin & Garvey Publishers.

Friedman, T. (2006). *The world is flat.* New York: Farrar, Straus and Giroux.

Furniss, T. (2006). *A history of space exploration.* London: Mercury Books.

Gadow, S. (1988). Covenant without cure: Letting go and holding on in chronic illness. In J. Watson & M. Ray (Eds.), *The ethics of care and the ethics of cure: Synthesis in chronicity.* New York: National League for Nursing.

Geertz, C. (1973). *The interpretation of cultures.* New York: Basic Books.

Gennaro, S. (2008). Celebrating 40 years of disseminating knowledge that improves global health. *Journal of Nursing Scholarship, 40*(1), 1–2.

Giddens, J. (2008). Achieving diversity in nursing through multicontextual learning environments. *Nursing Outlook, 56*(2), 78–83.

Giger, J., & Davidhizar, R. (2004). Transcultural nursing assessment and intervention (4th ed.). St. Louis: C.V. Mosby.

Giger, J., Davidhizar, R., Purnell, L., Harden, J., Phillips, J., & Strickland, O. (2007). American Academy of Nursing expert panel report: Developing cultural competence to eliminate health disparities in ethnic minorities and other vulnerable populations. *Journal of Transcultural Nursing, 18*(20), 95–102.

Glotz, P., & Bertsch, S. (2005). *Thumb culture: The meaning of mobile phones for society.* New Brunswick, NJ: Transaction Publishers.

Goodwin, B. (1994). *How the leopard changes its spots: The evolution of complexity.* New York: Simon & Schuster.

Goodwin, B. (2003). Patterns of wholeness: Holistic science. *Resurgence 1*(216), 12–14.

Griffiths, B. (1989). *A new vision of reality: Western science, Eastern mysticism, and Christian faith*. Springfield, IL: Templegate Publishers.

Grumme, V. (2015). Virtual presence. PhD Comprehensive Examination Final Paper. Submitted to Faculty, Florida Atlantic University, The Christine E. Lynn College of Nursing, Boca Raton, Florida.

Grumme, V., Barry, C., Gordon, S., & Ray, M. (Reviewed for publication.) *Advances in nursing science.*

Gutierrez, E., & Kendall, C. (2000). The globalization of health and disease: The health transition and global change. In G. Albrecht, R. Fitzpatrick, & S. Scrimshaw (Eds.), *The handbook of social studies in health & medicine*. Thousand Oaks, CA: Sage Publications.

Hannerz, U. (1993). *Cultural complexity: Studies in the social organization of meaning*. New York: Columbia University Press.

Hannerz, U. (1999). *Globalization and identity*. London: Wiley-Blackwell.

Harman, W. (1998). *Global mind change*. San Francisco: Berrett-Koehler Publishers, Inc.

Helman, C. (1994). *Culture, health and illness: An introduction for health professionals* (3rd ed.). Oxford: Butterworth/Heinemann.

Henderson, H. with Simran, S. (2006). *Ethical markets: Growing the green economy*. White River Junction, VT: Chelsea Green Publishing Company.

Heyman, J. (1999). United States surveillance over Mexican lives at the border: Snapshots of an emerging regime. *Human Organization, 58*(4), 430–438.

Hoffman, E. (2008). The Maslow effect: A humanist legacy for nursing. *American Nurse Today, 10*(3), 12–13.

Holland, D., & Quinn, N. (1987). *Cultural models in language and thought*. Cambridge: Cambridge University Press.

Jarvis, T., & Macdonald, S. (Eds..) (2014). *Cyberterrorism*. New York, NY: Springer Publishing Company.

Jennings, D., & Lowe, J. (2013). Photovoice: Giving voice to indigenous youth. *Pimatisiwin: a Journal of Aboriginal and indigenous community health, 11*(3), 521–537.

Johns, C., & Freshwater, D. (Eds.). (1998). *Transforming nursing through reflective practice*. Oxford: Blackwell Science.

Johns, C. (2007). *Engaging reflection in practice: A narrative approach*. Oxford: Blackwell Publishing Ltd.

Kaszycka, K., Strkalj, G., & Strzalko, J. (2009). Current views of European anthropologists on race: Influence of education and ideological background. *American Anthropologist, 111*(1), 43–56.

Kleinman, A. (1998). Do psychiatric disorders differ in different cultures? In P. Brown (Ed.), *Understanding and applying medical anthropology* (pp.185–196). Mountain View, CA: Mayfield Publishing Company.

Kluckhohn, C., & Kelly, W. (1945). The concept of culture. In R. Linton (Ed.), *The science of man in the world of crisis*. New York: Columbia University Press.

Kroeber, A. (1917). The superorganic. *American Anthropologist, 19*, 163–213.

Lauterbach, S., & Becker, P. (1996). Caring for self: Becoming a self-reflective nurse. *Holistic Nursing Practice, 10*(2), 57–68.

Leininger, M. (1970). *Anthropology and nursing: Two worlds to blend*. New York: John Wiley & Sons.

Leininger, M. (1978). *Transcultural nursing: Concepts, theories, and practices*. New York: John Wiley & Sons.

Leininger, M. (Ed.). (1981). *Caring: An essential human need*. Thorofare, NJ: Slack Incorporated.

Leininger, M. (Ed.). (1991). *Culture care diversity and universality: A theory of nursing*. New York: National League for Nursing Press.

Leininger, M. (1994). *Transcultural nursing: Concepts, theories, and practices*. New York: John Wiley. (Original work published 1978)

Leininger, M. (1995). *Transcultural nursing: Concepts, theories, research, and practice*. Columbus, OH: McGraw-Hill.

Leininger, M. (1996). Culture care theory. *Nursing Science Quarterly, 9*, 71–78.

Leininger, M., & McFarland, M. (2002). *Transcultural nursing: Concepts, theories, research, & practice* (3rd ed.). New York: McGraw-Hill Medical Publishing Division.

Leininger, M., & McFarland, M. (Eds.). (2006). *Cultural care diversity and universality: A worldwide theory of nursing* (2nd ed.). Sudbury, MA: Jones and Bartlett Publishers.

Libicki, M. (2007). *Conquest in cyberspace: National security and information warfare*. New York: Cambridge University Press.

Lindberg, C., Nash, S., & Lindberg, C. (2008). *On the edge: Nursing in the age of complexity*. Bordentown, NJ: Plexus Press.

Lipson, J., & DeSantis, L. (2007). Current approaches to integrating elements of cultural competence in nursing education. *Journal of Transcultural Nursing, 18*(1), 10S–20S.

Lipson, J., & Dibble, S. (2005). *Culture and clinical care.* San Francisco: The University of California Press.

Locsin, R., & Purnell, M. (2009). *A contemporary nursing process: The (un)bearable weight of knowing in nursing.* New York: Springer Publishing Company.

Lowe, J., & Nichols, L. (2014). Utilization of a Native American nursing conceptual framework: Implications for practice and research. *Australian Journal of Advanced Nursing, 31*(2), 13–22.

Lupul, M. (2005). *The politics of multiculturalism: A Ukrainian Canadian memoir.* Alberta: Canadian Institute of Ukrainian Study.

Mander J., & Goldsmith, E. (1996). *The case against the global economy.* London: Earthscan Ltd.

Maturana, H., & Varela, F. (1992). *Tree of Knowledge.* Boston: Shambhala Publication, Inc.

Mayeroff, M. (1971). *On caring.* New York: Harper & Row.

McFarland, M., & Wehbe-Alamah, H. (Eds.) (2015). *Leininger's culture care diversity and universality* (3rd. ed.). Burlington, MA: Jones & Bartlett Learning.

Meleis, A. (1996). Culturally competent scholarship: Substance and rigor. *Advances in Nursing Science, 19*(2), 1–16.

Miller, J., Leininger, M., Leuning, C., Pacquiao, D., Andrews, M., Ludwig-Beymer, P., & Papadopoulos, I. (2008). Transcultural nursing society position statement on human rights. *Journal of Transcultural Nursing, 19*(1), 5–7.

Milne, D. (1982). *The new Canadian constitution.* Toronto: James Lorimer & Company Publishers.

Miskin, F. (2008). *The next great globalization: How disadvantaged nations can harness their financial system to get rich.* Princeton, NJ: Princeton University Press.

Morse, J., Bottorff, J., Neander, W., & Solberg, S. (1991). Comparative analysis of conceptualizations and theories of caring. *Image: Journal of Nursing Scholarship, 23*(2), 119–126.

Morse, J., Solberg, S., Neander, W., Bottorff, J., & Johnson, J. (1990). Concepts of caring and caring as a concept. *Advances in Nursing Science, 13*(1), 1–14.

National Center for Complementary and Alternative Medicine. Retrieved August 12, 2008 from http://www.nccam.nih.gov

National Coalition of Ethnic Minority Nurse Associations (NCEMNA). Retrieved August 23, 2014 from http://www.ncemna.org

Newman, M. (1992). Prevailing paradigms in nursing. *Nursing Outlook, 40*(1), 10–14.

Newman, M. (2003). A world of no boundaries. *Advances in Nursing Science, 26*(4), 240–245.

Newman, M., Sime, M., & Corcoran-Perry, S. (1991). The focus of the discipline of nursing. *Advances in Nursing Science, 14*(1), 1–6.

Newman, M., Smith, M., Dexheimer-Pharris, M., & Jones, D. (2008). The focus of the discipline revisited. *Advances in Nursing Science, 31*(1), E16–27.

Nouwen, H. (1977). Compassion and the seven o'clock news. *The Sojourners, 6*(10), 15, 18.

Nouwen, H. (1979). *The wounded healer.* New York: Doubleday & Co., Image Books.

Omery, A., Kasper, C., & Page, G. (Eds.). (1995). *In search of nursing science.* Thousand Oaks: Sage Publications.

Pacquiao, D. (2007). The relationship between cultural competence education and increasing diversity in nursing schools and practice settings. *Journal of Transcultural Nursing 18*(10), 28S–37S.

Paley, J. (2001). An archaeology of caring knowledge. *Journal of Advanced Nursing, 36*(2), 188–198.

Parse, R. (1981). *Man-living-health: A theory of nursing.* New York: Wiley.

Parse, R. (1987). *Nursing science: Major theories, paradigms, and critiques.* Philadelphia: W.B. Saunders.

Parse, R. (1996). The human becoming theory: Challenges in practice and research. *Nursing Science Quarterly, 9*(2), 55–60.

Passel, J., & Cohn, D. (2008). Immigration to play lead role in future U.S. growth: U.S. population projections: 2005–2050. *Executive Summary, Pew Research Center, Social and Demographic Trends, February 11, 2008.* Retrieved May 24, 2009, from http://pewresearch.org/pubs/729/united_states-population-projections-27k

Peat, F. (2002). *From certainty to uncertainty: The story of science and ideas in the twentieth century.* Washington, DC: John Henry Press.

Peat, F. (2003). From physics to Pari: A continuing search for answers. *Resurgence, 1*(21), 24–26.

Pensky, M. (Ed.). (2005). *Globalizing critical theory (new critical theory)*. New York: Rowman & Littlefield Publishers.

Platt, C., & Platt, C. (2007). *Myspace to sacred space: God for a new generation*. Danvers, MA: Clearance Center.

Population projections for Canada, provinces, and territories. Population by age group and sex (2006–2031). Statistics Canada. Retrieved August 10, 2008 from http://www.statcan.ca

Postero, N. (2007). *Now we are citizens: Indigenous politics in postmulticultural Bolivia*. Stanford, CA: Stanford University Press.

Purnell, L., & Paulanka, B. (2008). *Transcultural health care: A culturally competent approach* (3rd ed.). Philadelphia: F. A. Davis Company.

Rachels, J. (2003). *The elements of moral philosophy* (4th ed.). Boston: McGraw-Hill.

Ray, M. (1981a). A study of caring within an institutional culture. Dissertation Abstracts International, 42(06). (University Microfilms No. 8127787).

Ray, M. (1981b). A philosophical analysis of care and caring within nursing. In M. Leininger (Ed.), *Caring: An essential human need*. Thorofare, NJ: Slack Incorporated.

Ray, M. (1989a). Transcultural caring: Political and economic visions. *Journal of Transcultural Nursing, 1*(1), 17–21.

Ray, M. (1989b). The theory of bureaucratic caring for nursing practice in the organizational culture. *Nursing Administration Quarterly, 13*(2), 31–42.

Ray, M. (1991). Caring inquiry: The esthetic process in the way of compassion, In D. Gaut & M. Leininger (Eds.), *Caring: The compassionate healer*. New York: National League for Nursing Press.

Ray, M. (1994a). Transcultural nursing ethics: A framework and model for transcultural ethical analysis. *Journal of Holistic Nursing, 12*(3), 251–264.

Ray, M. (1994b). Complex caring dynamics: A unifying model of nursing inquiry. *Theoretic and Applied Chaos in Nursing, 1*(1), 23–32.

Ray, M. (1997a). The ethical theory of existential authenticity: The lived experience of the art of caring in nursing administration. *Canadian Journal of Nursing Research, 29*(1), 111–126.

Ray, M. (1997b). Illuminating the meaning of caring: Unfolding the sacred art of divine love. In M. Roach (Ed.), *Caring from the heart: The convergence of caring and spirituality* (pp. 163–178). New York: Paulist Press.

Ray, M. (1998). Complexity and nursing science. *Nursing Science Quarterly, 11*(3), 91–93.

Ray, M. (2000). Bureaucratic caring revisited. In M. Parker (Ed.), *Nursing theories, nursing practice*. Philadelphia: F. A. Davis Company.

Ray, M. (2006). Marilyn Anne Ray's theory of bureaucatic caring: Part 1. In M. Parker (Ed.), *Nursing theories, nursing practice* (2nd ed., pp. 360–379). Philadelphia: F. A. Davis Company.

Ray, M. (2010a). *Transcultural caring dynamics in nursing and health care*. Philadelphia: F. A. Davis Company.

Ray, M. (2010b). *A study of caring within an institutional culture: The discovery of the Theory of Bureaucratic Caring*. Germany: Lambert Academic Publishing.

Ray, M. (2010c). Creating caring organizations and communities through communitarian ethics. *Journal of the World Universities Forum, 3*(5), 41–52.

Ray, M. (2011). Complex caring dynamics: A unifying model of nursing inquiry. In A. Davidson, M. Ray, & M. Turkel (Eds.), *Nursing, caring, and complexity science: For human-environment well-being* (pp. 31–52). New York: Springer Publishing Company.

Ray, M., & Turkel, M. (2014). Caring as emancipatory nursing praxis: The theory of relational caring complexity. *Advances in Nursing Science, 37*(2), 132–146.

Ray, M., & Turkel, M. (2015). The Marilyn Anne Ray's Theory of Bureaucratic Caring. In M. Parker & M. Smith (Eds.), *Nursing theories and nursing practice* (4th ed.). Philadelphia: F. A. Davis Company.

Ray, M., Turkel, M., & Marino, F. (2002). The transformative process for nursing in workforce redevelopment. *Nursing Administration Quarterly, 26*(2), 1–14.

Ringma, C. (2000). *Dare to journey with Henri Nouwen*. Colorado Springs, CO: Piñon Press.

Roach, M. (1987). *The human act of caring*. Ottawa, ON: Canadian Hospital Association.

Roach, M. (2002). *Caring, the human mode of being: A blueprint for the health professions* (2nd rev. ed.). Ottawa, ON: CHA Press.

Rogers, E. (2003). *Diffusion of innovations* (5th ed.). New York: Free Press.

Rogers, M. (1970). *An introduction to the theoretical basis of nursing*. Philadelphia: F. A. Davis Company.

Ryan, M., Carlton, K., & Ali, N. (2000). Transcultural nursing concepts and experiences in nursing curricula. *Journal of Transcultural Nursing, 11*(4), 300–307.

Sachs, J. (2005). *The end of poverty: Economic possibilities of our time*. New York: The Penguin Press.

Sahlins, M. (1976). *Culture and practical reason*. Chicago: University of Chicago Press.

Semotiuk, A. (2014). *A promise kept*. Charleston, SC: Create Space Independent Publishing Platform.

Simpson, S. (1989). Nursing and the culture at the end of the twentieth century. In M. Freilich (Ed.), *The relevance of culture* (pp. 189–197). New York: Bergin & Garvey Publishers.

Slatterly, F. (2004). *Where have all the nurses gone?: The impact of the nursing shortage on American healthcare*. Amherst, NY: Prometheus Books.

Smircich, L. (1985). Is the concept of culture a paradigm for understanding organizations and ourselves? In P. Frost, L. Moore, M. Louis, C. Lundberg, & J. Martin (Eds.), *Organizational culture*. Beverly Hills, CA: Sage Publications.

Smith, M. (2015). *Nursing theories and nursing practice* (4th ed.). Philadelphia, PA: F. A. Davis Company.

Smith, M., Turkel, M., & Wolf, Z. (Eds.) (2013). *Caring in nursing classics: An essential resource*. New York, NY: Springer Publishing Company.

Solecki, R. (1971). *Shanidar: The first flower people*. New York: Alfred A. Knopf.

Sorbello, B. (2008a). Finance: It's not a dirty word. *American Nurse Today, 3*(8), 32–35.

Sorbello, B. (2008b). Responding to a sentinel event. *American Nurse Today, 3*(10), 30–32.

Special issue (2007). Integrating cultural competence into nursing education and practice. *Journal of Transcultural Nursing, 18*(1), 5S–90S.

Special issue (2008). Caring in nursing education. *International Journal for Human Caring, 12*(2), 7–99.

Spector, R. (2004). *Cultural diversity in health and illness* (6th ed.). Upper Saddle River, NJ: Pearson Prentice Hall.

Spector, R. (2008). *Cultural diversity in health and illness* (7th ed.). Upper Saddle River, NJ: Prentice Hall.

Spikins, P. (2015). *How compassion made us human: An archaeology of stone age sentiment*. United Kingdom: Pen and Sword.

Statistics Canada. *2006 Canadian census*. Retrieved May 24, 2009, from http:/www12.statcan.ca/census-recensement/index-eng.cfm

Study: Canada's visible minority population in 2017. *The Daily*. Retrieved August 10, 2008, from http://www.statcan.gc.ca/daily-quotidien/050322/dq050322b-eng.htm

Swimme, B. (1996). *The hidden heart of the cosmos: Humanity and the new story*. Maryknoll, NY: Orbis Books.

Taylor, C. (1994). The politics of recognition. In A. Gutmann (Ed.), *Multiculturalism* (pp. 25–73). Princeton, NJ: Princeton University Press.

Teilhard, P. (1965). *Building the earth*. Denville, NJ: Dimensions Books.

Templeton, J. (1999). *Agape love*. Philadelphia: Templeton Foundation Press.

The 2005 workforce profile of registered nurses in Canada. The Canadian Nurses Association, Statistics Canada, September 2006.

The New American Bible (1970). New York: Catholic Book Publishing Co.

The Registered Nurse Population: Findings from the 2004 national sample of registered nurses. Retrieved August 9, 2008 from mhtml:file://D:\Nursing\2004

Thoma, H. (2003). All at the same time. Holistic science. *Resurgence 1*(216), 15–17.

Touhy, T., & Boykin, A. (2008). Caring as the central domain in nursing education. *International Journal for Human Caring, 12*(2), 9–15.

Tuan, M. (1998). *Forever foreigners or honorary whites? The Asian ethnic-experience today*. New Brunswick, NJ: Rutgers University Press.

Turkel, M. (2006a). What is evidence-based practice? In S. Beyea & M. Slattery (Eds.), *Evidence-based practice in nursing: A guide to successful implementation*. Marblehead, MA: HcPro Publishing.

Turkel, M. (2006b). Integration of evidence-based practice in nursing. In S. Beyea & M. Slattery (Eds.), *Evidence-based practice in nursing: A guide to successful implementation*. Marblehead, MA: HcPro Publishing.

Turkel, M. (2007). Dr. Marilyn Ray's theory of bureaucratic caring. *International Journal for Human Caring, 11*(4), 57–70.

Turkel, M., & Ray, M. (2000). Relational complexity: A theory of the nurse-patient relationship within an economic context. *Nursing Science Quarterly, 13*(4), 306–313.

Turkel, M., & Ray, M. (2001). Relational complexity: From grounded theory to instrument development and theoretical testing. *Nursing Science Quarterly, 14*(4), 281–287.

Turkel, M., & Ray, M. (2004a). A process model for policy analysis within the context of political caring. *International Journal for Human Caring, 7*(3), 17–24.

Turkel, M., & Ray, M. (2004b). Creating a caring practice environment through self-renewal. *Nursing Administration Quarterly, 28*(4), 249–256.

Turkel, M., & Ray, M. (2009). Caring for "not so picture perfect patients": Ethical caring in the moral community of nursing. In R. Locsin & M. Purnell (Eds.), *A contemporary nursing process: The (un)bearable weight of knowing persons* (pp. 225–229). New York: Springer Publishing Company.

Tylor, E. (1865). *Researches into the early history of mankind and the development of civilization.* London: J. Murray.

Tylor, E. (1871). *Primitive culture.* London: J. Murray.

Tylor, E. (1930). *Anthropology: An introduction to the study of man and civilization* (Vol. 1). London: Watts & Co.

U.S. Census Report. Retrieved August 9, 2008, from http://www.census.gov./pressrelease/www/releases/archives/population/012496.html

U.S. Census Bureau. (2000). U.S. Census Report. http://www.census.gov./press-, Retrieved August 10, 2008 from release/www/releases/archives/population/012496.html;

U.S. Census Bureau. (March 18, 2004). *U.S. Interim Projections by age, sex, race, and Hispanic origin,* Retrieved August 10, 2008 from http:www.census.gov/ipc/www/usintermin proj/

Visible minority. Retrieved August 9, 2008 from mhtml:file://D:\Nursing\Visible minority-Wikipedia, The free encyclopedia.mht

Watson, J. (1979). *The philosophy and science of caring.* Boston: Little, Brown and Company.

Watson, J. (1985). *Nursing: Human science and human care.* Norwalk, CT: Appleton-Century-Crofts.

Watson, J. (1988). *Nursing: Human science and human care: A theory of nursing.* New York: National League for Nursing.

Watson, J. (1999). *Postmodern nursing.* London: Churchill-Livingstone.

Watson, J. (2005). *Caring science as sacred science.* Philadelphia: F. A. Davis Company.

Watson, J. (2008a). *The philosophy and science of caring* (Rev. ed.). Boulder, CO: University Press of Colorado.

Watson, J. (2008b). *Assessing and measuring caring in nursing and health care* (2nd ed.). New York: Springer Publishing Company.

Wheatley, M. (1999). *Leadership and the new science.* San Francisco: Barrett-Koehler.

White, J. (1995). Patterns of knowing: Review, critique, and update. *Advances in Nursing Science 17*(4), 73–86.

Winslow, O. (2008). An older and more diverse nation by mid-century. Newsroom, Public Information Office, U.S. Census Bureau New, U.S. Department of Commerce. Released August 14, 2008. Retrieved May 24, 2009, from http:/www.census.gov/popest/archives/files/MRSF-01-US1.html

Zúñiga, D., & Pellow, D. (2008). The self-consciousness of placemaking. *Anthropology News 49*(9), 4–5.

Zwingle, E. (1999). Goods move. People move. Ideas move. And cultures change. *National Geographic, 196*(2), 12–36.

SELECT BIBLIOGRAPHY

Asante, M., & Gudykunst, W. (Eds.). (1989). *Handbook of international and intercultural communication.* Newbury Park, CA: Sage Publications.

Bonvillain, N. (2007). *Language, culture and communication* (5th ed.). Upper Saddle River, NJ: Prentice-Hall, Inc.

Boulding, E. (1988). *Building a global civic culture.* New York: Teachers College Press.

Corson, W. (1995). Priorities for a sustainable future: The role of education, the media, and tax reform. *Journal of Social Issues, 51*(4), 37–61.

Cuban Adjustment Act, 1966. Retrieved May 24, 2009, from http://www.state.gov/www/regions/wha/cuba/cuba_adjustment-act.html

Dienemann, J. (1997). *Cultural diversity in nursing.* Washington, DC: American Academy of Nursing.

Election Results of Canada. CSPAN, October 14, 2008.

Glynn, N., & Bishop, G. (1986). Multiculturalism in nursing: Implications for faculty development. *Journal of Nursing Education, 25*(1), 39–41.

International Journal for Human Caring, 1997 to present.

Healthy People 2020. http:www.healthypeople.gov. Retrieved January, 6, 2015.

Kaebnick, G. (2000). On the sanctity of nature. *The Hastings Center Report, 30*(5), 16–23.

Parfit, M. (1994). Powwow: A gathering of tribes. *National Geographic, 185*(6), 87–113.

Paterson, J., & Zderad, L. (1976). *Humanistic nursing.* New York: John Wiley & Sons.

Patient Protection and Affordable Care Act (Public Law, 111–148, 111th Congress, March 23, 2010). https://www/healthcare.gov. Retreived June 27, 2014.

Pluto. http://www.nasa.gov/new horizons, Retrieved, July 14, 2015.

Pope Francis. (2013). Evangelii Gaudium. Chapter 4, The inclusion of the poor in society (pp. 186–216). Retrieved from www.w2Vatican.va/content/francesco/en/apost_exhortations/documents/

Reidy, M., & Taggart, M. (1998). French Canadians of Quebec origin (pp. 155–178). In R. Davidhizar & J. Giger (Eds.), *Canadian Transcultural Nursing.* St. Louis: Mosby.

Scudder, T. (1999). The emerging global crisis and development anthropology: Can we have an impact? *Human Organization, 58*(4), 351–364.

Sherwood, G. (1997). Meta-synthesis of qualitative analyses of caring: Defining a therapeutic model of nursing. *Advanced Practice Quarterly, 3*(1), 32–42.

Singer, I. (1987). *The nature of love: The modern world.* Chicago: The University of Chicago Press.

Smith, M. (1999). Caring and the science of unitary human beings. *Advances in Nursing Science, 21*(4), 14–28.

Stiglitz, J. (2003). *Globalization and its discontents.* New York: WW Norton & Company.

Tarlow, S. (2000). Emotion in archaeology. *Current Anthropology, 41*(5), 713–746.

United Nations Millennium Development Goals, 2015. http:// www.undp.org. Retrieved January 5, 2015.

Vicenzi, A., White, K., & Bergun, J. (1997). Chaos in nursing: Make it work for you. *American Journal of Nursing, 97*(10), 26–32.

CHAPTER 2

The Essence of Caring

Human development and human fulfillment are achieved through the unfolding of the human capacity to care, through investment of the self in others; through commitment to something that matters. Caring is the human mode of being . . . . The capacity to care needs to be nurtured, and such nurturing is critically dependent on its being called forth by others. (Roach, 1987, p. 5)

Chapter Objectives

1. Define the meaning of caring from different etymological (meaning) perspectives.
2. Explore the caring concept within Florence Nightingale's philosophy and theory of nursing.
3. Identify the universality of caring in different disciplines: anthropology, theology, philosophy, ethics, education, political science, art, and nursing.
4. Review the concept of caring and caring science in contemporary nursing.
5. Explore the notion of caring practice wisdom (critical caring awareness, thought, and praxis).
6. Explain transcultural caring in professional nursing and its use as a science and application as one of the four dimensions of the Transcultural Caring Dynamics in Nursing and Health-Care Theory and Model.

Continued

KEY WORDS

Caring • nurturance • compassion • love • charity • ethics • justice • suffering • etymology of caring • caring science • transcultural nursing • transcultural caring • dynamic complexity • relational self-organization

Dimension of the Model

Essence of Caring

(Love, Empathy, Authenticity, Compassion, Co-Presence, Availability, Attendance, Communication)

The action of compassion/love as the mediating force to guide moral caring behavior and facilitate right action (justice or fairness) within the dynamics of culture

Figure 2–1: Dimension of the model: Essence of Caring.

At its essence, the profession of nursing combines the discipline of caring with the practice of caring. In other words, the nursing profession comprises the practice of caring for people who are in need or ill, along with the systematic study of caring in relation to disciplinary knowledge of the body, mind, and spirit and the transcultural context (Bishop & Scudder, 1991; Coffman, 2006, 2014; Leininger, 1991; McFarland & Wehbe-Alamah, 2015; Ray, 2010a, 2010b, 2010c; Smith, Turkel, & Wolf, 2013). Philosophy and/or theory often tie together the study of caring with the practice of caring. For example, a philosophy first inquires about the nature or meaning of an entity (something) (Heidegger, 1962) then unites it with concepts of history, universality, and generalizations of science, human science, and art. A philosophy of nursing addresses ways of being, knowing, and doing for a specific purpose. A theory expresses a purpose, explains, guides one's thinking, systematizes, refines, and, sometimes, predicts or verifies

the critical domains and phenomena/patterns of relationship within experience (Leininger, 1978). Specifically, nursing is a literal, philosophical, and theoretical response to a call from patients/clients or society (Paterson & Zderad, 1976, 1988). A nurse is called not only to care for and nurture sick individuals and alleviate suffering (Eriksson, 2006, 2007; Nightingale, 1969; Pfettscher, 2006; Roach, 2002) and to prevent illness and promote health (Dunphy, Winland-Brown, Porter, & Thomas, 2007) but also to fulfill a purpose for self, others, and society. Chinn (1994) remarked that the call to care is a willingness to be in relationship and responsive to others, to be in spirit and human existence together. As such, caring has several levels beyond mere concern for patients; it can be deeply relational, spiritual, and meaningful as one engages in the lives of others.

The goal of nursing practice is to be compassionate and to act justly by enhancing the well-being of others through knowledgeable caring actions (Ray, 1989a, 2010a, 2010b, 2010c, 2015; Ray & Turkel, 2014; Watson, 1985, 2005, 2008). These caring actions can be as rudimentary as smiling or touching, or as complex as preparing a 45-year-old stroke victim from another culture, for a life of rehabilitation and interdependency. Caring requires understanding human-environment relationships. Thus, caring requires understanding of the holistic nature of the patient (i.e., body, mind, and spirit), human relationships, diverse cultures, the nurse-patient relationship, and complex organizations. "The social organization of health and illness in the society determines the way people are recognized as sick or well, the way health or illness is presented to health-care professionals, and the way health or illness is interpreted by individuals" (Coffman,

2006, p. 125). Therefore, understanding complex human-environment relationships involves recognizing how the humanistic, social, ethical, and spiritual domains, along with the political, economic, legal, and technological domains, play a role in health and illness (Davidson, Ray, & Turkel, 2011; Ray, 1981a, 1989a, 1989b, 2001a, 2005, 2010a, 2010b, 2010c; Ray & Turkel, 2014, 2015).

Some scholars in nursing and philosophy have criticized the idea that caring is the essence of nursing (Crigger, 1997; Paley, 2001; Reverby, 1987). Such scholars argue that caring is too vague and exploits the caregiver or that nursing cannot lay claim to caring because caring is universal and is the focus of a number of other disciplines as well. The nursing philosopher Roach (1994, 1997, 2002) disagreed, stating the following:

> As the human mode of being, caring is not unique TO any particular profession. Caring does not distinguish one profession from other occupations or professions. Hence, the cure/care dichotomy sometimes used, for example, to distinguish medicine from nursing is a false dichotomy. As noted by Nouwen, 'care is the basis and precondition of all cure' [1974, p. 34]. Caring, rather may be considered unique IN nursing. . . . Caring alone embodies certain qualities, or it exists as the sole example of specific characteristics [in nursing]. In this one concept is subsumed the essential characteristics of nursing as a helping discipline, that is, all attributes used to describe nursing have their locus in caring. (Roach, 1997, p. 47)

Because caring is so universal and because it is so innate to nursing, it is incumbent upon nurses to understand its many dimensions and perspectives before caring for human beings from diverse cultures. This chapter begins with an historical overview of caring by exploring Nightingale's nursing perspective of caring, and a more philosophical history of caring in nursing. The chapter then reviews some general definitions of caring before examining the universality of caring as expressed in the following disciplines: anthropology, philosophy, theology, science, political science, art, and education. After looking at specific disciplines, the chapter returns to nursing and discusses more contemporary views of caring in nursing followed by transcultural caring experiences (i.e., case studies/stories).

❖ *Nursing Reflection*

Caring "as the human mode of being, caring is not unique TO any particular profession. Caring does not distinguish one profession from other occupations or professions. Hence, the cure/care dichotomy sometimes used, for example, to distinguish medicine from nursing is a false dichotomy. As noted by Nouwen, 'care is the basis and precondition of all cure' [1974, p. 34]. Caring, rather may be considered unique IN nursing.... Caring alone embodies certain qualities, or it exists as the sole example of specific characteristics [in nursing]. In this one concept is subsumed the essential characteristics of nursing as a helping discipline, that is, all attributes used to describe nursing have their locus in caring" (Roach, 1997, p. 47).

Keep in mind as you read that caring is one of the central dimensions of the Transcultural Caring Dynamics in Nursing and Health-Care Theoretical Model. A theoretical model facilitates understanding of cultural thought, language, and action (Holland & Quinn, 1987). By understanding caring from the perspective not only of nursing, but also of philosophy, ethics, anthropology, theology, and the other disciplines, nurses are better founded to practice caring in today's multidimensional, multidisciplinary, and multicultural world.

A History of Caring

The evidence of caring has been present since the beginning of human history. Human development depends on our capacity to care for ourselves and to care for others. Although caring is considered a universal phenomenon, contemporary nursing has recognized caring as the most distinguishing trait of humanness and has taken the leadership to professionalize it (Roach, 1997, 2002). The best place to begin a discussion on professional caring is with Florence Nightingale.

NIGHTINGALE'S PHILOSOPHY OF CARING

Caring in nursing began formally in the mid-1800s with the revolutionary work of Florence Nightingale (Dossey, 2000; Nightingale, 1969), a British woman who established the profession and integrated nursing care into an organized system.

Learn More

Nightingale is credited as founding professional nursing. Catholic nuns and Protestant deaconesses had already begun to establish the profession, however, in different European nations. In Europe at the time, nurse caring was tied to religious commitment, rather than professionalism. A group of dedicated and religious women bestowed works of mercy on the sick and needy (Donahue, 1985; Dossey, 2000). Moreover, Jeanne Mance, is considered to be the first lay-nurse of North America arriving in New France (Quebec) May 17, 1642, and the "mother" of professional nursing in Canada (Payer, 1992).

In Nightingale's time, the modern or mechanistic era of thought in Western civilization was reaching its pinnacle. The philosopher Descartes' view of the separation of matter and mind represented the mechanical worldview popular at the time (Tarnas, 1991). This worldview focused on mathematics, rationality, and objectivity. The worldview translated into medical practice, with its preference for the proof of hard science (Dossey, 2000). Despite this mechanistic climate, Nightingale did not confine herself to rational categories in creating her philosophy of care in nursing. Rather, she also looked to the universe as a causal whole, the person as a free agent, and the ideas of God and faith in her philosophy. Nightingale's own worldview (1969) underscored what we know today—that science is more than mechanism, objectivity, and determinism.

Indeed many of Nightingale's ideas parallel the ways of thinking present in 21st century science. Nightingale demonstrated the importance of:

1. Relationships, their dynamic nature, interconnectedness and patterns.
2. Empirical, quantitative studies and statistical and research-based practice.
3. Epidemiological record-keeping.
4. The participation of both nature and nurture in caring and health.
5. The relationship between science, nature, the environment, human action, and morals.
6. God, faith, spirituality and morality in practical action.
7. Being open to cross-disciplinary and cross-cultural practice and development.

Nightingale applied the knowledge and tools of science, such as empirical observation, measurement, and documentation in epidemiology (although she did not fully believe in the germ theory), to understand the environment and its affect on human beings. Into her caring philosophy, she introduced aesthetic and spiritual knowledge, the art of charity or "love of one's fellow man," and faith in God. She combined the environment or the reparative process of nature, such as the proper use of fresh air, light, warmth, cleanliness, and quiet, with charity and the work of God to create her essence of nursing (Calabria & Macrae, 1994; Dossey, 2000; Macrae, 2001; Nightingale, 1969, 1992; Pfettscher, 2006). At the same time, her scholarly orientation and focus on research and the organizational system afforded nursing its professionalism and credence in the scientific and social communities.

Nightingale as Transcultural and Transdisciplinary

Nightingale continues to be a role model today for the evolution of transcultural nursing. As a frequent world traveler, she came to appreciate culture, art, politics, and war. Nightingale spent 3 months "training" in Germany with the deaconesses of a Protestant religious community. She sought additional hospital training in Ireland and France with religious orders of nuns. After her training, in 1853, Nightingale became superintendent of an "Establishment for Gentlewomen in Distressed Circumstance during Illness" in London (Dossey, 2000; Dunphy, 2001).

In 1854, the Crimean War began, pitting Britain, France, and Turkey against Russia. The British government appointed Nightingale to head a group of women with no formal training to nurse on the diverse cultural front lines of battle. In the face of suffering, bloodshed, death, filth, hunger, and disorder, Nightingale rallied her nurses to make changes that would significantly reduce mortality rates. She focused first on cleanliness, food, and ventilation. She also kept meticulous records of the outcomes of care.

As the first transcultural nursing scholar and practitioner, Nightingale laid the foundation for the modern view of transcultural nursing advanced in the 20th century by the first nurse anthropologist, the late Dr. Madeleine Leininger (1970, 1978, 1991, 1997, 2002; Leininger & McFarland, 2002, 2006; McFarland & Wehbe-Alamah, 2015). In today's climate in which the cultures are more diverse, the conflicts more dangerous, the politics more contentious, and the economics more complicated, Nightingale's vision of nursing as improving health through caring, spirituality, increasing moral responsibility, and relationships with society and the environment, remain the same.

BASIS OF CARING IN CONTEMPORARY NURSING

Nightingale (1859/1969) laid the foundation for caring in nursing. Nursing theorists, such as Leininger (1970, 1977, 1978, 1981), Watson (1997, 1985, 1988, 2005, 2008), and Roach (1984, 1987, 2002) advanced caring as the essence of nursing. Leininger (1970, 1978) conceptualized transcultural care as foundational to her theory of transcultural nursing. Paterson and Zderad (1976, 1988) proposed developing humanistic nursing (caring) as a formal disciplinary basis of nursing. They stated that ". . . nursing is a responsible searching, transactional relationship whose meaningfulness demands conceptualization founded on a nurse's existential awareness of self and of other"(1976, p. 3). According to Paterson and Zderad, this transactional relationship is rooted in the dialogue, the call of the patient, and the response by the nurse. The disciplinary basis of caring in nursing was advanced at the First Conference on Caring at the University of Utah (1978), which has grown into the prestigious International Association for Human Caring (www.humancaring.org) featuring the quarterly publication, *International Journal for Human Caring*.

Other philosophies took this transactional relationship approach a step further to reflect the mutual or reciprocal nature of caring, and caring in the nurse-patient relationship (Boykin & Schoenhofer, 2001, 2008; Boykin, Schoenhofer, & Valentine, 2014; Davidson, Ray, & Turkel, 2011 ; Gadow, 1980, 1984, 1988, 1989; Gaut, 1979; 1981, 1984; *International Journal for Human Caring*, Volumes 1997-present; Leininger 1978, 1991; Mayeroff, 1971; Ray, 1981a, 1981b, 1989a, 1989b, 1994b, 1997a, 1998a, 2010a, 2010b, 2010c; Roach, 1984, 1987, 2002; Smith, Turkel, & Wolf, 2013; Watson, 1985, 1988; 1999, 2005, 2008; Zerwekh, 1997). Caring philosophies and theories provide an explanation of qualities of empathy, compassion, relatedness, and belongingness from different points of view not unlike the new approaches to science today (Briggs & Peat, 1989, 1999; Peat, 2002, 2003). Caring became so essential to nursing that researchers and theorists initially divided the types of caring into five philosophical categories: caring as a human trait, caring as a moral imperative, caring as an effect, caring as an

interpersonal interaction, and caring as a transcultural phenomenon (Morse, Solberg, Neander, Bottorff, & Johnson, 1990; Morse Bottorff, Neander, & Solberg, 1991; Morse et al, 1992a; Morse, Bottorff, Anderson, O'Brien, & Solberg, 1992b). Additional categories or metaphors have been integrated into the understanding of caring in nursing (Barnard & Locsin, 2007; Davidson & Ray, 1991; Davidson, Ray, & Turkel, 2011; Eriksson, 1997, 2006, 2007; Gaut, 1984; Locsin, 1995, 2001, 2005; Montgomery, 1993; Newman, Sime, Corcoran-Perry, 1991; Ray, 1981a, 1981b, 1984, 1989a, 1989b, 1998a, 1998b, 2001b, 2005, 2007, 2010a, 2010b, 2010c; Ray & Turkel, 2014; Roach, 1997; Sherwood, 1997; Smith, Turkel, & Wolf, 2013; Turkel & Ray, 2000, 2001; Watson, 2005, 2008, 2009; Watson & Ray, 1988).

PHILOSOPHICAL AND EMPIRICAL CATEGORIES OF CARING

- Caring as a human trait: refers to caring as the human mode of being, part of human nature and essential to human existence (see Boykin & Schoenhofer, 2001; Roach, 1987/2002).
- Caring as a moral imperative: refers to caring as a fundamental value of respect for person; there is adherence to a commitment of maintaining individual dignity and integrity (see Gadow, 1980, 1984, 1988; Ray, 1987, 1998b; Ray & Turkel, 2014; Turkel & Ray, 2009; Watson, 1988, 2005).
- Caring as an effect: refers to and extends from emotional involvement with empathic feelings for patient experience, feelings of concern, and dedication that motivates actions (see caring theories, and Morse et al, 1992a, 1992b; Ray 2010a, 2010b, 2010c).
- Caring as an interpersonal interaction: considered the *essence* of nursing. It is the experience within the nurse-patient relationship (see most caring theories but specifically Watson [1997, 2005]).
- Caring as a transcultural phenomenon: refers to the beliefs, values, attitudes, and behaviors that are transmitted from one culture group to another and involves the culture care universality and caring as culturally specific, including the culture of nursing (see Andrews & Boyle, 2007, 2015; Giger & Davidhizar, 2003; Leininger, 1970, 1978, 1991; Lipson & Dibble, 2005; McFarland, 2005; McFarland & Webhe-Alamah, 2015; Spector, 2003; and refer to the *Journal of Transcultural Nursing*).
- Caring as action: refers to caring as an intentional human activity that one is engaged in or

is occupied in doing. With knowledge, one must choose an action that is directed toward a goal (see Gaut, 1981, 1984; Ray's concepts of awareness, understanding, and choice illuminated in this book).

- Caring as communicative action and empowerment or praxis (critical reflection and social caring action regarding human rights and justice) (Ray, 1992, 2010c; Ray & Turkel, 2001, 2014; Sumner, 2008).
- Caring as an intervention: refers to specific nursing interventions, actions, or therapeutics or evidence-cased practice. Intervention is linked to the work, best practices, or evidence of nursing (being there, procedural and technical competence, knowledge, and skill [Smith, Turkel, & Wolf, 2013; Turkel, 2006a, 2006b]).
- Caring as an organizational culture: clarifies the meaning of caring in hospitals or other health-care agencies as the dialectic between humanistic, social, ethical, and spiritual phenomena and organizational cultural phenomena, political, economic, technological, and legal synthesized as bureaucratic caring theory (see Davidson, Ray, & Turkel, 2011; Ray, 1981a, 1984, 1989a, 1989b, 2001a, 2001b, 2005; Coffman, 2005, 2006, 2014; Ray, Turkel, & Marino, 2002; Ray, 2010a, 2010b, 2010c; Ray & Turkel, 2014; Turkel, 2007; Turkel & Ray, 2000, 2001, 2004a, 2004b, 2004c).
- Caring as technology: refers to the meaning of caring in relationship to technology, the virtual community—to machine technologies that support or sustain life, to computer technologies, to robotics (see Barnard & Locsin, 2007; Davidson, Ray, & Turkel, 2011; Heidegger, 1977; Locsin, 1995, 2001 Locsin & Purnell, 2009; Locsin, Purnell, Tanioka, & Osaka, 2011; Ray, 1987, 1994a,b,c,d; 1998b, 2001a, 2001b, 2007; Sandelowski, 1997, 2002; Swinderman, 2005, 2011; Wu & Ray, 2016).
- Caring as economics: refers to caring in terms of the integration between caring as love, education, and communication (interpersonal resources) in relation to the economic resources, goods, money, and services that affect decisions of nurses, patients, and administrators (see Buerhaus, 1986, 1994; Coffman, 2006, 2014; Ray & Turkel, 2014, 2015; Ray, Turkel, & Marino, 2002; Turkel & Ray, 2000, 2001).
- Caring as complex relational dynamics: reveals nursing as caring as dynamic, holistic, reciprocal,

transcultural, and emergent (the Theory of Relational Caring Complexity). It facilitates choice making of patients, caregivers, and administrators and drives change and creative ordering and reordering toward relational self-organization within complex human, institutional, and economic cultures (see Davidson & Ray, 1991; Davidson, Ray, & Turkel, 2011; Ray, 1989b, 1994a, 1994b, 1994c, 1994d, 1998a; Ray & Turkel, 2014; Turkel & Ray, 2000, 2001; Ray, Turkel, & Marino, 2002; Turkel 2006a, 2006b).

- Caring as a sacred science and art: illuminates nursing and caring as a spiritual practice, a wisdom phase where the connections among caring, loving, and experiencing the infinite become the meaning and process of facing our humanity as mystery, thus mirroring humanity of self and others back on itself and uniting us and the cosmic energy of love, as a unity (see Eriksson, 2006, 2007; Montgomery, 1993; Quinn, 1992; Roach, 1997, 2002; Ray, 1981b, 1997a, 1997b; Watson, 2005).

As the 20th century progressed, philosophers, such as Heidegger (1962) and Mayeroff (1971), and as the above categories defined in nursing illuminated, care and caring continued to be refined and clarified. In his book *On Caring* (1971), Mayeroff wrote the following:

> . . . *in order to care I must understand the other's needs and I must be able to respond properly to them, and clearly good intentions do not guarantee this. To care for someone I must know many things. I must know for example who the other is, what his powers and limitations are, what his needs are and what is conducive to his growth; I must know how to respond to his needs, and what my own powers and limitations are. Such knowledge is both general and specific. (p. 19)*

Mayeroff identified the major ingredients of caring as knowing, alternating rhythms, patience, honesty, trust, humility, hope, and courage. Mayeroff claimed that human beings find themselves by finding their place in the world. Humans discover where they belong through caring. He said that human beings are closer to a person or idea when they help it grow (Mayeroff, 1971). Watson (1988) revealed that nurses know the other through compassion/empathy in the "caring moment" through intentional consciousness and caring actions. In caring for others, humans help others to grow and can therefore find where they belong.

Definitions and Meanings of Caring

Reviewing historical perceptions and development of the concept of caring is one way to begin to grasp the essence of caring. Another component in the essence of caring is the word itself and its many meanings, connotations, and interpretations. Chapter 1 offered a brief overview of the meaning of caring in different contexts. This section will delve deeper into its many meanings in a variety of disciplines.

CARING AND COMPASSION IN CONTEXT

An effective place to start in defining a term is the dictionary (*The Concise Oxford Dictionary*, 8th ed., 1990), which defines care and caring as follows:

- *Care* (noun): (1) worry, anxiety; (2) serious attention, heed, caution; (3) a protection, charge.
- *Care* (verb): (1) feel concern for or about (nurture), (2) feel liking, affection for; (3) provide for; (4) look after.
- *Caring* (adjective): (1) compassionate, especially professional care with sick or elderly.

These definitions implicate compassion as one of the major thrusts of the concept of caring. Compassion involves suffering with and relieving others' pain by performing works of mercy (Fox, 1979). "The whole idea of compassion is based on a keen awareness of the interdependence of all living beings, which are all part of one another and all involved in one another" (Fox, 1979, introductory page, Merton, 1968). Compassion evokes a deeply felt awareness of oneness (Rohr, 2014). In nursing, Nightingale illuminates the spiritual essence of compassion—doing God's work (1969); Ray (1989b, 1991, 1997a) reveals compassion as human and divine, love and justice; and Watson (1985b, 1988, 2005, 2008) illustrates the core structure of compassion as harmony of body, mind, loving kindness, and spirit and transcendence.

Schumacher (1973/1999), Fox (1979), and Eisler (2007) referred to compassion and caring as an active presence in the universe and placed it within the public arena of work, technology, economics, the marketplace, and world nations. Thus, compassion is not just human personalism and inward but also must be directed outward; it is fraternal love and central to public moral decision making leading to justice making and healing society's social structures (Fox, 1979).

Ray (1981a, 1981b, 1984, 1989a, 1989b, 2001a, 2001b; Coffman, 2006) too wrote about the public meaning of caring (Coffman, 2006, 2014; Ray, 1981a, 1981b, 1984, 1989a, 1989b, 2001a, 2001b; Ray & Turkel, 2014, 2015). Ray's research revealed that organizational caring included not only the obvious social, spiritual, ethical, and humanistic aspects of caring but also economic, technological, legal, and political aspects. Caring was integrated universally throughout organizations and into their missions; caring was differentiated by the values of individual hospital units and by the nature of the bureaucracy, rather than by traditionally dictated caring versus noncaring roles. From this research, Ray advanced her defining Theory of Bureaucratic Caring, which concludes that caring in complex health-care organizations is a technological, economic, political, and legal tenet and a humanistic, ethical, spiritual, and social one (Ray, 2010a, 2010b, 2010c; Ray & Turkel, 2014, 2015).

THE MEANING OF CARING: A DISCIPLINARY STUDY

Caring has different meanings in different contexts. The following sections present perspectives of caring from a variety of disciplines outside of nursing.

Caring and Anthropology

Archaeologists have identified that human primates are united by a primordial empathy (Stein, 1989; Tarlow, 2000) and have interpreted the role that empathy and compassion play in the collective consciousness. Solecki (1971), an anthropologist who studied Neanderthal man, concluded that the two human characteristics most critical to human evolution were the human brain and the ability to care. While the brain has received a lot of attention from researchers and scientists, until recently, caring has not. Nevertheless, Solecki (1971) and Eisely (Roach, 1987, 2002) reported the appearance of

❖ *Nursing Reflection*

In caring for others, humans help others to grow and can therefore find where they themselves belong.

caring in Neanderthal man. Fossil remains located in their burial sites showed evidence of a handicapped man who would have required care from the community, despite being nonproductive (Solecki, 1971; Roach, 1987; Maguire, 2000). Currently, archaeologists are studying the concept of empathy. Paleontologists in Spain stated that ancestors of the Neanderthal, or pre-Neanderthals, *Homo heidelbergensis,* who lived 500,000 years ago, cared for the elderly and infirmed (Cosmos, University of Adelaide, 12 October, 2010). History (storytelling) unfolded in the fossil remains. These researchers discovered compassion in handling the dead, which also demonstrated caring—the evidence that material culture is rooted in emotional culture or a community of caring (Spikins, 2015). Caring as nurturing and loving behavior is a phenomenon unique to the emergence of man, and has been present throughout history.

The late Madeleine Leininger (1970, 1978, 1991), the first nurse-anthropologist and the founder of transcultural nursing, agreed with this finding. She asserted that caring for self and others is one of the oldest forms of human expression. Leininger remarked that "since the beginning of mankind, care appears to be the critical factor in bringing newborns into existence, stimulating individual growth, and in helping people to survive stressful experiences" (Watson, 1997, pp. xi-xii).

Caring and Theology and Spirituality

Caring spans all religions and spiritual beliefs, from Judaism to Islam to Christianity and other religions. Agape or altruistic or unconditional love is the most predominant force in relationships around the globe (Templeton, 1999).

Religion

Caring is a basic tenet of all major religions. In the Hebrew scripture, for example, God is revealed as the one who enters into a covenant with His people, restores the covenant, and fulfills the covenant relationship. The *Old Testament* covenant is not only the story of God's love and caring for human beings, but also demonstrates human beings' responsive caring for God (Farley, 1986; Ray, 1997a). Furthermore, this covenant instructs us to be compassionate and mindful of caring for others (Jeremiah, 3:33, *The New American Bible,* 1987).

In the Christian scriptures, the "fidelity of God is fulfilled in Jesus" (Roach, 1987, p. 16). Jesus

demonstrated that love is the greatest commandment and is an imperative for caring human relationships. Christianity teaches that humans can show their fidelity and commitment to God—and become worthy of belonging to God—by following the Word of Scripture, performing acts of mercy and healing, and by taking care of the sick and needy (Capra, Steindl-Rast, with Matus, 1991).

In Eastern religions, such as Buddhism, compassion and love also are expressed in concern and caring for others (Ray, 1994a, 2010a). Buddhism teaches that every aspect of Buddhist practice is designed to bring knowledge; Buddhists use physical appearance, supported by feelings, perception, and the mind, as the foundation for all existence. The state of insight is characterized by caring, a generous fearlessness that is not exclusionary or deceptive (Bhikkhu, 2005).

In the Islamic spiritual tradition, all action is taken in relation to Allah. Islam teaches that God is love and as expressed in the *Qur'an* (the holy book of Islam); God is seen as compassionate and merciful, and Islam encourages its followers to engage in works of charity (Armstrong, 2002; Jaoudi, 1993).

Native American spirituality embraces a caring philosophy that is both simple and profound. It emphasizes four objectives each day: learning something meaningful, teaching something meaningful, doing something meaningful for others without recognition, and respecting all living things. The essence of each of these goals, and of Native American spirituality, is caring for other beings (Templeton, 1999). The theologian Rohr (2014) stated that the "true self is compassion, love itself "(p. 46).

Spirituality

Caring theorists, such as Eriksson, Watson, Montgomery, and Ray each describe spirituality differently. For example, Eriksson describes a communion with and alleviating of suffering (Eriksson, 1997, 2006, 2007), while Watson envisions harmony of body, mind, and spirit (Watson, 1985, 2005). Montgomery describes transcending self, time, and space (Montgomery, 1993), while Ray perceives spirituality as the unfolding of Divine love (Ray, 1997a). All perspectives, to some extent, agree that spirituality encompasses the relationship of the human to mystery or to the infinite guiding force. One key purpose of spirituality is to discover belonging. For humans, belonging, often interpreted as the mutual process of love, is the most powerful, magnetic spiritual and universal force (Ray, 1994b, 2011).

Smith (1991) stated that the universe is permeated to its core by love. Merton (1985) declared that love calls forth our deepest creative power to appreciate meaning. Human beings love each other on a spiritual level but manifest this love through concrete actions of caring and compassion (Ray, 1991, 1997a, 2011, 2015; Watson, 2008). Humans possess true spiritual insight when they can love, and therefore care, beyond cultural boundaries (Merton, 1985). Smith (1991) remarked that the Golden Rule, doing unto others as you would have them do unto you, prevails in the contemporary global world and no theological or secular position claims predominance. The spirit of generosity and *caritas* (love or charity) is universal and must be encouraged (Templeton, 1999).

To some theorists and philosophers, belonging often goes beyond love. Belonging is the deepest quest of humanity in the search for meaning. Mayeroff (1971) pointed out that the experience of belonging emerges from mutual caring and need. Meaning and belonging are now the focus not only of a spiritual search but also of a scientific one. The notion that the whole is greater than the sum of its parts is a theological norm known to mystics for centuries and is applicable in the modern age (O'Murchu, 1997). Teilhard de Chardin (1960, 1965) discovered in his research of paleontological life forms, that science, philosophy, and religion converge as scientists ascertain that no fact exists in pure isolation from a vision of the whole. As life forms and cultures interconnect, complex patterns form, according to what fits, what is in harmony, what will grow, and what will die—in other words, according to what belongs. This sense of belonging, which lies at the heart of the new science, is also a central theme for spiritual scholars (Capra, Steindl-Rast, with Matus, 1991). It demonstrates the reach of the concept of caring in the universe.

❖ *Nursing Reflection*

Meaning and belonging are now the focus not only of a spiritual search but also of a scientific one.

Caring and Philosophy

Philosophy also has its own perception of the concept of caring (Marcel, 1949, 1951). Philosophy deals with the study of meaning. What does it mean to care? Blondel stated that "[t]he entry into philosophy is through the analysis of human life" (cited in Baum, 1971, p. 16). "Man is forever making free, individual choices...for the sake of fulfilling the necessary will or thrust at the core of his being...to become more truly himself. This is the logic of action" (Baum, 1971, pp. 16–17). The philosopher can explain caring by demonstrating the logic of a caring action (Gaut, 1984). By a careful analysis of action "there is a structure or necessity in all human action that becomes the key to understanding man's relationship to the whole of reality" (Baum, 1971, p. 16). To the philosopher, caring is not mere emotion; rather, it is decisive action. The action is logical when there exists agreement between the goal of the action and the means to accomplish the action.

Heidegger (1962), a prominent 20th century existential philosopher, claimed that to be is to care. Heidegger said that a person's essential relation to the world is present in the experience of care. He stated that care is what constitutes human existence; human conscience is the call to care, and the varieties of ways of being in the world are simply different ways of caring (Roach, 1987, 2002). Heidegger defined the human relationship with the earth as mutual caretaking. Humans dwell on the earth, take care of it, and the earth flourishes, as do the humans inhabiting it. In this view, caring for things and for the earth is a matter of decision (Henderson, 2006).

Another philosopher, Mayeroff (1971), viewed caring as a way for humans to grow through their relationships with other humans. As stated earlier, he identified the major ingredients of caring as knowing the other, alternating rhythms, patience, honesty, trust, humility, hope, and courage. He concluded that caring gives meaning and order to life. A life centered in caring enjoys a sense of belonging that stems from being needed by others.

Gaylin (1987, 1988), a philosopher and physician, stated that love and caring are essential constituents in human development. He reaffirmed the fundamental nature of care as a reciprocal loving process consisting of concern, worry, supervision, attention, and love.

Nightingale (1969) demonstrated the first nursing philosophy of care as composed of three elements: (1) assisting the reparative process of nature by putting patients in the best position for nature to act upon them, (2) practicing the art of charity, and (3) understanding the spiritual underpinnings of nursing. Nightingale's structure of the logic of nursing action reveals that by the act of caring for another, one grows and ultimately becomes whole and more integrated as a human being. Boykin and Schoenhofer (1993, 2001) call this notion "enhanced personhood" by being and becoming through caring.

Other nursing theorists have expanded upon Nightingale's philosophy of caring. Ray (1981b), for instance, articulated her philosophy on the essential nature of caring as "being there" authentic presence and oblative love. Ray views caring as a way of life through love, a way to live one's life with compassion for the well-being of others. Roach (1987/2002) also advanced a philosophy on the complex nature of caring. Her philosophy identified six "C's" of caring:

- Compassion: a way of living born out of awareness of one's relationship to all living creatures.
- Competence: the state of having knowledge, judgment, skills, energy, experience, and motivation to respond to the professional responsibilities.
- Confidence: the quality that fosters trusting relationships.
- Conscience: the informed medium through which moral obligation to others and the universe is personalized.
- Commitment: the complex affective response whereby one's desires and obligations converge with a deliberate choice to act in accordance with them.
- Comportment: communicative, symbolic behavior that signifies professional image, demeanor, showing respect, ways of interacting, speaking, dressing, and gesturing.

Watson's (1985, 1988, 2005, 2008) philosophy concentrated on human consciousness, imagination, and spirit as inner resources to promote health and healing. Watson elaborated on the transpersonal relationship—what entails protecting and enhancing human dignity, and strengthening body, mind, and spirit. In this sense, the caring moment is one where both the nurse and client are transformed.

Caring and Ethics

Ethics plays a role in understanding the essence of caring. Ethics is a *relational* concept and deals with what is good or right and what is evil or wrong. "Moral questions belong to the essence of the human condition" (van Tongeren, 1996, p. 177). Thus, "[m]oral concepts are embodied in and are partially constitutive of forms of social life" (MacIntyre, 1996, p. 1). The philosopher Kant believed that morality requires us to treat a person "always as an end and never as a means only" (Rachels, 1986, p. 115). Trust is a fundamental part of all human existence and the foundation of ethics (Logstrup, 1971). We trust that people will do the right thing so that our security and freedom are protected. Human relationships thus contain ethical issues involving trust, honesty, responsibility, respect, and love. Without ethics, which guides the way in which we live with others in terms of respectful conduct and protection of human dignity and human rights, cultures fragment, and societies disintegrate (Hirsh, 1976).

In the health-care arena, ethics deals with questions about how professionals should care (Griffin, 2002; Ray, 1994a, 1994b, 1994c, 2010a, 2010b, 2010c). Gilligan (1982) and Noddings (1984) acknowledged caring as the highest level of human development. A social caring ethic responds to principles of human rights and justice for all (Ray & Turkel, 2014). At the same time, a caring ethic includes the dictates of reason (Rachels, 1986). The nursing ethicist Gadow (1980, 1984, 1988) advanced the idea that care is an end in itself—the highest form of commitment to patients—and that the ethical role of the nurse is existential advocacy.

The biomedical model of ethics answers questions of how professionals should care and what is good in caring. The model is based upon the principles of beneficence (doing good), nonmaleficence (doing no harm), autonomy (allowing choice), justice (being fair), veracity (truth telling), and fidelity (devotion) (Burkhardt & Nathaniel, 2008, 2014; Beauchamp & Childress, 2001; Husted & Husted, 2001). Ethical questions arise in the context of caring, for instance, when health-care professionals determine how much autonomy to provide patients in decision making. Adding the element of culture often confuses such ethical questions. Often health-care professionals propose models of curing rather than caring, such as in the intensive care unit where there is conflict about end-of-life decisions, living wills, and "do not resuscitate" orders (Burkhardt & Nathaniel, 2014; Gadow,

1984, 1988; Ray, 1998b). In the past two or more decades, new views and policies to protect patients' safety in health-care organizations have unfolded, such as Health Insurance Portability and Accountability Act's (HIPAA) Privacy Rule (Page, 2004), evidence-based practice, root-cause analysis (Patient Protection and Affordable Care Act, United States Public Law, 2010; Turkel, 2006a, 2006b), and cultural competency (*Journal of Transcultural Nursing*, 2007, Supplement to Volume, 18, Number 1). A caring ethic is values-based (including cultural values), relational, intersubjective, intentional, contextual, and evolving. In practice, the ethics of caring is a moral ideal where the nurse/patient relationship is enhanced by mutual communication and effective decision making (Chase, 2004). The "good" character of the people involved in the ethical interaction becomes important in this activity.

Serving the "good" in ethics requires understanding the concept of "evil." Evil is the absence of good; caring and love are replaced by unwillingness. Saint Augustine asserts that by nature, creatures are good and that evil comes from freedom of choice. Evil is due to will, not to nature (Saint Augustine, 1958). Buber, the Jewish theologian, (1953, 1958) claimed that cultural moral "shoulds" and "should nots" appear in human conscience. Humans must make a conscious effort not to commit evil, but instead to restore the order of their being and to protect the unity of mind, will, and emotions. This effort is a form of self-care that Buber (1953, 1958, 1965) considers to be a form of God-care or the grace that illuminates and, thus, frees the person to share in the great act of higher conscience.

In her work, Nightingale addressed the presence of evil in the world. She viewed evil as part of God's universal law to teach persons, by their mistakes, the way to perfection in eternity (Calabria & Macrae, 1994). And Roach, in her treatise on the study of caring in nursing (1987/2002), commented that a nurse could not practice caring without a heightened state of moral awareness or conscience. The task of the caring ethicist is the interpretation of meaning of a moral dilemma, what can be gleaned from the fact that it confronts us, why it occurs to us as a dilemma, what constitutes it, and what meanings are beneath it (van Tongeren, 1996).

Studies in ethics continually reveal the importance of a heightened state of moral awareness in caring. In a quotation that perfectly portrays the importance of ethics to caring, the Native American spiritual leader Black Elk recorded:

> *One who walks a dark road is distracted,*
> *who is ruled by his senses and who lives for*
> *himself, rather than for his people.*
> (Templeton, 1999, p. 94)

Caring and Science

As stated earlier, science also emphasizes belonging as a critical component of humanity, and as the essence of caring. Human science is an approach to study beings (Morse, 1994; van Manen, 2014). It involves the methods of ethnography, grounded theory, phenomenology, and story, which study human beings in culture and society, respectively. Phenomenology, hermeneutics, and caring inquiry, three strongly philosophic human science approaches, portray the meaning of life experiences. Phenomenology uses reflective intuition to describe and clarify experience as it is lived and processed (Husserl, 1970). Hermeneutics interprets textual accounts of human experience (Ray, 1994b,c,d; Reeder, 1984; van Manen, 1990, 2014). Caring inquiry (Czerenda 2006; Ray, 1991, 2011, 2013; Teichler, 2000) uses the art of caring as an aesthetic journey to human understanding.

Human science reflects on and portrays the nature or meaning of being in the world. Reflection helps us to understand who we are and how we live in relationship to others and the environment. Reflection also helps us to live in a world where a lot is uncertain and to recognize that life is unfolding as we are living it. Human science emphasizes a deep investment in humanity, goodness, and interconnectedness.

There has been some integration of the philosophy of the human science into the natural sciences. The new sciences of complexity now evolving have come to terms with the concept of interconnectedness in the universe and belongingness in relationships. As demonstrated by our holistic solar system—changing, dynamic systems of planets, moons, asteroids, and comets creating order and disorder (Gleick, 1987, Goodwin, 2003)—chaos and wholeness are intertwined. Our entire universe is composed of organized chaotic systems within systems (Arntz, Chasse, & Vicente, 2005; Briggs & Peat, 1999; Davidson, Ray &, Turkel, 2011; Ray, 1998a). Capra (1975, 1997) one of the leaders in the new sciences of complexity, chaos theory, and holism, claimed that parts cannot be isolated in any living system; they arise from belongingness—interactions and relationships among parts that are properties of a whole. The character of the whole is always different from the sum of the parts.

The new sciences of complexity (Al-Khalili, 2003; Briggs & Peat, 1989; Byrne & Callaghan, 2013; Goodwin, 1994, 2003; Nicolis & Prigogine, 1989; Peat, 2002, 2003) establish the interconnectedness of life, characterized by relationship. Science is dynamic and transformative. Nicolis and Prigogine (1989) noted in their book, *Exploring Complexity*, that human science is more complex than physics and chemistry because of the processes discovered in the evolution of life and human cultures. The metaphor of chaos theory in science helps us to understand the subtlety that lies behind and within human and environmental encounters and the continuous process of change. Chaos is nature's creativity and brings with it "the apparently paradoxical feeling of an intimate, transcending faith or trust in a nurturing cosmos" (Briggs & Peat, 1999, p. 164).

Complex or dynamic relational activity is seen at the boundary between the evolving systems [what is emerging] at the edge of chaos. The elements of chaos are viewed as a growth process from which a new order emerges. It is a communication and an information system that, through a self-organizing process, feeds back on itself and coordinates system behavior through continuous mutual interaction.
(Ray et al, 1995, p. 49)

At the "edge of chaos" there is the possibility for disintegration or transformation through choice to self-organization (Davidson, Ray, & Turkel, 2011; Ray, 1994b; Lindberg, Nash, & Lindberg, 2008). "Self-organization in chaos theory, although seemingly without a goal, is influenced by creativity—a vision of a purposeful love, a purposeful God, a force or spirit of life expressing itself intelligently in the universe" (Ray, 1994b, p. 25). And, at the same time, self-organization is influenced by relational human caring. The human experience is likewise always changing. While human beings have had to deal with chaos throughout time, science has finally identified it as a fundamental force in the universe (Briggs & Peat, 1989, 1999; Peat, 2002).

This scientific shift incorporates the subjective role of the researcher in conducting the research. Scientists are both actors and spectators in discovering answers to their own questions. Another aspect of complex science not recognized in the past is that of anticipation (Rosen, 1988). Anticipation recognizes that the wholeness of the universe is brought forth as "knowledge-in-process" (Harman, 1998). Science is now anticipatory, emergent, and evolving, as opposed to stable and rigorous. Through complexity science, we understand that science cannot produce any complete and definitive understanding of reality. We understand that we do not fully understand. At the same time, we do know that all phenomena in the universe are interconnected through mind and matter. All other knowledge is merely anticipatory but relies on an undercurrent of caring (Ray, 1994b; Davidson & Ray, 1991; Davidson, Ray, & Turkel, 2011). Rosen expressed this notion of caring when he said, "We must let nature tell us what to do" (p. 29).

Science now recognizes belongingness, and therefore caring, as essential to universal existence. As participants in the universe, we seek to belong. We choose not just at the level of the mind but within a moral framework where choice making is a reflection of wisdom and understanding when people become aware that they share a common humanity, a common

Learn More

Rosen's (1988) notion of anticipation can be likened to the writing of Nightingale's theory in 1859 (republished in 1969, 1992); Dossey, (2000), a theory of nature in which she proclaimed that putting patients in the best condition for nature to act upon was the way for people to retain their vital powers. In addition, the idea of anticipation can be likened to the notion of the instillation of faith, hope, and love in Watson's (1985, 2005, 2008) caring philosophy in nursing, cocreation in relationships (Parse, 1995; Mitchell, 1999, 2006; Ray, 1991, 1994b; 1998a), expanded consciousness in Newman's (1986, 1994, 1997) theory, and the theory of relational complexity (relational self-organization) in Ray's and Turkel's (2000, 2001; Ray, Turkel, & Marino, 2002; Ray & Turkel, 2014) theory. All theories facilitate understanding of knowledge-in-process.

universe—in principle, relational caring, the action of love (Eriksson, 1997; Ray, 1994b).

> With the first landing on the moon in 1969, something changed in the collective consciousness of humanity. We began to perceive the earth differently, as a type of living creature rather than as dead, inert matter. We began to sense a unity within the whole cosmos (O'Murchu, 1997, p. 182). Teilhard de Chardin (1965) stated that "[t]he age of nations is past. The task before us now, if we would not perish, is to shake off our ancient prejudices, and to build the earth. (p. 54).

Caring and Education

Education helps to shape the moral character of community. To set forth a positive moral landscape, education specifically should attempt to foster relationships and caring, responsibility, and accountability. There are many challenges to our current education systems. Technology often supersedes one-on-one interpersonal time. Hostility rather than caring sometimes trumps positive academic relationships. Teachers are stretched to their limits in terms of classroom sizes, online demands, and professional responsibilities. And students are asked to focus on outcome-oriented research to support evidence-based practice. How can education nourish relationships of caring and moral good in such a climate (Bevis & Watson, 1989; Boykin & Parker, 1997; Coffman, 2006, 2014; France & Ray, 2014; Ray & Turkel, 2014, 2015; Turkel, 2007)?

Education in and of itself is a caring activity, a spiritual journey (Palmer, 1993; Ray 2010c; van Manen, 1990, 2014). At its heart, it requires a relationship between teacher and learner, and an obligation to impart and receive information. Education does not allow for indifference or denial of responsibility. Educators and nurse educators who model caring, establish environments of learning that reinforce mutual respect, self-care, self-reflection, and freedom of choice (Boykin, 1994; Boykin & Parker, 1997; *International Journal for Human Caring*, 2008, Volume 12, Number 4). Watson (1988) pointed out that in a teaching-learning environment, every human encounter offers opportunity for a caring moment that engages body, mind, and spirit. A moral caring, educational environment requires (Noddings, 1984):

- Modeling—development by example.
- Dialogue—reciprocal communicative interaction.

❖ *Nursing Reflection*

Educators, nurse educators, and practitioners of nursing who model caring establish environments of learning that reinforce mutual respect, self-care, self-reflection, and freedom of choice.

- Practice—fostering caring through multiple ways of knowing: empirical, ethical, aesthetic, personal, and sociocultural (Carper, 1978; Leininger, 1978, 1991).
- Confirmation—shaping and constructing an ethical ideal that involves transformation.

Caring education is a call for a decision to care; it is a philosophical, political, and moral act (Bevis & Watson, 1989; Moccia, 1986). To assist with this development, new tools for studying caring in education and practice have been advanced by a number of caring scholars (France & Ray, 2015; Watson, 2002, 2008, 2009).

Caring and Political Science

In the areas of political science and government, caring entails a move from progressivism to stewardship and reconciliation (Appleton, 2005; De Vries & Sullivan, 2006; Henderson, 2007; Lasch, 1991; Wolfe, 2011). Lasch commented that the world needs to replace the vision of endless economic expansion with a vision of mutual belongingness. In a society with limited resources, government needs to reorient and prioritize interconnectedness over individualism. An image of what humanity means is the foundation for every social, political, and economic choice (Ray, 1989b; Ray & Turkel, 2009, 2014; Turkel, 2007; Turkel & Ray, 2000, 2001).

Race, ethnicity, religion, and gender can identify and divide people, and lead to political struggle (Boulding 1988; Wolfe, 2011). Integrating diverse units into larger wholes is viewed as the key component of cultural, political, and economic modernity (Boulding, 1988). Transcultural caring is a process by which diverse people can be integrated into the larger whole. This sense of interconnectedness and oneness mandates limits to "progress at any cost" and calls for a heightened political attitude (communitarian ethic) described as hope, trust, and wonder, an assertion of the goodness of life through justice and civic virtue or prudence (Etzioni, 2004; Habermas, 1986; Henderson, 2007; Lasch, 1991; Ray, 2010c; White, 1996). Accordingly, a communitarian ethic manifesting prudence perfected by the virtue of love offers opportunity for public debate where subcultures gain "cultural capital" within the overarching cultural environment of a nation, and where the critique of social ethics calls for reformulation of what a "society considers public cultural truth" (White, 1996, pp. 214–215).

Caring and Art

Art can create harmony and beauty. Art connects the senses we feel when looking at or experiencing it, to the meaning and understanding that we attribute to it. Plato (cited in Rader, 1979) declared that the highest form of art is inspired by the pure eternal forms of goodness, truth, and love. The core of our human identity is love and trust, components of caring. Creativity is a paradox, "the function of a finite center that tends toward infinity" (Arieti, 1987, cited in Steiner, 1989, p. 413). Arieti (1987) noted that human beings, when aware of this finiteness in the infinite, try to decrease the unknown through creativity. Steiner (1989) revealed that the part of the human being that embraces creativity, also responds to beauty, searches for truth, values kindness and compassion, energizes lives, and accepts the responsibility to care (Bevis & Watson, 1989).

In her study of the art of nursing, Appleton (1991) proposed that giving "the gift of self" is central to nursing. She opined that caring as love is a personal sacrifice for the well-being of another. Ray's (1997b) study of the art of caring in nursing administration revealed an ethical theory of existential authenticity. The art of caring embodies the Platonic ideal; the administrator, through nurturing caretaking, modeling, and moral leadership, secures the good of all of her workers. In their study of creating a caring practice environment in hospitals, Turkel and Ray show that nurse and non-nurse administrators must provide opportunities for nurse self-care and facilitate trust and participation in decisions that affect the well-being of nurses and patients and the hospital organization (Ray, Turkel, & Marino, 2002; Turkel & Ray, 2004b, 2011). Shirey's (2005) analysis of nurturing in nursing administration addresses how the idea of nurturing the other is so critical to the art of nursing practice.

Contemporary Perceptions of Caring in Nursing

With that in mind, we arrive at the present day nursing perception of caring. Gaut (1984) aptly describes

caring, and her definition is especially relevant to transcultural caring: "As a word 'caring' does not have one determinate definition and a singular meaning in all contexts; rather it has a family of meanings and its meaning shifts across contexts [cultures] . . ."(p. 30).

In her analysis, Gaut (1984) expressed clearly that caring in nursing is a "mediated action accomplished through many activities" (p. 41). Purposeful activity, in Gaut's analysis, involves seeking the good of the other. Caring therefore becomes a moral activity. Action represents a grasp of reality. Truth or authenticity is present in the action of human beings (Baum, 1971).

Nursing researchers Benner, Tanner, and Chesla (1996, 2009) claimed that a human agent's grasp of and engagement in a nursing or caring situation determines the morality of that human agent in a nursing situation. Each level of advancement in practice—from beginner or novice to expert—represents not only theoretical and practical knowledge, but also experience and emotional response to nursing situations (Barry, Gordon & King, 2015). Through self-reflection, the ways of knowing and critical caring inquiry, these actions and experiences evolve into shared caring practice wisdom. Wisdom, according to Baum (1971), is only acquired through the human process of creating a spiritual-ethical culture, a process of understanding and enacting the virtue of compassion. Nightingale understood this when she recognized that spirituality formed the basis of all cultural phenomena. Spirituality in human cultural history is the necessary source of creativity in everyday aspirations, interactions, conflicts, and human becoming (Boulding, 1988; Ray, 1997b). Shared clinical wisdom in nurse caring is a complex, relational, moral, and spiritual process. To learn more about shared caring practice wisdom in a transcultural context, read the Transcultural Caring Experiences of Don and Gabriela at the end of the chapter.

CARING AS THE WAY OF MODERN NURSING

As technology continued to develop and concerns started to grow about its incidental decrease in human connectedness, the focus on caring in nursing intensified. In the mid-1970s, Leininger (1981) asserted that caring is the essence of nursing. She said (1978) that the "most unifying, dominant and central intellectual and practice focus of nursing is caring" and that "there is no discipline that is so directly and intimately involved with caring needs and behaviors than the discipline of nursing" (p. 13). Gaut's (1984) suggestion that caring has a family of shifting contextual meanings is in line with Leininger's (1991) Sunrise Theory of Culture Care Diversity and Universality and the many caring theories that have followed (Smith & Parker, 2015). Leininger (1995) however claimed that "culture care is the broadest, most holistic means to know, explain, interpret and predict nursing care phenomena to guide nursing care practices" (p. 104).

Roach (1987, 2002) highlighted caring as a human mode of being and the most consistently used concept to describe nursing since the evolution of the profession. Watson too revealed the critical role of caring in nursing science, education, and practice. Watson (1985, 1988, 1999, 2005, 2008) professed that caring is the aspiration of nursing, a moral ideal fostering protection and enhancement of human dignity and harmony of body, mind, and soul. Eriksson (1997, 2006, 2007), a nurse philosopher, remarked that caring is a way of living. According to Eriksson, caring is *caritas,* a deep human and professional communion, which requires being there in authentic presence, and reconciling suffering for others. "To have the courage to see your neighbor's suffering and to assume responsibility to alleviate it without just walking by, are the responses in which all care originates" (1997, p. 68). "Suffering and love are the deepest and innermost movements of the soul and the spirit and, therefore, they are the most fundamental processes of life and health" (1997, p. 75). Boykin and Schoenhofer

Learn More

As mentioned earlier, Roach (2002) created the six "Cs" of caring central to nursing: compassion, competence, confidence, conscience, commitment, and comportment. Communication enhanced the Cs list (Ray & Turkel, 2001; Turkel, 2004a, 2004b), and two additional Cs, culture and context (organizations) round out the dimensions of caring in contemporary nursing (Leininger, 1991; McFarland, 2006; Ray, 1989a, 2001a, 2001b, 2005; Coffman, 2006). Philosophers and theorists of caring (Parker, 2006) have influenced nursing curricula dedicated to advancing caring in education and practice.

(1993, 2001) identified nursing as caring and suggest that the goal of the nurse is to enhance life for self and others.

Emphasis on caring as central to nursing has steadily increased, and has captured a wider audience. Newman, Sime, and Corcoran-Perry (1991) concluded the following:

> ...the domain of inquiry is caring in the human health experience...the task of nursing inquiry will be to examine and explicate the meaning of caring in the human health experience to ascertain the adequacy of this focus for the discipline, and to examine the philosophic and scientific questions provoked by the focus statement. (p. 3)

Smith (1999, 2004) stated that nursing has had more than 20 years of systematic knowledge development in caring. Yet new researchers are continuing to elevate the concept of caring and are inviting more organized study of the phenomenon (see *International Journal for Human Caring*). Smith pointed out that Martha Rogers was one of nursing's leading critics of caring as the central focus of nursing. Smith performed an exhaustive study of caring and its relationship to Rogers' Science of Unitary Human Being conceptual system. Smith discovered that five constitutive meanings that represent the essential nature of the concept of caring were in fact present in Rogers' Science of Unitary Human Beings: manifesting intentions, appreciating pattern, attuning to dynamic flow, experiencing the infinite, and inviting creative emergence. Smith concluded that there actually was congruence between the idea of caring and love as central to nursing and Rogers'(1970; Barrett, 1990) conceptual system.

Ray's (1981b) philosophy symbolizes caring as co-presence and oblative love, giving, and receiving in response to need. "Caring is authentic presence, availability, attendance and communication which includes interest, acceptance, touch and empathy" (Ray, 1997b, p. 172). In the evolution of her thought, Ray argued that dynamic transcultural

❖ *Nursing Reflection*

Shared clinical wisdom in nurse caring is a complex, relational, moral, and spiritual process.

caring is the dominant mode of being for a trans-global world and nursing (Coffman, 2006, 2010, 2014; Ray, 1981a, 1981b, 1989a, 1989b, 1994a, 1994b, 1994c, 1997a, 1998a, 2005, 2010a, 2010b, 2010c; Ray & Turkel, 2001, 2010, 2012, 2014). Ray identified caring as an ontology (a way of being), epistemology (a way of knowing), teleology (has a purpose), and praxis (is a practice), and as complex caring dynamics, her ideas correlated with the new science of complexity (Davidson, Ray, & Turkel, 2011; Ray, 1994b, 1998a; Ray & Turkel, 2014). This position defines caring by holistic and transcultural means and includes the idea from complexity science that in complex caring dynamics there is recognition of the notion of the "edge of chaos," the point of creativity energy where disorder (disease, pain, suffering) that drives change toward a new order, is a choice point for healing, well-being and peaceful death—transformation or self-organization. In nursing, the choice point is transcultural, communicative spiritual-ethical caring that calls forth compassion, advocacy, respect, interaction, negotiation, and guidance—the process of relational caring self-organization (Davidson & Ray, 1991; Davidson, Ray, & Turkel, 2011; Ray, 1994b; Ray & Turkel, 2001, 2012, 2014). (See Figs. 2-2, 2-3, 2-4, and 2-5.)

TRANSCULTURAL CARING DYNAMICS

Transcultural Caring represents the author's current perception of the ontology and role of caring in nursing. The Essence of Caring (see Fig. 2-1) is one of the dimensions of the Transcultural Caring Dynamics in Nursing and Health-Care Theoretical

Figure 2–2: Classification system of caring.

Figure 2–3: Process of spiritual-ethical caring.

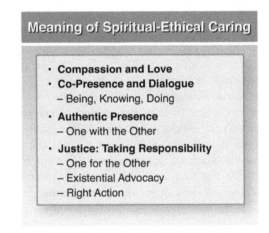

Figure 2–4: Meaning of spiritual-ethical caring.

Model (see Fig. 1-1). Keep in mind that the theory and model also includes three other dimensions: transcultural caring ethics, transcultural context, and universal (spiritual) sources. Transcultural caring is personal and mutual, and is defined as:

The relationship between charity and right action—between love as compassion and response to suffering and need, and justice or fairness in terms of doing what ought to be done within the dynamics of culture, or society. (Ray, 1989a, p. 19)

We live in a complex world and cultural beings create a variety of frameworks to find meaning in, and to understand and/or explain their afflictions, needs, conflicts, and suffering. The need for authentic

Ray's Transcultural Communicative Spiritual-Ethical CARING Tool for Cultural Competency

Transcultural communicative caring is a multidirectional way of caring in professional life that encourages transcultural communication (symbolic interaction, oral or linguistic interaction [or through an interpreter or video-conferencing]) to mutually understand the needs, suffering, problems, and questions of people that arise in culturally dynamic situations.

C: Compassion
  - Respond lovingly in authentic presence in person or via electronic communication by opening one's mind and heart to the other.
  - Act ethically by doing good, being fair, and facilitating choice.

A: Advocacy
  - Discern by discovering, ascertaining, distinguishing the vision of reality (worldview) of the other, and the contributions to the situation of the patient, family or significant other to facilitate mutual understanding and transformation.

R: Respect
  - Respect the culture (including the traditional or folk culture) of the patient and family, and the dynamics of the transcultural relationship of the patient, family, and community.

I: Interaction
  - Act competently by interviewing, listening, and manifesting transcultural knowledge and skill.
  - Ask questions to enhance the history and physical examination:
    - What do you think is causing your suffering/pain/problem?
    - How are you affected by the suffering/pain/problem?
    - What do you think may help or benefit you?

N: Negotiation
  - Mediate relationships and codevelop a plan of care by transcultural caring: allowing, recognizing, acknowledging, encouraging, affirming, confirming, and transforming the transcultural encounter.
  - Cocreate transforming self/life patterns by understanding the power within and the life-world patterns that promote connection of one to the other in community.
  - Mutually shape and devise a plan of care from the shared alliance (ethics of caring and responsibility [agreement, compromise, and understanding]) in choice-making with patients and family/significant others.

G: Guidance
  - Coeducate, codirect, advise, counsel, and inspire hope.

Figure 2–5: Ray's Transcultural Communicative Spiritual-Ethical CARING tool for culturally competent practice.

caring in the case of illness is apparent. The need to prevent illness and maintain health also should be apparent. Charity and right action, love and compassion are the responses to calls for care. Compassion and love known as *agape* (unconditional or limitless) and *oblative* (giving and receiving within the practice of caring in a spiritually committed sense) are oriented to upholding the values and engaging in the copresent relationship and the cointerpretation of meaning with the other. Love as *agape* illuminates the notion of ". . . longing for that which is good" for the other (West, 2007, p. 63). Transcultural caring acknowledges awareness of the depth of meaning of the nurse-patient relationship and highlights the importance of caring for people from different culture groups with different values, beliefs, attitudes, and behaviors. Transcultural caring facilitates opportunities for choice making that enhance self-organization—creativity, change, reconciling, and transformation in the patient and the nurse. In transcultural caring, nurses keep in mind spiritual-ethical behavior, a focus of attention on the meaning of the good, what is good to do, and what kind of good the nurse should try to promote (Alonso, 1996). Transcultural caring supports the notion that, in this discourse, the definition of culture is dynamic complexity. Thus, response to suffering can take different forms on the part of the patient and different professional forms.

❖ *Nursing Reflection*

Shared clinical caring wisdom in transcultural situations is critical thinking (self-reflection), and communicative spiritual-ethical caring (compassion and ethical interaction) to address diverse cultural beliefs, attitudes, and behaviors in cultural contexts. Transcultural spiritual-ethical caring communication assists in more meaningful, more respectful, more culturally sensitive interactions for the nurse, patient, and family to cocreate cultural competency by arriving together at choices for relational self-organization—healing, well-being, or a peaceful death. This culturally dynamic process can be facilitated by Ray's Transcultural Communicative Spiritual-Ethical CARING Tool (Ray & Turkel, 2001; see full discussion of the tool in Chapter 6).

In transcultural caring, the concepts of justice and fairness enter the picture. "The principle of justice places professional practices under the criteria of social ethics . . . from which the various needs and interests involved are coordinated with the available resources and possible courses of action" (Alonso, 1996, p. 203). From a social perspective, the caring obligation requires equal treatment of patients, attending to human rights, and working toward health care for all people. At this point in the history of the United States, justice and fairness may be difficult mandates. The "right" to health care is in process in the United States with the passage of the Patient Protection and Affordable Care Act (PPACA), Public Law 111-148, March 23, 2010 (www.healthcare.gov). The system calls for greater attention to access, compassion, and advocacy on the part of the health-care professional.

Transcultural caring entails evaluating what could or ought to be better in individual cultures and in society. As we have seen, transcultural caring operates on the interpersonal level and the societal level. In this sense, transcultural caring is a moral human activity that advances the moral character of interpersonal relationships and community life itself (Ray, 1989a, 2010a, 2010b, 2010c).

Summary

Our analysis of caring and science, theology, philosophy, ethics, education, political science, art, and nursing does not stratify the concept of caring, but rather unifies its meaning in the universe. The idea of belongingness in philosophy, science, and theology is present on any level, from the human relationship level, the cultural, to the spiritual one (Capra et al, 1991). All disciplines recognize that the more that is known, the more that everything is unknowable (Arntz et al, 2005); therefore life is mystery unfolding, revealed and hidden at the same time (O'Murchu, 1997). The following summarizes the essence of caring and transcultural caring in particular:

- Caring is the human mode of being.
- Caring is grounded in Roach's (2002) 6 Cs of commitment, compassion, conscience, confidence, competency, and comportment.
- Caring includes communication and context (the environment, organizations, and the universe).
- Caring is a human trait, moral imperative, human action and interaction, intervention, and transcultural phenomenon.

- Caring is the process that connects people, cultures, and societies and makes clear that underneath the separation created by professional disciplines, there lies a common need for belonging.
- Caring and love are the visible means that binds each of us together. "Love is the ultimate and highest goal to which man can aspire" (Frankl, 1959).
- Caring involves understanding of compassion as love and right action as justice in culturally dynamic nursing situations.
- Caring is dynamic, complex, and emergent, and thus is grounded in the new sciences of complexity (belongingness and interconnectedness).
- Caring forms the foundation for an ethical commitment to uphold the good of the other.

- Caring promotes a social and ethical obligation, responsibility, and accountability.
- Caring includes economical, technologic, legal, and political dimensions (the cultural context of society and organizations).
- Caring promotes respect for persons, animals, and the environment.
- Caring fosters spiritual-ethical communication/interaction that illuminates knowledge, skill, and transcultural and multicultural competency.
- Caring facilitates advocacy and mediation.
- Caring enhances choice making and relational self-organization.
- Caring guides others through counseling, codirection, and coeducation.

 ## Transcultural Caring Experiences

George

Read George's story for an illustration of contemplating the career choice of the profession of nursing and a life of caring.

George decided to enter the nursing program at St. Catherine's University. The School of Nursing included both an in-class and Web-assisted curriculum grounded in caring. In his first in-class hour, George learned that the course was dedicated to the study of caring and transcultural caring as the foundations of nursing as a discipline and profession. After introductions and going through the syllabus for the semester, the students were asked to reflect on their experiences of caring, compassion, love, justice, and culture. All these experiences were to be written without interaction or initial communication with classmates. Students could share their experiences at a seminar dedicated to Meaning and Interpretation of Caring at a future date if they chose to do so. Questions posed by the professor related to the nature of meaning, caring, love, compassion, suffering, empathy, ethics, the meaning of culture(s), multiculturalism, and transcultural interaction. George was experiencing an ethical dilemma. He is 19 years old. George came from an influential family from the Midwest, and is white and of Anglo-Saxon heritage. He had to persuade his parents to allow him to attend nursing school. He was raised as an only child and had a few close relatives.

George's Self-Meditation

How could he, George, embrace the notion of caring and transcultural caring in nursing? George thinks that the idea of love or love itself should be left for personal relationships and not professional relationships. George did, however, believe that right action is ethical and public and should be supported by professional nurses and other professions, especially politicians. George spent time in reflection. He thought about the choice he made to enter nursing. He got nervous and thought that he had made the wrong choice when he found out that the whole program focused on caring and transcultural caring, which he did not really understand. George did not want to share these thoughts at all. However, at the same time, George wanted to communicate how uncomfortable he was about the whole caring idea.

Classmate Maria's Reflection

Maria, 10 years George's senior and from the Hispanic culture, is concerned about George's lack of participation in class. His body language suggests that he is "disinterested." Maria wants to help George because she is so committed to nursing. She waited many years to have the chance to attend nursing school after marriage and having two children. She waits until the class is over before she approaches him. Maria believes that caring is an important part of nursing and just being human. She is committed to the ideals of the nursing program developed at St. Catherine's University.

Questions for Transcultural Caring Analysis

Reflect on the meaning of caring and your vision of transcultural caring for nursing.

- What do you believe about caring from a general point of view, from a nursing perspective, and from a transcultural perspective?
- What does it mean to you to be viewed as a cultural being and a multicultural being?
- Given your concern about George, how would you approach him? What would you say to him?
- What experiences in Maria's life present her with challenges and understanding of George's situation?
- Does George have a right to remain silent, not to participate in dialogue in the remaining classes especially when he chose to become a student in a school of nursing with a caring curriculum?
- What do you think about freedom of choice?
- Should a curriculum be dedicated to philosophical and theoretical ideas that highlight meaning, love, compassion, nurturance, personal, and professional growth and rights of others?
- What do you think about pairing compassion with hospitals, technology, economics, politics, and so forth?
- Do you think that caring is or should be a widespread phenomenon in the culture at large? Should it be central to other professional groups?
- Do you think that building a transcultural and transethical society is the way to go in nursing or in the culture as a whole?
- What are your thoughts about the "right to health care" through private and government-funded or -supported insurance programs?

Further Reflective Analysis and Questions

Your Model of Maria's Caring Action

- After reflecting on the meaning of caring and transcultural caring to you, to your understanding of caring in nursing, and to a curriculum dedicated to caring, create a transcultural caring narrative and or model for engaging with George.

- Present an analysis of the conversation that you would have with George about nursing, his values, and his response to your caring.

Don

Read Don's story for an illustration of sharing transcultural caring wisdom.

Don, an Anglo-American, has been a registered nurse for 6 years. He graduated from the University of Arizona, School of Nursing. He has lived in Tucson since graduation and worked in critical care for 4 years and oncology for 2 years. Desiring a new and deeper caring and spiritual challenge, he chose to work on the Navajo (or Dine, a name the Navajo call themselves, which translates to "the people") reservation with Native Americans, also known as American Indians or indigenous Americans (Lowe & Nichols, 2014). Don moved from Tucson to become a member of a community health team on the Shiprock Navajo Reservation in the four corners area of Utah, Arizona, Colorado, and New Mexico.

Don loved living on the Navajo Indian reservation, although he had a period of adjustment to his new culture. The changes in location, the Navajo culture, symbols, rituals, societal organization, the different needs, and the changes in living conditions (poverty in his view) all took some adjustment. The culture and spiritual expression was indeed different than his own. He had special housing accommodations living with the other members of the health-care community. Don was happy to work with Native Americans in their own environment. Although he had experience caring for Native Americans at the University Hospital in Tucson, this experience was much richer on the reservation. With each day, he was becoming more familiar with the meaning of Navajo culture and life for the Navajo people.

Recently, Don met a new patient named Joe. Joe had just returned to the reservation after 20 years of working in Santa Fe, New Mexico, assisting artists to sell their wares. Joe was particularly proud to have sold some of the Native American goods from the reservation. Joe was anxious to engage with the "native universe" once again. He loved the idea of connecting back to the land and nature but also was worried about all the social and political changes on the reservation. Throughout his adulthood, Joe smoked more than a pack of cigarettes a day and drank alcohol regularly, usually whiskey. Joe had been previously diagnosed with lung cancer and had taken a course of treatment (i.e., radiation and chemotherapy) in Albuquerque. He decided not to participate in the treatment program anymore after physicians told him that his cancer had spread to the liver, hip bone, and rib cage.

When Joe returned to the reservation, he immediately felt a sense of identity and peace. He moved in with his sister and her two teenaged children, who recently moved into a small house from the Hogan (traditional Navajo dwelling) where they had lived. Joe found that he had to reintegrate back into the community because he needed community support to help his sister care for him. Joe encouraged visits from the medicine man (discovernavajo.com; Locke, 2005)—the spiritual leader of his tribe. He knew he would receive strength to deal with his future.

As his nurse, Don was assigned to do home visits with Joe. At the same time, Joe began to participate in healing ceremonies with the medicine man on a regular basis to learn more about his Navajo spiritual culture and for his own personal well-being. Joe was concerned that he was coming to the end of his life. Joe was reluctant to discuss his interaction with the medicine man with Don.

As a caring, holistic, and transcultural nurse, Don genuinely wanted to learn everything about the Navajo culture and about the healing ceremony. As a white man, he also was aware of the sacredness of the ceremony and the privacy of the healing rituals. He knew the healing rituals relieved Joe's pain and suffering for a period. Don gave expert care to Joe—cared for him physically, by giving him back rubs, administered his pain medications, and talked with him about his artwork and the successes he had at marketing Indian art. He loved to listen to Joe's stories and trust was building between the two men. Don had great respect for the Navajo and all Indian cultures and beliefs but he really wanted to witness the healing ritual. He knew that it would be a great privilege if Joe would allow him to be present for it. After about 1 month, Joe told Don that he wanted Don to meet the medicine man who was caring for him. After conferring, Joe said he would ask the medicine man if he would like to meet Don.

Questions for Transcultural Caring Analysis

You are reflecting upon Don and Joe's stories and the experience of caring for a Native American person in his home on the reservation.

- What does culture or multiculturalism mean to you?
- Contemplate your own beliefs, attitudes, and behaviors toward people of different cultures, toward caring for them.
- How would they affect your personal and professional relationship with a patient, such as Joe and his family?
- What is the meaning of the "native universe" to you? What does it mean to Don and Joe? (Although you learned a little about native peoples in an anthropology course, you know that you would have to study the subject and perhaps talk with native people and nurses. You would have to study the dimensions of nursing in the Native American culture—"holism, trust, connection respect, traditions, caring and spirituality" [Lowe & Nichols, 2014, p. 14].)
- What is interconnectedness of body, mind, and spirit (holism) in Indian culture (Lowe & Crow, 2009; Weaver, 1999)?
- How can nurses bridge the gap between traditional health and healing beliefs and Western cultural beliefs?
- How can a cancer care nurse benefit from more transcultural caring knowledge?
- What "end-of-life" caring practices are acceptable in the Navajo culture?

- How do Navajo "end-of-life" caring practices differ from your own or what you have experienced in your own family?
- What is end-of-life care and spiritual wisdom of Native Americans? How would you help Joe with his cancer? What does the healing presence of the medicine man mean in Native culture and the community? Is it right to want to observe spiritual rituals of the medicine man?
- Don is a "White" man and nurse in the Navajo community. How will you implement transcultural caring? Does it mean that you never "impose" any of your beliefs on Joe? How would *you* engage in a participatory relationship? How would you encourage transcultural spiritual-ethical communicative caring? What does that process mean to you?
- You are interested in how Joe may have been treated when he lived and worked off the reservation, how he was probably "marginalized" by the culture as a whole. What does marginalization mean to you?
- What do you think life off the reservation is like for native people? (Think about what you learned in American history, how the Indians were treated, and what happened to the people and lands. You contemplate what it is like learning firsthand about the people who have lived the experience.)
- Do nurses really care for people from the patients' perspectives, from the patients' views of the world, from patients' knowledge of caring and caring practices or patterns?

Further Questions for Reflection

- Contemplate the policies of the Indian Health Services (IHS) of the U.S. Department of the Interior Bureau of Indian Affairs (BIA). How do you know if policies differ on reservations of diverse tribal groups? What is the meaning of a social ethic of transcultural caring for North American Indians? How many Indian tribes are there? How many Alaskan Native cultures are there? What is the native universe in North America? Does it differ between Canada and the United States?

Gabriela

Gabriela was working in Lisbon, Portugal. She was born there. Her family emigrated from Portugal when Gabriela was about 10 years old, first to London, England, then to Washington, DC. Her father worked for an international banking company. Over the course of time in the United States, Gabriela became fluent in English. She was fluent in Portuguese and Spanish. Gabriela completed a bachelor of science degree in nursing from a values-based, globally focused university. Gabriela did a study abroad in Madrid, Spain in her junior year, during which she worked in a clinic caring for immigrant families, mainly from Africa. In her senior year, Gabriela was initiated into *Sigma Theta Tau*, the International Honor Society of Nursing. Their scholarly publication *Journal of Nursing Scholarship* was one more thing that persuaded her to pursue global nursing. Gabriela was particularly interested in global health care in Africa because she had a connection through her birth country, and especially after she heard about the United Nations Development Millennium Goals 2015 and the post-2015 development agenda (see http://www.un.org/mdg.goals). She also was attracted to the new approaches to health care by the World Health Organization (WHO) and the commitment of WHO to taking health into all policies. (See information on the 8th Global Conference on Health Promotion, June 2013, http://www.who.org). As a student, Gabriela became aware of the nursing goals of the International Council of Nurses (ICN). Gabriela decided to return to Lisbon and work in a hospital. She loved working in maternal-child nursing and took a course of study in nurse-midwifery. After completing her education and gaining some experience in assisting with the births of babies and caring for families, she wanted to go to Africa. One of the countries of interest to her was Mozambique, which was explored by Vasco da Gama and colonized by Portugal in the early 1500s. The history of the country fascinated her, from the Bantu-speaking (the common language of Swahili) people to other tribal people who migrated from the West to the Mozambique coast, and to the influence of the Arabs. Mozambique was in a unique geographical position, flanked by Tanzania, Malawi, Zambia, Zimbabwe, Swaziland, and South Africa, six of the 54 countries of sub-Saharan Africa. The people speak many languages, primarily Swahili; Portuguese; and, in some populated areas, English. Gabriela was very concerned about the level of poverty for the more than 21 million people, and the state of health of women and children in the country. There was a growing need for improving maternal-child care, especially in the rural regions. Gabriela learned that the UN and WHO were supporting a program to educate nurse midwives in Maputo, the capital of Mozambique, to not only provide general midwifery care but also to do cesarean sections to save the lives of women and babies in rural Mozambique. She wanted to be a part of this program. After receiving permission from the Maputo provincial authorities, Gabriela embarked on a life of service with other nurse midwives to assist rural women who were suffering from lack of health care and education. She put all her transcultural nursing and midwifery skills into action, assisting mothers in the birthing process, performing cesarean sections, and educating the women about their health, including HIV/AIDS, the health of their children, adequate nutrition, clean water, sanitation, family relationships, educational pursuits, and productive work. (Adapted in part from *Birth of a Surgeon* Data [Wide Angle PBS TV Program], Mozambique, July 22, 2008.).

Transcultural Caring Questions for Analysis

- What are your thoughts about transcultural nursing and global health care?
- How does global health compare with public health?
- Does nursing in the United States and Canada have a moral obligation to participate in ethical and social caring, not only caring for the needs of people in one's own country but also, caring for the needs of people of the world?
- What is the state of maternal-child care in Africa and around the world? Are there different statistics affecting different countries of Africa? Compare and contrast the state of health care, maternal-child health care between United States and Mozambique?
- What are the maternal health statistics of countries of the West and Africa?
- What are the responsibilities of nurse-midwives? What are some of the new responsibilities that are advanced by the UN Millennium Goals 2015 and post-2015 and the WHO to meet the needs of women and maternal-child health in rural sub-Saharan Africa?
- What is the difference between nurse-midwives and lay midwives in the West?

Further Questions for Reflection

- What is the maternal and infant mortality rate in Mozambique, Africa? Compare and contrast those statistics with statistics in the United States, and in Western nations, and Asia, especially China and Japan. Where do the United States and Canada fall in terms of maternal and infant mortality?
- What is the state of education for children and women in Africa? What is the state of nursing education?
- What is the state of general health care, sanitation, and clean water resources in Mozambique?
- What are the linguistic patterns in Mozambique? How many languages/dialects exist in Africa? Why is English a dominant language in sub-Saharan Africa?
- What is the state of hunger and general poverty in Mozambique and in other countries of Africa?
- What is the state of HIV and AIDS in Mozambique? How does this statistic compare with other nations in sub-Saharan Africa? Are HIV/AIDS medications available? Who is assisting with this public health and global problem?
- What is the proportion of the country of Mozambique that does not have sustainable access to clean drinking water and sanitation?
- What is the state of conflict, war, ethnic hatred, and ethnic cleansing in Mozambique and in some other African nations? Why do you think this is going on? What histories of colonization contributed to the state of African affairs?
- How are African nurses as members of the International Council of Nurses addressing problems within Africa?
- What is the state of health and human rights in terms of female genital cutting (i.e., female circumcision or mutilation) and the politics of intervention in this practice in Africa? What is the role of professional nurses and health-care professionals in global health? Is this issue prevalent in other nation states? Is intervention transcultural caring?

- What is the Transcultural Nursing Society Position Statement on Human Rights (Miller et al, 2008) (see http://www.tcns.org)?
- Who is the director-general of the WHO? How long is the term of office?
- What is nursing's role in WHO? What does a collaborating agency of the WHO mean?
- What is nursing's role within the UN?
- What is the ICN?

Further Reflective Analysis

Your Model of Gabriela's Caring Action

- After reflecting on the meaning of caring and transcultural caring to you and to your understanding of caring in nursing, create a transcultural caring narrative and/or model for engaging with the nursing community of Maputo, Mozambique to assist rural African pregnant women, and children.
- Present an analysis of an e-mail/online conversation that you would have with the Secretary-General of the World Health Organization (WHO) about transcultural nursing and caring values and practices.

References

Al-Khalili, J. (2003). *Quantum: A guide for the perplexed.* London: Weidenfeld & Nicolson.

Alonso, A. (1996). Seven theses on professional ethics. *Ethical Perspectives: Rethinking professional ethics, 3(4)*, 200–206.

Andrews, M., & Boyle, J. (2007). *Transcultural concepts in nursing care* (5th ed.). Philadelphia: Lippincott Williams & Wilkins.

Appleton, C. (1991). *The gift of self: The meaning of the art of nursing.* PhD Dissertation, University of Colorado Health Sciences Center, School of Nursing, Denver, Colorado. Volume 52–12B# 9215314.

Appleton, C. (2005). *Playing with fire: The meaning of reconciling.* [PhD Dissertation]. Fort Lauderdale, FL:. Nova Southeastern University.

Arieti, S. (1987). *Creativity.* New York: Basic Books.

Armstrong, K. (2002). *Islam: A short history* (Revised and updated). New York: The Modern Library.

Arntz, W., Chasse, B., & Vicente, M. (2005). *What the bleep do we know!?* Deerfield Beach, FL: Health Communications, Inc.

Augustine, Saint. (1958). *City of God.* (G. Walsh, Z. Demetrius, G. Monahan, & D. Honan, Trans.). New York: Doubleday.

Barnard, A., & Locsin, R. (Eds.). (2007). *Technology and nursing: Practice, concepts and issues.* Hampshire, United Kingdom: Palgrave MacMillan.

Barrett, E. (1990). *Visions of Rogers' science-based nursing.* New York: National League for Nursing.

Barry, C., Gordon, S., & King, B. (2015). *Caring in the nursing situation.* New York: Springer Publishing Company.

Baum, G. (1971). *Man becoming.* New York: Herder and Herder.

Beauchamp, T., & Childress, J. (2001). *Principles of biomedical ethics* (5th ed.). Oxford: Oxford University Press.

Benner, P., Tanner, C., & Chesla, C. (1996). *Expertise in nursing practice: Caring, clinical judgment, and ethics.* New York: Springer Publishing Company.

Benner, P., Tanner, C., & Chesla, C. (2009). *Expertise in nursing practice: Caring, clinical judgment, and ethics.* New York: Springer Publishing Company.

Berman, P. (2004). *Terror and liberalism.* New York: W.W. Norton and Company.

Bevis, E., & Watson, J. (1989). *Toward a caring curriculum: A new pedagogy for nursing.* New York: National League for Nursing.

Bhikkhu, B. (2005). *Handbook for mankind.* Thailand: National Buddhism Office.

Birth of a Surgeon [Wide Angle Television Program]. (July 2008). New York: Public Broadcasting System (PBS). Retrieved August 3, 2008, from Public Broadcasting System (PBS) at http://www.pbs.org/wnet/wideangle/episodes/birth-of-a surgeon/data-mozambique and the UN Millennium Development Goals.

Bishop, A., & Scudder, J. (1991). *Nursing: The practice of caring.* New York: National League for Nursing Press.

Boulding, E. (1988). *Building a global civic culture*. New York: Teachers College Press.

Boykin, A. (Ed.). (1994). *Living a caring-based program*. New York: National League for Nursing Press.

Boykin, A., & Parker, M. (1997). Illuminating spirituality in the classroom. In M. Roach (Ed.), *Caring from the heart: The convergence of caring and spirituality* (pp. 21–33). New York/Mahwah, NJ: Paulist Press.

Boykin, A., & Schoenhofer, S. (1993). *Nursing as caring: A model for transforming practice*. New York: National League for Nursing Press.

Boykin, A., & Schoenhofer, S. (2001). *Nursing as caring: A model for transforming practice* (2nd ed.). Sudbury, MA: Jones and Bartlett Company.

Briggs, J., & Peat, F. (1989). *Turbulent mirror*. New York: Harper & Row, Publishers.

Briggs, J., & Peat, F. (1999). *Seven lessons of chaos: Timeless wisdom from the science of change*. New York: HarperCollinsPublishers.

Buber, M. (1953). *Good and evil*. New York: Charles Scibner's Sons.

Buber, M. (1958). *I and Thou* (2nd ed.). New York: Collier Books, MacMillan Publishing Company.

Buber, M. (1965). *The way of man: According to the teaching of Hasidism*. London: Routledge and Kegan Paul.

Buerhaus, P. (1986). The economics of caring, challenges, and new opportunities for nursing. *Topics in Clinical Nursing, 8*(2), 13–21.

Buerhaus, P. (1994). Economics of managed competition and consequences to nurses: Part 1. *Nursing Economics, 12*(1), 10–17.

Burkhardt, M., & Nathaniel, A. (2008). *Ethics issues in contemporary nursing* (3rd ed.). Clifton, Park, NY: Thompson, Delmar Learning.

Calabria, M., & Macrae, J. (Eds.). (1994). *Suggestions for thought by Florence Nightingale: Selections and commentaries*. Philadelphia: University of Pennsylvania Press.

Capra, F. (1975). *The tao of physics*. Berkeley, CA: Shambhala Press.

Capra, F. (1997). *The turning point: Science, society and the rising culture*. New York: Bantam.

Capra, F., Steindl-Rast, D. with Matus, T. (1991). *Belonging to the universe*. San Francisco: HarperSanFrancisco.

Carper, B. (1978). Fundamental patterns of knowing. *Advances in Nursing Science, 1*, 1–13.

Chase, S. (2004). *Clinical judgment and communication in nurse practitioner practice*. Philadelphia: F. A. Davis Company.

Chinn, P. (1994). Developing a method for aesthetic knowing in nursing. In P. Chinn & J. Watson (Eds.), *Art and aesthetics in nursing*. New York: National League for Nursing Press.

Coffman, S. (2006). Marilyn Anne Ray: Theory of bureaucratic caring. In A. Marriner Tomey & M. Alligood (Eds.), *Nursing theorists and their work* (6th ed., pp. 116–139). St. Louis: Mosby Elsevier.

Coffman, S. (2014). The theory of Bureaucratic Caring. In M. Alligood (Ed.), Nursing theorists and their work (8th ed., pp. 98–119). St. Louis: Elsevier.

Cosmos, The science of everything. University of Adelaide, Science Magazine, October 12, 2010. Retrieved July 1, 2014, from ww.cosmosmagazine.com/news/early-cave-dwellers-took care-elderly

Crigger, N. (1997). The trouble with caring: A review of eight arguments against an ethic of care. *Journal of Professional Nursing, 13*(4), 217–231.

Czerenda, A. (2006). *"The show must go on": A caring inquiry into the meaning of widowhood and health for older Indian widows*. Doctor of Nursing Science Dissertation. Boca Raton, FL: Florida Atlantic University.

Davidson, A., & Ray, M. (1991). Studying the human-environment phenomenon using the science of complexity. *Advances in Nursing Science, 4*(2), 73–87.

Davidson, A., Ray, M., & Turkel, M. (Eds.) (2011). *Nursing, caring, and complexity science: For human-environment well-being*. New York: Springer Publishing Company.

De Vries, H., & Sullivan, L. (2006). *Political theologies: Public religions in a post-secular world*. New York: Fordham University Press.

Donahue, M. (1985). *Nursing: The finest art*. St. Louis: The CV Mosby Company.

Dossey, B. (2000). *Florence Nightingale: Mystic, visionary, healer*. Philadelphia: Lippincott Williams & Wilkins.

Dunphy, L. (2001). Florence Nightingale: Caring actualized: A legacy for nursing. In M. Parker (Ed.), *Nursing theories, nursing practice*. Philadelphia: F. A. Davis Company.

Dunphy, L., Winland-Brown, J., Porter, B., & Thomas, D. (2007). *Primary care: The art and science of advanced practice nursing* (2nd ed.). Philadelphia: F. A. Davis Company.

Eisler, R. (2007). *The real wealth of nations: Creating a caring economics.* San Francisco: Berrett-Koehler Publishers, Inc.

Eriksson, K. (1997). Caring, spirituality and suffering. In M. Roach (Ed.), *Caring from the heart: The convergence of caring and spirituality* (pp. 68–84). New York/Mahwah, NJ: Paulist Press.

Eriksson, K. (2006). *The suffering human being.* (K. Olsson & C. Peterson, Trans.). Chicago: Nordic Studies Press.

Eriksson, K. (2007). Becoming through suffering: The path to health and holiness. *International Journal for Human Caring 11*(2), 8–16.

Etzioni, A. (2004). *The spirit of community.* New York: Crown Publishers, Inc.

Farley, M. (1986). *Personal commitments.* San Francisco: Harper & Row, Publishers.

Fox, M. (1979). *A spirituality named compassion and the healing of the global village: Humpty Dumpty and us.* Minneapolis: Winston Press.

France, N., & Ray, M. (2014). Studying caring science in nursing: The foundation of the discipline and profession of nursing at Florida Atlantic University. In K. Vaiyda (Ed.), *Nursing for the curious: Why study nursing?* Australia: University of Canberra.

Frankl, V.(1959). *Man's search for meaning.* New York: Pocket Books.

Gadow, S. (1980). Existential advocacy: Philosophical foundation of nursing. In S. Spicer & S. Gadow (Eds.), *Nursing: Images and ideals, opening dialogue with the humanities* (pp. 79–101). New York: Springer.

Gadow, S. (1984). Touch and technology: Two paradigms of patient care. *Journal of Religion and Health, 23*(1), 63–69.

Gadow, S. (1988). Covenant without cure: Letting go and holding on in chronic illness. In J. Watson & M. Ray (Eds.), *The ethics of care and the ethics of cure: Synthesis in chronicity.* New York: National League for Nursing.

Gadow, S. (1989). Clinical subjectivity: Advocacy with silent patients. *Nursing Clinics of North America, 24*(12), 535–541.

Gaut, D. (1979). *An application of the Kerr-Soltis model to the concept of caring in nursing education.* Doctoral Dissertation, University of Washington, Seattle, WA. (Dissertation Abstracts International, 1981, University Microfilms No. 7927790.)

Gaut, D. (1981). Conceptual analysis of caring: Research method. In M. Leininger (Ed.), *Caring: An essential human need* (pp. 17–24). Thorofare, NJ: Charles B. Slack, Inc.

Gaut, D. (1984). A theoretic description of caring as action. In M. Leininger (Ed.), *Care: The essence of nursing* (pp. 27–44). Thorofare, NJ: Slack Incorporated.

Gaylin, W. (1987). *Rediscovering love.* New York: Penguin Books.

Gaylin, W. (1988). *Feelings: Our vital signs.* New York: HarperCollins.

Giger, J., & Davidhizar, R. (2003). *Transcultural nursing: Assessment and Intervention* (4th ed.). St. Louis: Mosby.

Gilligan, C. (1982). *In a different voice.* MA: Harvard University Press.

Gleick, J. (1987). *Chaos: Making a new science.* New York: Penguin Books.

Goodwin, B. (1994). *How the leopard changed its spots: The evolution of complexity.* New York: Simon & Schuster.

Goodwin, B. (2003). Patterns of wholeness. *Resurgence, 1*(216), 12–14.

Griffin, D. (2002). *The emergence of leadership: Linking self-organization and ethics.* London: Routledge.

Habermas, J. (1986). *The theory of communicative action,* Vol. 2 (T. McCarthy, Trans.). Boston: Beacon Press.

Harman, W. (1998). *Global mind change* (2nd ed.). San Francisco: Berrett-Koehler, Publishers.

Heidegger, M. (1962). *Being and time* (J. Macquarrie & E. Robinson, Trans.). San Francisco: HarperSan Francisco.

Heidegger, M. (1977). *The question of technology and other essays.* (W. Lovitt, Trans. and with an Introduction). New York: Harper & Row, Publishers.

Henderson, H., with Simran, S. (2006). *Ethical markets: Growing the green economy.* White River Junction, VT: Chelsea Green Publishing Company.

Henderson, H. (2007). Alternative futures. *Spirituality & Health, 10*(2), 69–71, 92–93.

Hirsh, N. (1976*). Ethics and human relationships.* New York: Carlton Press.

Holland, D., & Quinn, N. (1987). *Cultural models in language and thought.* Cambridge: Cambridge University Press.

Husserl, E. (1970). *The crisis of European sciences and transcendental phenomenology* (D. Carr, Trans.). Evanston, IL: Northwestern University Press.

Husted, G., & Husted, J. (2001). *Ethical decision making in nursing and healthcare: The symphonological approach.* New York: Springer Publishing Company.

International Journal for Human Caring, 12(2), pp. 7–95. (Special Issue on Caring in Nursing Education and Practice).

International Journal for Human Caring, 1997 to present.

Jaoudi, M. (1993). *Christian and Islamic spirituality.* New York: Paulist Press.

Journal of Transcultural Nursing, 18(1), 7S-90S. (Supplement to Volume1) (Special issue: Integrating cultural competence into nursing education and practice)

Lasch, C. (1991). *The true and only heaven: Progress and its critics.* New York: W.W. Norton, & Company.

Leininger, M. (1970). *Nursing and anthropology: Two worlds to blend.* Columbus, OH: Greyden Press.

Leininger, M. (1977). The phenomenon of caring. Caring: The essence and central focus of nursing. *American Nurses' Foundation,* March 1977, 2:14.

Leininger, M. (1978). *Transcultural nursing: Concepts, theories, and practices.* New York: John Wiley and Sons.

Leininger, M. (Ed.). (1981). *Caring: An essential human need.* Thorofare, NJ: Charles B. Slack, Inc.

Leininger, M. (Ed.). (1991). *Culture care diversity & universality: A theory of nursing.* New York: National League for Nursing Press.

Leininger, M. (1995). *Transcultural nursing: Concepts, theories, research, and practice.* Columbus, OH: McGraw-Hill College Custom Series.

Leininger, M. (1997). Overview and reflection of the theory of culture care and the ethnonursing research method. *Journal of Transcultural Nursing, 8*(2), 32–51.

Leininger, M. (2002). Culture care theory: A major contribution to advance transcultural nursing knowledge and practices. *Journal of Transcultural Nursing, 13*(3), 189–192.

Leininger, M., & McFarland, M. (2002). *Transcultural nursing: Concepts, theories, research and practice* (3rd ed.). New York: McGraw-Hill.

Leininger, M., & McFarland, M. (2006). *Culture care diversity & universality. A worldwide nursing theory* (2nd ed.). Sudbury, MA: Jones and Bartlett Publishers.

Lindberg, C., Nash, S., & Lindberg, C. (2008). *On the edge: Nursing in the age of complexity.* Bordentown, NJ: Plexus Press.

Lipson, J., & Dibble, S. (2005). *Culture & clinical care.* San Francisco: University of California Press.

Locsin, R. (1995). Machine technologies and caring in nursing. *Image: Journal of Nursing Scholarship, 27*(3), 2001–2003.

Locsin, R. (Ed.). (2001). *Advancing caring, technology, and nursing.* Westport, CT: Auburn House.

Locsin, R. (2005). *Technological competency as caring in nursing.* Indianapolis, IN: Sigma Theta Tau International.

Logstrup, K. (1971). *The ethical demand* (T. Jensen, Trans.). Philadelphia: Fortress Press.

Locke, R. (2005). *The book of the Navajo.* Los Angeles, CA: Mankind Publishing Company (Holloway House Publishing Group). (Original work published 1976)

Lowe, J., & Crow, K. (2009). Utilization of a Native American Nursing conceptual framework to transform nursing education. *International Journal for Human Caring, 13*(3), 56–64.

Lowe, J., & Nichols, L. (2014). Utilisation of a Native American nursing conceptual framework: Implications for practice and research. *Australian Journal of Advanced Nursing, 31*(2), 13–22.

MacIntyre, A. (1996). *A short history of ethics.* New York: Simon & Shuster.

Macrae, J. (2001). *Nursing as a spiritual practice: A contemporary application of Florence Nightingale's views.* New York: Springer Publishing Company.

Maguire, D. (2000). Population, consumption, ecology: The triple problematic. In T. Hessel & R. Ruether (Eds.), *Christianity and ecology: Seeking the well-being of earth and humans* (pp. 403–427). Cambridge MA: Harvard Center for Study of World Religions, Distributed by Harvard University Press.

Malik, K. (2014). *The quest for a moral compass:* A global history of ethics. London: Melville House.

Marcel, G. (1949). *The philosophy of existence* (M. Harari, Trans.). New York: Philosophical Library.

Marcel, M. (1951). *The mystery of being.* (G. Frazier, Trans.). (Vol. 1). Chicago: Regnery.

Mayeroff, M. (1971). *On caring.* New York: Harper-CollinsPublisher.

McFarland, M. (2006). Madeleine Leininger, Culture care theory of diversity and universality. In A. Marriner Tomey & M. Alligood (Eds.), *Nursing theorists and their work* (pp. 472–496). St. Louis: Mosby Elsevier.

Merton, T. (1968). *Conjectures of a guilty bystander.* New York: Doubleday Image.

Merton, T. (1985). In N. Stone & P. Hart (Eds.), *Love and living.* San Diego: Harcourt Brace Jovanovich Publishers.

Miller, J., Leininger, M., Leuning, C., Pacquiao, D., Andrews, M., Ludwig-Beymer, P., & Papadopoulos, I. (2008). Transcultural nursing society position statement on human rights. *Journal of Transcultural Nursing, 19*(1), 5–7.

Mitchell, G. (1999). Evidence-based practice: Critique and alternative view. *Nursing Science Quarterly, 12*(1), 30–35.

Mitchell, G. (2006). Rosemarie Rizzo Parse: Human becoming. In A. Marriner Tomey & M. Alligood (Eds.), *Nursing theorists and their work* (6th ed.) (pp. 522–559). St. Louis: Mosby Elsevier.

Moccia, P. (1986). *New approaches to theory development.* New York: National League for Nursing Press.

Montgomery, C. (1993). *Healing through communication: The practice of caring.* Newbury Park, CA: Sage Publications.

Morse, J. (Ed.). (1994). *Critical issues in qualitative research methods.* Thousand Oaks, CA: Sage Publications.

Morse, J. Anderson, G., Bottorff, J., Yonge, D., O'Brien, B., Solberg, S., & McIlveen, K. (1992a). Exploring empathy: A conceptual fit for nursing practice? *Image: Journal of Nursing Scholarship, 24*(4), 273–280.

Morse, J., Bottorff, J., Anderson, G., O'Brien, B., & Solberg, S. (1992b). Beyond empathy: Expanding expressions of caring. *Journal of Advanced Nursing, 17,* 809–821.

Morse, J., Solberg, S., Neander, W., Bottorff, J., & Johnson, J. (1990). Concepts of caring and caring as a concept. *Advances in Nursing Science, 13,* 1–14.

Morse, J., Bottorff, J., Neander, W., & Solberg, S. (1991). Comparative analysis of conceptualizations and theories of caring. *Image: Journal of Nursing Scholarship, 23*(2), 119–126.

Newman, M. (1986). *Health as expanding consciousness.* St. Louis: Mosby.

Newman, M. (1994). Theory for nursing practice. *Nursing Science Quarterly, 7,* 153–157.

Newman, M. (1997). Evolution of the theory of health as expanding consciousness. *Nursing Science Quarterly, 10,* 22–25.

Newman, M., Sime, M., & Corcoran-Perry, S. (1991). The focus of the discipline of nursing. *Advances in Nursing Science, 14*(1), 1–6.

Nicolis, G., & Prigogine, I. (1989). *Exploring complexity.* New York: WH Freeman.

Nightingale, F. (1969). *Notes on nursing: What it is and what it is not.* New York: Dover.

Nightingale, F. (1992). *Notes on nursing.* Philadelphia: J. B. Lippincott Company. (Commemorative Edition)

Noddings, N. (1984). *Caring: A feminine approach to ethics and moral education.* Los Angeles: University of California Press.

Nouwen, H. (1974). *Out of solitude.* Notre Dame: Ave Maria Press.

O'Murchu, D. (1997). *Quantum theology: Spiritual implications for the new physics.* New York: The Crossword Publishing Company.

Page, A. (Ed.). (2004). *Keeping patients safe: Transforming the work environment of nursing* (Institute of Medicine Report). Washington, DC: The National Academics Press.

Paley, J. (2001). An archaeology of caring knowledge. *Journal of Advanced Nursing, 36*(2), 188–198.

Palmer, P. (1993). *To know as we are known: Education as a spiritual journey.* San Francisco: HarperSanFrancisco.

Parker, M. (Ed.). (2006). *Nursing theories, nursing practice* (2nd ed.). Philadelphia: F. A. Davis Company.

Parse, R. (1995). *Illuminations: The human becoming theory in practice and research.* New York: National League for Nursing Press.

Paterson, J., & Zderad, L. (1976). *Humanistic nursing.* New York: Wiley.

Paterson, J., & Zderad, L. (1988). *Humanistic nursing.* New York: National League for Nursing Press.

Payer, T. (1992). Jeanne Mance. *Fresiq: Bulletin officiel de la fondation de recherché in sciences infirmieres du Quebec, 3*(1), 1.

Peat, F. (2002). *From certainty to uncertainty.* Washington, DC: Joseph Henry Press.

Peat, F. (2003): From physics to Pari: Holistic science: A continuing search for answers. *Resurgence, 1*(216), 24–26.

Pfettscher, S. (2006). Florence Nightingale. In A. Marriner Tomey & M. Alligood (Eds.), *Nursing theorists and their work*. St. Louis: Mosby.

Quinn, J. (1992). Holding sacred space: The nurse as healing environment. *Holistic Nursing Practice, 6*(4), 26–35.

Rachels, J. (1986). *The elements of moral philosophy*. New York: Random House.

Rader, M. (1979). *A modern book of esthetics* (5th ed.). New York: Holt, Rinehart and Winston.

Ray, M. (1981a). *A study of caring within an institutional culture*. Doctoral dissertation, University of Utah, Dissertation Abstracts International, 1981 (University Microfilms No. 81-27-787).

Ray, M. (1981b). A philosophical analysis of caring in nursing. In M. Leininger (Ed.). *Caring: An Essential Human Ingredient* (pp. 25–36). Thorofare, NJ: Slack Incorporated.

Ray, M. (1984). The development of a classification system of institutional caring. In M. Leininger (Ed.), *Care: The essence of nursing and health* (pp. 95–112). Thorofare, NJ: Slack Incorporated.

Ray, M. (1987). Technological caring: A new model in critical care. *Dimensions of Critical Care Nursing, 6*, 166–173.

Ray, M. (1989a). Transcultural caring: Political and economic visions. *Journal of Transcultural Nursing, 1*(1), 17–21.

Ray, M. (1989b). The theory of bureaucratic caring for nursing practice in the organizational culture. *Nursing Administration Quarterly, 13*(2), 31–43.

Ray, M. (1991). Caring inquiry: The esthetic process in the way of compassion. In D. Gaut & M. Leininger (Eds.), *Caring: The compassionate healer* (pp. 181–189). New York: National League for Nursing Press.

Ray, M. (1992). Critical theory as a framework to enhance nursing science. *Nursing Science Quarterly, 5*(3), 98–101.

Ray, M. (1994a). Transcultural nursing ethics: A framework and model for transcultural ethical analysis. *Journal of Holistic Nursing, 12*(3), 251–264.

Ray, M. (1994b). Complex caring dynamics: A unifying model for nursing inquiry. *Theoretic and Applied Chaos in Nuring, 1*(1), 23–32.

Ray, M. (1994c). Communal moral experience as the research starting point for health care ethics. *Nursing Outlook, 42*(3), 104–109.

Ray, M. (1994d). The richness of phenomenology: Philosophic, theoretic, and methodologic concerns. In J. Morse (Ed.), *Critical issues in qualitative research methods* (pp.116–135). Newbury Park, CA: Sage Publications, Inc.

Ray, M. (1997a). Illuminating the meaning of caring: Unfolding the sacred art of divine love. In M. Roach (Ed.), *Caring from the heart: The convergence of caring and spirituality*. New York: Paulist Press.

Ray, M. (1997b). Existential authenticity: An ethical theory of nursing administrative caring art. *Canadian Journal of Nursing Research, 29*(1), 111–126.

Ray, M. (1998a). Complexity and nursing science. *Nursing Science Quarterly, 11*(3), 91–93.

Ray, M. (1998b). A phenomenologic study of the interface of caring and technology in intermediate care: Toward a reflexive ethics for clinical practice. *Holistic Nursing Practice, 12*(4), 69–77.

Ray, M. (2001a). The theory of bureaucratic caring. In M. Parker (Ed.), *Nursing theories, nursing practice* (pp. 421–431). Philadelphia: F. A. Davis Company.

Ray, M. (2001b). Complex culture and technology: Toward a global caring communitarian ethics of nursing. In R. Locsin (Ed.), *Advancing technology, caring, and nursing* (pp. 41–52). Westport, CT: Auburn House.

Ray, M. (2006). The theory of bureaucratic caring (2nd ed.). In M. Parker (Ed.), *Nursing theories, nursing practice* (pp. 360–379). Philadelphia: F. A. Davis Company.

Ray, M. (2007). Technological caring as a dynamic complexity in nursing practice. In A. Barnard & R. Locsin (Eds.), *Perspectives on technology and nursing practice*. United Kingdom: Palgrave.

Ray, M. (2010a). *Transcultural caring dynamics in nursing and health care*. Philadelphia: F. A. Davis Company.

Ray, M. (2010b). *A study of caring within an institutional culture: The discovery of the Theory of Bureaucratic Caring*. Germany: Lambert Academic Publishing.

Ray, M. (2010c). Creating caring organizations and communities through communitarian ethics. *Journal of the World Universities Forum, 3*(5), 41-52.

Ray, M. (2013). Caring inquiry: The esthetic process in the way of compassion. In M. Smith, M. Turkel, & Z. Wolf (Eds.). *Caring in nursing classics: An essential resource* (pp. 339–345). New York: Springer Publishing Company.

Ray, M. (2015). Rootedness in holistic nursing: The ontologic mystery and structure of caring. *Beginnings*, *35*(2), 12–14.

Ray, M., DiDominic, V., Dittman, P., Hurst, P., Seaver, B., Sorbello, B., & Stankes-Ross, M. (1995). The edge of chaos: Caring and the bottom line. *Nursing Management, 26*(9), 48–50.

Ray, M., & Turkel, M. (2001). Culturally based caring. In L. Dunphy & J. Winland-Brown (Eds.), *Primary care: The science and art of advanced practice* (pp. 43–55). Philadelphia: F. A. Davis Company.

Ray, M., & Turkel, M. (2009). Relational caring questionnaires. In J. Watson (Ed.), *Assessing and measuring caring in nursing and health science* (2nd ed.). New York: Springer Publishing Company.

Ray, M., & Turkel, M. (2010). Marilyn Anne Ray's theory of Bureaucratic Caring. In M. Smith & M. Parker (Eds). *Nursing theories and nursing practice* (3rd ed.). Philadelphia: F. A. Davis Company.

Ray, M., & Turkel, M. (2012). A transtheoretical evolution of caring science within complex systems. *International Journal for Human Caring, 16*(2), 28–49.

Ray, M., & Turkel, M. (2014). Caring as emancipatory nursing praxis. *Advances in Nursing Science, 37*(2), 132–146.

Ray, M., & Turkel, M. (2015). Marilyn Anne Ray's Theory of Bureaucratic Caring. In M. Parker & M. Smith (Eds.). *Nursing theories and nursing practice* (4th ed.). Philadelphia: F. A. Davis Company.

Ray, M., Turkel, M., & Marino, F. (2002). The transformative process for nursing in workforce redevelopment. *Nursing Administration Quarterly, 26*(2), 1–14.

Reeder, F. (1984). Philosophical issues in the Rogerian science of unitary human beings. *Advances in Nursing Science, 8*(1), 14–23.

Reverby, S. (1987). *Ordered to care: The dilemma of American nursing, 1850–1945*. Cambridge: Cambridge University Press.

Roach, M. (1984). Caring, The human mode of being: Implications for nursing. In *Perspectives on Caring: Monograph 1*. Toronto: University of Toronto, Faculty of Nursing.

Roach, M. (Ed.). (1997). *Caring from the heart: The convergence of caring and spirituality*. New York: Paulist Press.

Roach, M. (2002). *The human act of caring: A blueprint for the health professions* (Rev. Ed.). Ottawa: Canadian Hospital Association Press. (Original work published 1987)

Rogers, M. (1970). *An introduction to the theoretical basis of nursing*. Philadelphia: F. A. Davis Company.

Rohr, R. (2010). *Silent compassion: Finding God in contemplation*. Cincinnati, OH: Franciscan Press.

Rosen, R. (1988). The epistemology of complexity. In J. Kelso, A. Mandrell, & M. Schlesinger (Eds.), *Dynamic patterns in complexity*. Singapore: World Scientific.

Sandelowski, M. (1997). (Ir)reconcilable differences? The debate concerning nursing and technology. *Image: Journal of Nursing Scholarship 29*(2), 169–174.

Sandelowski, M. (2002). Visible humans, vanishing bodies, and virtual nursing: Complications of life, presence, place, and identity. *Advances in Nursing Science, 24*(3), 58–70.

Schumacher, E. (1999). *Small is beautiful: Economics as if people mattered*. Point Roberts, WA: Hartley & Marks Publishers. (Original work published 1973)

Sherwood, G. (1997). Meta-synthesis of qualitative analysis of caring: Defining a therapeutic model of nursing. *Advanced Practice Nursing Quarterly, 3*(1), 32–42.

Shirey, M. (2005). Nurturance: Concept clarification and theory for nursing administration practice. *International Journal for Human Caring, 9*(3), 65–72.

Smith, H. (1991). *The world's religions*. San Francisco: HarperSanFrancisco.

Smith, M. (1999). Caring and science of unitary human beings. *Advances in Nursing Science 21*, 14–28.

Smith, M. (2004). Review of research related to Watson's theory of caring. *Nursing Science Quarterly, 17*(1), 13–25.

Smith, M., & Parker, M. (2015). Nursing theories and nursing practice (4th ed.). Philadelphia: F. A. Davis Company.

Smith, M., Turkel, M. & Wolf, Z. (2013). *Caring in nursing classics: An essential resource*. New York: Springer Publishing Company.

Solecki, R. (1971). *Shanidar: The first flower people*. New York: Alfred A. Knopf.

Spector, R. (2003). *Cultural diversity in health and illness* (6th ed.). Upper Saddle River, NJ: Prentice Hall Health.

Spikins, P. (2015). *How compassion made us human: An archaeology of stone-age sentiment*. United Kingdom: Pen and Sword.

Stein, E. (1989). *On the problem of empathy* (W. Stein, Trans.). Washington, DC: ICS Publications.

Steiner, G. (1989*). Real presence*. London: Faber and Faber.

Stone, N., & Hart, P. (Eds.). (1985). *Thomas Merton, love and living*. New York: Harcourt Brace Jovanovich, Publishers.

Sumner, J. (2008). *The moral construct of caring in nursing as communicative action*. Saarbrücken, Germany: VDM Verlag Dr. Müller.

Swinderman, T. (2005). *The magnetic appeal of nurse informaticians: Caring attractor for emergence*. Doctor of Nursing Science Dissertation. Boca Raton, FL: Florida Atlantic University.

Tarlow, S. (2000). Emotion in archaeology. *Current Anthropology, 419*(5), 713–746.

Tarnas, R. (1991). *The passion of the western mind*. New York: Ballantine Books.

Teichler, E. (2000). *The amazon at midlife: The meaning of movement through women's life transitions*. PhD Dissertation, Denver, CO: University of Colorado.

Teilhard de Chardin, P. (1960). *Le divine milieu*. New York: Harper & Row Publishers.

Teilhard de Chardin, P. (1965). *Building the earth*. Dimensions Books.

The Concise Oxford Dictionary (8th ed.). (1990). Oxford: Oxford University Press.

Templeton, J. (1999). *Agape love: A tradition found in eight world religions*. Philadelphia: Templeton Foundation Press.

The New American Bible. (1987). Nashville, TN: Thomas Nelson Publishers.

Turkel, M. (2006a). What is evidence-based practice? And integration of evidence-based practice in nursing. In S. Beyea & M. Slattery (Eds.), *Evidence-based practice in nursing: A guide to successful implementation*. Marblehead, MA: HcPro Publishing.

Turkel, M. (2006b). Integration of evidence-based practice in nursing. In S. Beyea & M. Slattery (Eds.), *Evidence-based practice in nursing: A guide to successful implementation*. Marblehead, MA: HcPro Publishing.

Turkel, M. (2007). Dr. Marilyn Ray's theory of bureaucratic caring. *International Journal for Human Caring, 11*(4), 57–70.

Turkel, M., & Ray, M. (2000). Relational complexity: A theory of the nurse-patient relationship within an economic context. *Nursing Science Quarterly, 13*(4), 306–313.

Turkel, M., & Ray, M. (2001). Relational complexity: From grounded theory to instrument development and theoretical testing. *Nursing Science Quarterly, 14*(4), 281–287.

Turkel, M., & Ray, M. (2004a). A process model for policy analysis within the context of political caring. *International Journal for Human Caring, 7*(3), 17–24.

Turkel, M., & Ray, M. (2004b). Creating a caring practice environment through self-renewal. *Nursing Administration Quarterly, 28*(4), 249–256.

Turkel, M., & Ray, M. (2009). Caring for the "not so picture perfect patient": Ethical caring in the moral community of nursing. In R. Locsin & M. Purnell (Eds.), *A contemporary nursing process: The (un)bearable weight of knowing persons* (pp. 225–249). New York: Springer Publishing Company.

Van Manen, M. (1990). *Researching lived experience*. Albany, NY: State University of New York Press.

Van Manen, M. (2014). *Phenomenology of practice*. Walnut Creek, CA: Left Coast Press.

Van Tongeren, P. (1996). Ethics: Tradition and hermeneutics. *Ethical Perspectives: Rethinking Professional Ethics, 3*(4), 175–183.

Watson, J. (1985). *Nursing: Human science, human care*. Norwalk, CT: Appleton-Century-Crofts.

Watson, J. (1988). *Nursing: Human science, human care*. New York: National League for Nursing.

Watson, J. (1997). *The philosophy and science of caring*. Boston: Little, Brown and Company.

Watson, J. (1999). *Postmodern nursing and beyond*. London: Churchill Livingstone.

Watson, J. (2005). *Caring science as sacred science*. Philadelphia: F. A. Davis Company.

Watson, J. (2008). *Nursing: The philosophy and science of caring* (Rev. Ed.). Boulder, CO: University Press of Colorado.

Watson, J. (2008). *The philosophy and science of caring* (2nd rev. ed.). Boulder, CO: University Press of Colorado.

Watson, J. (Ed.). (2009). *Assessing and measuring caring in nursing and health science*. (2nd ed.). New York: Springer Publishing Company.

Watson, J., & Ray, M. (1988) (Eds.). *The ethics of care and the ethics of cure: Synthesis in chronicity.* New York: National League for Nursing.

Weaver, H. (1999). Transcultural nursing with Native Americans: Critical knwledge, skill, and attitudes. *Journal of Transcultural Nursing, 10*(3), 197–202.

West, C. (2007). *The love that satisfies.* West Chester, PA: Ascension Press.

White, R. (1996). Communitarian ethic of communication in a postmodern age. *Ethical Perspectives: Rethinking Professional Ethics, 3*(4), 207–218.

Wolfe, A. (2012). *Political evil: What it is and how to combat it.* New York: Vintage Books.

Wu, C. J., & Ray, M. (2016 in press). Technological caring for healthcare complexities of patients with cardiac disease comorbid with diabetes. International *Journal for Human Caring, 20*(2).

Zerwekh, J. (1997). The practice of presencing. *Seminars in Oncology Nursing, 13*(4), 260–262.

Select Bibliography

Boykin, A. (Ed.). (2004). *Living a caring-based curriculum.* New York: National League for Nursing Press.

Griffin, G., & Griffin, J. (1973). *History and trends of professional nursing* (7th ed.). St. Louis: CV Mosby Company.

Smith, B. (1998). *On the origin of objects.* Cambridge, MA: MIT Press.

Swanson, K. (1999). What is known about caring in nursing science. In A.S. Hinshaw, S. Fleetham & J. Shaver (Eds.), *Handbook of clinical nursing research* (pp. 31–60). Thousand Oaks, CA: Sage.

Tarlow, S. (1999). *Bereavement and commemoration: An archaeology of mortality.* Oxford: Blackwell.

Teilhard de Chardin, P. (1967). *On love.* New York: Harper & Row Publishers.

United Nations Development Goals, 2015, and post-2015 development agenda. Retrieved September 21, 2014 from http://un.org/mdg.goals

Wall, B. (1971). *Love and death in the philosophy of Gabriel Marcel.* Washington, DC: University Press of America.

Wolin, R. (2005). Jurgen Habermas and post-secular societies. *The Chronicle Review*, Section II, *LII* (5), B16–B17.

World Health Organization, Health in every policy. Retrieved September 21, 2014 from www.who.org/Finland

CHAPTER 3

Transcultural Caring Ethics

We are discussing no small matter, but how we ought to live.
Socrates in Plato's *Republic* (ca. 390 B.C.) (Rachels, 2003)

Chapter Objectives

1. Illuminate the search for transcultural ethical understanding.
2. Outline Western ethical theories.
3. Describe the good and evil or the shadow side of conscience.
4. Outline the process of moving forward in transcultural ethics.
5. Describe ethical relativism and universalism.
6. Describe transcultural ethical caring.
7. Advance transcultural caring ethics.
8. Explore transcultural caring experience: Ruth.
9. Explore transcultural caring experience: Letitia.

KEY WORDS

Nursing • caring • ethics • moral • good • evil • right • human rights • cultural rights • duty • obligation • universalism • cultural relativism • beneficence • nonmaleficence • autonomy • justice • fairness • transcultural ethics • transcultural caring ethics • moral blurring • moral blindness • health-care systems • codes of ethics

Dimension of the Model

Transcultural Caring Ethics
(The Good, Commitment/Trust,
Respect, Fidelity, Integrity,
Beneficence/Nonmaleficence, Justice/Truth,
Autonomy, Human Rights, Cultural Rights,
Rights of Nature)
The knowledge shaping moral caring
experience that facilitates transcultural
ethical caring

Figure 3–1: Dimension of the model: Transcultural caring ethics.

"*E*thics is concerned with human actions" (MacIntyre, 1996, p. 85). Ethics thus is concerned with human character or virtue (Rachels, 2003). "Ethics is defined as a code of conduct developed and reinforced in terms of what is good and right (or moral) in character and behavior" (Ray, 1998, p. 72). Ethics and morality deal with questions of how people ought to live in society (Burkhardt & Nathaniel, 2013; MacKinnon & Fiala, 2014; Rachels, 2003). The terms translate to mean rules or norms, suggesting dignity for human persons (human rights) and justice and right action in human communities/environment (Ahlquist, 2003; Anderko, Chalupka, & Anderko, 2014; Lange, 2005; Ray, 2010a, 2010b, 2010c; Ring, 2014; Roach, 2002). Ethics demands serving the good and being responsible for others, known as the ethical demand (Logstrup, 1997). Ethics as inquiry about the nature of good and evil (beneficence and maleficence respectively) in society studies ways of being (character and virtue), rules, and action about people as they relate together (Rachels, 2003). Overall, ethics encourages the virtue of personal fidelity and commitment to a truth (see Fig. 3-1), such as, "Fear God and keep his commandments; for this is the whole duty of man" (Ecclesiastes, 12:13, *The New American Bible*, 1987); the absolute moral law is followed by everyone without exception in all circumstances for all time (the "categorical ought"), such as: "reason requires that we never lie" (Kant, 1959); or selfless devotion to a cause, "first the Good (the affirmation of truth), *then* the risk of Evil (as perversion of the Good)" (Badiou, 2001, p. xiii). Consequently, moral behavior is an exercise *in* virtue that "manifests human excellence" (MacIntyre, 1996, p. 80).

Thus, ethics and moral behavior encompass historical traditions and beliefs about the nature of good and evil, character or virtue, and right and wrong conduct. As a social and cultural phenomenon, ethics and morals identify a code of rules that are learned, examined, and applied with reason and caring throughout life (Bosek & Savage, 2006; Burkhardt & Nathaniel, 2008, 2013; Lange, 2005; Leininger, 1990, 1995; Rachels, 2003; Ray, 2010c; Roach, 2002). A further example of a universal truth in professional nursing is caring, "a moral ideal whereby the end is protection, enhancement, and preservation of human dignity" (Watson, 1985, p. 29).

The Search for Ethical Understanding

Some moral concepts change as social life changes, and moral concepts come to life as people and groups relate to each other in sociocultural life. In essence, moral concepts are partially representative of forms of sociocultural life. One central way in which we may identify one form of sociocultural life as distinct from another is by identifying differences in moral concepts (MacIntyre, 1996). This notion becomes important as globalization expands and cultures interface more frequently. For example, changes in the modern global arena have brought forth critical moral concerns in relation to cultural and religious differences, human rights, cultural (including socioeconomic-political) rights, poverty, health care, HIV/AIDS, the rights of nature (i.e., the environment, agriculture, water, air, sanitation), migration, refugees, homelessness, gender and personal relationships, treatment of animals, electronic communication patterns, pornography and human trafficking, terrorism, war, and peace (MacKinnon & Fiala, 2014). As representative forms of sociocultural life, new questions are raised (Callahan, 2001; Davis & Dickinson, 2004; Leininger, 1995). Over time, "[i]n any culture, accepted duties sometimes clash, and deeper, more general principles are needed to arbitrate between them" (Midgley, 1993). In global culture, increasingly there is a breakdown of unified moral rules that may have been established in any one culture (Berman, 2004; Wolfe, 2012).

Today, questions revolve around how moral rules will be used, what will be required to understand them, and how will they be evaluated (Ahlquist, 2003). As such, contemporary ethics as a branch of philosophy that deals with understanding continues to investigate theories established over time, especially Western ethical theories, and to develop new theories about the nature of right and wrong, duty, obligation, freedom, virtue and most significantly, how the environment, human rights, justice, and transcultural forms of relating are cocreated, change, and can be understood.

ETHICAL THEORIES

There are various theories that, although sometimes controversial (MacKinnon & Fiala, 2014; Rachels, 2003), provide an understanding of the foundations of morality and help to facilitate the understanding of ethical dilemmas and questions. Many theories have been advanced in moral philosophy in Western and Eastern cultures, and although Eastern philosophies are studied or practiced in the West, we are most familiar with ethical theories that originate in the West (they will be highlighted at this point; the religious and ethical traditions of Eastern philosophies/theories are addressed in Chapter 5).

A theory is a guide or a synthesis of concepts used to explain complex phenomena. A brief overview of theories that contribute to knowledge of ethics in nursing and health care and lay the foundation for transcultural ethics in the dynamic global world are as follows:

- Divine Command Theory
- Natural Law
- Ethics in Ancient Greece
- Medieval and Renaissance Ethics
- Christian Ethics
- Kantian Ethics (Deontology)
- Utilitarianism
- Virtue Theory

Learn More

Ethical Theories
- Divine Command Theory
- Natural Law
- Ethics in Ancient Greece
- Medieval and Renaissance Ethics
- Christian Ethics
- Kantian Ethics (Deontology)
- Utilitarianism
- Virtue Theory
- Biomedical Ethics
- Ethics of Care/Caring
- Transcultural Ethics
- Transcultural Caring Ethics

- Biomedical Ethics
- Ethics of Care/Caring
- Transcultural Ethics
- Transcultural Caring Ethics (see information as chapter progresses)

Divine Command Theory

In the major theistic traditions, including Judaism, Christianity, and Islamic God is conceived as a lawgiver who has laid down rules that we are to obey. The idea of the tree of knowledge of good and evil was revealed by God in Genesis, 2:9 in the *Old Testament*. The theory about the nature of right (the moral life) and wrong (the immoral life) became known as the Divine Command Theory. The Ten Commandments (rules) were given to Moses (Exodus, 20:1–17, *The New American Bible*, 1987) in the Hebrew Scripture *(Old Testament)*, followed through by Jesus, the Son of God, in Christian Scripture *(New Testament)*, and expressed by Allah through the prophet, Mohammed in the *Qur'an*. People are created as free agents so they may choose to accept or reject God's commandments. Believers are held accountable to the commandments and specifically on the "day of judgment" at the end of life. Atheists (those who do not believe in God) have rejected the theory. Believers asked questions similar to the Greek philosophers: "Is conduct right because God commanded it; or does God command it because it is right?" These questions have been central to the study of philosophy ever since (Rachels, 2003, pp. 50–51).

Natural Law

The Natural Law theory is perceived of as rational order with values and purposes built into its very nature. Natural law pertains to the ordered structure of the world governed by cosmic reason and by divine decree. Natural law is thus differentiated from human legislation. On the one hand, the natural law provides direction for human conduct as a precondition of a person's natural development, and on the other hand, natural law is a set of rules ordered by God and transmitted to human beings by way of the Ten Commandments and also, by way of revelation through the exercise of conscience (Haldane, 1993).

❖ *Nursing Reflection*

Reflect upon your own religious or spiritual background and how it guides your moral actions.

❖ *Nursing Reflection*

Reflect upon what you believe about the structure of the world and how you would reason the meaning of the natural world and your place in it.

Ethics in Ancient Greece

Western ethical theories seeking rational or logical understanding of the principles of human conduct began with the ancient Greeks, namely Socrates, Plato, and Aristotle around the 5th and 4th centuries B.C. Greek ethics revolved around two main themes: happiness (i.e., *eudaimonia*, the good life) and virtue (i.e., *arête*—wisdom, justice, courage, moderation, piety, or right behavior). The focus of ethics for Plato first was on discovering ethical truths through rational *introspection;* and, second, on the need for a *consensus* among people about public and private values. For Socrates and later Aristotle, the focus of ethical insight was located in the experience of life itself, and that truth can be discovered through logical arguments. "A position is only as good as the arguments that support it" (Rowe, 1993, p. 130), and the principle of choice is the midpoint between two extremes, virtue or vice (MacIntyre, 1996). This ethical legacy has been left to the modern world.

Medieval and Renaissance Ethics

The earliest origins of medieval philosophy, the period from the 2nd to the 5th centuries after the Greek and Roman periods, was advanced by the Catholic church fathers who interpreted Judeo-Christian scriptures (Haldane, 1993). Natural law appeared within this period. The theory of moral law was addressed by Saint Augustine wherein he said that, "God endows each man [woman] with a conscience whereby he [she] may know the moral

law" (Haldane, 1993, p. 136). The moral rules are written in the *Bible*, and accordingly, a person has a desire to perfect oneself in the truth, that is "to love God with all one's heart, soul and mind" (Saint Augustine, 1958).

Medieval and renaissance ethics extended throughout the time span and reached fulfillment in the 11th to 16th centuries. These ethics are connected with the dominant philosophical tradition of Scholasticism, primarily of Saints. Anselm and Thomas Aquinas, and authors of primarily two religious orders, the Dominicans and the Franciscans. Saint Thomas Aquinas, considered one of the great philosophers of the past and present, wrote 15 volumes called the *Summa Theologiae* that synthesized the Greek thought of Aristotle and Catholic doctrine into a reasoned Christian philosophy. Aquinas held a rationalistic view of ethical/moral thinking illuminating natural law (rational order and purposeful tendencies built into its nature) as discoverable by the use of right reason. Aquinas integrated this rational thought of Aristotle with the Christian theology of God as providing supernatural assistance through revelation and grace, thus making it possible for supernatural transformation of the goal of virtue from the state of human flourishing to that of blessedness (eternal union with God) (Haldane, 1993, pp. 141–142). "The virtues [goodness, trust, honesty, humility, courage, fidelity, etc.] are both an expression of and a means to obedience to the commandments of the natural law, and to the natural virtues are added the supernatural virtues of faith, hope, and love" (MacIntyre, 1996, p. 118).

Christian Ethics

Christian ethics is a way of life appropriate to those who accept the Christian faith. Christian faith accepts the reality of God and the God that is disclosed not only in the *Old Testament* but also specifically in the ministry of Jesus outlined in the *New Testament*. The life of Jesus exemplifies teachings of the Kingdom of God (Preston, 1993, pp. 94–95). In the teachings of Jesus, the ethical conduct that is central is the Golden Rule, "Do unto others as you would

❖ *Nursing Reflection*

Reflect upon how you have developed ethical and moral insight from personal and family values and how you have developed the concepts of the good and virtuous. Consider the evolution of logical argument in your own behavior in your personal life and professional responsibilities.

❖ *Nursing Reflection*

Reflect upon the meaning of conscience, reason, and the virtues that you deem important in your personal and professional lives.

have them do unto you" (Matthew, 7: 12, *The New American Bible*, 1987). Love of self and others, including our enemies, and forgiveness is the thrust of the message. At the same time, the idea of justice or treating others rightly despite how one is treated is emphasized. The Sermon on the Mount (the Beatitudes) (Matthew, 5:3–10) outlines the teachings of Jesus and the rewards that will be attained in eternal life. In the *New Testament* scripture, often good was wrought from evil. Love in word, will, and action is the essence of the message (Preston, 1993). "Love as motivation does not give detailed content to ethical decisions. That requires knowledge and discernment, a combination of skills and perceptiveness" (Preston, 1993, p. 98).

The focus on love in Christian ethics has not always produced right action throughout history. All major groups of Christians at some time or another have persecuted each other, and other religious or secular groups. There is a concerted effort being made in contemporary Christian culture to concentrate on promoting the dignity of all people by dialoguing together to address and heal past injustices, and an attempt to cocreate healing, peace, and harmony in a pluralistic world (Preston, 1993).

Kantian Ethics

Kant is considered one of the foremost European philosophers of the 18th century. Kant argued against the claims of the rationalist views advanced by the Greek thinkers, such as Plato and Aristotle; and Christian philosophers, such as Saint Thomas Aquinas. He argued against the proofs of the existence of God but did claim that his moral theory could be used as a lens for interpreting scripture. Kant argued that we can "know" without referring to *particular* experiences. Respect for persons and the idea that *moral rules are absolute regardless of one's wants or desires* is the foundation of Kantian ethics. Kant believed that people may never be used as means to an end. "This is the ultimate law of morality" in

Kant's philosophy (Rachels, 2003, p. 130). Kant believed in the commitment to human freedom (the ability to act autonomously), to the dignity of human beings (persons have intrinsic worth), and to the view that moral obligation derives neither from God, nor from human authorities, communities, preferences, or desires for happiness of human agents (the principle of utilitarianism), but from reason. The moral demand or moral law in Kant's deontology (deon meaning the study of the principle of duty) follows a reasoned view: "the rightness or wrongness of an act depends upon the nature of the act and not on the consequences that occur from it" (Burkhardt & Nathaniel, 2008, p. 541). Categorical "oughts" are binding on people who are rational agents. Kant's Categorical Imperative states "that no action can be judged as right which cannot reasonably become a law [universal] by which every person should always abide" (Burkhardt & Nathaniel, 2008, p. 540). Kant, however, had a dual and paradoxical view of human beings (O'Neill, 1993, p. 180). Kant's Kingdom of Ends exemplified this notion wherein each person is autonomous and self-legislates; each person is both a rule maker and is bound by the rule that is made (O'Neill, 1993, p. 179). Kant's ethics remains the most influential attempt to justify *universal* moral principles as absolute without reference to what one prefers (utilitarianism) or to a theological framework (O'Neill, 1993).

❖ *Nursing Reflection*

Reflect upon the meaning of absolute moral rules or laws. Are there absolute moral rules in contemporary multicultural society? Are there or should there be absolute moral rules in nursing, such as, for example, no lying, no deception, or keeping promises under any circumstance? Do you think that respect for others and the idea of human dignity are primary virtues in life and society? How does Kant's theory vary from a theory of virtue or character? What is the difference between a value and virtue? How important is respect in professional nursing situations in treating others as rational (choice-making) beings? What does autonomy mean to you? What does it mean in professional nursing? How would the mentally ill be viewed in the Kantian theory?

❖ *Nursing Reflection*

Reflect upon concepts of compassion, love, mercy, and justice in your personal life and in professional nursing situations. Are love and compassion above and beyond the call of professional duty (Rachels, 2003, p. 109)? Can one do evil in the perceived name of good?

Social Contract Theory

In this theory, morality does not depend on God, moral facts, or altruism but morality should be understood as something that arises from, for example, self-interests or selfishness According to the philosopher, Hobbes, four basic facts exist in human life:

1. There is equality of need for survival, food, clothing, and shelter.
2. There is scarcity—we have to work hard for things to survive.
3. There is equality of power but who will get the goods of this earth when goods are scarce.
4. There is limited altruism to assist people who cannot care for themselves because we essentially care for ourselves and are selfish. (Rachels, 2003, p. 142).

In this theory, moral rules are rules that are necessary if people are to gain the benefits of social living. The rules revolve around the fact that we must be able to count on each other, so as not to harm each other deliberately, to rely on people to keep their agreements or contracts, and to share resources. "Morality consists in the set of rules governing how people are to treat one another, that rational people will agree to accept for their mutual benefit, on the condition that others follow those rules as well" (Rachels, 2003, p. 145). Thus, we must agree upon rules to govern relationships with one another with enforceable power and ways vested in the state to keep those rules (the social contract theory).

Utilitarianism

Utilitarian Theory, advanced initially by philosophers Bentham and Mill, holds that (1) actions are to be judged right or wrong solely by virtue of their consequences, (2) in assessing consequences, the only thing that matters is the amount of happiness or unhappiness that is created, and (3) each person's happiness counts the same (Rachels, 2003, p. 102). In essence, "Right actions are those that produce the greatest possible balance of happiness over unhappiness, with each person's happiness counted as equally important" (Rachels, 2003, p. 103). This theory, also known as consequentialism, draws upon the idea that people can be used as means to an end (Rachels, 2003). Each person's welfare is equally important to determine whether an action is right and right actions are the ones that produce the most good. Happiness as the one ultimate good and unhappiness as the one ultimate evil is known as hedonism. Arguments against the consequentialist

❖ Nursing Reflection

What moral rules are you bound to follow in your society to maintain the social contract with the public? Is there a difference between a social contract and a covenant? Is nursing a contract or covenant with the public? What is the meaning of the state nursing license or Certificate of Competence (Canada) as a social contract? What moral rules are there in the profession of nursing and how are they justified (see State Registered Nurse licensing rules, the Codes of Ethics of the Canadian Nurses Association, American Nurses Association, and the International Council of Nursing; Transcultural Nursing Society Position Statement on Human Rights)? Are there social contract rules that, as a nursing, medical, or pharmacy professional, we do not have to follow; under what conditions (in your reflection, consider abortion or contraceptive medications and if they have become a part of a wider social contract)? Do universal rules apply to a culturally diverse world?

notion of happiness reveal that happiness is a response we have to the attainment of things that we recognize as good, independently, and in their own right (Rachels, 2003, p. 104). The Utilitarian Theory has been argued within the theory of economics and has a direct affect upon health care and public health with their foci on the greatest good for the greatest number, and on outcomes.

Virtue Ethics

The character of the human being and character itself must be taken into consideration in a theory of Virtue Ethics. In classic Greek thought and ethics, Aristotle in 325 B.C. was concerned with virtue, with the good of human beings and what makes someone a virtuous person (Pence, 1993). At the same time, the virtuous life for the early Greeks was associated with reason. In essence, the virtuous life was inseparable from reason or practical wisdom (Rachels, 2003, p. 173). With the coming of Judeo-Christian life and thought, right living was following the precepts of God and the Divine Commandments. For Christians, following Divine Law also meant engaging the theological virtues of faith, hope, and love (Rachels, 2003) reinforced by Christ.

❖ *Nursing Reflection*

Do Kant's ethics and the Utilitarian Theorycollide? If it is true that we use Utilitarian Theory in public civic life, health care, and public health (the greatest good for the greatest number), how do the ideas of personal, individual human rights coexist (Rachels, 2003, pp. 106–107)? What is meant by the Constitution of the United States, orthe rule of law, the Amendments to theConstitution, or the Canadian Charter ofRights in terms of Utilitarian Theory? Another question raised in the Utilitarian Theory relates to the idea that it focuses on the future, the consequences (what will happen), rather than also looking at the past. How do facts of the past that may be relevant to determining a person's obligation to another play a role in determining caring for a patient or making health and nursing policy (see the Codes of Ethics and the principles outlined in The Joint Commission? What does the idea of choicefor the good of the other mean to you? Would you focus on consequences or on the individual freedom and autonomy? How do these ideas play a role in evidence-based practice or outcomes-oriented approaches in nursing practice today?

Examples of general virtues are: compassion, courage, self-control, generosity, justice, fairness, loyalty, patience, fidelity, thoughtfulness, truthfulness, prudence, and self-discipline. Overall, virtue ethics encompasses the nature of how one should *be* in the world rather than what one ought to do (Burkhardt & Nathaniel, 2008).

After the Renaissance period (14th to 16th centuries), in philosophical ethics, the notion of Divine Law was replaced with what is referred to as its secular equivalent, the Moral Law. Virtue ethics has challenged Kantian and Utilitarian ethics (Beauchamp & Childress, 2001), especially since the mid-1950s. In the health sciences, Pellegrino has made virtue ethics central to the philosophy of medicine and the roles of physicians and nurses (Burkhardt & Nathaniel, 2008). From a nursing perspective, ". . . Florence Nightingale thought that virtue was an important

trait of the good nurse" (Burkhardt & Nathaniel, 2008, p. 45). Virtue and virtuous acts have been highlighted throughout the history of nursing and lay the foundation for the ethics of care and caring.

Biomedical Ethics

Biomedical ethics exemplifies a number of ethical principles: beneficence, nonmaleficence, autonomy, veracity, confidentiality, justice, and fidelity Beauchamp & Childress, 2001; Burkhardt & Nathaniel, 2013; Edge & Groves, 1994; MacKinnon & Fiala, 2014; Veatch, 1977). "Ethical principles are basic moral truths that guide deliberation and action" in medicine and nursing and are grounded in ethical theories (see descriptions in this section) (Burkhardt & Nathaniel, 2008, p. 53). Biomedical ethics presuppose the ethical principle of respect for persons (see Codes of Ethics of the American Nurses Association [2001, 2015], Canadian Nurses Association [2008], International Council of Nurses [2006]. **Beneficence** is to do good and requires nurses to act in ways that benefit or are good for patients. Nurses are obligated to act beneficently—what is morally and legally demanded by nursing's professional role (Burkhardt & Nathaniel, 2008, 2013). Beneficence or the good in the nursing role and practice is complex in that nurses are required to have scientific, ethical, humanistic, and aesthetic and personal knowledge of and competency in holism: nurse-patient relationships; body, mind, and spiritual well-being of the patient; cultural differences; and how the context (i.e., economic, legal, technological, and political [power issues]) of health-care organizations are integrated into or affect the well-being of patients, family members, or significant others (American Nurses Association, Code of Ethics for Nursing (2015), wwwnursingworld.org/codeofethics; Carper, 1978; Leininger, 1991, 1995; Ray, 1989b, 2001, 2006; Ray & Turkel, 2014, 2015). Promoting the well-being of

❖ *Nursing Reflection*

What virtues are important in nursing? What makes a virtuous nurse? What is the difference between being and doing in nursing, and between being virtuous and acting ethically in practice? Should there be a consistency between one's essential nature and what a nurse does or ought to do in practice? Do nurses employ reason along with virtue in the practice of nursing? How?

patients under these circumstances requires a type of supererogation or what is known as "above and beyond the call of duty." It also requires incorporation of virtue and caring ethics (see theories in this section). Nurses must always be alert to medical orders and their own behavior that can contradict beneficent acts. **Nonmaleficence** is a principle that requires nurses to act in such a way that no deliberate harm, risk of harm, and harm that relates to doing no harm in the wake of doing good. The first principle of the Hippocratic oath of medicine is to do no harm (Burkhardt & Nathaniel, 2008, pp. 60–62). Weighing a potential harm against a potential benefit is a constant ethical reasoning and caring process in nursing. **Autonomy** means to facilitate the freedom for self-governance or self-organization in patients with the assistance of family members or significant others. Often there is a critique of the principle of autonomy or self-governance in cultures, such as in Native American culture, where decisions are more communally based (Lowe & Nichols, 2014; Smith-Morris, 2007). Allowing choice, working with the patient, family, and community to cocreate what is needed for health and well-being is a primary nursing role. Nurses are to be advocates of the patient through *knowledgeable* caring, which means that within the principle of autonomy, there should be no coercion, paternalism, thoughtlessness, and deception. **Veracity** is an ethical principle that relates to telling the truth. "Truthfulness is widely accepted as a universal human virtue. . . .[t]ruth-telling engenders trust" (Burkhardt & Nathaniel, 2008, p. 65). In terms of relational caring, trust is one of the most important ways of being (Hilsenbeck, 2006; Ray, Turkel, & Marino, 2002). Although a relational concept, within the notion of trust there is appreciation for the independent existence of the other and requires "letting go" or the relinquishing of control over the other; "it includes an element of risk and a leap into the unknown, both of which take courage" (Mayeroff, 1971, p. 27) for truth-telling. When there is a perception of mistrust, people hold back on disclosing their secrets or information and the adage of "seeking one's own counsel" is the actual truth. Veracity in health care requires patience and courage to communicate openly and seek understanding of patient and family needs. Confidentiality is linked with privacy and refers to the right an individual has to personal information or secrets that are disclosed to others, especially health-care professionals. The ethical principle of confidentiality demands that one does not disclose private or secret information about another person with whom one has been entrusted (Burkhardt & Nathaniel, 2008, pp. 66–68; see Health Insurance Portability and Accountability Act [HIPAA], United States, Public Health Law 104-199). Respect for persons is the foundation of the principle of confidentiality. **Justice** is "the ethical principle that relates to fair, equitable, and appropriate treatment in light of what is due or owed to persons, recognizing that giving to some will deny receipt to others who might otherwise have received these things" (Burkhardt & Nathaniel, 2008, p. 73). Justice issues relate to the distribution of the greatest good to the greatest number. In health care and public health care in particular, the principle focuses on distribution of goods, money, and services (distributive justice). In nations that have a universal health-care system, the principle of justice in the distribution of health-care goods and services is more equitable than in nations that do not; however, health is an ever-demanding and evolving concept, so equal distribution is an ideal rather than an achieved end in itself. The important thing about justice is fairness. How does one be fair to the other when there is an equal or greater demand for goods and services? It requires an attitude and belief in caring, a way of giving and often giving up for the other. In a family situation, a mother may have to attend to one child's needs over the other in a particular situation. In nursing, on a unit when there is an equal demand for care and nurse caring and staffing ratios are minimal, often choices have to be made such that the more ill patient or the patient or family member in the greatest need will get the attention at a particular time. Resource allocation of goods, money, and services and interpersonal resources require sacrifice, thoughtfulness, communication, and advocacy for direct nurse-patient care, organizational management, and health and social policy development. **Fidelity** is an ethical principle that relates to faithfulness and keeping promises. In nursing, the principle of fidelity means loyalty to the patient within the nurse-patient relationship (Burkhardt & Nathaniel, 2008). Nurses make promises to their patients by means of the social contract of a nursing license or certificate of competence and as they care for the patients. Nurses must do everything in their power to be a patient advocate. With the rise of individualism in culture and perceived lack of mutual trust between nurse and health-care organizations, institutional loyalty has been seriously jeopardized (Ray, Turkel, & Marino, 2002; Turkel & Ray, 2004).

❖ *Nursing Reflection*

What is a principle? Why do we have ethical principles in nursing, medicine, or health care? What are the personal and professional codes of ethics that motivate your ethical thinking and behavior? How have you developed principled behavior in your life and professional education or practice? Have you found a way to clarify your values and principles to be more cognizant of biomedical principles? What principles are priorities in nursing practice? How do you identify with the biomedical principles when you are in a nursing situation or educational facility? Are there times when ethical principles are jeopardized in educational settings or in nursing practice? Do patients trust nurses, physicians, or administrators? Do nurses trust patients, physicians, or administrators?

Ethics of Care/Caring

In philosophy, the Ethics of Care emerged during the feminist movement within the latter part of the 20th century. Feminist ethics illuminated women's basic moral orientation to that of caring for others—compassion and taking care of others in an interpersonal way (Chinn, 2013; MacKinnon & Fiala, 2014; Rachels, 2003). Gilligan (1982), one of the first women and leading scholars of her time, engaged in a critique to correct the misperceptions in psychology by illuminating the motives, the growth, and development of morality of women and women's moral commitments. The ethical principles that emerge from most of these feminist theories of care show the dynamics of relationships and the concept of responsibility to the other—the good is equated with caring for others. "Care becomes the self-chosen principle of a judgment that remains psychological in its concern for relationships and response but becomes universal in its condemnation of exploitation and hurt" (Gilligan, 1982, p. 74). Even though the focus of modern feminine psychology and ethics is oriented to a new approach to feminine moral development, many ideas are based upon theological and human virtues of classical and medieval periods. What is new is the focus of attention on relationship, the call, and response of one person to the other, and care as central to moral development in women.

This orientation illustrates how important the meaning of care and caring was to the survival of human beings, as has been identified in anthropology (Leininger, 1978, 1991, 1995; Tarlow, 2000). The orientation to care and caring illuminates the relational idea of respect for self and other human beings. The character traits of caring capture the *meaning* of a truly good human being, one who cares and is responsible for others. At the same time, a caring human being is one who is conscious of the potential for selfishness in the individual self but lives in accordance with a moral code that enhances a sense of belonging to others, the world, and the universe at-large (Capra, Steindl-Rast with Matus, 1991).

The ethics of care and caring in nursing became prominent with the evolution of the concept of caring in nursing and also, at the same time, the ethics of care theme advanced in psychology. A guiding moral framework of ethical caring (enhancement and protection of human dignity, alleviation of suffering, and the nursing event/situation) in nursing was advanced by many theorists of caring (Davidson, Ray, & Turkel, 2011; Eriksson, 1997, 2006; Leininger, 1990; Ray, 1994a, 1994b, 1997, 1998, 2007, 2010a, 2010b, 2010c; Roach, 2002; Watson, 1988, 2005, 2008). Although complex and even paradoxical, evaluation and research have shown that in nursing situations, nurses integrate both the ethics of principle/duty and reason *and* the ethics of caring, healing, and responsibility (Cooper, 1991; Hilsenbeck, 2006; Ray, 1987, 1998, 2007; Roach, 2002). Within this synthesis, there usually is creative moral tension that facilitates insight into and understanding of moral confusion and moral chaos, and the agonizing vulnerability in relation to the complexity of ethical decision making in the nursing situation (Chase, 2004; Gadow, 1989). Nursing continues to contribute to the understanding of caring as a moral enterprise—a value, virtue, intentional act, reason, and practical wisdom—a call and response and responsibility to self, others, the environment, and the universe.

Transcultural Ethics

Transcultural ethics is very complex and dynamic. Each individual is a collage and integration of diverse values, beliefs, attitudes, and behaviors that make up human experience. Culture relates to patterns of learned behaviors and values that are interpreted and shared among members of a designated group and usually transmitted to others of their group through time (Leininger, 1978, 1990, 1991).

❖ *Nursing Reflection*

What does an ethic of care and caring mean to you? How do you practice an ethic of care and caring with patients? What do healing and responsibility for the other mean to you? Is caring a universal principle and a culturally relative way of being? Do you find it hard to practice an ethic of care/caring in nursing today? What creative tension have you experienced between a set of principles, such as beneficence, autonomy, justice, and compassion or mercy? What principles and virtues do you find difficult? Are you ever morally confused about what to do in nursing situations? Have you experienced moral conflict, blurring, or moral blindness (Gadow, 1988, 1989; Ray, 1998; Turkel & Ray, 2009) when it comes to a difficult ethical situation in nursing or health care? Have you seen immoral behavior in nursing or medical practice, outright wrong actions? How have you dealt with observable or your own silent moral problems? Are there gray areas in nursing ethics either in the classroom or in nursing practice situations of potential cheating or deceiving the patient or the organization, truth telling, and promise keeping?

Ethics is grounded in consciousness and conscience, which underscores beliefs about why we exist. Ethics is humanistic and principle-based and reveals a broader religious or spiritual purpose of reasons why we exist and how we should relate to and act with each other. Ethics is associated with respect for persons and moral action in the lifeworld and in living with others (American Nurses Association Code of Ethics with Interpretive Statements, 2001, 2015, www.nursingworld.org/codeofethics). The immediate purpose of transcultural ethics is to "hear the other" and "learn from the other" with mutual respect. This validates the idea that all people are cultural beings and have diverse values, beliefs, and attitudes. As cultural beings relate, transcultural ethics offers a framework within which to interact. The conscience in which this ethics illuminates strives to mitigate disrespect or elements of misconduct and to propagate the good, purpose, truth, and beauty within the interactions of all people and in nursing, nurses and patients, families or community groups.

In today's challenging global culture, transcultural ethics seeks to understand differences in people in interaction with others. Transcultural ethics validates the idea of increasing and learning compassion and reaching out to alleviate suffering—to help human beings by meeting needs and trying to secure human rights (individual or communal), and do what is just for others (Dalai Lama 1999; Hirsch, 1976; Leininger, 1991; Martin, 2015; Rachels, 2003; Ray, 1989a, 1994a, 2010a, 2010b, 2010c; Ray & Turkel, 2014; Singer, 1993; Watson, 2005; Wielenberg, 2005). Buchanan, in the *Hastings Center Report* on ethics across cultures, stated that "[h]uman rights, by definition, are rights we have simply by virtue of our humanity, regardless of differences in our cultures, and regardless of when or where we live" (1996, p. 26). However, while it is true that all humans are endowed with human rights, differing cultures determine the meaning of human rights, and how they are granted. Human rights have differed historically, religiously, culturally, and traditionally. This theory and model of dimensions of Transcultural Caring Dynamics in Nursing and Health Care—the essence of caring, transcultural ethics, transcultural context (persons in the sociocultural environment), and universal (spiritual) sources—provides a foundation for awareness, understanding, and choice making (Ray, 2010a) and can be considered a human rights theory, enacting humane, just, and right action. Thus, on the individual and community levels, transcultural ethics mediates conflicts of conscience. From a universal perspective, ethical theories, including Transcultural Caring Dynamics in Nursing and Health Care, help to resolve basic human rights conflicts through compassion, argumentation, and reasoned choice.

Transcultural ethics is consistent with transcultural caring and thus transcultural caring and transcultural caring ethics are defined as follows: the relationship between charity and right action, between love as compassion and response to suffering and need, and justice or fairness in terms of doing what ought to be done within [the dynamics of] a culture or society (Ray, 1989a, p. 19). Culture, made up of beliefs, attitudes, values, principles, codes, standards, and rules of behavior, varies even within a given cultural community. What are the new codes of ethics for social media? Should there be ethical rules and regulations related to human-to-human contact through media outlets? How ethical should we be obligated to be? What are the ethical and legal implications for communications/social media (Patterson & Wilkins, 2013; Pember & Calvert, 2012)? Every individual experiences life differently and conscience forms not only because of cultural orientation, but also from life experience.

NURSING REFLECTS ON THEORIES OF ETHICS

Adopting a specific ethical theory or framework is extremely difficult because each has its own advantages and disadvantages and own interpretations (Benjamin & Curtis, 1992). A holistic approach in nursing challenges us to appreciate the relationship among body, mind, spirit, and the cultural/multicultural context, and the different ethical theories, including the Theory of Transcultural Caring Dynamics in Nursing and Health Care, and how to use theories and Codes of Ethics to review critical value domains in and for nursing and health care and health policy. The American Nurses Association (ANA) has completed a review of their 2001 version of the Code of Ethics for Nurses. New Codes of Ethics by the ANA

❖ *Nursing Reflection*

Reflect upon the transcultural and multicultural environment of today. Is there a difference between general ethical theories and transcultural ethics? Should there be? How does one respond to the call to "learn" compassion and engage in compassionate conversation so that the community of voices can be "heard"? How does a nurse continually accept the challenge of respect for all persons all over the world to protect and enhance human dignity? Do you think transcultural ethics and transcultural ethical caring can be viewed as supererogation (going beyond the call of duty or obligation) in its commitment to all people of the world? How is reason used in transcultural ethical and human rights' situations? How would you as a nurse deal with a situation where you see unethical behavior by a nurse or physician colleague toward a person of another culture? What is your moral obligation? How would you as a nurse "reinvent community" (i.e., familial, educational, social media, organizational, or municipal community) to promote transcultural caring ethics (i.e., sociocultural change, improved human rights, health care, social, or health policy)?

will be ready for use by professionals in 2015 (see www.nursingworld.org/codeofethics).

Ethical theories are associated with religion, rational thought, or may be considered naturalistic. Religiously oriented ethics deal with virtue, the theological or Godlike virtues and principles, the notion of the good, of faith, hope, and love and other character virtues or principles that illuminate personal and communal relationships. Rational ethics deals with principles of moral reasoning followed by a fundamental agreement of what is good, moral, or lawful in society (Rachels, 2003; Wielenberg, 2005). In the theory of natural law or natural ethics, the world is considered a rational order with values and purposes *built into* its very nature and accounts for values and virtues of the good, such as charity, hope, sacrifice, and humility in terms of the *meaning* of good and evil, and right and wrong. It can be considered humanistic and/or theological morality. Natural law from a theological perspective not only deals with elements of human rationality but also responds to the unchanging, eternal law of the divine (Buckle, 1993), which in contemporary ethical terms is illuminated as "human beings created by love, for love, to love" (Roach, 2002, p. 3).

Burkhardt and Nathaniel (2008, 2013) claim that the ethics of ". . . moral reasoning is the historical basis for the creation, evolution and the practice of nursing" (p. 4). In this view, relationships are implied but the focus is on the nature of moral thinking and the matter of weighing reasons and being guided by them. Nevertheless, ". . . not every reason that may be advanced is a good reason. There are bad arguments as well as good ones, and much of the skill of moral thinking consists in discerning the difference" (Rachels, 2003, p. 12). The difference for nursing lies in the ethics of caring in its many forms of understanding (see Chapter 2). Roach (2002) claimed that caring is not unique to nursing but unique *in* nursing because caring in nursing is the locus of all attributes used to describe nursing (p. 39). The theme of nursing is relational and first of all addresses a common starting point of being present to and for the other in compassion for the purposes of doing good, being fair or just, allowing choice, alleviating suffering, and doing no harm. Even with the complexities of the economic, political, and technological influences on the professional practice of nursing, it is inherent then that all moral reasoning would flow from the premise of caring. Caring thus is a human and rational mode of being and action.

The contemporary Eastern philosopher and ethicist, the Dalai Lama (1999), has called the world community back to social responsibility through the development of a wider sense of compassion, or caring. Compassion is a humanistic and divine concept. Compassion is a value for and a way of behaving; compassion is a means of expression of a purposeful way of being; compassion is knowledge of the other, a perspective on the differences and commonalities of people in society. Compassion is "a call to imitate God's particular way of being with us, God-with-us" in love (Roach, 2002, p. 51). It is the theme of this chapter and book to examine this wider sense of compassion through knowledge and understanding of the meaning of transcultural caring ethics (Ray, 1989a, 1989b, 1994a, 2001, 2005).

Evaluate the ethical theories that have been presented. In doing so, consider the following questions:

- How would you evaluate the theories in relation to the contemporary nursing practice and health-care system of today?
- What ethical theories would you embrace?
- What is the importance of the ethics of virtue and the ethics of caring? How do they compare with the ideas of Nightingale and the caring theorists?
- How does one deal with potential unethical actions in nursing situations that border on wrongdoing and outright evil?
- Can an ethic of care/caring be used to evaluate economics and political power in health-care organizations, in social media communication, and in overall health care and health policy, for example, in the United States?
- Compare and contrast the advances (research and development) in the ethics of principle and the ethics of care and caring in philosophy, psychology, transcultural studies, and nursing. Are they the same or do they differ?

Good and Evil: The Ethical Conflict

"Ethical [and moral] behavior is the result of ethical decision making, requiring qualities of ethical commitment, consciousness, conscience, and competency" (Ray, 1998, p. 72). Ethics, and specifically, morality, incorporates what people *believe* about "the good" and how they should act. Ethics encompasses the rules that govern what is right, and the willingness of people to choose correctly. Morality is difficult to define but encompasses the behavior or the act, essentially how one lives or ought to live in society or culture, the moral community (Rachels, 2003, Ray, 2010c).

Ethics also examines evil, considered the opposite of good in behavior. Evil means acting out of line with socially, lawfully, or religiously accepted rules or codes of conduct. Although the general meaning of ethics addresses the notion of the good of society, conflicts arise within ethics in terms of questions of what *is* the "good" and why we should obey rules at all (Rachels, 2003). In searching for how one ought to live in society, it inherently leads to the Golden Rule as Smith (1991) pointed out, "Do unto others as you would have them do unto you" (Matthew, 7:12, *The New American Bible*, 1987). This common rule lies at the base of morality (Midgley, 1993) and is the foundation for shared solutions and potential reconciliation of ethical conflict.

❖ *Nursing Reflection*

For nursing, caring is the essence of the profession. Caring is a *moral* ideal whereby "protection, enhancement and preservation of humanity for the restoration of inner harmony and potential healing" is the goal (Watson, 1985, p. 58). Transcultural caring ethics in nursing relates to caring and is "the relationship between charity and right action—between love as compassion and response to suffering and need, and justice or fairness [right action] in terms of doing what ought to be done within [the dynamics of] culture or society" (Ray, 1989a, p. 19). The ethical demand of transcultural caring ethics is authenticity, humility, and sacrifice in the care and responsibility of and for the other. By knowledgeable caring presence and caring competency (i.e., awareness, knowledge, and understanding) of the other's holistic needs (i.e., body, mind, and spirit), the transcultural caring nurse evokes, mediates, directs, and facilitates with the patient and family, and other professionals, reasoned moral choice (Ray, 1994a, 1994b) toward transcultural understanding and self-organization or transformation to improved health, healing, or a peaceful death.

THE IDEA OF THE GOOD

The idea of the "good" is historical and traditional. The good is considered both an infinite good, the invisible other, an I-Thou relationship that exists in individual conscience, and a societal good that expresses the choices made to protect human dignity within the moral community (Turkel & Ray, 2009). Thus, the good is cultural, religious, and oriented to rules or ways of life. In religiously grounded ethics, God or a higher power, or the Buddha, is considered the source of all good. God or a higher power represents the ultimate good, the Creator, the invisible other, the One who loves. According to religiously grounded ethical decrees, "the good demands the whole, not only the whole of man's [women are implied in this quote] outlook but his whole work, the whole man, together with the fellow-men who are given to him" (Bonhoeffer, 1949, p. 193).

Nonreligious ethical decrees also call for a holistic outlook and call forth charity and right action (Wielenberg, 2005). The holistic, the indivisible whole, relates to the whole of creation as good where a human being not only exists as an individual (i.e., body, mind, and spirit) but also as a member of a community of people who all belong and are all situated in the universe (Bonhoeffer, 1949; Capra, Steindl-Rast with Matus, 1991). Bonhoeffer (1949) stated that we inquire about good, "not at all by abstracting from life, but by looking deeply into life" (p. 214). Looking deeply into life to seek the good also illuminates the constructs of meaning, purpose, truth, and beauty (Gadamer, 1986). Frankl (1963) reminded us in his book on *Man's Search for Meaning* that the human spirit can rise above degeneracy and dehumanization, a horror that he experienced in a concentration camp during World War II. By being able to contemplate the love of his wife when they were separated by the Nazis, Frankl had a belief in human goodness, a belief in the meaning and purpose of life. He understood that love is the ultimate and highest goal to which man can aspire. Understanding that the salvation of man is through love and in love and that there is a spiritual energy that generates order and wholeness despite the immorality that he endured in the concentration camp, Frankl recognized that he could "send light into the darkness." He believed that love was the meaning, purpose, truth, and beauty of life; in essence, authentic love is what is beautiful, and therefore it is the good (Kadinsky, 1977).

The Evolution of the Idea of the Good

Complex societies and institutions, including the institution of the family, are the major centers where organized patterns and rules of behavior are established for the evolution of a good society. Societal ethics encompasses matters of human rights and justice, what is fair in collective society. At the same time, to be a good society or to have good institutions, the society or institution must be led by good people who are connected by a desire to serve the good of humankind (Bellah, Madsen, Sullivan, Swidler, & Tipton, 1991; Wielenberg, 2005). The fact that we belong to communities and exist within webs of relationships and social systems makes apparently straightforward rules of ethics more complex. Constant social changes challenge ethical rules and rules of law of the past. Ethics involves conscience, a discovery of who we are as individuals and what our responsibility is to other individuals, society, and to the universe as a whole. "Conscience comes from a depth which lies beyond a man's own will and his own reason and it makes itself heard as the call of human existence to unity with itself" (Bonhoeffer, 1949, p. 242). Conscience has an authority itself and judges actions—affecting the good, purpose, truth, and beauty—based on the risk they pose to inner peace and unity within. In a spiritually oriented conscience, unity with the self is not just egoism (the authority of self-centeredness) but is unity with God or a higher power illuminating the law of love of God and neighbor. In this sense, responsibility for the other is not only bound by principles that have been advanced to sustain a social order, but also, to God or a higher power who "sees" the heart and who has ordained a set of commandments, especially the commandment of love (Bonhoeffer, 1949). (This idea will be taken up again in Chapter 5: Universal Sources.)

An Example of the Good in Nursing

The good in and of nursing is holistic, relational, and caring. It represents what Bonhoeffer (1949) claimed that the good demands: the whole, not only the whole of a person's attitude but whole work, the whole person, together with other persons who are given to him or her in a period of time or situation. *This notion of the "good" is represented in the following story of an Army nurse, Lauren, caring for a soldier during the Iraq war.*

A combat casualty patient wounded by a roadside bomb less than 30 minutes earlier has just arrived in the field hospital situated in the Green Zone in Baghdad. A 21-year-old soldier, Matthew, is crying out, moaning with pain. His eyes speak of unspeakable suffering, sorrow, confusion, and terror. His left leg has been blown off by an improvised explosive device (IED) and his right leg is lifeless; his right temporal region is caved in and is still bleeding after the medics tried to stop the hemorrhaging at the battle scene. Lauren, morally conflicted but never hardened by what she has experienced in the combat zone, speaks to him softly, telling him that they will call his wife; she touches his chest gently and soothes his face as best she can, while giving him a morphine injection and then trying to get the IV blood hanging. Lauren cries while wiping Matthew's tears away. Matthew's eyes tell her that he trusts her and her colleagues who are setting up for surgically stabilizing the area of the left leg that was blown off by the IED and the possibility of an emergency amputation of his right leg, and stabilization of the head wound. She reassures Matthew that everyone in the room is there for him, helping him, working for him, and praying for him (knowing that they probably cannot save what remains of his one leg). The U.S. Air Force C17 flight crew is on their way to air evacuate him to Germany for further orthopedic and neurologic surgery, a family reunion, and occasions for healing of the body, mind, and spirit.

❖ *Nursing Reflection*

Lauren cares for the whole person within a nursing situation. She gives her whole self, her whole attitude in the wholeness of the work of caring. Although sad, Lauren recognizes that in war, there is both good and evil. She is heartened that Matthew will be going home soon. Her sense of love and caring in the midst of tragedy and loss awakened souls to the fragility of life and the life-giving nature of the meaning of the "good" in nursing.

THE IDEA OF EVIL

Along with the notion of the good, the presence of evil has been identified. Evil is the opposite of good or maleficence; it as an unwillingness to choose correctly or rightly and creates a crisis of conscience (inner peace and unity) and possible devastating effects or outcomes. Evil is considered the dark side of the call of conscience to do good, or the dark side of the self or what the psychiatrist, Jung called the shadow side (Sanford, 1988). The philosopher, Badiou (2001) claimed that evil is dishonesty or fatigue that besets devotion to a truth or selfless devotion to a cause. Evil as a perversion of a truth can take three forms: (1) betrayal, rejection of a truth, (2) delusion, confusion by mere pretense but assuming authenticity, and (3) overpowerment, imposing total power of a truth, the absolute commitment to one's *own* believed truth. Evil thus is a perversion of truth or the good as humans relate together. As ever-present in human lives, evil is a constant threat because of its power to possess and destroy the human soul, or overshadow human beings by disengagement with or causing harm to others. Conflict within the self or the consequence of the dark side of the soul contributes to suffering in the world (Sanford, 1988). Evil resides in various forms of ethical tension as moral distress or chaos, moral blurring, and moral blindness (Gadow, 1980, 1988, 1989). As an ever-present conflict, evil not only is centered in the self but also—as human beings interrelate, cultures evolve, and globalization increases—is centered in groups and sociopolitical environments that have a major effect on the lives of other human beings and on societies. Thus communities of conflict often overshadow communities of caring. Conflict itself has its roots in racial, ethnic, and gender identities, including sociopolitical and economic differences; class struggles; and different religious beliefs or interpretations of beliefs, virtual relationships, and general personal opinions or prejudices about people and things in everyday life (Appleton, 2005; Boulding, 1988; Chinn, 2013).

The Evolution of the Idea of Evil

Throughout history, increasing integration of different culture groups into national societies and now transnational or global societies grew out of the perceived need to take advantage of certain economic, technological, strategic, and military opportunities (Huntington, 1973). Historically, enculturation (cultural adaptation) emerged from war or oppression in many nation-states but at the same time, because of commands to follow a particular societal line of thinking, the results of oppression may still be felt in many nations or regions of the world. Buried under years of transgenerational fear, misunderstanding, and hostility, divisions among people continue bringing forth further conflict, thoughts of war, and even the eruption of war itself. Major conflicts leading to wars, crime, abandonment, or even widespread disease are considered consequences of evil or the shadow side of the good. Unfortunately, this type of evil too can be done in the name of good—often through miscast notions of religion (Boulding, 1988; Dalai Lama, 1999). Events in the Darfur region of the Sudan, Nigeria, and Iraq (for example, terrorism, ethnic hatred, and ethnic and religious cleansing) show signs of the miscast notions of religion. These events reveal the "shadow side" of those exerting misguided power and authority over others. Consequently, specific tribal groups who represent a different religion became targets for war fighting and are driven from their homes, displaced, raped, left to starve, or killed.

From an ethical point of view, rather than following rules of conduct and law based upon human rights, freedom, acceptance, and tolerance for others to cocreate a good society, bad leaders have turned what could be a good into an evil. Globalization, changes in world economic trade treaties, migration, and increased attention given to cultural differences and cultural identities offer *new* opportunities for studying and understanding the nature of conflict or protracted conflict whether it is historical, ethnic, personal, religious, political, or economic (Appleton, 2005). Social and political change, albeit fragile, in Northern Ireland provides an example of how protracted religious conflict can be lawfully and ethically reconciled after years of hostility. Ethical theories and transcultural ethical caring knowledge help in the effort to understand.

The Idea of Maleficence in Nursing

Nurses frequently are challenged ethically in practice (Benner, Tanner, & Chesla, 2009; Burkhardt & Nathaniel, 2008, 2013; Gadow, 1988a, 1988b; Ray, 1994b). Moral confusion, moral blurring, moral blindness (Gadow, 1989), and even evil can result. The legal consequence of nursing practice is closely aligned with the moral consequence because of the social contract (professional trust and licensure) that nurses have with the public. Ethically, nurses often present a picture of agonizing vulnerability and

moral distress (pain and suffering), and many "silently" cry for help as do their patients as moral crises ensue (Gadow, 1988; Ray, 1998, 2007; Turkel & Ray, 2004, 2009). This picture is becoming more evident in hospitals and in community health centers every day. In the United States, for example, the health-care system is strained, bringing to light ethical dilemmas related to economics or the cost of a technological health-care delivery system, access to care, increased morbidity, changing illness patterns of patients, the nurse shortage, nurse staffing, and patient safety and quality of care (Aiken, Clarke, Sloane, Sochalski, & Silber, 2002; Clarke, Rockett, Sloane, & Aiken, 2002; Lynn & Redman, 2005; Sherwood & Drenkard, 2007). Ethical issues that were never reported in the past, such as what is referred to as horizontal violence or bullying to members of one's own profession (Longo, 2007) and drug addiction and impairment of nurses (Dittman, 2007) are becoming more apparent. Additionally, the increased use (and potential abuse) of technology, and the overwhelming suffering and health needs of vulnerable people from diverse cultures and socioeconomic groups have affected the moral voice of nursing (Bailey & Elliott, 2014; Beidler, 2005; Leininger, 1991; Leininger & McFarland, 2006; McFarland & Wehbe-Alamah, 2015; Ray, 1998, 2007, 2010a, 2010c; Ray & Turkel, 2014; Ray, Turkel, & Marino, 2002; Turkel & Ray, 2004, 2009; Wu & Ray [in press]). Often, nursing, medical, and administrative professionals overlook the cries of nurses and patients. As a consequence, moral distress (pain and suffering), moral blurring (confusion and disillusionment), or moral blindness (ignoring one's individual conscience or institutional obligation to act ethically and legally) looms. The loss of insight into the meaning of professional caring and compassion, and its aspiration and responsibilities to be fair to others with right action has resulted in many decisions that are considered ethically questionable, wrong, or evil (Gadow, 1988, 1989; Ray, 1998, 2007). This moral quandary calls for increased knowledge and skill related to the meaning of good and evil.

Examples of Maleficence, Neglect, or Malpractice in Nursing Using Badiou's Outline of Evil

1. **Betrayal, rejection of a truth**
   Example 1: A nurse in a busy Emergency Department lets a patient or patients wait for hours for care with little communication, and then when she finally interacts with

the patient(s), she provides very little care. This nurse claims to be devoted to caring for others.

❖ *Nursing Reflection*

In this example, reflect upon the morality of causing harm and suffering by noncaring and moral blindness (*negligence*).

Example 2: A nurse does not wash her hands with soap or an alcohol sanitizer. She drops and contaminates intravenous tubing and then inserts the tubing into the patient's intravenous bag or vein.

❖ *Nursing Reflection*

In this example, reflect upon the morality of potentially harming patients, inflicting suffering, and potentially causing infection or even death by poor aseptic practices (*malpractice*).

2. **Assuming authenticity but deluding oneself by merely pretending**
Example 1: A nurse working in the Emergency Department shows preference for and provides a higher level of care for wealthier or higher socioeconomic class patients and ignores poverty-stricken or ethnically different or vulnerable patients. This nurse claims to care equitably for patients.

❖ *Nursing Reflection*

In this example, reflect upon the morality of the effect of ignoring the needs of one group of patients in favor of another (*class care and malpractice*).

Example 2: A nurse steals a patient's narcotic pain medication to feed her own addiction and replaces the pain medication with normal saline, gives the altered pain medication to the patient, and charts it as the right drug and correct dose. She then continues caring for that patient.

❖ *Nursing Reflection*

In this example, reflect on the morality of deliberately lying to and deceiving a patient, the tension between an impaired nurse who is legally licensed to practice nursing (*the culture of impairment and agonizing vulnerability of nurses committing malpractice*).

3. **Overpowerment, imposing total power of *a* truth**
Example 1: A nurse administrator who knows that he should be supporting staff nurses, justifies to the chief executive and operational officers that because of higher stress levels inherent in their jobs, *only* physician-economic desires should be recognized and should take precedence over staff nurse and patient care needs.

❖ *Nursing Reflection*

In this example, reflect upon the morality of intentionally hurting and deceiving one's own colleagues for personal gain (horizontal [nurse-nurse] *violence*).

In these examples, the nurses chose to act unethically and chose to harm the patient or, on the part of the nurse administrator, nurses. It is not just the nursing situation that is the issue, but also, the ethical *choice* is the key to understanding whether or not an event is ethical or unethical (MacIntyre, 1996, p. 65). The concern in ethics or moral behavior is the process of recognizing, witnessing, and judging (Ratzinger, 2007). In the process of choice making, there is a polarity on the axis between rightness and wrongness on which conduct lies and the inherent attraction of one pole and aversion of the other (Saint Thomas Aquinas, in Haldane, 1993, p. 135). It is both the *intentionality within*, the compassion and fairness in our approach to the patient, family, nurse, or community, and *what we choose* that provides the grounds for doing good or evil or harm in nursing events or situations. As patient safety issues mount in the contemporary health-care system (Aiken et al, 2002; Clarke et al, 2002; Cronenwett et al, 2007; Page, 2004; Ray & Turkel, 2014; Turkel & Ray, 2004, 2009), evaluation of the moral tone of professionals (i.e., nurses, nurse and non-nurse administrators, allied health personnel, and physicians) and organizational policies, and the meaning of compassionate *and* reasoned choice as primary elements of ethical conscience and action will require more reflection, increased education, dialogue, and understanding.

The Search for Understanding Through Transcultural Ethics and Transcultural Ethical Caring

How do we embrace transcultural ethics in our society and in health care? The core of transcultural ethics assumes that all discourse and interaction is transcultural because of the strengths of and differences in values, beliefs, and attitudes of individuals and groups within local and global societies. Because of the diversity in culture within and outside of communities and nations, and in health care, transcultural ethics involves questions related to how people ought to live with others who share the same lifeworld yet may hold different views of that lifeworld in what is meaningful and important (Ray, 1994a, 2001, 2010a, 2010b, 2010c). Transcultural ethics, transcultural caring, and transcultural ethical caring share the same fundamental characteristics: respect for all persons and a sense of compassion, justice, and clinical and cultural wisdom (Ray, 1994a, b; Benner, Tanner, & Chesla, 2009). To reiterate, transcultural caring is defined as:

> the relationship between charity and right action—between love as compassion and response to suffering and need, and justice or fairness in terms of doing what ought to be done within [the dynamics of] a culture or society. (Ray, 1989a, p. 19)

Compassion is not only feeling for the other but is a way of being and knowing. Compassion is personal and mutual. It is "becoming the other" through openness, dialogue, and understanding of suffering and need (Ray, 1992). Justice as fairness is similar to the way in which John Rawls examined justice in his theory. As the moral basis of society, fairness is where society has "the obligation to structure itself in such a way that there are equal liberties and opportunities to social goods" (Ray, 1989a, p. 19). Transcultural caring overall is the process of valuing in what could be better in nursing, health care, and world society or culture. It is a process of

human activity to facilitate in society a sense of a "just mutuality" (i.e., social justice facilitated through individual and collective ethical action) to build a better culture where one is, and to help build the global civic culture (Ray, 1989a, p. 19; Ray & Turkel, 2014). The global civic culture demands an ethical foundation because each of us is responsible for the other. As the ethicist, Logstrup (1997) expressed, "we hold the other's life in our hands!" (Watson, 2005).

Culture, made up of beliefs, attitudes, values, principles, codes, standards, and rules of behavior, varies within a given cultural community. Every individual experiences life differently and conscience forms because of knowledge—independent of experience, and dependent on experience. Increased globalization and communication mandates the need to incorporate a deeper understanding of ethics as transcultural ethics (Floridi, 2014; Ray, 2010a, 2010b, 2010c). Boulding (1988) remarked that the building of the global civic culture could only be achieved by understanding the historical diversity of values in culture but, at the same time, understanding the things that have united cultures. An example of what unites diverse cultures within democratic societies is freedom, a fundamental principle that must exist and be guaranteed by institutions to give voice to what people really want and ought to want to sustain a good society (Bellah et al, 1991; Habermas, 1986). People of diverse religions claim that love is the fundamental virtue that unites, and is the ultimate purpose of all true knowledge. Both are true. In the process of evolution in building the global civic culture, questions about what will happen to cultural differentiation arise. Can different cultures retain cultural identity and differentiation within a common core of community?

Modernity has created unique issues in cultural identity. On the one hand, people desire to interrelate with others, which will influence change in ideas and traditions. On the other hand, people continue to desire to retain their past ways of thinking and acting. The electronic media have a powerful effect on traditional lifeways in different cultures, especially in how the youth are influenced through popular culture (Davis & Dickinson, 2004; Ingraham, 2007; Yapple & Korzenny, 1989). Thus, the electronic media have worldwide significance (Floridi, 2014). Views of modern culture vary—some supportive, others critical. Media promotes increased communication and understanding on the one hand, and wrong information and exploitation on the other. White (1996) suggests in his communication ethics that there should be a commitment to "developing a language in the public media wherein moral issues and moral claims of different people" can be presented, and where there is "respect for the diversity of interpretation within subcultures" (White, 1996, pp. 216–217).

The mosaic of multiculturalism in many parts of the world reflects the notion of dynamic complexity, demonstrating that overall culture can be defined more as a choice. Although choice plays a major role in what is accepted or rejected from a cultural point of view, cultural identity, and its changing definitions (which are discussed in Chapter 4), remains critical as to how one views the self and one's cultural heritage and one's relationships. How, when, and to what extent do history and tradition remain a part of diverse peoples as they move about the world? History in the United States reveals that most immigrants adapted to the American culture based upon the beliefs in the unique Constitution and Amendments, rights, and freedoms and the rule of law. More recently, many immigrants, although drawn to the United States for various reasons, desire to retain their own cultural and linguistic traditions rather than acculturate into the historic culture (Tuan, 1998). For example, in south Florida, many Cuban Americans and people from other Latin American cultures chose to speak only Spanish. In other areas of North America, many culture groups isolate themselves in enclaves where close relationships protect them from a culture that may be perceived as harmful. The challenge is cocreating transcultural ethics in a global civic culture that appreciates, honors, and understands that ethical and moral values, norms, codes, principles, sanctions, rights, responsibilities, and obligations are *"culturally constituted and expressed* within meaningful living contexts" (Leininger, 1990, p. 64). Therefore, transcultural ethics always must address the living context, the universality, and diversity within interrelating cultures (Leininger, 1991, 1995; Leininger & McFarland, 2006 Martin & Ray [in press]; McFarland & Wehbe-Alamah, 2015).

UNIVERSALISM AND RELATIVISM IN TRANSCULTURAL ETHICS

Is it possible to create a common standard of ethics and human rights to satisfy all cultures globally? The fundamental idea behind human rights is that because of the kind of beings we are, that is human beings, we are entitled to be treated in certain ways (Ray, 2010a, 2010c). Most would agree with the basic principle of respect for and protection of human dignity (and cultural value differences are foundational to human rights). Philosophers of ethics refer to these notions as *principle-based universalism* and *cultural relativism*. Ethical universalism deals with principles; there are some moral rules that *all* cultures and societies have in common, because those rules are necessary for a society to exist (Rachels, 2003, pp. 16–26). For example, caring is a universal principle because caring is necessary for survival. Nevertheless, caring is expressed differently in diverse cultures (cultural and ethical relativism). For cultural understanding in nursing, Leininger addressed the issue of cultural universalism and diversity in her theory of nursing (Leininger, 1978, 1991; Leininger, & McFarland, 2006; McFarland & Wehbe-Alamah, 2015). Universalism highlights what is common in culture and diversity deals with what is culturally specific. Diversity of expression of caring is considered culturally relative from an ethical perspective and deals with the fact that different cultures have different moral codes. Some moral codes are based upon social conventions, such as types of dress, rather than on reasoned standards. Because of the integral cultural component to human rights, basic human rights should change now that our universe is globally pluralistic. The question becomes, in light of all of the global differences, exactly how should human rights change? Laws are enacted to prevent or diminish immorality or a sense of wrongdoing in a society. A rule of law is based upon rules that flow from the human heart and the collective will to act justly (*Nuremberg*, PBS TV Program, September 23, 2007). For example, laws against murder or terror facilitate social order in a society and provide a sense of security for members of a society. In a culturally diverse world, are laws against murder or terror universal? Is there a universal notion that all human beings can experience security, and can rights to security protect all cultures? Whose beliefs prevail? Does each culture have to tolerate the others' individual and social practices? In other words, are ethical universalism and ethical relativism reconcilable?

Reconciliation is possible. What should change for all cultures is finding a way to acknowledge cultural differences through a process of transcultural caring (i.e., compassion and fairness) that highlights increased awareness, sensitivity, insight, and communication—listening, dialoguing, and seeking understanding for the continuous development of respect, identity, and self-organization of individuals, groups, communities, and societies. Thus, transcultural caring attempts to reconcile ethical universalism and cultural relativism because transcultural caring embraces universality in principles, like respect for persons and protection of human dignity, while addressing tolerance tempered with moral reason. The ethicist, Rachels (2003) reminds us that tolerance is a virtue, "[b]ut there is nothing in the nature of tolerance that requires you to say that all beliefs, all religions, and all social practices are equally admirable. . . . If you did not think that some were better than others, there would be nothing for you to tolerate" (p. 29).

To criticize a cultural practice is not to condemn a whole culture; it means that cultures are a mixture of good and bad practices (e.g., democracy, human rights, and the rule of law along with human trafficking, child pornography, and ethnic cleansing).

The ongoing fragility of crosscultural understanding is well illustrated by the dominant global discourses of political conflict of the present time which once again use cultural difference—whether it be focused on ethnicity or on religion—as a convenient way of demonizing others and justifying war, terrorism and other forms of political violence.
(Reuter, 2005, p. 8)

Overall, the key is transcultural ethical caring: compassion, and understanding of and focus on what unites instead of what separates. Thus, transcultural ethical caring entails working with, not independently of, different culture groups to create and transform human rights and ethical understanding.

Transcultural Caring Ethics in Nursing

Transcultural caring incorporates love as compassion, and justice and fairness toward right action within the dynamics of complex, dynamic cultures (Ray, 1989a, 1999). Gadow (1980) claimed that, through caring for the other, the nurse has the ethical responsibility to help the patient and family members understand the meaning of his or her need, suffering, illness, or difficulty. Nurses do address problems but as the practice of nursing advances within the complexities of the technological and socioeconomic age of health care, the patient

❖ *Nursing Reflection*

Transcultural ethics illuminates the following:

* Respect the dignity of all people.
* Promote the good of all people.
* Honor all people through compassion and justice.
* Value language differences.
* Acknowledge complexity of religious, spiritual, and humanistic values.
* Seek understanding of dynamic relationships related to ethnohistorical evolution of people in world cultures.
* Seek understanding of the transmission of diverse values (purposes of existence) and learned behaviors and rules of law in cultures.
* Promote communitarianism (listening to and learning from the other; encouraging all people to have a voice at the "table").
* Negotiate and facilitate the alleviation of conflict and strife in culture.
* Develop covenants and rules of law, human rights, and cultural rights that promote rights to liberty and equality regardless of race, color, sex, language, religion, national or social origins, property, and birth status. (Excerpted in part from The United Nations Universal Declaration of Human Rights, 1948; and the Transcultural Nursing Society Position Statement on Human Rights, 2008).
* Protect the rights of nature (the environment).
* Promote individual and public health and well-being of all people.

and others most dear to them must be more involved in the decisions that affect his or her life. Nurses, patients, and family members are being called upon to focus on *deep values* within a continually changing cultural context. The context is continually shaped and transformed by the values and moral interactions of the nurse-patient relationship (Ray, 1994b, 2010a, 2010b, 2010c). To put it more simply, the nurse must be aware of the *meaning* underlying the relationship and the interaction. Nurses must be advocates—act on behalf of patients—especially if the patient is from a different culture. When nurses are called upon to care for and communicate with a patient, they are in fact being called to act as moral agents for the patient

(Sumner, 2008). As *moral agents*, caring (Roach, 2002) involves:

- Compassion (feeling for patients and advocating on their behalf)
- Commitment (keeping promises to patients)
- Conscience (facilitating morally "right" choices)
- Confidence (engaging intraprofessional and interprofessional integrity)
- Competence (possessing nursing knowledge and skill)
- Comportment (acting responsibly, humanely, and ethically in communicative interaction)

Nurses may take this moral agency of caring for granted in their everyday professional actions, but as moral agents, nurses ultimately have the power to facilitate choices of patients, family members, and physicians for health, healing, well-being, or a peaceful death.

Overall, transcultural caring ethics involves trust. Being a trusted person by acting trustworthily in all transactions opens the heart and mind more deeply to the spiritual-ethical values, in essence to living compassionately. Then ". . . everything has is reasons, its place, importance, and relevance in this divine work" (De Caussade, 1983, p. 101). Thus, **transcultural ethical caring actions** incorporate the following:

1. Cocreating trust.
2. Living compassionately (relational caring).
3. Acting humbly.
4. Respecting people of diverse religious and spiritual beliefs.
5. Preserving lifeworld values of the good, purpose, meaning, truth, and beauty.
6. Communicating wisely (See the Transcultural Communicative Spiritual-Ethical CARING Tool as an example in Chapters 2 and 6).
7. Refining culturally diverse attitudes through dialogue and communicative action.
8. Thinking critically by an informed conscience and attitude.
9. Encouraging creativity and potentialities.
10. Acting justly through a mutual fairness.
11. Refining laws (social justice and human rights through collective ethical action).
12. Accepting uncertainty (transcultural dynamics).
13. Renewing education with knowledge of caring and moral principles.
14. Protecting and restoring the environment (human-environment well-being).
15. Facilitating reasoned choice (understanding the universality of principles and diversity of cultural relativism).
16. Transforming the public sphere (openness and dialogue within organizations and local, regional, national, and global communities).

TRANSCULTURAL ETHICAL CARING ACTION IN THE AGE OF COMPLEXITY

The age of complexity manifests a shift in consciousness. "As a global community, we are in the middle of a transition from the industrial to the information age, and this transformation is reflected and reflected in everything around us" (Bar-Yam, 2004, p. 13). Everything is interconnected. We are becoming aware of problems of the human condition—over- or underdevelopment, abuse of the environment, poverty, cultural illness, unequal health-care distribution leading to health-care disparities, and so forth. As health care and the organizational and global contexts become more complex, health-care professionals need to examine what values should endure and should reflect a way to solve complex problems in a complex world (Bar-Yam, 2004; Majumder, 2005). There is a call from people of the world to deepen an understanding of compassion and become more compassionately involved in and responsible for each other's lives. Nursing is slowly responding to the call by initiating transcultural nursing and transcultural ethical caring action in practice. However, cocreating trust and living compassionately in the world of health care and in nursing practice will take much education. The "living out" of the call of compassion is where the difficulty lies. Love and compassion require creativity and originality. Morris (in Kurzweil, 2005) stated, "[t]he meaning of life is creative love. Not love as an inner feeling, as a private sentimental emotion, but love as a dynamic power moving out into the world and doing something original" (p. 485).

We know what original and creative ideas mean to science in developing new understanding about the universe, but what do they mean to advancing transcultural human caring relationships in nursing? The moral tone that exists challenges us to reflect upon how we shape and are shaped by the interactions of our moral societal and professional communities, the choices that we make or cocreate, and the various cultural (professional and ethnic) meanings associated with the nature of what it means to be human and humane in today's complex clinical environments. There is something tremendous at stake in all that we do in professional practice, for example, in the ethics of "high tech and high touch," the illness and health patterns of culturally diverse people, and the moral questioning of the economic value of health care. We are all transcultural beings, struggling with competing voices from within, differences in values from without, and commonalities of desiring to live in moral communities. The heritage of nursing is concern about others, and the health, and well-being of others in times of vulnerability, suffering, and need. Transcultural ethical caring encompasses not only compassion, the biomedical principles of beneficence, nonmaleficence, and autonomy, but also justice of what meanings prevail in the sociocultural context—the technological, the political, the economic, and legal dimensions of institutional and societal systems (Coffman, 2006; Ray, 1989b, 2001, 2006, 2010c).

In health-care institutions, ethics in general is a challenge. "Since the time of Hippocrates, it has been a fundamental ethical tenet of the medical profession (at least in the West) that the physician [or nurse] is not to harm his or her patient" (Buchanan, 1996, p. 29). Doing no harm takes priority in *most* nursing and health-care situations. However, nurses care for patients and families amid severe ethical challenges. Nursing care is not just associated with the nurse-patient relationship but also, the economic, technological, and political domains. Organizations are corporate. Even the legal aspects of health care are having a bigger effect in quality of care, patient safety, malpractice, and lawsuits. More and more, health care and even health itself is being defined from a societal level. Health is not simply the consequence of a physical, mental, or spiritual state of being. Health also is associated with the social organization of health and illness in a society, the health-care system (Coffman, 2006, 2014). The human condition has been elevated to the sociocultural domain. It is no longer an individualistic endeavor (Arendt (1958/1998; Ray, 2010c). Multiple paradoxes and subsequent possibilities for disintegration or positive transformation are emerging in human society and subsequently in the health-care system. In health care, administrators and nurses have not spent enough time examining different value domains, especially how nursing is affected by the movement from primarily an individualistic, patient-centered, or even a care-based health-care system to a personal-mutual or communal transcultural health-care system that incorporates not only the humanistic dimension but all the dimensions of the sociocultural context, the political, legal, technological, and economic (Ray & Turkel, 2014, 2015). Because of the complexity of the modern world, nursing practice in hospitals reveals a "suffering moral community," primarily because of the affect of challenging ethical issues with corporate politics, economics, and the issues of the use and abuse of information technology and lifesaving technologies (Ray, 1998, 2007; Turkel & Ray, 2004, 2009). These organizational cultural changes (Ray, Turkel, & Marino, 2002; Ray & Turkel, 2014), and other issues, such as horizontal violence (Longo & Sherman, 2007), chemical dependency in the workplace (Dittman, 2007), and patient safety challenges (Cronenwett et al, 2007), have negatively affected nursing. Nurses and other health-care professionals are involved in situations where technology and economic decisions trump decisions that are considered humanistic and ethical. Autonomous decisions that patients and family members make may be counter to a nurse's or physician's own values or ethical and cultural learning. Nurses are often in conflict with physician care decisions. The conflict frequently arises at the end of life where technology continues to make ethical decisions more complex. Sometimes, moral blurring or moral blindness to complex clinical situations makes the morally "right" decision difficult to discern, such as the choice between palliative care and the continuation of life using life-supportive technologies (Ray, 1998). Ethical actions among members of the moral community become more and more important. In such situations, nurses always must demonstrate compassion and caring for patients, despite their own moral confusion. Rethinking professional ethics to determine what is the morally "right" approach depends not only upon using compassion, and right reason with ethical principles, such as beneficence and autonomy, but also incorporating ways the nurse as a transcultural ethicist is a "culture broker," mediating between the patient and family, physician, and the organizational system to try to enact cultural justice or fairness in choice making (Leininger & McFarland, 2006; Ray, 1989a, 1998, 2007, 2010a, 2010b, 2010c). The dynamics of the lived cultural context of moral interaction of the patient, family or significant others, nurses, and physicians continues to call forth virtues of trust, respect, fidelity, and integrity, the foundation of transcultural communicative caring. Truth comes to life within a committed and educated moral community (Ray & Turkel, 2014; Turkel & Ray, 2009).

RETHINKING PROFESSIONAL NURSING ETHICS AS TRANSCULTURAL ETHICAL CARING

Nursing education requires specific attention to the ethics and meaning of quality caring practice or best practices. Nursing must seek excellence in caring by studying theories and principles of ethics and seeking understanding of cultural values, beliefs, and values to show respect for all people of the world. The ethical principles of biomedical and social ethics—explored earlier in the chapter—are described in Codes of Ethics for Nurses (see codes of ethics from the American Nurses Association [2015]; The Patient Care Partnership [replacing the American Hospital Association's Patient's Bill of Rights, 2003]; Canadian Nurses Association [2008], International Council of Nurses [2006], cited in Burkhardt & Nathaniel, 2013).

Nursing reinforces the transcultural ethical caring actions by principles and the value of cultural specificity or relativism in the Code of Ethics for Nurses with Interpretative Statements (2001, 2015; www.nursingworld.org/codeofethics). The universal ethical principle is respect for human dignity, followed by the ethically relativistic notion of establishing a relationship with individual persons to provide nursing care regardless of lifestyle, race, gender, value system, or religion. Reconciliation through transcultural ethical caring is understood by the following code): "The nurse respects the worth, dignity, and rights of all human beings irrespective of the nature of the health problem. . . . . Nursing care aims to maximize the values that the patient has treasured in life and extends supportive care to the family and significant others . . ." (The Nature of Health Problems, 1:3. Code of Ethics for Nurses with Interpretive Statements, ANA, 2015, p. 7; new guidelines will be forthcoming at www.nursingworld.org/codeofethics). Moreover,

> *Nurses have four fundamental responsibilities: to promote health, to prevent illness, to restore health and to alleviate suffering. The need for nursing is universal. Inherent in nursing is respect for human rights, including cultural rights, the right to life and choice, to dignity and to be treated with respect. . . .*
> (The International Council of Nurses Code of Ethics for Nurses [in Burkhardt & Nathaniel, 2008, p. 537])

As nurses embrace education for quality and patient safety as well as how to use social media for nursing care locally and globally (Cronenwett et al, 2007; Ess, 2013), the interrelationship between transcultural caring ethics and evidence-based practice will become more apparent. "Best practices" will include more attention to cultural diversity, vulnerability, caring, and human and patient rights (Turkel, 2006a, 2006b). For example, the Patient Care Partnership, 2003, formerly the American Hospital Association's: A Patient's Bill of Rights, and the Transcultural Nursing Society Position Statement on Human Rights, (Miller et al, 2008) incorporate transcultural caring ethics. Thus, traditional ethical principles of beneficence, nonmaleficence, autonomy, fairness, and fidelity will be reinforced with transcultural ethical caring and human rights components. As a moral agent and codeterminant of health care with the patient and family members or significant others, nurses will be sensitive to the individual ethnic culture of the patient and the cultural context—the sociocultural environment from which the patient hails. Countries, communities, and health-care organizations also determine how health is interpreted by means of their political, economic, technological, and legal systems, and the macroculture.

TRANSCULTURAL CARING ETHICS: THE PRESENT AND THE FUTURE

Transcultural Nurses Participating in Ethics Committees

Ethics committees are formed to deal with difficult ethical problems in health-care organizations. By engaging a diverse group of professionals, including physicians, nurses, clergy, social workers, and lawyers in collective moral reasoning, patients and families can have reasonable confidence that complex health-care needs will be evaluated with care. At this stage in ethics committee development there is a need for more awareness of the cultural diversity of patients, and the organization as a cultural entity (including how technology, and electronic data sources are used) in today's health care in North America. As nurses take their positions as "transcultural ethicians" (transcultural ethical caring brokers) on ethics committees and in the rooms of patients, the breadth of caring ethics and transcultural caring ethics in particular will demonstrate the seriousness of the cochoice-making role of nurses and patients. As cochoice makers, patients' contributions to their own health care by using their own data-gathering techniques from the Internet or other sources will be honored to help them codecide with family/significant others and health-care professionals in health-care matters. "Morality is, first and foremost, a matter of consulting reason" (Rachels, 2003, p. 12). Moral thinking and moral conduct are a matter of weighing reason and being guided by them [moral thinking and conduct] (Rachels, 2003) and at the same time taking into consideration culture and human caring. Facilitating compassionate and reasoned choice in the age of complexity is the ultimate goal. Although the ethics of caring is taken for granted in most health-care situations, human experience with respect to the meaning of caring must be a significant part to the weighting of moral issues. Within this context, then, the new ethics of compassion, human patient rights, cultural rights, and cultural justice will become central to understanding morally right action in choice making (Ray, 2010a, 2010c; Ray & Turkel, 2014).

Transcultural Ethical Caring Challenges in Local, National, and Global Communities

In rethinking professional ethics, cultural rights and social and cultural justice need to be constantly interpreted and reinterpreted on personal, societal, or communal levels. Questions surface in relation to receiving and providing health care that overall affect patients, families, and health-care professionals. Ethical questions about whether or not health care is a right or a privilege arise in some societies. Socioeconomic issues prevail—who will pay for health care, what type of care can or will be made available, who will provide the care, who is justified to receive care, what resources are available to provide care, where care will be provided, and how much information legally and ethically can be transmitted electronically, for example, via the virtual world and robotics (Davidson, Ray, & Turkel, 2011). These questions raise all health-care transactions from the microculture or personal culture to the macrocultural level and thus demonstrate that *all* questions or concerns are ethical and transcultural. Although the need for health care is personal and moral transactions emerge between the person and physician or nurse (the microculture), every transaction also is at the macrocultural level. "[H]ealth [and health care] is intimately connected to the way people (including nurses) in a cultural group, an organizational culture, or a bureaucratic system construct reality and

give and find meaning" (Coffman, 2006, p. 125). For example, in Canadian health care, though interpersonal between a patient and nurse or patient and physician, there also is a social contract between the patient and the government; health care is a right for all citizens. Hence, the meaning of health must be understood within a broader cultural context—a microcultural context or the individual's beliefs and a health professional's care practices for the most part become coexistent with a macrosociocultural context. Thus, the meaning of health is associated with the social, ethical, political, economic, technological, and legal dimensions of a cultural or societal system and reinforces the need for understanding cultural meanings of health and, thus, transcultural caring ethics (Coffman, 2006; Ray, 1994a, 2005; Ray & Turkel, 2014, 2015).

Habermas (1986; Wolin, 2005), a proponent of discourse or what is referred to as communication ethics, believes that to be convincing, moral reasoning needs a broader public discourse that should possess the give and take of argumentation through communicative reasoning so that mutual understanding can result. "A communitarian communication ethic is much more attentive to the undercurrents of dissatisfaction and the sense of injustices among peripheral groups [vulnerable persons or ethnic minorities] . . . arising out of an awareness of identity and one's human dignity" (White, 1996, p. 215). Finding common ground through reasoning by collaborative argumentation is fundamental to how differences of opinion or conflicts of values are resolved or reconciled. It is the basis for transcultural understanding. Someone or some community of people have to take the risk to begin the process. As Habermas (in Wolin, 2005) emphasized, "The give and take of argumentation, as a learning process, is indispensable. Through communicative moral reasoning, we strive for mutual understanding and learn to assume the standpoint of the other [empathy and compassion]" (p. B16). Habermas's views give rise to transcultural ethical caring as a dominant disciplinary focus for the future of sociopolitical interaction in health-care organizations and global communities.

Communicative ethical-spiritual caring action becomes even more complex as multicultural societies interact. Different cultures and different languages interface with different points of view. Can moral reasoning lead to agreement within complex communicative interaction, especially now with more and more electronic communication? Often, heated emotion arises and overpowers reason. Who will mediate ethically? Who are the moral agents? Today, when human-to-human interaction is considered too complex or fails, many situations are reconciled by the law to exact fairness or justice. There is a call for the growth and development of the meaning of transcultural ethical communication at micro and macro levels where the voice of the people can be heard and all information can be defended, and negotiated by the moral voices of professionals and even politicians. For example, the Transcultural Nursing Society Position Statement on Human Rights (Miller et al, 2008) promotes health care, human rights, and cultural rights. Transcultural nurses are professionally focused on the universality of caring, and preserving and maintaining individual and collective human rights of people to advance knowledge of cultural illness and health, cultural freedoms, and cultural justice. The *Journal of Transcultural Nursing, Journal of Nursing Scholarship, International Journal of Human Caring, International Journal of Nursing Studies,* and others have committed themselves to improving the health of people in the world through communicating research and transcultural practices in publications. Thus, transcultural ethical caring is the challenge to the world community. The ethics of caring for the other calls forth new ways to understand conflict and to learn the art, science, and skill of reconciling and peacemaking (Appleton, 2005; Chinn, 2013). As health-care professionals committed to compassion, nurses are in a unique position to facilitate healing, reconciliation, and peace worldwide.

Summary

- Transcultural caring is both universal (common to all humanity) and relative (culturally specific) across cultures.
- Caring is necessary for human survival, which makes it universally necessary and acceptable.
- Transcultural caring is committed to holism (body, mind, and spirit), compassion, justice (fairness), truth in relationships, human rights, and cultural rights.
- Transcultural caring ethics illuminates respect for persons and preservation of and responsibility for human dignity.
- Transcultural caring incorporates cultural patterns in the care experience through the events, organizational environments, behaviors, signs, symbols, and the experience of transcultural communication and moral action.
- Transcultural caring ethics incorporates the codes of ethics for nurses nationally and internationally, including national and international human rights documents.
- Transcultural caring ethics illuminates that we share a common humanity, thus acknowledging universal principles of ethics while seeking understanding of diverse cultural mores.
- Transcultural caring ethics acknowledges that love (compassion and mercy) takes priority over a purely principle- or duty-based ethical response.
- Transcultural caring ethics illustrates that moral thinking and caring knowledge coincide with action and practice.
- Transcultural caring ethics illuminates respect for persons and preservation of and responsibility for human dignity.
- Transcultural caring ethics is creative and original, calling forth new ways to facilitate hearing, listening to, advocating for, and choice making in relation to how we ought to live with the members of communities who share the same lifeworld but hold different views of human virtues, ethical principles, cultural values, and religious beliefs (Martin & Ray [in press]; Ray, 1994a, 1994b).
- Transcultural caring ethics acknowledges the nurse as a moral 'agent who advocates and facilitates reasoned choices toward health, healing, well-being, or self-organization with the patient, family, other professionals, and members of communities (national and global).

Transcultural Caring Experiences

Ruth

Ruth is the head nurse of the emergency room (ER) in a hospital in Jerusalem, Israel. Ruth has received a call that a person named Mohammed Jahoudi will be coming to the ER by ambulance. It was confirmed by the military that the ambulance was arriving in a few minutes and that the patient will be accompanied by military police. The diagnosis is a bullet wound to the right temporal region. The military official did not reveal the seriousness of the trauma. From the moment Ruth received the telephone call and information, she felt conflicted. She knew that the patient was a Palestinian, wounded at an Israeli checkpoint near the West Bank. She also knew Palestinian people had been patients at the hospital in the past and were cared for by staff and medical and nursing students who were Jewish. *[The university schools of medicine and nursing student population include all faith communities, Jewish, Christian, and Islam, in the education process.]* Ruth was well aware of the peace negotiations over many years that have been taking place between the Jews and Palestinians.

Ruth recognized that she had to ask more questions to get prepared for the emergency patient. How critical was the patient? What type of scans would be necessary to determine the degree of the trauma? How should she talk with her staff about this situation? Would the patient be able to communicate? Could she get an interpreter on site? How would she notify a family member if she could? When should she notify the neurological team? Would the patient need a ventilator? The operating room and intensive care unit personnel may have to be alerted for possible future care.

Ruth "got herself together" and knew in her heart that she had to care for her patient and ask the right questions. She had to deal with her own conflict. After all, the patient was a human being and she knew that the universal code of nursing ethics is respect for persons. She thought, "What if my father had been in the same situation and was taken to a hospital or clinic in the West Bank?" She hoped that someone, especially a nurse, would care for him.

Questions for Transcultural Ethical Caring Analysis

You, as an ER nurse, are reflecting on Ruth's experience. Reflect upon and describe your feelings and thoughts in this transcultural ethical caring situation.

- How would you feel if you were Ruth? What is your initial reaction? Would you feel conflicted or morally confused?
- How do you view yourself as an ethical being, an ethical professional?
- What is the meaning of transcultural caring ethics in this nursing situation? Outline what transcultural ethical issues prevail.
- What neurological problems may be present with a gunshot wound or trauma to the brain?
- How would you lead a team of professionals in an ER with diverse values, beliefs, and attitudes to care for a culturally diverse patient with head trauma?
- What is the International Code of Ethics for Nurses? What is the Israeli Nursing Code of Ethics?

Further Reflective Questions

- What religious, political, and economic issues could prevail when caring for a patient from a region within the country where there may be differences of belief and attitudes?
- Could you relate any part of this story to a nursing situation in your hospital or clinic in terms of culturally diverse patients or the not so picture-perfect patient (see Turkel & Ray, 2009)?
- How do you think you would reconcile the issue of cultural difference yourself?
- What are the central tenets of the religions in Israel (Judaism, Christianity, and Muslim [Islam]) (see Chapter 5)?
- Are health-care professionals called to stricter ethical behavior than others? What human and cultural rights should be honored? What choices would you make?

Further Questions and Thoughts for Discussion
- Investigate what the transcultural phenomena are in Israel, the West Bank, and Gaza Strip according to history, tradition, politics (including the military), and religion by searching the literature or the Internet.
- Briefly describe the meaning of transcultural or religious conflict in this context. (Explore the literature or the Internet.)
- What potentially new political approaches to living peacefully in Jerusalem, Israel, and Palestine are being supported and negotiated? By whom?
- After reflecting on the issues outlined above, create a transcultural ethical caring narrative and model for continuing education in an ER.

Letitia

Letitia works in the intensive care unit (ICU) of a public hospital as a registered nurse. She is deeply rooted in her African American culture. Last year, she married her husband, Raul, a Latino man with culturally diverse roots in Puerto Rico. Just this evening, Letitia was thinking that they should go to Puerto Rico for their first anniversary.

In her professional role on the ICU, Letitia occasionally is asked to fill the role of a charge nurse on nights, 7 p.m. to 7 a.m. She has a little more than 2 years of experience with an associate's degree in nursing (ADN) and is taking a course for her bachelor of science in nursing (BSN) at the local university. The ICU is busy. It is the only inner city hospital that takes care of the needs of the city's vulnerable patients of a lower socioeconomic status and different minority groups. One evening Letitia was assigned to Mr. Stover, a 61-year-old patient on a ventilator with a diagnosis of multisystem failure from chronic alcoholism and other complications. Mr. Stover has no family and no religion noted on the chart. The nurse from the day shift reported that "he was failing fast." His temperature was up, his blood pressure was low, and his pulse barely palpable. He is on intravenous feedings with a number of medications added to enhance his cardiac and renal systems, and his blood pressure and respiratory failure. Letitia is scared. She has taken care of only a few dying patients before. She cannot believe that he could have no family or significant others to be with him. Also, Letitia is already busy with other critically ill patients. There are three other nurses on duty in the ICU. They have their own patients. The unit often is identified as lacking warmth and sensitive team relationships. After getting her assignment, the charge nurse notified Letitia that she would be getting an admission of a very ill 75-year-old patient with an abdominal infection after surgery, Mr. Rodriquez, who does not speak English very well. He is diagnosed with methicillin-resistant *Staphylococcus aureus* (MRSA). He is going to go into an isolation bed at the west end of the ICU with full universal precautions. Letitia is even more frightened now because Mr. Rodriquez is very ill with what the doctor thinks is a nosocomial infection. Letitia does not believe that Mr. Rodriquez should be in the ICU at all since the ICU should be a dedicated clean environment for critically ill patients. She is afraid of transferring any infection to Mr. Stover, to her husband at home, or to herself for that matter. Letitia does not know what to do. She has mixed feelings about the nursing situation. Letitia also thinks that perhaps she should have learned some Spanish from her husband. She would like to run away. She is getting to the "end of her rope," getting burned out, and thinking about maybe going to another hospital, another unit, or going to school full-time, this time perhaps in business—something else that would be better for her personal and professional well-being.

However, tonight she knows she cannot do that. Her patients need her compassionate caring. She does love to care for patients and help them as best as she can. She will now have to be there for Mr. Stover and talk softly with him, give him some kind of hope. She will be the only person he has at the end of his life. She wonders if she could get a chaplain to help her. She knows that maybe she will have to remove the ventilator if she can talk to the doctor to assess the quality of life of Mr. Stover and whether or not it is wise to keep him on a ventilator. At the same time, Letitia knows too that she must admit Mr. Rodriquez.

The charge nurse and hospital need her to fulfill her obligation as a staff nurse. Letitia knows there is a staffing crisis in the public hospital and so many more sick and disenfranchised patients are coming for care.

The hospital and the ICU in particular, are overloaded. Now, the hospital administration has decided to put infectious disease cases in the ICU. Letitia is confused but reflects quickly on her plight, says a prayer, and decides to get to work, first to see Mr. Stover and make sure he knows she is there for him.

Letitia will have to then mask, gown, and glove herself and see how she can get Mr. Rodriquez settled into his isolation room even though he cannot understand English very well. She knows that she must be very careful with aseptic technique so that she does not transfer bacteria to Mr. Stover, to herself, or to any other person on the unit. She has to be careful with laboratory personnel so that they maintain universal precautions. Letitia decides that she will have to bring many issues to the attention of her nurse manager, and the chief nursing officer as soon as possible.

Questions for Transcultural Ethical Caring Analysis

You as an ICU nurse are reflecting on Letitia's experience. Letitia is an African American nurse married to a Puerto Rican American. She is engaged in transcultural nursing and transcultural communicative ethical-spiritual caring. Reflect on how you feel after reading Letitia's story.

- What is your initial reaction to this nursing situation? What is the agonizing vulnerability of Letitia in this ethical situation? What does it mean to be morally confused, or morally conflicted or blurred, in clinical nursing situations? (See Gadow (1989); Ray (1998). Turkel & Ray, 2009)
- What are your thoughts about having to be a charge nurse and leaving it "all up to you?" What is a moral tone of the hospital? Should a patient with MRSA be placed in an ICU? What political and economic issues prevail in this experience?
- How would you communicate your thoughts from a transcultural ethical caring view, recognizing the cultural diversity of Letitia and her patients, and that the hospital is a small organizational culture?
- How would you care for Mr. Rodriquez from a transcultural caring/ethical caring perspective? Briefly describe the transcultural ethical conflicts that are presented, including issues of language differences.
- What are your thoughts and feelings about caring for a patient who is at the end of life, on a ventilator, and alone? Is the ICU a technological caring culture? How would you care for Mr. Stover at the end of life? Should Mr. Stover be transferred to a palliative care unit or its equivalent?

Further Questions for Reflection

- What are universal precautions? How do you think you would reconcile the transcultural ethical issues presented in a hospital? Reflect upon and describe your feelings about the culture of this hospital organization. What kind of issues are going on in this hospital, nursing management, and nursing situations? What ethical choices would you make with the hospital managers?
- How would you as a nurse manager evaluate HCAHPS (Hospital Consumer Assessment of Health Care Providers and Systems) Survey Scores? How would you use the National Database for Nursing Quality Indicators (NDNQI; United States quality data to improve nursing quality)? How would you as a nurse manager implement a unit and hospital department for patient (and nurse) safety and quality?
- How would you assess the "resilience" phenomenon of nurses and other professionals in terms of their health and safety? What is "compassion fatigue," and why does it occur?
- Should nursing administrators be called to stricter ethical behavior than others? Is there an issue of horizontal violence in this ethical situation?
- What human and nursing rights and patient rights may be violated in this nursing situation? (See Transcultural Nursing Society Position Statement on Human Rights, the Codes of Ethics for nurses, and information from the American Hospital Association and the Joint Commission.)
- What ethical choices would you make with your patients? Do you agree with Letitia?
- What do you think about a hospital that puts patients with infectious diseases in the ICU? Is this a common practice in the United States?
- What are the historical, traditional, political, and ethical challenges that face nursing in health-care systems? How do they vary from country to country? Are the codes of ethics universal in the international communities of nurses?

Further Discussion of Infectious Diseases, and Patient and Nurse Safety

- What is MRSA, or CRE (carbapenem-resistant Enterobacteriaceae)?
- How does a patient get MRSA or CRE? What does nosocomial infection mean? What about the possibility of transferring this infection to self and family members.
- What are universal precautions? Do nurses have an **ethical responsibility** to do frequent hand washing or use an alcohol disinfectant when in the hospital and going from patient to patient when providing care? Are gowns enough to put over a uniform? What about your shoes? How are they protected? What germs are being carried from work to home or any other environment? What does one do when one goes home after caring for a patient with MRSA?
- What are all the ethical issues related to wound infections and infections of any kind in hospital, for example, not only MRSA and CRE but *Clostridium difficile* (C-diff), and vancomycin-resistant enterococcus (VRE) ? (See the Centers for Disease Control and Prevention's Web site and the Internet related to these infectious diseases and others.)
- What does a "root-cause analysis" entail in a hospital? What does doing a "sepsis panel" mean?
- How morally conflicted or morally confused would you feel if you were faced with this assignment in the ICU?
- After reflecting on the issues outlined above, create a transcultural ethical caring narrative and model of analysis that you would use to develop continuing education in the ICU and hospital at-large related to what evolved from this complex transcultural ethical caring situation.

References

Ahlquist, D. (2003). *G.K. Chesterton: The apostle of common sense*. San Francisco: Ignatius Press.

Aiken, L., Clarke, S., Sloane, D., Sochalski, J., & Silber, J. (2002). Hospital nurse staffing and patient mortality, nurse burnout, and job dissatisfaction. *Journal of the American Medical Association, 288*(16), 1987–1993.

American Nurses Association. (2001). *Code of ethics for nurses with interpretive statements*. Washington, DC: ANA. www.nursingworld.org/codeofethics

American Nurses Association. (2015). Code of ethics for nurses with interpretive statements (Rev. ed.). Washington, DC: ANA. Retrieved August 12, 2015 from http://www.nursingworld.org/codeof ethics.

Anderko, L., Chalupka, S., & Anderko, C. (2014). Climate change: An ecocentric values-based caring approach. International Journal for Human Caring, 18(2), 33–37.

Appleton, C. (2005). *The experience of reconciling conflict*. PhD dissertation, Nova Southeastern University, Ft. Lauderdale, FL.

Arendt, H. (1998). *The human condition*. Chicago: The University of Chicago Press. (Original work published 1958)

Augustine, St. (1958). *City of God* (Intro. by E. Gilson) (Trans. by G. Walsh, D. Zema, G. Monahan, & D. Honan). New York: Doubleday, Image Books.

Badiou, A. (2001). *Ethics: An essay on the understanding of evil*. London: Verso.

Bailey, D., & Elliott, R. (2014). Living in the shadow of humanity: Environmental respiratory threats to migrant backstretch workers employed at thoroughbred racetracks. International Journal for Human Caring, 18(2), 25–32.

Bar-Yam, Y. (2004). *Making things work: Solving complex problems in a complex world*. Boston: NECSI, Knowledge Press.

Beauchamp, T., & Childress, J. (2001). *Principles of biomedical ethics* (3rd ed.). New York: Oxford University Press.

Beidler, S. (2005). Ethical issues experienced by community-based nurse practitioners addressing health disparities among vulnerable populations. *International Journal for Human Caring, 9*(3), 43–50.

Bellah, R., Madsen, R., Sullivan, W., Swidler, A., & Tipton, S. (1991). *The good society*. New York: Alfred A. Knopf.

Benjamin, M., & Curtis, J. (1992). *Ethics in nursing* (3rd ed.). New York: Oxford University Press.

Benner, P., Tanner, C. & Chesla, C. (2009). *Expertise in nursing practice: Caring, clinical judgment, and ethics* (2nd ed.). New York: Springer Publishing Company.

Berman, P. (2004). Terrorism and liberalism. New York: W. W. Norton & Company.

Bonhoeffer, D. (1949). *Ethics*. New York: MacMillan Publishing Company.

Bosek, M., & Savage, T. (2006). *The ethical component of nursing education*. Philadelphia: Lippincott Williams & Wilkins.

Boulding, E. (1988). *Building a global civic culture*. New York: Teachers College Press.

Buber, M. (1958). *I and Thou*. New York: MacMillan Publishing Company.

Buchanan, A. (1996). Judging the past: The case of the human radiation experiments. *Hastings Center Report, 26*(3), 25–30.

Buckle, S. (1993). Natural law. In P. Singer (Ed.), *A companion to ethics* (pp. 161–174). Malden, MA: Blackwell Publishers.

Burkhardt, M., & Nathaniel, A. (2008). *Ethical issues in contemporary nursing* (3rd ed.). Clifton Park, NY: Thomson.

Burkhardt, M., & Nathaniel, A. (2013). Ethics and issues in contemporary nursing (4th ed.). Stamford, CT: Cengage Learning.

Callahan, D. (2001). Doing good and doing well. *Hastings Center Report, 31*(2), 19–21.

Capra, F. Steindl-Rast, D., with Matus, T. (1991). *Belonging to the universe*. San Francisco: HarperSanFrancisco.

Carper, B. (1978). Fundamental patterns of knowing in nursing. *Advances in Nursing Science, 1*(1), 13–24.

Chase, S. (2004). *Clinical judgment and communication in nurse practitioner practice*. Philadelphia: F. A. Davis Company.

Chinn, P. (2013). Peace and power (8th ed.). Burlington, MA: Jones & Bartlett Learning.

Clark, C. (2014). Seeing civility. American Nurse Today, 9(7), 18, 20–21.

Clarke, S., Rockett, J., Sloane, D., & Aiken, L. (2002). Organizational climate, staffing, and safety equipment as predictors of needlestick injuries and near-misses in hospital nurses. *Association for Professionals in Infection Control and Epidemiology, 30(4)*, 207–216.

Code of ethics for nurses with interpretive statements. (2001). American Nurses Association. Washington, DC: American Nurses Association.

Code of ethics for registered nurses. (2008). *Canadian Nurses Association/Association des infirmières et infirmiers du Canada. Ethical Research Guidelines* (Centennial ed.). Ottawa, ON: Canadian Nurses Association. Retrieved June 2, 2009, from http://www.cna-nurses.ca/CNA/documents/pdf/publications/Code of Ethics_2008_e.pdf

Code of ethics for nurses (ICN). (2006). Geneva, Switzerland: International Council of Nurses. Retrieved June 2, 2009, from http://www.icn.ch/icncode.pdf

Coffman, S. (2006). Marilyn Anne Ray, Theory of bureaucratic caring. In A. Marriner Tomey & M. Alligood (Eds.), *Nursing theorists and their work*. (6th ed., pp. 116–139). St. Louis: Mosby-Elsevier.

Coffman, S. (2014). Marilyn Anne Ray, Theory of bureaucratic caring. In M. Alligood (Ed.), Nursing theorists and their work (8th ed.). St. Louis: Elsevier.

Cooper, C. (1991). Principle-oriented ethics and the ethic of care: A creative tension. *Advances in Nursing Science, 14*(2), 22–31.

Cronenwett, L., Sherwood, G., Barnsteiner, J., Disch, J., Johnson, J., Mitchell, P., Sullivan, D., & Warren, J. (2007). Quality and safety education for nurses. *Nursing Outlook, 55*(3), 122–131.

Dalai Lama. (1999). *Ethics for the new millennium*. New York: Riverhead Books.

Davis, G., & Dickinson, K. (2004). *Teen TV*. London: BFI Publishing.

De Caussade, J. (1983). *The sacrament of the present moment* (K. Muggeridge, Trans.). New York: HarperSanFrancisco.

Dittman, P. (2007). *The lived experience of male nurses who have successfully rehabilitated from chemical dependency through the state of Florida's intervention project for nurses*. PhD dissertation, Florida Atlantic University, Boca Raton, FL.

Edge, R., & Groves, J. (1994). *The ethics of health care*. New York: Delmar Publisher, Inc.

Eriksson, K. (1997). Caring, spirituality and suffering. *Caring from the heart: The convergence of caring and spirituality* (pp. 68–84). New York: Paulist Press.

Eriksson, K. (2006). *The suffering human being*. Chicago: Nordic Studies Press.

Ess, C. (2013). Digital media ethics. United Kingdom: Palgrave McMillan, Polity.

Frankl, V. (1963). *Man's search for meaning*. New York: Washington Square Press.

Gadamer, H. (1986). *The relevance of the beautiful.* Cambridge: Cambridge University Press.

Gadow, S. (1980). Existential advocacy: Philosophical foundation of nursing. In S. Spicer & S. Gadow (Eds.), *Nursing: Images and ideals, opening dialogue with the humanities* (pp. 79–101). New York: Springer.

Gadow, S. (1988). Covenant without cure: Letting go and holding on in chronic illness. In J. Watson & M. Ray (Eds.), *The ethics of care and the ethics of cure: Synthesis in chronicity* (pp. 5–14). New York: National League for Nursing.

Gadow, S. (1989). Clinical subjectivity: Advocacy with silent patients. *Nursing Clinics of North America, 24,* 535–541.

German, K., & Drushel, B. (2011). The ethics of emerging media. New York: Continuum.

Gilligan, C. (1982). *In a different voice.* Cambridge, MA: Harvard University Press.

Habermas, J. (1986). *The theory of communicative action: Reason and the rationalization of society* (Vol. 1). Boston: Beacon.

Habermas, J. (1987). *The theory of communicative action: Lifeworld and systems: A critique of functionalist reason* (Vol. 2., T. McCarthy, Trans.). Boston: Beacon Press.

Haldane, J. (1993). Medieval and renaissance ethics. In P. Singer (Ed.), *A companion to ethics.* Malden, MA: Blackwell Publishing.

Hilsenbeck, J. (2006). *Unveiling the mystery of covenantal trust: The theory of the social process between the nurse manager and the chief nursing officer.* PhD dissertation, Florida Atlantic University, Boca Raton, FL.

Hirsch, N. (1976). *Ethics and human relationships.* New York: Carlton Press. Center for Disease Control and Prevention—Emerging Infectious Diseases. Retrieved August 12, 2015 from http://www.cdc.gov/eid.

Huntington, S. (1973). Transnational organizations in the world politics. *World Politics, 25*(3), 333–334.

Ingraham, L. (2007). *Power to the people.* Washington, DC: Regnery Publishing, Inc.

Kadinsky, W. (1977). *Concerning the spiritual in art* (M. Sadler, Trans.). New York: Dover Publications, Inc.

Kant, I. (1959). *Foundations of the metaphysics of morals* (L Beck, Trans.). Indianapolis: Bobbs-Merrill.

Kurzweil, R. (2005). *The singularity is near.* New York: Viking Press.

Lange, B. (2005). *The clarity-parity community nursing practice framework: A critical ethnographic study of women in recovery returning to community.* DNS dissertation, Florida Atlantic University, Boca Raton, FL.

Leininger, M. (1978). *Transcultural nursing: Concepts, theories, and practices.* New York: John Wiley and Sons.

Leininger, M. (Ed.). (1990). *Ethical and moral dimensions of care.* Detroit: Wayne State University Press.

Leininger, M. (Ed.). (1991). *Culture care diversity & universality: A theory of nursing.* New York: National League for Nursing Press.

Leininger, M. (Ed.). (1995). *Transcultural nursing: Concepts, theories, research and practice* (2nd ed.). Columbus, OH: McGraw-Hill.

Leininger, M., & McFarland, M. (Eds.). (2006). *Culture diversity & universality: A worldwide theory of nursing* (2nd ed.). Sudbury, MA: Jones & Bartlett.

Logstrup, K. (1997). *The ethical demand.* Notre Dame, IN: University of Notre Dame Press.

Longo, J. (2007). Horizontal violence among nursing students. *Archives of Psychiatric Nursing, 21,* 177–178.

Longo, J., & Sherman, R. (2007). Leveling horizontal violence. *Nursing Management, 38*(3), 34–37, 50–51.

Lowe, J., & Nichols, L. (2014). Utilization of a Native American conceptual framework: Implications for practice and research. *Australian Journal of Advanced Nursing, 31*(2), 13–22.

Lynn, M., & Redman, R. (2005). Faces of the nursing shortage: Influences on staff nurses' intentions to leave their positions of nursing. *Journal of Nursing Administration, 35*(5), 264–270.

MacIntyre, A. (1996). *A short history of ethics.* A Touchstone Book. New York: Simon & Schuster.

Martin, M. B. & Ray, M. (in press). Enhancing the role of the transcultural nurse in the global environment. In M. McFarland & H Wehbe-Alamah (Eds.). Transcultural nursing: Concepts, theories, research and practice (4th ed.). New York: McGraw-Hill Global Education Holdings.

MacKinnon, B., & Fiala, A. (2014). Ethics: Theory and contemporary issues (8th ed.). Stamford, CT: Cengage Learning.

Majumder, M. (2005). Respecting difference and moving beyond regulation: Tasks for US Bioethics commissions in the twenty-first century. *Kennedy Institute of Ethics Journal, 15*(3), 289–303.

Martin, M. (2015). The 2015 Millennium development goal, Number 3 and Gender equality.

Mayeroff, M. (1971). *On caring.* New York: HarperPerennial.

McFarland, M., & Wehbe-Alamah, H. (2015). Leininger's culture care diversity and universality: A worldwide nursing theory (3rd ed.). Burlington, MA: Jones & Bartlett Learning.

Midgley, M. (1993). The origins of ethics. In P. Singer (Ed.), *A companion to ethics* (pp. 3–13). Malden, MA: Blackwell Publishing.

Miller, J., Leininger, M., Leuning, C., Pacquiao, D., Andrews, M., Ludwig-Beymer, P., & Papadopoulos, I. (2008). Transcultural nursing society position statement on human rights. *Journal of Transcultural Nursing, 19(1)*, 5–7.

Nuremberg [TV Program]. Public Television System, September 23, 2007.

O'Neill, O. (1993). Kantian ethics. In P. Singer (Ed.), *A companion to ethics* (pp. 175–185). Malden, MA: Blackwell Publishing.

Page, A. (2004). *Keeping patients safe: Transforming the work environment of nurses.* Washington, DC: The National Academies Press.

Patterson, P., & Wilkins, L. (2013). Media ethics (8th ed.). New York: McGraw-Hill Humanities/Social Sciences/Languages.

Pember, D., & Calvert, C. (2012). Mass media law (18th ed.). New York: McGraw-Hill Humanities/Social Sciences/Languages.

Pence, G. (1993). Virtue ethics. In P. Singer (Ed.), *A companion to ethics* (pp. 240–248). Malden, MA: Blackwell Publishing.

Preston, R. (1993). Christian ethics. In P. Singer (Ed.), *A companion to ethics* (pp. 91–105). Malden, MA: Blackwell Publishing.

Rachels, J. (2003). *The elements of moral philosophy* (4th ed.). Boston: McGraw-Hill.

Ray, M. (1987). Technological caring: A new model in critical care. *Dimensions of Critical Care Nursing, 6*, 166–173.

Ray, M. (1989a). Transcultural caring: Political and economic visions. *Journal of Transcultural Nursing, 1(1)*, 17–21.

Ray, M. (1989b). A theory of bureaucratic caring for nursing practice in the organizational culture. *Nursing Administration Quarterly, 13(2)*, 31–42.

Ray, M. (1992). Critical theory as a framework to enhance nursing science, *Nursing Science Quarterly, 5(3)*, 98–101.

Ray, M. (1994a). Transcultural nursing ethics: A framework and model for transcultural ethical analysis. *Journal of Holistic Nursing, 12(3)*, 251–264.

Ray, M. (1994b). Communal moral experience as the starting point for research in health care ethics. *Nursing Outlook, 42*, 104–109.

Ray, M. (1997). Illuminating the meaning of caring: Unfolding the sacred art of divine love. In M. Roach (Ed.), *Caring from the heart: The convergence of caring and spirituality* (pp. 163–178). New York: Paulist Press.

Ray, M. (1998). A phenomenological study of the interface of caring and technology in intermediate care: Toward a reflexive ethics for clinical practice. *Holistic Nursing Practice, 12(4)*, 69–77.

Ray, M. (1999). Transcultural caring in primary health care. *National Academies of Practice Forum, 1(3)*, 177–182.

Ray, M. (2001). Complex culture and technology: Toward a global communitarian ethics of nursing. In R. Locsin (Ed.), *Advancing technology, caring, and nursing*. Westport, CT: Auburn House.

Ray, M. (2006). The theory of bureaucratic caring. *Nursing theories and nursing practice* (2nd ed., pp. 421–431). Philadelphia: F. A. Davis Company. (Original work published 2001)

Ray, M. (2007). Technological caring as a dynamic of complexity in nursing. In A. Barnard & R. Locsin (Eds.), *Technology and nursing: Practice, concepts and issues* (pp. 174–190). New York: Palgrave Macmillan.

Ray, M. (2010a). Transcultural caring dynamics in nursing and health care. Philadelphia: F. A. Davis Company.

Ray, M. (2010b). A study of caring within an institutional culture: The discovery of the theory of Bureaucratic Caring. Germany: Lambert Academic Publishing.

Ray, M. (2010c). Creating caring organizations and cultures through communitarian ethics. Journal of the World Universities Forum, 3(5), 41–52.

Ray, M., & Turkel, M. (2014). Caring as emancipatory praxis: The theory of relational caring complexity. Advances in Nursing Science, 37(2), 132–146.

Ray, M., & Turkel, M. (2015). Marilyn Anne Ray's Theory of bureaucratic caring. In M. Smith (Ed.), Nursing theories and nursing practice (4th ed.). Philadelphia: F. A. Davis Company.

Ray, M., Turkel, M., & Marino, F. (2002). The transformative process in workforce redevelopment. *Nursing Administration Quarterly, 26*(2), 1–14.

Reuter, T. (2005). Towards a global anthropology. *Anthropology News, 46*(7), 7–8.

Ring, W. (2014). Climate 911: A call to action for health professionals. International Journal for Human Caring, 18(2), 43–44.

Roach, M. (2002). *The human act of caring* (2nd revised ed.). Ottawa: Canadian Hospital Association.

Rowe, C. (1993). Ethics in ancient Greece. In P. Singer (Ed.), *A companion to ethics* (pp. 121–132). Malden, MA: Blackwell Publishing.

Sanford, J. (1988). *Evil: The shadow side of reality.* New York: Crossroad.

Sherman, R. (2013). Building a sense of community on nursing units. American Nurse Today, 8(3), 32–34.

Sherwood, G., & Drenkard, K. (2007). Quality and safety curricula in nursing education: Matching practice realities. *Nursing Outlook, 55*(3), 151–158.

Singer, P. (Ed.) (1993). *A companion to ethics.* Malden, MA: Blackwell Publishing.

Smith, H. (1991). *The world's religions.* San Francisco: HarperSanFrancisco.

Smith, M., Turkel, M., & Wolf, Z. (2013). Caring in nursing classics: An essential resource. New York: Springer Publishing Company.

Smith-Morris, C. (2007). Autonomous individuals or self-determined communities? The changing ethics of research among Native Americans. *Human Organization, 66*(3), 327–336.

Socrates [quote]. In J. Rachels (2003). *The elements of moral philosophy* (4th ed., p. 1). Boston: McGraw-Hill.

Sumner, J. (2008). *The moral construct of caring in nursing as communicative action.* Saabrüken, Germany: VDM Verlag Dr. Müller.

Tarlow, S. (2000). Emotion in archaeology. *Current Anthropology, 419*(5), 713–746.

The New American Bible. (1987). Nashville: Thomas Nelson Publishers.

The patient care partnership: Understanding expectation, right and responsibilities. American Hospital Association. Atlanta, GA: AHA Services, Inc.

The United Nations Universal Declaration of Human Rights (Articles 1-30)(1948). Office of the High Commissioner for Human Rights, Geneva, Switzerland. Retrieved June 3, 2009, from http://www.un.org/en/documents/udhr/

Transcultural Nursing Society Position Statement on Human Rights (2008*). Journal of Transcultural Nursing, 19*(1), 5–7.

Tuan, M. (1998). *Forever foreigners or honorary whites.* New Brunswick: Rutgers University Press.

Turkel, M. (2006a). What is evidence-based practice? In M. Turkel (Ed.), *Evidence-based practice in nursing: A guide to successful implementation.* Marblehead, MA: HcPro Publishing.

Turkel, M. (2006b). Integration of evidence-based practice in nursing. In M. Turkel (Ed.), *Evidence-based practice in nursing: A guide to successful implementation.* Marblehead, MA: HcPro Publishing.

Turkel, M., & Ray, M. (2004). Creating a caring practice environment through self-renewal. *Nursing Administration Quarterly, 28*(4), 249–254.

Turkel, M. & Ray, M. (2009). Caring for "not so picture perfect patients": Ethical caring in the moral community of the hospital. In R. Locsin & M. Purnell (Eds.), *A contemporary nursing process: The (un)bearable weight of knowing* (pp. 225-249). New York: Springer Publishing Company.

Veatch, R. (1977). *Case studies in medical ethics.* Cambridge, MA: Harvard University Press.

Watson, J. (1985). *Nursing: Human science, human care.* Norwalk, CT: Appleton-Century-Crofts.

Watson, J. (1988). *Nursing: Human science, human care.* New York: National League for Nursing Press.

Watson, J. (2005). *Caring science as sacred science.* Philadelphia: F. A. Davis Company.

Watson, J., & Ray, M. (Eds.). (1988). *The ethics of care and the ethics of cure: Synthesis in chronicity.* New York: National League for Nursing.

White, R. (1996). Communitarian ethic of communication in a postmodern age. *Ethical Perspectives, 3*(4), 207–218.

Wielenberg, E. (2005). *Value and virtue in a Godless universe*. Cambridge: Cambridge University Press.

Wolfe, A. (2012). Political evil: What it is and how to combat it. New York: Vintage Books.

Wolin, R. (2005). Jurgen Habermas and post-secular societies. *The Chronicle of Higher Education,* September 23, 2005, Section B, B16–B17.

Wu, C. & Ray, M. (in press). Technological caring for complexities of patient with cardiac disease comorbid with diabetes. International Journal for Human Caring, 20(2).

Yapple, P., & Korzenny, F. (1989). Electronic mass media effects across cultures. In M. Asante & W. Gudykunst (Eds.), *Handbook of international and intercultural communication* (pp. 295–319). Newbury Park, CA: Sage Publications.

CHAPTER 4

Transcultural Context for Transcultural Nursing

We are all connected. We are entangled; if you want to call it quantum entanglement, fine. But we are entangled. And there is no real separation between us, so that what we do to another, we do to an aspect of our self. None of us are [is] innocent in that regard. There's something out there we don't like; we can't really turn our backs on it because we are all co-creators somehow or another. And we have to do the right things to try to get the future that is best for all of us. That's our responsibility as co-creators. . . .
William Tiller, *What the Bleep Do We Know!?* (2005, p. 226)

Chapter Objectives

1. To appreciate the changing image of cultural reality at the global crossroad.
2. To identify social structural characteristics, which symbolize categories of social information of the person in communal, social, virtual, organizational, and global contexts.
3. To examine the person in the transcultural context.

Continued

KEY WORDS

Culture • transcultural context • social structural characteristics • rituals • symbols • multiculturalism • identity • panidentity • e-dentity/virtual • race • diversity • ethnicity

Chapter Objectives—cont'd

4. To appreciate the concept of transculturality (interculturality).
5. To present the meaning of transcultural nursing/caring.
6. To appreciate the call and meaning of transcultural communicative spiritual-ethical caring.
7. To present and promote thought and discussion on a transcultural caring experience: Mary.

KEY WORDS—cont'd

- panethnicity • caring
- personal-mutual community • transculturality (interculturality) • social organizations • transcultural nursing • transcultural caring • transcultural communicative spiritual-ethical caring

Dimension of the Model

Transcultural Context

(Person in Family/Society/Culture–Political, Economic, Educational, Legal, Technological, Ecological, Health-Care Systems)

The diverse identity and personal/ethnic/cultural/ multicultural values, beliefs and attitudes about relationships, symbols, rituals guiding transcultural experience in social, communal, health-care and global cultural systems

Figure 4–1: Dimension of the model: Transcultural Context Dimension.

The theorist, Harman (1998) stated that we are living through one of the most phenomenal times in history. Scientific and technological changes are occurring at a rapid rate. And resource development, competition, conflict/war, and cooperation are changing the global political and economic landscapes. Cultures are integrating and emerging in new and dynamic ways, and at the same time, cultures are tearing apart. These changes bring into question the meaning of identity and the position and responsibility of the person in the family, community, organization, society, culture, the virtual culture, and world—the transcultural context (see Fig. 4-1). The Universal Declaration on Cultural Diversity (UDCD) by the United Nations' Educational, Scientific, and Cultural Organization (UNESCO) declared that culture is the common heritage of humanity and is expressed locally and distinctly by diverse groups (Chernela, 2006). While the composition of culture is changing at such a rapid rate, the desire to maintain connection to specific cultural/ethnic identity

and traditions remains strong. Cultures survive because of genetic heritage, loyalty to traditions, reciprocal cooperation, and willingness of people to care and make social sacrifices for each other (Dunbar, Knight, & Power, 1999). The transcultural context is a reflection of these phenomena—a mutual human-environment process that is historical and relational—continually evolving and emerging.

Within the transcultural context, ethnic or cultural traditions and social organization are represented symbolically through social categories or structures, such as kinship (i.e., genetic/family heritage/lineage), language/linguistic, religion/spirituality, political, economic, legal, technological (including the virtual community), educational, ecological/environment, agricultural, and health care to explain, understand, or deal with the society and world. Embedded within the structures of social organization (i.e., social, cultural, psychological, and spiritual) are stories about people in community and culture throughout history around the globe. Culture as community or community as culture refers to a philosophy, a family, a family of choice, a group, a locality, a place, or virtual space where people give and receive love and caring, and find meaning (Cohen, 1985; Day, 2006; Delanty, 2003; Kirkpatrick, 1986; Leininger & McFarland, 2006; McFarland & Wehbe-Alamah, 2015; Lipson & Dibble, 2005; Ray, 2001a, 2001b, 2010a, 2010b, 2010c; Rheingold, 2002; Smith & Liehr, 2014; Wolf, 2014). The social organizational structures of community interface with each other and illuminate the social reality. For instance, kinship structure relates to heritage, family, relatives, and close relationships within societies, and religion structure relates to systems of belief. Encounters within and among different ethnic groups/cultures have generated both conflict and good will with respect to the diversity of beliefs, symbols, and meanings of these various social structures. These encounters and decisions made

Learn More

Examples of social realities include:

- Language or linguistic structure identifies how people communicate;
- Iconographic art relates to cultural signs and symbols;
- Technological structure, including the virtual structure, relates to what humans create for survival and progress;
- Economic structure speaks of exchange of goods, services, money, or their equivalents;
- Legal structure determines rules and laws;
- Political structure determines how people govern to live together;
- Education structure determines how people informally and formally teach, learn, grow, and develop; and
- Health-care structure relates to cultural beliefs and systems of health, illness, healing, care or caring, dying, and death.

according to these encounters have determined the course of history.

Change binding us on a global scale has revealed the connectedness of all cultures and the search for a deeper meaning to living together (i.e., transculturality or interculturality) (Leininger & McFarland, 2006; McFarland & Wehbe-Alamah, 2015; Postero, 2007). Because history has revealed that ethnic groups engage in conflict and peaceful resolution in the evolution of culture, anthropologists ask, "[t]o what degree are humans innately or primarily aggressive and violent or, conversely, pacific and cooperative . . .?" (Bonta, 2007, p. 13). What are the social, cultural, and psychological structures that foster conflict and nonviolence that make the restoration of harmony in communities possible (Bonta, 2007; Chinn, 2013; Davidheiser, 2007)?

Despite aggression and conflict and competition for resources, for the most part, people in diverse cultures recognize that cooperation among groups is necessary for survival. Now, recognition of our common humanity, along with appreciation of multiple traditions, has sparked a movement toward more consideration of what is valuable and what should be valued in local and global cultures (Werner & Bell, 2004). The public eye now is turned toward social equity, human rights, peace and justice, economic viability of all people, and ecological protection and safety. Despite what seem

to be irresolvable crises in so many parts of the world, there is a quest for building public trust in world communities (Ray, 2010c). This chapter will highlight our current transcultural context—the person in family and community—within the perspective of the changing image of reality, including identity, culture, multiculturalism, race, ethnicity and panethnicity, and the virtual community. The chapter also will present transcultural nursing ideas and transcultural communicative spiritual-ethical caring ideals. These factors will help nurses in grappling with, participating in, and understanding local and global nursing and health-care issues, changing forms of cultural knowledge in the world, and the need for transcultural nursing and communicative spiritual-ethical caring.

Transcultural Context

The transcultural context illuminates the interrelationship between the person and the other. For example, it illuminates the interrelationship between person and environment, person and nature, person and society, and person and the cosmos. Persons hence are intimately related to and are one with their environment—the mutual human-environment process (Davidson, Ray, & Turkel, 2011). There is a personal-mutual meaning to relationships, communities, and cultures. "On the one hand, we look outward and attempt to see the world for what it is, and on the other hand we look inward to grow in understanding of ourselves" (Thoma, 2003, p. 15). The new sciences of complexity, including the social sciences, technology, and spirituality, reveal a changing vision of reality— we are all connected; we are part of an unbroken circle of the oneness of the universe; we are all linked together coherently but each doing *different* things at *different* paces (Ho, 2003). Rather than a focus on individuals as independent particles or bits of information as independent, there is a focus on the inseparable web of relationships (Bar-Yam, 2004; Newman, Smith, Dexheimer-Pharris, & Jones, 2008; Ray & Turkel, 2014; Smith, 1996). "The properties of the parts can be understood only by the dynamics of the whole" (Capra, Steindl-Rast, with Matus, 1991, p. xii). The whole, while difficult to describe, is more than the sum of its parts. It is dynamic, and always open to possibilities, emerging and unfolding (Bar-Yam, 2004). Energy as cosmic mystery, force, or oneness is a significant component of the new science and is always emerging. Energy within the network of relation-ships can be created at each local point and can be transferred or spread over entire systems, or the universe itself. In the arena of human and spiritual relationships, energy is viewed as the oneness of God, as love, and as caring (Dalai Lama, 1999; Merton, 1985; Newman et al, 2008; Ray, 1994a, 1997; Teilhard de Chardin, 1957, 1959, 1965; *The New American Bible*, 1970; Watson, 2005). Energy relates to belongingness and is concerned with ". . . a reality greater than myself, whether it is a love re-lationship, a community, a religion, or the whole universe" (Capra et al, 1991, p. 14). Thus, human-ity, science, and spirit are no longer separated. "It isn't a question of science bringing spirituality in. Wolf (2005) states that "it's more a question of ex-panding the circle within which both science and spirituality lie, so that the kind of question we can ask can be looked at from the different points of view that both science and spirituality bring to the table" (Wolf in Arntz, Chasse, & Vicente, 2005, p. 210). "To make known the unknown is the rally-ing cry of science [including the social world and spirituality]" (Arntz et al, 2005, p. 210).

CHANGING VIEWS OF THE TRANSCULTURAL CONTEXT FROM THE PHILOSOPHY OF SCIENCE

Changing views of the philosophy of science facili-tate deeper understanding of the changing image of reality as transcultural, technological, dynamic, and emerging. What do we mean by the transcultural context? We know that it encompasses the personal and mutual or the idea of connectedness of person,

❖ *Nursing Reflection*

Transcultural Context
Persons are intimately related to and are one with their environment—the mutual human-environment process. There is a personal-mutual meaning to relationships, communities, and cultures. "On the one hand, we look outward and attempt to see the world for what it is, and on the other hand we look inward to grow in understanding of ourselves" (Thoma, 2003, p. 15). Our image of reality is always dynamic, emerging, and open to possibilities as we engage in transcultural human relationships.

family, community, society, and the world. To an-swer this question more specifically in the modern world, we will turn to metaphysics, a branch of philosophy that deals with reality. What is the metaphysical reality (matter and energy/force)? What is the nature of being or person (ontology), how do we know (epistemology), and what is "re-ality" that lies beyond the physical (the transcen-dent)? Answers demonstrate that the paradigm shifts over time. Harman (1998) declared that three metaphysical principles of reality underlie science. "Each age had its own characteristic worldview, its characteristic paradigm, and one ultimately leads to another" (Arntz, et al, 2005, p. 29).

- In earlier centuries, the first metaphysical perspective—matter and energy, capacity of a force—dealt with matter or material giving rise to mind. At the same time, there was an appreciation of the "oneness" of all (Halper, 2005).
- In the middle ages, the second metaphysical perspective acknowledged the dualistic nature of matter and mind. Mind was considered divided from body (mind-body split) or humanity was divided from nature.
- In the new and third metaphysical perspective, the mind gives rise to matter (Harman, 1998, pp. 29–30); "mind and matter are one and the same" (Arntz et al, 2005, p. 241). "Every sense experience, thought, action and interaction plays out on the field of consciousness" (Arntz et al, 2005, p. 77). Patterns emerge in consciousness from the cellular, to networks of interaction, to collective memory. Human beings, the world, and everything in it are highly complex (Bar-Yam, 2004; Newman et al, 2008). For example, look at the human body: consciousness is not now consid-ered to be located only in the brain but the brain is a *reservoir* for awareness, understanding, and choice (intentional consciousness). "Quantum computations in our brains connect our conscious-ness to the funda-*mental* [sic] universe" (Arntz et al, 2005, p. 138), the human-environment integral relationship. The brain is designed to magnify these quantum effects (interactions of the cortex and proteins that control behavioral action of everything) and project them upward to larger and larger processing elements; the brain is like a com-puter, an information processing system (Arntz et al, 2005; Smith, 1996). In nursing, Margaret Newman claimed that health was expanding con-sciousness. Unfolding consciousness is a process

that will occur regardless of what actions nurses perform; however, nurses assist clients in getting in touch with what is going on in their lives and in what way they can facilitate the process through caring, pattern recognition, and being open to possibilities (Newman, in Brown & Alligood, 2014).

To explain the idea of consciousness, we will examine this third perspective more fully. The third perspective has been coined as the new sciences of complexity but its roots return to early Greek and Biblical thought (Briggs & Peat, 1989; Halper, 2006). Complexity sciences include various theories, such as the quantum, chaos, holography, and string theories, and concepts, such as consciousness, expanding consciousness (Newman, 1994), belongingness, interconnectedness, uncertainty, dynamism, patterns of relationship, self-organization, and emergence (Bar-Yam, 2004). This change in perspective—the ascent to consciousness—yields a personal-mutual or personal-environmental-global connection including a spiritual connection. "The world as part of our minds is no longer considered lifeless matter . . . but arises from a field that looks more like information, intelligence or consciousness than like matter" (Arntz et al, 2005, p. 19). In this ascent to consciousness, personalization of the mind is thus, relational. The person as a central being is brought into association with other minds. Because the universe as part of our minds, is no longer considered lifeless matter but arises from a field that is even more subtle than energy, we belong; it is information, intelligence, consciousness, and even love (Arntz et al, 2005; Newman et al, 2008; Ray, 1981a, 1989a, 1997; Smith, 1999; Watson, 2005). The personalized energy of the mind is in communion and communication *with* the other, persons and nature—the global mind (Capra et al, 1991; Harman, 1998; Goodwin, 2003). Teilhard de Chardin (1959) stated that "[t]o be fully ourselves . . . we must advance—towards the 'other'" (p. 263). We belong to the other, the plants, animals, the environment, and the universe. "We all belong together in this great cosmic unity" (Capra et al, 1991, p. 15).

Persons who advance toward the other in the mutual human-environment (transcultural) process have developed structures of cultural knowledge that form our identity, ethnic or cultural or multicultural traditions, and transcultural relationships, which can unite or divide. As living history and tradition, culture and transculturalism provide guidance on how we should live when we share a common humanity with similar and disparate values (Ray, 1989a, 1994b, 2010a, 2010b, 2010c). As such, culture cannot be found in *particular* cultures nor in specific interactions but in an *emergent process*—sets of possibilities that are cocreated when people engage in personal responsibility and moral accountability through mutual dialogue and questioning. (See the essence of the theory of "Transcultural caring dynamics in nursing and health care" and its interacting dimensions, where everything is emerging by means of awareness, understanding, and choice—Chapters 1–6.) Teilhard de Chardin (1965) concluded, "[t]he peoples of the earth, the 'natural units of humanity' must achieve earthly Harmony through the very variety of their racial [and ethnic] characteristics—characteristics which reciprocally enrich one another" (p. 13).

To build the earth, world culture is faced with ". . .putting man [human beings] back into the center of the picture (p. 186). . . . to transfigure the agonizing immensity of the world into a center of loving energy" (Merton, 1985, p. 191). Human persons must address the meaning of personal and collective identities, the meaning of caring and sacrifice that holds people together, to comprehend the making of modern identity. Teilhard de Chardin claimed that this energy is love; it is not just the ascent to consciousness in the modern sense but the ascent to a superconsciousness, where "the laws of love are directed not merely to the fulfillment of his own will but rather to the transcendent and mysterious purposes of the Spirit, i.e., the good of all men [human beings and animals]" (Merton, 1985, p. 193). Spiritual and ethical superconscious demands that people begin a new life because "the burden of the old has now become an unbearable accumulation of fatigue, mistakes, betrayals, evasions, disappointments" (Merton, 1985, p. 195), as well as ". . . violence, hatred and revenge" (p. 213). There is the need in individual and world culture to recover humility, authenticity and forgiveness, "to be renewed, transformed and liberated from selfishness and grow in transcultural caring: love (compassion) and justice" (Ray, 1989a, 2010a, 2010c). To illustrate this idea, Merton (1985) stated the following:

> . . . men [and women], nations, and societies are [must be] willing to make the enormous sacrifices required if they are to communicate

intelligibly with one another, understand one another, cooperate with one another in feeding the hungry millions [literally and figuratively] and in building a world of peace (p. 219).

THE ONE AND THE MANY

The scientific and theological paradigm shifts are extending to the social sciences and are affecting all cultures (Byrne & Callaghan, 2014; Lemkow, 1990; O'Murchu, 1997). The universe and the people in it as interconnected living beings are part of the emergence of the new conceptions of reality. People are at the heart of the choice to change, to transform. "The key is new knowledge" (Arntz et al, 2005, p. 49) and understanding. The Buddha reminded us that "[w]hat we think we become" (p. 85). What has been so dominant in the past was the Cartesian notion of mind-body dualism—separateness of mind from matter, the observer from what is observed, science from religion, and so forth (Harman, 1998). Now scholars are recognizing that humans are integrally involved in a mutual human-environment process (Rogers, 1970). The human as a microcosm reflects the macrocosm of the "other" as a whole and vice versa (other humans or the universe). There is a similarity of patterns and archetypes that connect. We are intimately connected with what we encounter or observe. The physicist, Capra revealed, "the human is an image of the totally created reality" (1991, p. 115). Personhood or the identity of person now is defined through relationships, self-awareness, or consciousness of the other as related to oneself (Capra et al, 1991). Axelrod (1984) remarked that as we go forward together in the world we must enlarge the specter of the future. Our future can be understood within a caring perspective within the transcultural context. Our future as a transcultural reality, a participatory process, is cocreated through mutual respect and cooperation. Mutual respect in a transcultural context comes by way of transcultural caring (i.e., love, compassion, and justice) if we believe that the future is sufficiently important relative to the present. Because of the new reality of belongingness and interconnectedness in the global world of today, there is an ethical demand (transcultural spiritual-ethical caring communication) for increasing *awareness*, dialogue, and *understanding* to facilitate *choices* that will help heal and transform persons in their environments and cultures—the center of the theoretical model articulated in this book.

Nursing's Contribution to Understanding the Changing Image of Reality

In nursing, Rogers (1970, 1994; Smith, 1999, 2011) was a leader in science and highlighted the irreducibility of humans and the environment, human-environment integrality in her theory of nursing, the science of unitary human beings (SUHB). This *unitive* theory gave nursing an understanding that the mutual human-environment process is relational, pandimensional, open-ended (unfolding and emerging), and pattern seeing. It is more than seeing the person as a part, rather as a whole, more than the sum of the parts (Phillips, 1994). Other theorists and scholars followed in Rogers' footsteps, such as Newman (1986; Newman et al, 2008; Pharris, 2005), who developed the theory of health as expanded consciousness; Parse, who advanced the theory of human becoming (Parse, 1998, 2005); and Davidson (Davidson & Ray, 1991; Davidson, Ray, & Turkel, 2011), who integrated complexity sciences and the SUHB.

In her theory of nursing: *Culture Care Diversity and Universality: A Worldwide Theory of Nursing*, Leininger (1978, 1991, 1997a, 1997b; Leininger & McFarland, 2006; McFarland & Wehbe-Alamah, 2015) identified the united nature of persons and their cultural context, human community, or environment. The person is a cultural/multicultural being and is connected to the context through transcultural interactions. We share a common humanity, and transcultural care, as Leininger stated, is the

❖ *Nursing Reflection*

Personhood or the identity of person now is defined through relationships, self-awareness, or consciousness of the other as related to oneself (Capra et al, 1991). In nursing, Boykin and Schoenhofer (2001) illuminate personhood as a process of living grounded in caring; persons are whole and complete in the moment; and personhood is enhanced through participating in nurturing relationships with caring others. Transcultural caring is the universal reality that connects one with the other (Coffman, 2006, 2014; Leininger, 1991; Leininger & McFarland, 2006; McFarland & Wehbe-Alamah, 2015; Ray, 1989a, 1989b, 2005, 2010a, 2010b, 2010c; Ray & Turkel, 2014).

universal that connects. To be is to care. The existential philosopher Heidegger (1962) stated that "[t]he totality of Being-in-the-world as a structural whole has revealed itself as care" (p. 231). Care and caring are necessary for human survival, and culture care values and beliefs are embedded in religious, kinship, political, cultural, economic, technological, and historical dimensions. While care is a universal reality for cultural survival, patterns, forms, expressions, and processes of care vary among all cultures of the world. Leininger's theory helped nursing to recognize that caring is the essence of nursing and that when caring for people, nurses need to understand how people are intimately connected with their cultural context, their ethnic and religious traditions, the changing global community, and the environment. Nurses also must be aware of how human beings have constructed categories or structures of cultural knowledge to make sense out of or construct meaning of the world in which they/we live.

The Meaning of Seeking Understanding of Global Culture and Community

How do people come to identify themselves as belonging to a particular culture, a community, and to the global community that is ever changing? Many people actually feel disengaged from communities that matter, such as at home and work and national and international communities that affect their lives. In the United States especially, individualism is considered a very important value; in the East, communalism is a more important value. In more recent analyses of community and an understanding of consciousness as the "global mind," there is acknowledgment that human beings relate both individually *and* communally, that is, relationally—the person is always situated in community, a transcultural context (Cohen, 1985; Day, 2006; Delanty, 2003; Kirkpatrick, 1986; Leininger, 1991; Rogers, 1970, 1994).

What does it mean to be a member of a culture, a community, a transcultural context? How do human beings feel accepted, loved, and cared for? How do others influence them? What facilitates growth and change in a dynamic and complex world of diversity of values in human society as a whole? As science, theology, and other disciplines are accepting the notion of consciousness and experience into their philosophies and research, how will the "global

mind" (consciousness) direct the new reality of the meaning of culture as whole, caring, dynamic, and emergent? "No phenomenon in science is more complex, spans a wider range of possible states, or is harder to predict than human social behavior," stated Vallacher and Nowak (1994, p. xv). "The way we think about people is often complicated, sometimes confusing and never static" (Vallacher & Nowak, 1994, p. 269). Consciousness and the transcultural context are *living* history.

PROCESSES WITHIN THE DYNAMIC TRANSCULTURAL CONTEXT

"Social and cultural practices, involving work, ideas, projects, beliefs, duties, choices, regrets, fears, both derive from and produce the situation that currently happens to envelop us" (Davies, 2006, p. 9). When culture, which is always dynamic, is developed, cocreated, and enhanced by human beings in relationship, it becomes transcultural. Cultural manifestations address how meaning is cocreated transculturally among people of diverse cultures. How the structures and processes of cultural knowledge can be more understood to determine what is valuable and what should be valued are expressed in ordinary life (Werner & Bell, 2004). Cultural manifestations, such as customs, rituals, words or stories, myths, images or art, food or culinary art, and musical compositions, are illuminated as signs or symbols to convey the meaning of something and communicate information in a culture (Womack, 2005).

Cultural Practices: Customs, Rituals, Signs, Symbols

Cultural practices illuminate customs, signs, rituals, and symbols. Often these practices are characterized as *folk*, indigenous, or traditional. *Customs* are "cultural group behavioral patterns or observances that may be established by tradition, social habits, and religious precepts and they are differentiated from specific legal mandates" (Winick, 1970, pp. 148-149). They are enforced by ethical, religious, or social disapproval if there are violations to customary practices. "Both symbols and signs [and rituals] communicate information through images, words, and behaviors" (Womack, 2005, p. 3). *Signs* convey meaning but have a more fixed meaning or one possible meaning in specific contexts. Signs give direction, such as religious signs that signify the action an individual would take to God's will in specific contexts (Womack, 2005). *Rituals* are the prescribed order of customary cultural practices and observances. Rituals are generated over time, provide stability, indicate change, and impart security to people in diverse cultures, for example, birth, marriage, and death rituals observed in all cultures (Womack, 2005, p. 4). "*Symbols* [italics added] are above all a means of communication" (Womack, 2005, p. 1). Symbols are indefinite expressions or manifestations of cultural behavior and knowledge and have multiple levels of meaning. As such, "[sy]mbols are the language of religion, magic, and expressive culture, including art, literature, theater, music, festivals, and sporting events" (p. 1). Symbols that express diverse meanings produce action, such as in nursing, the symbol of the stethoscope around the neck replacing the nurses' cap as a symbol of status and authority. Through collective memory of its rituals, signs, and symbols, culture becomes history and tradition (Wolf, 2014). Bee (1974) stated that all cultures are in a process of sociocultural change. Culture thus encapsulates the past in the present meaning, a "sense" of history by gathering knowledge from humans in the social and cultural practices (i.e., rituals, symbols, and signs) of the world (Davies, 2006).

Emergence and Sociocultural Behavior

Social behavior is always emerging in transcultural contexts. People facilitate understanding by teaching and learning how information is generated and how to use it. In the past, information was transmitted on a much smaller scale, thus cultures were bound and insular. The electronic age of information and communication, however, has revealed the rapidity with which information can be disseminated. Information can be volatile and stable at the same time in global relationships depending on how it is received and what choices are made. Thus, how we process information is paradoxical—on the one hand, information can create conflict to some and stability to others. Either one can become an adaptive state depending on the choices that are made. For example, terrorists adapt to the information that can disrupt stable social behavior. Stimulation from information in this case is agitating. On the other hand, transcultural communicative caring information that supports and reassures a social group can be calming and cocreate unity or a sense of trust and wholeness, even harmony. In the dynamics of information sharing in local and global cultural change, how does one decipher the truth? Philosophers, theologians, and scientists claim that collectively, we have to be open to new ideas, analyze them, reflect on the past, and

ethically do the right things to cocreate a future that will be best for all of us (Arntz et al, 2005). Information can be used for good or bad. "Justice [fairness] is the great transformer of earlier misused power that culminated into unresolvable, interpersonal conflicts" (Appleton, 2005, p. 138).

Doing the right thing begins by seeking understanding of how information is clustered and how people network. To cocreate "right" futures calls for aspiring to "a culture of participatory civility where people learn to listen, contribute to, and respond on the merits [of dialogue, public policies] in an atmosphere of mutual respect" (Fishkin, 1992, p. 190). As Rawls (1971; Ray, 1989a; Ray & Turkel, 2014) stated, justice must be distributive so that equal liberty is open to all citizens (locally and globally), and subsequently all citizens have the same basic rights that apply to everyone equally. That component of justice is highlighted in the meaning of transcultural caring as compassion and love and justice as fairness and right action within culturally dynamic communities (Ray, 1989a, 2010a).

A leading social philosopher, Habermas, claimed that people mature through socialization and communication. His theory of communicative action, of shared understanding using reason and knowledge related to social, political, and economic conditions, addressed moral consciousness, the necessity of the claim to truth (doing good), the claim to truthfulness (seeking goodness), and the claim to rightness of how people mutually relate and interact (Habermas, 1995; Ray, 1992, 1999a; Sumner, 2006, 2008). When there is consideration for what it means to be human, and there is negotiated discourse, the discourse is moral (communicative ethics). "Through communicative reason, we strive for mutual understanding and learn to assume the standpoint of the other [compassion and empathy]" (Habermas 2006; Wolin, 2006, p. B16). Problems or misunderstanding often emerge when, in the course of communication, the many languages and interpretations within and among cultures interrupt reasoned discourse. Integration of cultures at such a rapid rate in many parts of the world, especially the West and especially with immigration, opens up the need for continual dialogue about the meaning of communicative interactions within the complexity of the lifeworld.

Transcultural Context as Dynamic

Everything is transcultural. As we know, the transcultural context highlights the person in family, community, and society including technology, organizations, and culture. The transcultural context is complex, dynamic, and emergent. The call to communicative action and the need for transcultural communicative caring ethics reflects a deepening of consciousness in humanity and the world; it is an integration of compassion and justice; it is reinforcement of the meaning of the personal and the mutual; it is a plea to serve the good of all people. As the personal and the mutual become more understood as one and the same, we recognize that what happens to any one of us happens to everyone. We are responsible for self and others and the whole universe.

Understanding structures of experience within patterns of diverse cultures illuminates the interconnectedness of all, and the social systems that are emerging. Structures of social experience form social structures or categories of experience and become institutionalized as norms that can guide and serve the overall good of a society, individual and collective cultures, nation-states, and the global community. The social structure unfolds to reveal the person within family and community not only as social, cultural, ethical, educational, and spiritual entities but also as political, economic, legal, technological, educational, and environmental entities within changing cultural systems. Understanding these structures of experience can come through deep reflection, appreciation, and knowledge of world societies and the need for human caring and justice. Social interaction is cocreated and shaped by history, traditions including religions, political power, laws, cultural energy, and ethical responses to the meaning of the "good" society. Within each society, there is a quest for illumination, recognition, and understanding of diverse values within diverse cultures and races.

As the dynamics of relationship are changing through the dynamics of different forms of cultural and or multicultural learning, destructive patterns of relational energy can create negative energy that ignores the transcultural meanings of what makes a good society or world culture. We can think of the terror created after the experience of September 11, 2001, in the United States where people of many cultures, religions, and countries were affected (Berman, 2004). The event challenged personal understanding and collective consciousness and views of good and evil. It transformed American cultural politics; it caused fear and isolation and retaliation in the form of war, but also opened up room for a national examination of where the American culture is now and where it is going (Sherman & Nardin, 2006). Did the evaluation lead to greater understanding? Knowledge of transcultural energy for good or bad can infuse communities with understanding of the inseparable relationship between the individual and the world. All cultures have a face and a heart. Actions can be manifested by reactions leading to prolonged conflict, violence, and potentially warlike responses or to a deeper understanding of what happens within networks of relationships. The resolution of conflict comes only when all parties finally come to awareness and understanding of our inseparable natures and begin to acknowledge the face and heart of the other. Although difficult, taking the standpoint of the other with compassion, empathy, and justice is crucial for any conflict resolution. The social philosopher, Taylor, reported that in the modern world, the religious notion of agape, which is love that is altruistic, unconditional, and unlimited (Templeton, 1999) will strengthen the idea of serving the good in society to cocreate a better world despite the uncertainty and complexity of all our worlds (1989, p. 516). Furthermore, Habermas (2006; Wolin, 2006) recognized that a new postsecular (postmaterial) moral, political, and economic world is emerging. However, now that ethical, religious, and spiritual views are visibly considered in the realms of the political and economic, they must always be examined within a context of openness and suspension of anyone's particular religious or spiritual conviction as the path to truth. The intrinsic worth of each person and the diversity of meaning of *all* views need to be respected and honored. Habermas stated that it is necessary that this extraordinary type of understanding be supported and sustained. As an example, conflict emerged during and after the election in 2007 in Turkey when there was the potential to bring Islamic-inspired rule back to Turkey, which was under a democratic secular rule of law. On July 30, 2008, the court ruled on the constitutionality of the country's ruling government elected in 2007 declaring it not a threat to Turkish democracy. At the same time, the court restrained the potential for steering the country in a too religious direction (Tavernise in *New York Times*, Europe Online, July 31, 2008). Thus, cultural or multicultural recognition is supported within cultural and political affiliations and must be sustained through transcultural communicative spiritual-ethical caring (Ray, 1989a, 1994a, 2010a, 2010b, 2010c; Taylor, 1994).

Transcultural Caring as Communicative Spiritual-Ethical Caring

Transcultural nurses support the ideal of communicative spiritual-ethical caring with its focus on compassion and justice within a position of cultural dynamics. Transcultural caring is at the essence of nursing (Ray, 1989a, 1999b, 2010a, 2010b, 2010c; Ray & Turkel, 2014). Transcultural caring as the ideal acknowledges the face and heart of the other as the norm. It is the ground of transcultural communicative spiritual-ethical caring, a spiritual and ethical way of being. For example, professional transcultural nurses engage with patients, the community, and the world community; they seek and serve the good as trusted members of the human community. As a human "face and heart" in a suffering world, nurses reveal compassion and act justly, conveying unconditional love and truth. Transcultural caring nurses speak to understanding humans in need of physical, emotional, and spiritual care given with profound respect and competence for healing, health, well-being, or a peaceful death. Thus, transcultural communicative spiritual-ethical caring is all encompassing.

Derivation of Identities

Caring has been identified by archaeologists as one of the central foundational processes in cultural evolution. Throughout history, identities have been formed in and through the creation of relational communities (Leininger, 1970, 1978, 1991; Ray, 1981a,b, 1989a,b, 1981a, 1981b, 1989a, 1989b, 1994a, 1994b, 2010a, 2010b, 2010c). In contemporary culture, the concept of identity has many components. People derive their identities from a variety of sources: biomedical and genetic bases, kin and family, lineage, family of choice, ethnicity, workplace, religious groups, professional roles, and small and extended communities, including virtual communities. Identity also can be derived from other sources, such as gangs or cult membership, socioeconomic strata, and diverse caste systems (Morris, 2012). Revolutions in technology, for example, positron emission tomography (PET) scans and other brain-mapping technologies, have identified the idea of biomedical personhood or "picturing identity" by making known the biological activity of human beings at the molecular level (Dumit, 2004). Furthermore, computer and Internet technology have illuminated identity as *e-dentity,* a fusion of reality and virtual space (Peer, 2007). Identities

determine the extent to which people are healthy or ill, learn, grow, develop and cocreate relationships, and enjoy the "fruits of the earth."

In the making of modern identity, Taylor (1989) defined identity in terms of what it means to be a person, a self, or a human agent (p. 3). Taylor asked, "What underlies our own dignity?" and "What makes our lives meaningful or fulfilling?" (p. 4). These questions raise the concept of identity to the moral realm, to the level or relationships, where personal accountability and mutual responsibility must be taken into consideration.

Identity in the modern world is complex (Byrne & Callaghan, 2014). It is related to race—black, Asian, white (Rushton, 1999). It is related to gender or health and illness. It is related to the person as a human agent embedded within a culture, community, or nation. At the same time, identity is connected to the global culture through multiple forms of technology (information), and communication (e-dentity), travel, or migration. Technological identity in the form of robots or the human-humanoid connection is taking shape (Campling, Tanioka, & Locsin, 2007; Floridi, 2014; Kurzweil, 2005; Locsin, Purnell, Tanioka, & Osaka, 2011). As global complexity proliferates, especially over immigration, resource issues, resource "grab," sustainability, and "Best Practices" (Economy & Levi, 2014), we also are aware of a shift from agricultural and commercial forms of existence developed over millennia to ecommerce—economies of possibility with or without specific localities but always with access to and from a person in a technological space or community. Community and/or culture thus is space and place and symbolic and representational.

The new economic and technological vision of reality has raised new questions and influenced new forms of understanding about the meaning of selfhood, personhood, and culture(s). There are paradoxical views related to new definitions of marriage and family, new definitions of health and happiness, changing views of human connectedness with nature, the virtual community, searches for a deeper spirituality, and a quest for universal harmony. In this rapid evolution of modern identity, there are questions and contradictions related to human rights, cultural rights, religious rights, animal rights, environmental rights, health rights, and border and transnational rights. What should be valued in societies or cultures? What is the relationship between "self-determination" within a culture and seeking the good of people of the whole world? What is the meaning of ethnicity and culture? How do culturally diverse people with different beliefs, values, and attitudes about the world and life experiences accept each other and live together?

ETHNICITY, RACE, RACIALIZED ETHNICITY, PANIDENTITY, MULTICULTURALISM

To live together, questions abound about what it means to be indigenous/Aboriginal (first people), racial, tribal, ethnic, and cultural (Byrne & Callaghan, 2014; Chernela, 2006). Universally and locally, culture is multifaceted. Issues of the status and significance of race and interracial/ multiracial relationships; identity and panidentity, ethnic identification and ethnic loyalty; ethnicity and culture or multiculturalism lead to questions of cultural preservation, cultural safeguarding, cultural protection, and cultural enhancement. Multiculturalism and the politics of recognition, immigration, and changing nature of communities and nation-states become more visible. Should there be acculturation or cultural assimilation in various nation-states, as has been advanced in the West, or should there be an idea called cultural emergence (openness to sets of possibilities)? What do people of diverse cultures or nations do when the powerful overtake the powerless, when violence for the sake of violence looms? How can voices best be heard? It is true that the questions have begun to be answered in scientific, religious, and some political communities. A special transcultural dynamic is arising that gives rise to seeking dialogue, seeking understanding, and seeking humane answers (Habermas, 1994, 1995, 2006; Habermas in Wolin, 2006). However, at the same time, all people are wrestling with questions of the meaning of race, ethnicity, and culture, of what it means to be human and cultural today (Carrere, 2006; Dauer, 2006). People wrestle with different ideologies, religious beliefs, cultural histories, and individual and collective rights.

Sometimes people do not like each other for different reasons. Often geographical boundaries and resources for development or protection are in dispute (Economy & Levi, 2014). Specific cultural identities are being challenged with the rise of economic modernity and the permeation of technology. Cultural identities as dynamic and multifaceted show that "[a]t any given moment you have many 'components' that make up your identity" (Lustig & Koester, 2000, p. 6). Thus, culture contains a variety of categorical identities that include genetics, race, kinship, lineage,

ethnicity, class, religion, sexuality, and nationality. The idea is similar to emergence and the unfolding of possibilities within the context of the new science. Meaning continually unfolds and emerges as the minds and hearts of human beings are interpenetrated by each other.

Race and Lineage in Kinship Structure

Rushton (1999) states that because of the history of discrimination, inequality, violence, and dominance perpetrated by the white race against the black race over centuries, there was no greater taboo in the modern world than to speak about race and its differences. Arguments arose. "On the one side were those who argued for the demise of the concept, claiming that it was of little use in the study of human variation and, further, was burdened with negative sociopolitical implications" (Kaszycka, Štrkalj & Strzalko, 2009, p. 43). However, race, in the discipline of anthropology, was and continues to be studied and communicated. Over time, the concept of

❖ *Nursing Reflection*

In adoptive relationships, there are special challenges about *lineage*. Today, many adoptive children are from different races, heritages, linguistic forms, cultures, and countries. In the past in Western culture, adoptive children were often from their home countries and did not know they were adopted. Subsequently, they did not learn about their biological family, or get to know them in person. The legal records were sealed. Today, the law has changed to respond to the quest for knowledge of one's ancestors and lineage as a part of one's identity, biomedical and genetic history, and history in general. Many people are seeking to know who their biological parents are, contacting them by telephone or e-mail, and getting to know them interpersonally. For nurses, although a sensitive topic for an individual patient or family, it is important to know about lineage in relation to the health record—the transcultural assessment and planning to provide relevant transcultural nursing care. Although patients may be reluctant to share such deep personal information, using transcultural communicative caring knowledge and skill will assist in cocreating best practices and transcultural caring competence.

race was thought to be socially constructed, "a set of ideas about human difference rather than an irrevocable fact of human biology" (Thompson, 2006, p. 6). As such, *all* ideas beyond the idiosyncratic are 'social constructs' insofar as they are shared cultural knowledge" (Thompson, 2006, p. 6). Challenges to the anthropological consensus about race as socially constructed are emerging; the term *social construct* now is thought to be poorly descriptive of the phenomenon it seeks to describe because race too is a biological fact. In recent history, there are at least three specific biological races (subspecies of human beings): Asian, black, and white (formerly referred to as Oriental, Negro, and Caucasian, respectively), (Rushton, 1999). Multiracial subspecies of human beings are emerging as diverse races blend. Race and biology are significantly linked (Hartigan, 2006). Race is about division and difference, about genetic inheritances and culturally dynamic learned behaviors. Leroi (2004) stated that race helps us to speak sensibly about genetic differences, to understand genetic inheritance, to trace or identify genetic inheritances, and to isolate genes. On the other hand, Thompson (2006) states that race should be viewed as more than biology. Thompson declared that race should be understood as *lineage*, connecting people through lines of descent where one's lineage (from each parent and other ancestors) emphasizes the plural inheritances that make up each of us as individuals. Plural inheritances from ancestral lineage(s) show that we are all a part of the chronicle of history (Johanson & Shreeve, 1989). Hartigan (2006) further claimed that not only do we need to understand lineage, but we also need to reexamine the cultural significance of race. Race matters culturally through a host of dynamic processes of moral, social, linguistic, political, economic, and legal elements (Hartigan, 2006). As a result, race links the ancestral lineage, cultural perceptions, and categorical identities, and influences how we relate and view each other and the world.

Racialized Ethnicity

The term *racialized ethnicity* acknowledges the problematic nature of ethnicity for individuals who reside at the racial margins by: (1) recognizing the extension of racial meaning to ethnicity, a concept intended to signify cultural distinctions; and (2) considering the personal, social, and political struggle that often takes place between their self-defined identity (ethnic or otherwise) and socially imposed racial identity"

(Tuan, 1998, p. 23). Racialized ethnicity also leads to issues in health care and in nursing situations where often, by thought and action, nurses pigeonhole people who are a blend of diverse races and cultures (plural inheritance) into one specific ethnic group with specific traits. Nursing care then may be inappropriate unless persons are asked their cultural preferences and what has meaning for them.

Many other examples of acceptance of the struggle with race and ethnicity as self-defined and socially defined are experienced in different regions of the world. As an example, in the Caribbean culture of Puerto Rico, plural inheritance or mixed lineages from black and white races, including native Aboriginals, are manifest. People have intermingled and intermarried and a new blended and special "Hispanic" culture within multicultures has emerged. Also, the complexity of race and ethnicity can be witnessed in the intermingling of the Asian and white and black races (Asian racial groups from diverse cultures of Asia, such as China, Japan, Korea, Thailand, and others). People from the white and black races and diverse cultures of many regions of the world have intermingled and blended. Racialized ethnicity shares a complex lineage within defined kinship structures and is changing the meaning of kinship in general.

Global society—and the cultural ramifications of race—mandates that come to our awareness and understanding about belongingness challenges how we make choices that respect and honor the other. Seemingly contradictory but important as we go forward in a global world, Pollock (2006) states that we must be absorbed in "rejecting false notions of human difference, engaging lived experiences shaped along racial lines, enjoying versions of such differences, and constantly critiquing and challenging systems of racial inequality built upon these notions of difference" (p. 8). "Antiracism requires not treating people as race group members when such treatment harms, and treating people as race group members when such treatment assists" (Pollock, 2006, p. 10).

THE MEANING OF MULTICULTUALISM AND THE CHANGING NATURE OF THE MEANING OF ETHNICITY AND PANETHNICITY

Multiculturalism recognizes diversity of cultures in complex societies united by mutual respect (Habermas, 1994; Postero, 2007) and is continually under evaluation in a geopolitical world.

Multiculturalism is a mosaic of many cultures. As the meaning of identity is changing to represent a global encirclement, there is a transformation from individualism to communitarianism, from cultural singularity to interconnectedness. Both the personal and the mutual are integrated. The concept of multiculturalism will embody different meanings at different times. It is constantly being critiqued. Generally, multiculturalism relates to the multiethnic and multiracial makeup of societies and refers to respect for the rights and identities of others, respect for, and openness to universal human potential (Habermas, 1994). Nation-states today, for the most part represent a multicultural perspective or multiple identities, called in the political realm by Postero (2007) *identity politics,* and called by Taylor (1994) the *politics of recognition,* wherein diverse groups, tribes, or communities live together under a rule of law established by governmental decree or state intervention.

Most forms of multiculturalism specifically recognize formerly marginalized groups, ensuring their individual rights as citizens, and in some cases granting collective rights as groups. The concept is called *managed multiculturalism* (Postero, 2007). Some examples include:

- Legal changes that made rights to bilingualism the law in Canada;
- Governmental/legal changes for the Inuit (Eskimo) people of Canada gave territorial rights to their own northern territory, called Nunavut;
- Governmental decrees for the Australian Aboriginal people gave recognition for no development on symbolic Aboriginal sites within municipal geographical areas of Australia;
- Increased legal and tribal rights are under evaluation for First Nations (Aboriginal) peoples of Canada or Native Americans in the United States.

The call to address multiculturalism for honoring Aboriginal rights, tribal and religious traditions, and immigration status needs is becoming increasingly louder, especially in the Western democracies.

Individual and Collective Rights in Multiculturalism

Individual rights, on the one hand, and universal or collective rights on the other hand, complicate the challenge of the meaning of culture in particular and multiculturalism in general. Some people state that multiculturalism bends toward the loss of a universal rule of law or a moral ideal. Often there is a concern for whose morality prevails. Does multiculturalism mean to respect the rights of a cultural group within a nation-state as a whole or to respect the rights of individual members of a cultural group who challenge specific rules of law within nation-states? Attention has been paid, in the past, more to the latter (Taylor, 1991). Merton (1985) and others are concerned about narcissism where everything is centered on the affirmation of the limited desires and needs of a few. As reported and enacted in some countries, however, there is a call for the universal or collective ethno-political view that encourages a more balanced reciprocity of all peoples (Taylor, 1994). The focus is on collective identity recognition as the new political cultural behavior. "The struggle for recognition can find only one satisfactory solution, and that is a regime of reciprocal recognition among equals" (Taylor, 1994, p. 50). Despite this struggle for public recognition or the need for equitable distribution of justice, the challenge of multiculturalism or now postmulticulturalism, is not only understanding the need for and politics of recognition but also encouraging the taking of responsibility to <u>care</u> for human beings, and being accountable for the laws or decrees that can sustain or potentially destroy a people. The notions of multiculturalism without culture (Phillips, 2007), postmulticulturalism, or "beyond multiculturalism" welcomes "interculturality" (Postero, 2007) or transculturality, which signals a move to recognizing the dynamics of a common humanity, an interactive process of mutual respect, caring, and consistent dialogue among people who share differences of culture, traditions, and language. Rights to self-determination, religious and cultural beliefs, security, health, and well-being, which must be freely given, must be protected by a legal obligation within a nation-state (Fishkin, 1992; Hamacher, 2006). However, often the obligatory stance is imposed from outside pressures, for example, the United Nations or some other world governing body, such as the European Union or the World Health Organization. In transcultural nursing, the protection of human rights is a commitment, freely given, to respect the rights of all peoples from all cultures to enjoy their full potential, including the highest attainable standard of health, and an obligation to safeguard human rights and quality health care through the discovery and implementation of culturally competent care (Douglas et al, 2011; Miller et al, Transcultural Nursing Society Position Statement on Human Rights, 2008; Rosenkoetter & Nardi, 2007).

Political Recognition Of Transculturality/ Interculturality

In the modern world, the proliferation of conflict and war signals a focus slanted more toward fear of cultural differences rather than acknowledgment of the sharing of a common humanity. Gutmann (1994), however, reported that the future now must speak to intercultural political recognition by "pointing to the possibility that some form of constitutional democracy may offer such a politics based not on difference—class, race, ethnicity, gender, or nationality—but rather on democratic citizenship of equal liberties, opportunities, and responsibilities for individuals" (p. xii). In many ways, this ideal is similar to Rawl's theory of justice (Rawls, 1971; Scherer, 2006) "where each society has the obligation to structure itself in such a way that there are equal liberties and opportunities to social goods" (Ray, 1989a, p. 19). Democratic citizenship involves equal liberties, opportunities, and responsibilities for all individuals and gives voice to the uneasy relationship between individual autonomy and its relationship with collective identity (Appiah, 1994). Thus, within interculturality or transculturality, the meaning of multiculturalism, ethnicity, and panethnicity is becoming clearer and is evolving. Under a modern interpretation, interculturality, or transculturality includes multiculturalism, postmulticulturalism, or multiculturalism without culture (Phillips, 2007; Postero, 2007). The concept of ethnicity has moved toward the notion of panethnicity, and as it relates to transculturality or interculturality, it is the choice to construct a cultural base that reflects more commonality than difference based upon recognition, equal protection, rules of law, and genuine care and concern for the other. Within the world community, however, sectarian violence or tyranny and its proliferation in many parts of the Middle East, Africa, the United Kingdom, Europe, and the Americas foster a fear, and justly so, that ideas of transculturality and democratic citizenship with equal liberties are not possible unless serious changes are made in religiously inspired violence (Berman, 2004; Wolfe, 2011).

Panethnic Choice

When understanding panethnicity, transculturality or interculturality, it is important to keep in mind that ethnicity, although seemingly fixed in some communities, is continually evolving; it involves choice making. Culture and ethnicity used to be determined

❖ Nursing Reflection

The concept of ethnicity has moved toward the notion of panethnicity; it relates to transculturality or interculturality; it is the choice to build local and global cultures that reflect more commonality than difference based upon recognition, equal protection, rules of law, and genuine transcultural caring and concern for the other. *Transculturality (interculturality)* combines the following:

- Awareness of transcultural and intercultural needs and desires
- Openness to the meaning of relatedness as belongingness and interconnectedness,
- Openness of the meaning of relatedness as compassion and justice
- Engagement of spiritual reflection (i.e., faith, hope, and love)
- Openness to the other as similar to ourselves
- Recognition of a common humanity with diverse expressions of beliefs, values, and attitudes
- Implementation of the ethics of respect for persons in the personal-mutual sense of community within the mutual human-environment process
- Cocreation of transcultural communicative spiritual-ethical caring action committed to understanding diverse cultural beliefs, values, and attitudes and actions
- Evaluation of democratic ideals of liberty and equality or other ideals that function or should function within good governments and societies
- Enactment of mutual choice making to serve all equitably
- Openness to possibilities
- Emergence of new patterns of caring interaction

by geographical or symbolic boundaries. Physical and symbolic boundaries used to mark the beginning and end of a culture or community. When integrating to the new world after immigration, many people had a concern about the effects of enculturation, acculturation, or assimilation (articulated as sociocultural change) (Bee, 1974), the melting pot, or the potential loss of one's specific cultural identity to the dominant political cultural identity of a community or nation-state. Ethnic groups thus created small cultures or enclaves in communities based upon their own culturally specific values, beliefs, attitudes, language, music, foods, and behaviors for the purposes of love, care, and support. In the developed world, ethnicity now involves openness and flexibility regarding cultural traditions and elements. "Ethnic boundaries that mattered most in the past have undergone a fundamental transformation" (Alba, 1990). However, there does appear to be more commitment in some regions of the world to fundamentalist beliefs, producing more ethnic and religious boundaries, including conflict and violence (Toft, 2005). Contact on the one hand can either restrict communication and understanding or improve it. Flexibility on the other hand in social interaction improves communication and understanding and is always open to possibilities for continuous cocreation. Friendships among groups and marriages between different ethnic groups that were frowned upon in the past have become more commonplace (Tuan, 1998). As Nagel (1991, 1994, 1995; Tuan, 1998) reported ". . . we construct culture [ethnicity] by picking and choosing items from the shelves of the past and the present" (Nagel in Tuan, 1998, p. 65). Rather than focusing on ethnic differences, there is recognition of similarity grounded in common experiences and recognition of a common humanity that is linking people together. Despite many media reports that highlight dissension around the world, people are engaging in ". . . 'ethnic options,' the ability to choose whether or not ethnicity will matter in their lives" (Tuan, 1998, p. 5). Now that boundaries are becoming blurred, especially in the United States, Canada, Australia, and Europe, identifying ethnicity for the most part takes a conscious choice and an effort (Byrne & Callaghan, 2014; Tuan, 1998). Moreover, as communication becomes instantaneous throughout the digitalized world, and international travel becomes more accessible, cultural (ethnic) identification continues to dissolve, evolve, and emerge.

Choice is the new approach to ethnicity, panethnicity, and transculturality. Choice determines what happens when conflicts emerge in the families, organizations (e.g., business and health care), local communities, or the globe. In a world of pluralism and integration of cultures, questions arise as to whether or not ethnic communities can maintain their identities after losing much of their cultural distinctiveness to communitarianism (Etzioni, 1993). However, today many ethnicities/cultures are bound by religion and sectarianism and not necessarily separated by national or international boundaries or loyalties. With rapid change on the horizon, ethnic traditional values are challenged. Often fear and subsequent conflict or war breaks out. The need to understand the personal-mutual meaning of community becomes more apparent. Taylor (1994) remarked that an erosion of or changes to identifying with ancestral tradition and ethnic cultures may parallel the desire for recognition of differences and an increase in the politics of recognition. New cultural meaning thus is being driven by human as well as political and religious recognition. Social interaction, integration, and digital communication have helped to advance global interconnectedness through technological communication and economic interdependence. The idea of culture as panethnic and transcultural supports a world where emergent culture is more dynamic and open, yet at the same time, insular and conflicting. Taylor (1991) stated that large complex economic and technological societies have to be guided by bureaucratic rationality, by awareness and cocreative action of what it means to be human, ethical, political, economic, religious, and technical in an interconnected world. We are left with the questions: What is the meaning of cultural dynamism? What does the world community want to emerge?

Building the Global Civic Culture

The building of the global civic culture acknowledged by Teilhard de Chardin (1965), Boulding (1988), and Ray (1989a; Turkel & Ray, 2009) is only possible with awareness, understanding and choice (the center of the Theory and Model of Transcultural Caring Dynamics). And with that choice, the dynamics of transculturality are emerging. The theory of chaos, a subset of the science of complexity and the new science perspective, examines order within disorder at the communication choice point. This is the "do or die" point. At this point, choice is between one of two options: disorganization and potential disintegration or transformational unity and relational self-organization (Ray, 1994b, 2011). Cocreative choice and communicative spiritual-ethical caring are keys to choice making; the ethical communicative caring relationship is the means to transformation, to the personal-mutual idea of community (Etzioni, 1993; Kirkpatrick, 1986; Ray, 1989a, 2010c). All people then must be active participants in the communicative caring activity. "We are all in it together." The future of community is personal and mutual, individual and collective, rather than individualistic or socialistic. It is continuously changing and transforming. The old view of a disengaged, self-responsible person accrediting personhood as nonsituated and self-centered or self-sufficient (Taylor, 1989) has given way to a recognition of personhood as unique and shareable (Brencick & Webster, 2000), personal and mutual, self and other, cultural and transcultural. Subsequently, *transculturality (interculturality)* in the age of complexity combines the following (Boulding, 1988; Habermas, 1995; Marcel, 1952; Ray, 1989a, 1994a 2010a, 2010c; Teilhard de Chardin, 1959, 1965):

- Awareness of transcultural and intercultural needs and desires
- Openness to the meaning of relatedness as belongingness and interconnectedness
- Openness of the meaning of relatedness as compassion and justice
- Engagement of spiritual reflection (i.e., faith, hope, and love)
- Openness to the other as similar to ourselves
- Recognition of a common humanity with diverse expressions of beliefs, values, and attitudes
- Implementation of the ethics of respect for persons of the personal-mutual sense of community within the mutual human-environment process
- Cocreation of transcultural communicative spiritual-ethical caring action committed to understand diverse cultural beliefs, values, and attitudes and actions
- Evaluation of democratic ideals of liberty and equality or other ideals that function or should function within good governments and societies
- Enactment of mutual choice making to serve all equitably
- Openness to possibilities
- Emergence of new patterns of caring interaction

Progress in Transculturality

Can there be progress toward "multiculturalism without culture," interculturality, and transculturality? Transculturality implies relationality. The struggle for individual, isolated ethnic and religious identity resulting in conflicts, war, and terrorism seems to mar the path to the inevitability of panethnicity and transculturality. Increased conflict, however, ensues at times of great progress among cultures (Appleton, 2005). It can be growth producing or stifling. Now

that we are at the global crossroads, nation-states are challenged with the changing meaning of culture, cultural beliefs, and values and attitudes that members of specific societies hold. The mark of civilization or the building of a global civic culture is the refusal to share in the degradation or destruction of any people (Boulding, 1988; Saint Augustine, 1958; Sherman & Nardin, 2006; United Nations Millennium Development Goals, and Beyond, 2015 and post 2015). People who have engaged in military activities, even wars that are recognized as just wars, are affected by the destruction of humanity and community, the earth, and the universe. They understand, often more than others, that societies must be built on accepting differences of values and being open to highlighting the commonality of and protection of all humanity (Into the furnace of war, oanderson@libraryofsocialscience.com). Understanding transculturality will unfold more peacefully when we recognize contributions of every human being and her place in society (Taylor, 1991). In our new global and multicultural reality, it is necessary to engage in sincere political and religious interaction and dialogue and economic understanding at all levels. Taylor remarked that even in our human frailty and predicament of cultural misunderstanding "we . . . still need to see ourselves as part of a larger order that can make claims on us" (Taylor, 1991, p. 89).

Progress in Sociocultural Systems

In his treatise on the understanding of cultural patterning and progress Bee remarked, "contradictions and incompatibilities between patterns seem to be the rule rather than the exception" (1974, p. 14). The philosopher Hegel (1977; Bee, 1974; Inwood, 2008; Stace, 1955) noted that progress unfolds only through the conflict or opposition generated by contradictions (paradoxes), the dynamic of the dialectic: thesis, antithesis, and synthesis. "Every sociocultural system (thesis) tends to generate its own internal contradictions (antithesis); this leads to conflict, which can only be resolved by the alteration of the given system (synthesis). The new system then becomes the thesis, and the process begins again" (Hegel, in Bee, 1974, p. 31). Thus, connectedness, conflict, choice, and transformation are hallmarks of change or continual emergence. Whether or not we integrate any of the terms, such as multiculturalism, postmulticulturalism, or transculturality, the fusion and intermingling of races and religious and ethnic groups or cultural groups of any affiliation must speak to how we, as committed people, are prepared for the claims that now are being made on us as a global community (Economy & Levi, 2014). The new claim is to build the earth or the global civic culture (Boulding, 1988). Building the earth thus is "leading to the direct establishment of an equally common form, not merely of language, but of morality and ideals" (Teilhard de Chardin, 1965, p. 78).

By way of explanation, Hegel's philosophy of opposition, change, and transformation can help us to understand today's global culture. The force of human consciousness (i.e., ethics, morality, and spirituality) is now a major factor in understanding social relationships. Nothing can be looked at as purely objective and material but must be viewed as unitary and integral, the integral nature of the human and the environment/culture (Davidson, Ray, & Turkel, 2011; Leininger, 1991; Rogers, 1970). The quote at the beginning of the chapter highlighted the idea of entanglement and cocreation. Tiller (in Arntz et al, 2005) claimed, "we have to do the right things to try to get to the future that is best for all of us. That's our responsibility as co-creators" (p. 226). This inclusive view emphasizes for scientists, politicians, theologians, and health-care professionals that we must recognize that the others are ourselves. The decision to cocreate society from a relational point of view relates to caring action. Cocreating meaning is dynamic thinking, creative tension that calls for the virtue of humility to clear the way to create a space for any voice and at the same time, for a commitment to some judgment of our own (Palmer, 1993). The ascent to a moral and spiritual consciousness reinforces the personal-mutual-spiritual connection. The deeper meaning of transculturality or interculturality is communicative spiritual-ethical caring—the human and spiritual-ethical discipline of carefully listening to the other's reality and participating in the dynamic energy that ". . . draws us into faithful relationship with all of life" (Palmer, 1993, p. 125).

Transcultural Nursing

Nursing has always recognized the importance of human connectedness and ethical and spiritual relatedness. The central tenet of nursing is caring, a phenomenon that unites humanity across cultures. Nurse caring actions therefore are transcultural (Leininger, 1978, 1991; Leininger & McFarland, 2006; McFarland & Wehbe-Alamah, 2015, Ray,

1981a, 1989a, 1998, 1999b, 2005 , 2010a, 2010b, 2010c; Ray & Turkel, 2014, 2015; Roach, 1987/2002; Sherwood, 1997; Turkel, Ray & Marino, 2002; Watson, 1979, 1988, 2005, 2008). As a transcultural discipline, nursing is dynamic. In addition, as in all cultures, nursing is a culture that is continually seeking the deeper meaning of itself as it interfaces with people from diverse cultural backgrounds and other professional cultures in a global world.

The mother of modern nursing, Nightingale (1860/1969) pointed to the complexity of nursing as a reparative discipline. She formulated the idea that nature/ecological environment is the healer and the nurse is the facilitator of the healing. Nightingale's philosophy is well grounded in the new metaphysic where the person and nature are considered one. Nightingale looked at nature as God's work and the nurse as acting in conjunction with nature (God) to facilitate well-being. Thus, the idea of nursing as a mutual human-environment process was born. This idea was later advanced by Martha Rogers (1970, 1994) within the science of unitary human beings.

Nurses were awakened to the specific idea of nursing as a culture and nursing as transcultural by the late Madeleine Leininger, the first nurse-anthropologist (1970, 1978, 1991; Leininger & McFarland, 2006, McFarland & Wehbe-Alamah, 2015). Leininger reinforced the idea of transcultural nursing development in her theory, *Culture Care Universality and Diversity: A Theory of Nursing*. Leininger's scholarship demonstrated how nursing care is culturally and transculturally connected by the fact that:

- First, people are interconnected. To improve outcomes, it is necessary to provide culturally relevant and competent care and to provide such care, it is necessary to seek to understand people of all cultures.

- Second, the meaning of health is affected by cultural lifeways, such as genetic, kinship and lineage systems, generic, traditional or folk health-belief systems, the scientific health-care system, care practices, the construction of language and communication, and the elements of the social structure: the educational, political, legal, economic, technological, agricultural (nutritional), ecological/environmental systems (Coffman, 2006, 2014; Davidson, Ray, &

Turkel, 2011; Helman, 1997; Leininger, 1978, 1991; Leininger & McFarland, 2006; Ray, 1981a, 1989a,b, 2005, 2010a, 2010b, 2010c; Ray & Turkel, 2014, 2015).

Leininger's theory shows how the social structure in any culture influences cultural care for competent and relevant care choices and outcomes (i.e., culture care preservation and maintenance, culture care accommodation and negotiation, and culture care repatterning and restructuring). Other scholars followed in the footsteps of Leininger to advance understanding of the nature of transcultural nursing, nursing and anthropology, cultural relevance, and cultural competence. Through theory construction and/or application, and research in practice of multiple cultures, texts exemplifying the diversity of cultures by other transcultural nursing scholars emerged (see the Theory and Model of this book, Transcultural Caring Dynamics in Nursing and Health Care, and Transcultural Nursing Society Scholars, www.tcns.org).

TRANSCULTURAL SOCIAL AND HEALTH-CARE ORGANIZATIONS

The person in a family, community, society, and culture make up the social organization. People are embedded within challenging and dynamic transcultural structures: ecological, linguistic, artistic, ethical, religious, political, economic, educational, legal, technological, and health care where patterns of social interaction emerge. These structures represent, in part, the lifeworld and lifeways not only of a person within a particular cultural context but also of the human family. Organizations as particular social organizational structures or contexts are created for different purposes, such as for banking, technology-transfer, education, and health care (Morgan, 1998; Zimmerman, Lindberg, & Pisek, 2001). Organizations as small cultures/transcultural contexts with specific purposes represent small cultural communities where diverse values and beliefs, rituals, and symbolism are cocreated and shared through interaction. Hospital or community health organizations exist for the purposes of meeting the health, healing, and caring needs of people. The social organization or arrangement of health and illness, largely determines how persons are recognized as sick or well, how illness or health is presented to health-care professionals, and the way in which health is interpreted by the individual or culture group of which

one is a part (Coffman, 2006, 2014; Helman, 1997). Value differences in all people including nurses play a significant role in relation to responses. Awareness of values, understanding value differences, and facilitation of choices for patients and families ground the profession of nursing transculturally. Professional groups including nurses, physicians, administrators, other health-care professionals, and support personnel form professional or social cultures, formally and informally within the culture of a health-care organization. Thus, there are cultures within a culture. The groups may be from diverse multicultural/ ethnic or religious cultures or others who are adopting dominant cultural lifeways. Professionals construct their work-life realities into patterns of behavior for specific purposes that are cultural in nature. They have values, beliefs, attitudes, and behaviors that are generated within a group and passed on from one generation to the next. Cultures are sustained and grow precisely because the values, beliefs, traditions, and rituals are transmitted from one group to another over time (Wolf, 2014).

Nurses and physicians, while having similar goals of caring for patients for health and well-being, have different approaches to care practices. Physicians focus more on diagnosis, pharmacological, intervention, and cure, while nurses focus more on assessment, planning, and implementing care. Meaning associated with these values is embedded within these groups and begins in the respective educational programs. Meaning also becomes embedded within organizational health-care cultures as a whole. Differences in meaning illuminate conflicts of values of professionals and also of patients, and much of organizational problem-solving requires continual interpretation of the meaning of goals established by external and internal value systems, and social interaction among all groups.

While professionals and other members of a health-care community represent their own multicultural backgrounds, as a collective group, they are a macrocosm of the complexity of the universal culture that has been cocreated by history and groups of people who make up a particular nation as they live and work together. Complex problems in organizations are solved by people who determine better ways to solve them and can be from any level of the organizational strata, not just from the executive level. Most organizational cultures are slow to change despite that new people might bring forth innovations in technology and management. Challenges to an existing culture are not always welcome. There is an unwillingness to change and conflict can emerge. As we have learned, it is out of conflict that change or transformation comes forth (Ray, 2010a, 2010b, 2010c). We have all witnessed the challenges to implementing electronic health records (EHRs) from handwritten documentation into hospitals in North America (Campling, Ray, & Lopex-Devine, 2011; Swinderman, 2005, 2011). Innovations emerge most often only when there are talented people doing research, and enough people are respecting, accepting, and supporting the people and new ways to do things. As a consequence, there is acceptance of an innovation among diverse groups when each person has a stake in the process and outcome; the demand is high; there is no alternative; and when there is a diffusion of innovation in the society as a whole such as implementation of the computer worldwide (Rogers, 2003; Turkel & Ray, 2012).

Transcultural nursing and health care in hospitals or community health agencies slowly is being implemented in health-care organizations. It is not necessarily because people in hospitals are totally committed to transcultural nursing and caring goals, but because so many diverse culture groups in the professional ranks and patients exist and are engaged in social interaction; and because of the demand from outside accrediting organizations like the Joint Commission.

Organizational social and health-care cultures illuminate the following:

- Dynamical beliefs, values, and attitudes of diverse people (i.e., professionals and patients) that are created and cocreated by and in human consciousness, consciences, cultures, and social interactions.
- Social interaction includes ways of being and knowing, including caring as a fundamental way of being, modes of thought (i.e., reason, intuition, imagination, will), feelings, norms, ideologies, communicative actions.
- Social interaction among groups reveals patterns of diverse cultural meaning (e.g., information and dynamic energy).
- Horizons of meaning emerge through continuous cocreation.
- Dynamic energy from the interplay between and among people can emerge as a set of possibilities that elicits understanding or misunderstanding,

depending upon awareness, knowledge, understanding, and choice.

- Values emerge for what is considered valuable in local and world cultures.
- Constant struggle is a natural part of shared relationships (Appleton, 2005). Struggle or conflict occurs when balances of power (dynamic energy) or competition for power and meaning of what is valuable in relationships are tilted too much in one direction or another. What is valuable in relationships is symbolic of diverse cultural values, human values, belief in the value of self and others, religious beliefs, and visions about the meaning of the lifeworld. It is are carried within the imagination and behavior of human beings (Werner & Bell, 2004; Wolfe, 2011).
- Multiple generations trying to work together in organizations can choose to act positively with or negatively against another. Choosing to act negatively toward another is now referred to in nursing as "horizontal violence" (bullying), emotional violence, hostility, and aggression toward others due to lack of understanding, will, ethics, and transcultural skills (Longo, 2007; Longo & Sherman, 2007).
- Seeking understanding or seeking good demands ethical choice making.
- Choosing to communicate and act in an ethical caring manner to understand people, as life unfolds within hospital systems or any other system, is required to cocreate balance, harmony, healing, and sets of possibilities.
- As transcultural relationships and communicative spiritual-ethical caring are more understood, conflict can be more understood.
- Transformation occurs when there is mutual respect and opportunities for choice making in the design, development, health, and healing possibilities of self and others.
- All people, whether in positions of leadership or in general nursing practice positions, can begin to transform practice, organizations, and even societies.

History is full of the stories of relationships revealing conflict and balance, war and peace, and misunderstanding and agreement. Locating the meaning of the personal-mutual meaning of community, the recognition of a common humanity within diverse relationships, helps in the identification of what is needed transculturally for continuity of understanding, negotiation, and choice making.

THE CALL AND RESPONSE OF TRANSCULTURAL COMMUNICATIVE SPIRITUAL-ETHICAL CARING FOR NURSING/HEALTH CARE

Transcultural communicative spiritual-ethical caring practice is relational and contextual and open to possibilities (Ray, 2001a, 2001b; Ray & Turkel, 2001, 2014, 2015). Trans-cultural nurses seek understanding and facilitate the transformation to health, healing, and well-being through communicative spiritual-ethical caring in any or all transcultural contexts. Organizations today have people from multiple cultures and multiple generations interacting—patients, nurses, social workers, administrators, physicians, and other support personnel. As these diverse cultures with diverse values integrate to form panethnic and multicultural identities in organizations, transcultural communicative spiritual-ethical caring becomes clear.

Nursing practice involves nurse and patient relationships, care patterns, and the organizational context wherein there are identified health-care problems of patients and the different ways in which individual or groups of patients respond to illness, health, and healing. The need for continual understanding of complex transcultural relationships within systems is critical. As Leininger reinforced, culture care patterning with her vision of the meaning of culture care universality and diversity, the discipline opened nurses to understanding relatedness and interconnectedness, the person as a cultural/multicultural being, and existing within a cultural/transcultural/multicultural context. With knowledge of transcultural nursing philosophy and theory, nurses come to understand how the kinship and lifeways of people, and the political, economic, technological, legal, educational, religious, and traditional and scientific health-care systems influence patient and nurse perceptions of suffering and pain, health, and illness. The process of transcultural communicative spiritual-ethical caring requires understanding of the many facets of caring as ethical, spiritual, and physical and how caring is integrated with the sociocultural and organizational system environments (Coffman, 2006, 2014; Ray, 1989a, 1989b, 2005 2010a, 2010b, 2010c; Ray & Turkel, 2001, 2014, 2015). The mutual or relational process of interpretation of cultural patterns occurs through listening, communicating, negotiating, and renegotiating to arrive at the meaning of cultural health and illness, and suffering and dying. Thus, transcultural communicative spiritual-ethical caring that respects all persons first and foremost, followed by caring actions that exemplify cultural sensitivity, appreciation, understanding, and competency, helps nurses and organizations to progress and prosper despite the uncertainty and complexity of their worlds.

Transcultural caring is the promise of modern nursing. Transcultural communicative spiritual-ethical caring illuminates the need for culturological assessment for diverse cultural pattern seeing, appreciation, and interpretation for all participants in the nurse-patient and professional relationship, and the health-care environment.

Transcultural communicative spiritual-ethical caring incorporates the following:

- Copresence: being present to the other with love and compassion.
- Respect: acting with respect and honor to preserve, protect, and enhance human dignity.
- Compassion: sympathizing and empathizing with the other as a multicultural/ transcultural being.
- Commitment: promise keeping, attention, and dedication to the patient and significant others.
- Conscience: being and acting ethically through caring values and principles.
- Justice: being fair to the patient to facilitate right action.
- Confidence: believing in the self and the other.
- Competence: being skilled in nursing tasks and engaging transcultural understanding of the other.
- Comportment: examining one's intention and behavior and dress to understand symbolic interaction.
- Advocacy: negotiation and guidance in a mutual human-environment process.
- Sociocultural context of an organization: understanding the meaning of caring as interplay among the humanistic, social, ethical, and spiritual dimensions of professionals and patients and the social, political, economic, legal, and technological dimensions of the organizational culture (Coffman, 2006, 2014; Ray, 1981a, 1989b, 2001a, 2001b, 2005, 2010a, 2010b, 2010c; Ray & Turkel, 2012, 2014, 2015; Turkel, 2007).
- Communication: engaging the other in relationships and communication by facilitating choice making and transcultural communicative spiritual-ethical caring action.
- Language: using language and/or interpreters for patient and family understanding and choice making.

Transcultural caring as a complex, transcultural, relational process, grounded ethically and spiritually, is even more complex as the world deals with ideas of multiculturalism or transculturality in the global environment. At the same time that transcultural caring can be considered the promise of modern nursing, it is the promise of modern identity in the global culture to deal with the dynamic problems that a global community brings forth. Even with the advent of e-dentity, transcultural communicative spiritual-ethical caring is an imperative to develop trust and confidence when one does not see a person face-to-face. As this knowledge grows, professional nurses will emerge as having competency to educate not only nurses in the profession itself but also others in transcultural ethical communication and choice making around the world.

Love and caring are synonymous (Ray, 1981b; Watson, 2005). The idea of being able to "see good" is fundamental to transcultural caring (Ray, 1994b; Leininger & McFarland, 2006). Watson (1988) stated that the goal of human caring is "the protection, enhancement and preservation of the person's humanity which helps to restore inner harmony and potential healing" (p. 58). Transcultural communicative spiritual-ethical caring knowledge has to do with fulfilling the promise implicit in a caring profession—placing demands upon a nurse who has a sense of self-in-relation to the other to respect the other, uphold human dignity, and act as a moral caring person. Transcultural nursing sheds light on respecting the other by the connection between nursing as care and caring, and health care and culture (Leininger & McFarland, 2006; McFarland & Wehbe-Alamay, 2015). The contribution of transcultural nursing and caring to understand the theories and practices of health care and caring in particular is continually unfolding. Insights from research target understanding of complex cultures, complex systems, and complex people. As such, appreciating and reclaiming nursing as caring and claiming transcultural caring for the present and future is significant to transformation of the local and global understanding of nursing and health.

Summary

This chapter made the following points:

- The person is embedded in a transcultural context that is dynamic and emergent.

- As the world has become more global, the nature of the personal-mutual meaning of community has emerged from strictly individualism and communalism.
- The personal is the mutual and the mutual is the personal. We are each responsible to and for each other.
- Meaning is revealed in transcultural contexts, the social structural characteristics of collective and organizational systems—such as kinship, social, ethical, religious, spiritual, educational, ecological/environmental, political, economic, technological, and legal systems—that illuminate our common humanity and diversity of values, beliefs, attitudes, and behaviors.
- The notion of culture is dynamic and continually emerging from a focus on individual cultures to multiculturalism, postmulticulturalism, and beyond multiculturalism.
- Panidentity, panethnicity, racialized ethnicity, and multiculturalism command our attention to understand the politics of recognition as an ethical and communicative spiritual-ethical caring enterprise without which achievement of understanding a panethnic world is impossible.
- Transculturality or interculturality has been recognized as a new perspective on multiculturalism.
- Transcultural conflict or opposition can be what also fosters choice toward transformation within diverse cultures, organizations, and nation-states.
- Nursing is a transcultural caring discipline.
- Transcultural caring is the essence of nursing.
- Transcultural communicative spiritual-ethical caring is necessary for negotiating choice and transformation to health, healing, and harmony.
- Transcultural caring is the modern identity of nursing.
- Transcultural caring is a spiritual and ethical enterprise illuminating compassion, love, and justice.
- Seeing the good and seeking the good of all people is a continuous ethical demand.
- Transcultural communicative spiritual-ethical caring is the modern identity of the global world.
- Transcultural caring fosters awareness, appreciation, understanding, and interpretation of cultures, multicultures, and transculturality (interculturality).
- Transcultural caring using communicative caring ethics facilitates transcultural competence (i.e.,

awareness, understanding, and mutual choice making).

• Transcultural caring in nursing facilitates transformation and relational self-organization (i.e., health, healing, well-being, and peaceful death).

In conclusion, persons are endowed with human dignity and the ability to choose. As culture emerges toward transculturality and transcultural caring, we are aware that wise choices are connected by authentic conscience, a spiritual and ethical self, and a personal/mutual meaning of community. There is a perennial wisdom to be found through exploration and identification of the deepest part of ourselves

(Harman, 1998). Wisdom is associated with knowledge, information, intelligence, instruction, intuition, understanding, caring, and love, which is considered what is deepest in the self, a transcendent center (Teilhard de Chardin, 1965). Transcultural caring as compassion through love is the energy of the universe; it is what unites living beings because it joins them by what is deepest in them; the personal is the mutual, the self is "the other and the many" (Teilhard de Chardin, 1959). Transcultural nursing in particular has a commitment to the knowledge and skill through transcultural spiritual-ethical caring to contribute to and facilitate health, healing, and progress toward communal well-being and transculturality.

Transcultural Nursing in Practice
Transcultural Caring Experience

Mary, RN, CNO

Mary is a chief nursing officer in a busy public hospital in a major city in the United States. She is responsible for 850 nurses who work on all units of the hospital during a 24-hour day. In the past few years, there has been a nursing shortage and about 250 nurses have been hired in the hospital from different multicultural and multilingual backgrounds or countries, such as India, Philippines, England, Canada, Jamaica, Haiti, and Mexico. Not only can these new hires alleviate the problems caused by the nursing shortage, but they also can help to provide better care for a multicultural patient population.

Mary is concerned about quality of care and good patient and health outcomes. She is preparing for a spontaneous visit at any time from the Joint Commission. Mary would like to see that the hospital is designated as a center of excellence and eventually receive magnet status from the American Nurse Credentialing Center, Magnet Recognition Program (www.nursingworld.org/ancc/magnet.html). Recently, Mary has been informed that there is friction and outright conflict between nurses educated in nursing programs in the United States and nurses educated elsewhere, and friction with some patients of diverse cultures. Nurse managers on some of the units, primarily the medical-surgical floors, reported more cases of conflict. The main issues have come from Medical Unit 1 and Surgical Unit 2. On Medical Unit 1, 10 Filipino nurses have formed a strong group, and the whole unit of nurses is not interacting well. The Filipino nurses report that they are experiencing hostility from American nurses. On Surgical Unit 2, the full-time American nurses stated that they are upset that there is a problem with nurses from Jamaica and Haiti, especially giving discharge-planning instructions to patients and families because of their differences in cultural values and their accents. Patients and their family members claim that they could not understand the nurses from different heritages.

Although discussion of racial issues is more subdued, racial discrimination has been identified by the four Haitian and five Jamaican nurses on Surgical Unit 2. Two of the Jamaican nurses are now American citizens but most of the nurses from the two Caribbean islands have legal work documents. Mary and her nurse managers have encountered some challenges with diverse nurse and patient cultural groups in the past, but now, the challenges seem to be much more difficult to discuss and resolve.

NURSE MANAGERS IN THE UNITS

Toby is the nurse manager on Medical Unit 1 and Jane is nurse manager on Surgical Unit 2. Both managers are relatively new to nursing administration and have been at the hospital for about 3 years. Toby has a bachelor of science degree in nursing (BSN) from a university in the northeastern United States, and Jane is earning a master of science (MSN) degree from a local university. Both managers are Caucasian. Neither nurse has worked with Filipino or Caribbean nurses in the past. The managers have come to the executive committee meeting with Mary and other nurse managers for help in dealing with the transcultural issues that are developing on the units. Mary asked if any of the managers has experience in transcultural issues or in conflict management. Maria Elena, born in Mexico and now living in Los Angeles, said that she was educated at the University of Utah, where a course in transcultural nursing highlighted Leininger's theory of cultural care diversity and universality, and other cultural theories. Although very busy in the outpatient department, Maria Elena volunteered to begin a continuing education course to assist nurses on transcultural nursing and transcultural competence throughout the entire hospital. At the request of Mary, the chief nursing officer, Maria Elena also has agreed to attend meetings with representatives of various cultural groups and the nurse managers from Medical Unit 1 and Surgical Unit 2.

REFLECTION: OVERVIEW AND QUESTIONS FOR ANALYSIS OF MARY'S TRANSCULTURAL CARING EXPERIENCE

The hospital is a complex transcultural social and health-care organization. As this chapter has identified, there are many changes occurring in American culture because of multiculturalism and immigration. Families, communities including organizations, and societies and geographical areas are ethnically, culturally, and multiculturally dynamic. Values, beliefs, and attitudes are diverse, creating relational and intercultural behavioral challenges. Organizations are becoming multiracial, multiethnic, and even panethnic. Hospitals are no different. The United States and other nations are involved in economic interdependence and globalization. Languages other than English are the order of the day. Communication and information technology and the virtual community are changing the face of the nation. In the Western health-care system, there is a critical shortage of nurses. Nurses from developing countries are recruited to respond to the nursing shortage.

QUESTIONS FOR ANALYSIS OF MARY'S TRANSCULTURAL CARING EXPERIENCE

- Reflect upon the transcultural nursing situation and the nursing shortage, and what Maria Elena is going to have to analyze to attend a meeting with the chief nurse, Mary, and unit nurse managers, Toby and Jane, and representatives from the diverse cultural groups.
- What other information will Maria Elena need to develop to present an educational workshop(s) on transcultural nursing in the hospital? Who should be included?
- Can you identify what patterns of leadership are present in the hospital organization in Mary's story?
- What is the transcultural makeup of the organization and the nurses?
- What is transcultural nursing and transcultural caring? (Include definitions from this book and your own thoughts. Also, check all resources available in print and online.)
- What is the Joint Commission and what is expected from the Joint Commission of regulations related to cultural competence in hospitals and other health-care organizations?
- What can you interpret from the facts and communication patterns from the transcultural nursing experience in the hospital presented?
- Are there rights to privacy about race and ethnic backgrounds in complex organizations, and especially in hospitals? What does HIPAA in health-care organizations mean?

FURTHER QUESTIONS FOR REFLECTION

- What is the meaning of conflict in the organizational culture, in nursing, and on the units? How is it resolved? In this transcultural caring experience, was conflict addressed in the organization in the past?
- Do you think there could be potential transcultural conflict and horizontal violence (incivility or bullying) among the nurse managers and their staff? Is there potential conflict between the nurse managers and the chief nursing officer? Why?
- How do you think Maria Elena should be supported by the chief nursing officer and the nurse managers? What is transcultural communicative spiritual-ethical caring?

- How will Maria Elena gather data related to the conflicts that are arising on the units, especially the units where the transcultural issues were first witnessed? How should racial issues be dealt with? How should language differences be dealt with?
- What kind of transcultural educational workshop(s) should Maria Elena design? Look up the assumptions and elements of Leininger's transcultural nursing theory of Culture Care Diversity and Universality. Examine the meaning of organizations as small cultures with respect to the meaning of human cultures, identity, panidentity, panethnicity, multiculturalism, and transculturality (interculturality). Look up Ray's theory of Bureaucratic Caring, and review the Theory and Model of Transcultural Caring Dynamics in Nursing and Health Care as well as information from the chapters outlined in this book. Examine the various diverse cultures that have been identified in this project from many transcultural nursing texts.
- What transcultural educational concepts should be included for transcultural relevancy and competency in nursing practice? (See the work of Dr. Mary Martin in transcultural nursing staff development.)
- What are your thoughts about health as expanding consciousness and other emerging ideas of the human-environment relationship and transcultural context in nursing, such as Davidson et al, Newman, Parse, Rogers, Smith, and so forth?

Additional Questions for Transcultural Evaluation within Nursing, Hospitals, and Culture as a Whole

- Identify the central ideas related to the nursing shortage in the United States and the Western world. Why has this occurred? Seek information from literature, Web sites of professional organizations, demographics of the West, and your own opinion.
- List potential patterns of conflict that you may have identified in your nursing practice, and from this transcultural nursing/caring experience or any other transcultural nursing experience. (See Sherman, 2012, 2013.)
- What are the dominant patterns of multiculturalism in the United States? Why are there so many conflicts?
- What are the dominant multicultural patterns of culture in Canada? Why are there so many conflicts? What is "compassion fatigue"?
- What are the cultural patterns of Filipinos in the United States? What is the history of the Philippines and the United States? (See Ray, 2013.)
- What are the different countries that make up the Caribbean community?
- What is meant by Afro-Caribbean culture? Compare and contrast cultures and languages as well as religious practices and patterns of Puerto Rico, Haiti, and Jamaica and other islands that may be familiar to you. (See Archibald, 2011.)
- What are the religions and the religious patterns of Caribbean culture?
- Compare and contrast indigenous/Aboriginal cultures and Afro-Caribbean culture. (As an example, see Lowe & Nichols, 2014, in regard to Native American culture and Archibald, 2013, in regard to Afro-Caribbean culture.)
- Compare and contrast the potential culture groups and multicultural or panethnic groups in large metropolitan cities, such as New York City, NY, Los Angeles, CA, in the United States, and Vancouver, BC and Toronto, ON in Canada.
- What is the meaning of health care in a multicultural environment today? Does it vary among Western democracies or in other countries of the world? (See the works of Boyle and Andrews; Douglas, Giger, and Davidhizar; Horn, entire issue of the *Journal of Transcultural Nursing* 10(1), 5–74, 1999; Kavanaugh and Kennedy; Leininger, Leininger and McFarland, McFarland & Webhe-Alamah; Lipson and Dibble, Purnell and Paulanka, Spector, Ray, the United Nations Millennium Development Goals, 2015 and post 2015; Wenger, and World Health Organization statistics for examples.)

REFERENCES

Alba, R. (1990). *Ethnicity in America: The transformation of white America*. New Haven, CT: Yale University Press.

Andrews, M., & Boyle, J. (2007). *Transcultural concepts in nursing care* (5th ed.). Philadelphia: Lippincott Williams & Wilkins.

Appiah, K. (1994). Identity, authenticity, survival. In A. Gutmann (Ed.), *Multiculturalism* (pp. 149–163). Princeton, NJ: Princeton University Press.

Appleton, C. (2005). *The experience or reconciling*. PhD Dissertation, Nova Southeastern University.

Archibald, C. (2011). Cultural tailoring for an Afro-Caribbean community: A naturalistic approach. *Journal of Cultural Diversity, 18*(4), 114–119.

Arntz, W., Chasse, B., & Vicente, M. (2005). *What the bleep do we know!?* Deerfield Beach, FL: Health Communications, Inc.

Axelrod, R. (1984). *The evolution of cooperation*. New York: Basic Books, Inc, Publishers.

Bar-Yam, Y. (2004). *Making things work: Solving complex problems in a complex world*. Boston, MA: Knowledge Press.

Bee, R. (1974). *Patterns and processes: An introduction to anthropological strategies for the study of sociocultural change*. New York: The Free Press.

Berman, P. (2004). *Terrorism and liberalism*. New York: W. W. Norton & Company.

Bonta, B. (2007). Peaceful societies today-news, reviews and clues. *Anthropology News, 48*(7), 13–14.

Boulding, E. (1988). *Building the global civic culture*. New York: Teachers' College Press.

Boykin, A., & Schoenhofer, S. (2001). *Nursing as caring: A model for transforming nursing practice*. Boston: Jones & Bartlett.

Boykin, A., Schoenhofer, S., & Valentine, K. (2014). *Health care system transformation for nursing and health care leaders: Implementing a culture of caring*. New York: Springer Publishing Company.

Brencick, J., & Webster, G. (2000). *Philosophy of nursing*. Albany: State University of New York Press.

Briggs, D., & Peat, F. (1989). *The turbulent mirror*. New York: Harper & Row, Publishers.

Brown, J., & Alligood, M. (2014). Health as expanding consciousness. In M. Alligood (Ed.), *Nursing theorists and their work*. St. Louis: Elsevier.

Byrne, D., & Callaghan, G. (2014). *Complexity theory and the social sciences: The state of the art*. New York: Routledge.

Campling, A., Tanioka, T., & Locsin, R. (2007). Robots and nursing: Concepts, relationship and practice. In A. Barnard & R. Locsin (Eds.), *Technology and nursing: Practice, concepts and issues* (pp. 73–90). United Kingdom: Palgrave MacMillan.

Capra, F., Steindl-Rast, D., with Matus, T. (1991). *Belonging to the universe*. San Francisco: HarperSanFrancisco.

Carrere, E. (2006). *Creating a human world*. Scranton, PA: University of Scranton Press.

Chernela, J. (2006). A call to words. *Anthropology News, 47*(4), 6–7.

Chinn, P. (2013). *Peace and power: New direction for building community* (8th ed.). Burlington, MA: Jones & Bartlett Learning.

Coffman, S. (2006). Marilyn Anne Ray: Theory of bureaucratic caring. In A. Marriner Tomey & M. Alligood (Eds.), *Nursing theorists and their work* (pp. 116–139). St. Louis: Mosby-Elsevier.

Coffman, S. (2014). Marilyn Anne Ray, the theory of bureaucratic caring. In M. Alliigood (Ed.), *Nursing theorists and their work* (8th ed.) (pp. 98–119). Elsevier.

Cohen, A. (1985). *The symbolic construction of community*. New York: Routledge.

Dalai Lama. (1999). *Ethics for the new millennium*. New York: Riverhead Books.

Dauer, S. (2006). Possible anthropological contributions. *Anthropology News, 47*(4), 6.

Davidheiser, M. (2007). Overview of peace and conflict resolution study and practice. *Anthropology News, 48*(7), 11–12.

Davidson, A., & Ray, M. (1991). Studying the human-environment phenomenon using the science of complexity. *Advances in Nursing Science, 13*(2), 73–87.

Davidson, A., Ray, M., & Turkel, M. (Eds.)(2011). *Nursing, caring, and complexity science: For human-environment well-being*. New York: Springer Publishing Company.

Davies, M. (2006). *Historics*. New York: Routledge.

Day, G. (2006). *Community and everyday life (The new sociology)*. New York: Routledge.

Delanty, G. (2003). *Community*. New York: Routledge.

Douglas, M. (1999). Editorial [Transcultural Nursing]. *Journal of Transcultural Nursing, 10*(1), 5. [First editorial publication with new Editor of the *Journal of Transcultural Nursing* with Sage Periodicals Press).

Douglas, M., Uhl-Pierce, J., Rosenkoetter, M. et al. (2011). Standards of practice for culturally competent care. Update. *Journal of Transcultural Nursing, 22*(4), 317–333.

Dumit, J. (2004). *Picturing personhood: Brains, scans and biomedical identity.* Princeton: Princeton University Press.

Dunbar, R., Knight, C., & Power, C. (Eds.). (1999). *The evolution of culture.* New Brunswick, NJ: Rutgers University Press.

Dzurec, L., Kennison, M., & Albataineh, R. (2014). Unacknowledged threats proffered "in a Manner of Speaking": Recognizing workplace bullying as shaming. *Journal of Nursing Scholarship, 46*(4), 281–291.

Economy, E., & Levi, M. (2014). *By all means necessary: How China's quest is changing the world.* Oxford: Oxford University Press.

Espinoza, C., Ukeja, M., & Rusch, C. (2010). *Managing the millennials.* New York: Wiley.

Etzioni, A. (1993). *The spirit of community.* New York: Crown Publishers, Inc.

Fishkin, J. (1992). *The dialogue of justice: Toward a self-reflective society.* New Haven: Yale University Press.

Floridi, L. (2014). *The fourth revolution: How the infosphere is reshaping human reality.* London: MacMillan Palgrave: Polity.

Giger, J. & Davidhizar, R. (2003). *Transcultural nursing: assessment and intervention* (4th ed.). St. Louis: Mosby.

Goodwin, B. (2003). Patterns of wholeness. *Resurgence, 1*(21), 12–14.

Gutmann, A. (1994). *Multiculturalism.* Princeton, NJ: Princeton University Press.

Habermas, H. (1994). Struggles for recognition in the democratic constitutional state. In A. Gutmann (Ed.), *Multiculturalism* (pp. 107–148). Princeton: Princeton University Press.

Habermas, J. (1995). *Theory of moral consciousness and communicative action.* Cambridge, MA: The MIT Press.

Habermas, J. (2006). On the relations between the secular liberal state and religion. In H. de Vries & L. Sullivan (Eds.). *Political theologies: Public religions in a post-secular world* (pp. 252-260). New York: Fordham University Press.

Halper, E. (2006). *One and many in Aristotle's metaphysics: The central books* (Vol. 2). Las Vegas, NV: Parmenides Press.

Hamacher, W. (2006). The right not to use rights. In H. de Vries & L. Sullivan (Eds.). *Political theologies: Public religions in a post-secular world* (pp. 671–690). New York: Fordham University Press.

Harman, W. (1998). *Global mind change* (2nd ed.). San Francisco: Berrett-Koehler Publishers, Inc.

Hartigan, J. (2006). Saying "socially constructed" is not enough. *Anthropology News, 47*(2), 8.

Hegel, G. (1977). *Hegel: The essential writings* (Ed. with intro. by F. Weiss). New York: Harper Perennial.

Heidegger, M. (1962). *Being and time.* (J. Macquarrie & E. Robinson, Trans.). San Francisco: HarperSanFrancisco.

Helman, C. (1997). *Culture, health and illness* (3rd ed.). Oxford: Butterworth Heinemann.

Ho, M. (2003). Dance of life: Holistic science. *Resurgence, 1*(216), 18–19.

Horn, B. (1995). Transcultural nursing and child-rearing of the Muckleshoots. In M. Leininger (Ed.), *Transcultural nursing: Concepts, theories, research & practices* (2nd ed., pp. 501–515). New York: McGraw-Hill, Inc. *Into the furnace of war. Library of Social Sciences.* Retrieved Newlsletter/Blog, oanderson@libraryofsocialscience.com

Inwood, M. (2008). *Hegel: Philosophy of mind, translated with introduction and commentary* (Trans. by W. Wallace & A. Miller). New York: Oxford University Press, Inc.

Johanson, D., & Shreeve, J. (1989). *Lucy's child: The discovery of a human ancestor.* New York: Avon Books.

Journal of Transcultural Nursing, 10(1), 5–74. [Entire Issue on Transcultural Nursing].

Kaszycka, K., Štrkalj, G. & Strzalko, J. (2009). Current views of European anthropologists on race: Influence of educational and ideological background. *American Anthropologist, 111*(1), 43–56.

Kavanaugh, K., & Kennedy, P. (1992). *Promoting cultural diversity: Strategies for health care professionals.* Newbury Park, CA: Sage Publications.

Kirkpatrick, F. (1986). *Community: A trinity of models.* Washington, DC: Georgetown University Press.

Kurzweil, R. (2005). *The singularity is near.* New York: Viking.

Leininger, M. (1970). *Anthropology and nursing: Two worlds to blend.* New York: John Wiley & Sons.

Leininger, M. (1978). *Transcultural nursing: Concepts, theory and practices.* New York: John Wiley & Sons.

Leininger, M. (1991). *Culture care diversity and universality: A theory of nursing.* New York: National League for Nursing Press.

Leininger, M. (1997a). Transcultural nursing research to transform nursing education and practice: 40 years. *Image: The Journal of Nursing Scholarship 29*(4), 341–354.

Leininger, M. (1997b). Transcultural spirituality: A comparative care and health focus. In M. Roach (Ed.), *Caring from the heart: The convergence of caring and spirituality.* New York: Paulist Press.

Leininger, M., & McFarland, M. (Eds.). (2006). *Culture care diversity & universality: A worldwide theory of nursing* (2nd ed.). Sudbury, MA: Jones and Bartlett.

Lemkow, A. (1990). *The wholeness principle: Dynamics of unity within science, religion & society.* Wheaton, IL: Quest Books.

Leroi, A. (2004). *Mutants: On genetic variety and the human body.* New York: Viking.

Lipson, J., & Dibble, S. (2005). *Culture and clinical care.* San Francisco: The University of California Press.

Locsin, R., Purnell, M., Tanioka, T., & Osaka, K. (2011). Human rights and humanoid relationships in nursing and complexity science. In A. Davidson, M. Ray, & M. Turkel (Eds.), *Nursing, caring, and complexity science: For human-environment well-being.* New York: Springer Publishing Company.

Longo, J. (2007). Horizontal violence among nursing students. *Archives of Psychiatric Nursing, 21,* 177–178.

Longo, J., & Sherman, R. (2007). Leveling horizontal violence. *Nursing Management, 38*(3), 34–37, 50–51.

Lowe, J., & Nichols, L. (2014). Utilisation of a Native American nursing conceptual framework: Implications for practice and research. *Australian Journal of Advanced Nursing 31*(2), 13–22.

Lustig, M., & Koester, J. (2000). *Among us: Essays on identity, belonging, and intercultural competence.* New York: Longman.

Marcel, G. (1952). *Man against mass society.* Chicago: Henry Regnery Company.

Martin, M. (2015). Gender equality and empowerment of women in Arab countries: A transcultural caring perspective. *International Journal for Human Caring, 19*(1), 13–18.

McFarland, M., & Wehbe-Alamah, H. (2015). *Leininger's culture care diversity and universality: A worldwide*

theory of nursing (3rd ed.). Burlington, MA: Jone & Bartlett Learning.

Merton, T. (1985). *Love and living* (Eds. N. Stone & P. Hart). New York: Harcourt Brace Jovanovich Publishers.

Miller, J., Leininger, M., Leuning, C., Pacquiao, D., Andrews, M., Ludwig-Beymer, P., & Papadopoulos, I. (2008). Transcultural Nursing Society position statement on human rights. *Journal of Transcultural Nursing, 19*(1), 5–7.

Morgan, G. (1998). *Images of organization.* San Francisco: Berrett-Koehler Publishers, Inc.

Morris, E. (2012). Respect, protection, faith, and love: Major care constructs identified within the subculture of selected urban African American adolescent gang members. *Journal of Transcultural Nursing 23*(2), 262–269.

Morse, J., Bottorff, J., Neander, W., & Solberg, S. (1991). Comparative analysis of conceptualizations of caring. *Image: The Journal of Nursing Scholarship, 23,* 119–126.

Nagel, J. (1991). The political construction of ethnicity. In N. R. Yetman (Ed.), *Majority and minority: The dynamics of race and ethnicity in American life* (pp. 76-86). Boston: Allyn & Bacon.

Nagel, J. (1994). Constructing ethnicity: Creating and recreating ethnic identity and culture. *Social Problems, 41,* 152-176.

Nagel, J. (1995). American Indian ethnic renewal: Politics and the resurgence of identity. *American Sociological Review 60,* 947-965.

Newman, M. (1986). *Health as expanding consciousness.* St. Louis: Mosby.

Newman, M., Smith, M., Dexheimer-Pharris, M., & Jones, D. (2008). The focus of the discipline. *Advances in Nursing Science, 31*(1), E16-27.

Nightingale, F. (1969). *Notes on nursing: What it is and what it is not.* New York: Dover. (Original work published 1860)

O'Murchu, D. (1997). *Quantum theology: Spiritual implications of the new physics.* New York: The Crossword Publishing Company.

Palmer, P. (1993). *To know as we are known: Education as a spiritual journey.* San Francisco: HarperSanFrancisco.

Parse, R. (1998). *The human becoming school of thought: A perspective for nurses and other health professionals.* Thousand Oaks, CA: Sage.

Parse, R. (2005). The human becoming school of thought. In M. Parker (Ed.), *Nursing theories, nursing practice* (pp. 227–262). Philadelphia: F. A. Davis Company.

Peer, C. (2007). Theatre grad brings fantasy to life. *McMaster Times*, Fall Edition, 28.

Pharris, M. (2005). Margaret A. Newman: Health as expanding consciousness. In M. Parker (Ed.), *Nursing theories, nursing practice* (pp. 263–286). Philadelphia: F. A. Davis Company.

Phillips, A. (2007). *Multiculturalism without culture*. Princeton: Princeton University Press.

Phillips, J. (1994). The open-ended nature of the science of unitary human beings. In M. Madrid & E. Barrett (Eds.), *Rogers' scientific art of nursing practice*. New York: National League for Nursing Press.

Pollock, M. (2006). Everyday antiracism in education. *Anthropology News, 47*(2), 9–10.

Postero, N. (2007). *Now we are citizens: Indigenous politics in postmulticultural Bolivia*. Stanford, CA: Stanford University Press.

Purnell, L., & Paulanka, B. (2008). *Transcultural health care: A culturally competent approach* (2nd ed.). Philadelphia: F. A. Davis Company.

Rawls, J. (1971). *A theory of justice*. Cambridge: Harvard University Press.

Ray, M. (1981a). A study of caring within an institutional culture. *Dissertation Abstracts International, 42*(06) (University Microfilms No. 8127787).

Ray, M. (1981b). A philosophical analysis of caring within nursing. In M. Leininger (Ed.), *Caring: An essential human need* (pp. 25–36). Thorofare, NJ: Charles B. Slack, Inc.

Ray, M. (1989a). Transcultural caring: Political and economic visions. *Journal of Transcultural Nursing, 1*(1), 17–21.

Ray, M. (1989b). The theory of bureaucratic caring for nursing practice in the organizational culture. *Nursing Administration Quarterly, 13*(2), 31–42.

Ray, M. (1992). Critical theory as a framework to enhance nursing science. *Nursing Science Quarterly 5*(3), 98–101.

Ray, M. (1994a). Complex caring dynamics: A unifying model of nursing inquiry. *Theoretic and Applied Chaos in Nursing, 1*(1), 23–32.

Ray, M. (1994b). Transcultural nursing ethics: A framework and model for transcultural ethical analysis. *Journal of Holistic Nursing, 12*(3), 251–264.

Ray, M. (1997). Illuminating the meaning of caring: Unfolding the sacred art of divine love. In M. Roach (Ed.), *Caring from the heart: The convergence of caring and spirituality* (pp. 163–178). New York: Paulist Press.

Ray, M. (1998). Complexity and nursing science. *Nursing Science Quarterly, 11*, 91–93.

Ray, M. (1999a). Critical theory as a framework to enhance nursing science. In E. Polifroni & M. Welch (Eds.), *Perspectives on philosophy of science in nursing* (pp. 382–386). Philadelphia: Lippincott.

Ray, M. (1999b). Transcultural caring in primary health care. *National Academies of Practice Forum, 1*(3), 177–182.

Ray, M. (2001a). The theory of bureaucratic caring. In M. Parker (Ed.), *Nursing theories, nursing practice* (pp. 421–431). Philadelphia: F. A. Davis Company.

Ray, M. (2001b). Complex culture and technology: Toward a global caring communitarian ethics of nursing. In R. Locsin (Ed.), *Advancing technology, caring, and nursing* (pp. 41–52). Westport, CT: Auburn House.

Ray, M. (2005). The theory of bureaucratic caring. In M. Parker (Ed.), *Nursing theories, nursing practice* (2nd ed., pp. 360–379). Philadelphia: F. A. Davis Company.

Ray, M. (2010a). *Transcultural caring dynamics in nursing and health care*. Philadelphia: F. A. Davis Company.

Ray, M. (2010b). *A study of caring within an institutional culture: The discovery of the Theory of Bureaucratic Caring*. Germany: Lamber Academic Publishers.

Ray, M. (2010c). Creating caring organizations and cultures through communitarian ethics. *Journal of the World Universities Forum, 3*(5), 41–52.

Ray, M. (2011). Complex caring dynamics: A unifying model of nursing inquiry (pp. 31–52). In A. Davidson, M. Ray, & M. Turkel (Eds.), *Nursing, caring, and complexity science: For human-environment well-being*. New York: Springer Publishing Company. (Reprinted with revisions from original article in Theoretic and Applied Chaos in Nursing (1994).

Ray, M., & Turkel, M. (2014). Caring as emancipatory nursing praxis: The Theory of Relational Caring Complexity. *Advances in Nursing Science, 37*(2), 132–146.

Ray, M., & Turkel, M. (2015). Marilyn Anne Ray's Theory of Bureaucratic Caring. In M. Smith (Ed.), *Nursing theories and nursing practice* (4th ed.). Philadelphia: F. A. Davis Company.

Ray, M., & Turkel, M. (2001). Culturally based caring. In L. Dunphy & J. Winland-Brown (Eds.), *Primary care: The art and science of advanced practice nursing* (pp. 43–55). Philadelphia: F. A. Davis Company.

Ray, M., & Turkel, M. (2012). The transtheoretical evolution of caring science within complex systems. *International Journal for Human Caring, 169*(2), 28–49.

Ray, M., Turkel, M., & Marino, F. (2002). The transformative process for nursing in workforce redevelopment. *Nursing Administration Quarterly, 26*(2), 1–14.

Rheingold, H. (2002). *Smart mobs: The next social revolution.* Cambridge, MA: Basic Books.

Roach, M. (2002). *The human act of caring: A blueprint for the health professions* (rev. ed.). Ottawa: Canadian Hospital Association Press. (Original work published 1987)

Rogers, E. (2003). *Diffusion of innovations* (5th ed.). New York: Free Press.

Rogers, M. (1970). *An introduction to the theoretical basis of nursing.* Philadelphia: F. A. Davis Company.

Rogers, M. (1994). The science of unitary human beings: Current perspectives. *Nursing Science Quarterly, 2,* 33–35.

Rosenkoetter, M., & Nardi, D. (2007). American Academy of Nursing expert panel on global nursing and health: White paper on global nursing and health. *Journal of Transcultural Nursing, 18*(4), 305–315.

Rushton, J. (1999). *Race, evolution & behavior.* New Brunswick, NJ: Transaction Publishers.

Saint Augustine. (1958). *City of God* (G. Walsh, D.B. Zema, G. Monahan, & D. J. Honan, Trans.). New York: Image Books.

Scherer, M. (2006). Saint John: The miracle of secular reason. In H. de Vries & L. Sullivan (Eds.), *Political theologies: Public religions in a post-secular world* (pp. 341-362). New York: Fordham University Press.

Sherman, D., & Nardin, T. (Eds.). (2006). *Terror, culture, politics.* Bloomington: Indiana University Press.

Sherman, R. (2012). What followers need from their leaders. *American Nurse Today, 7*(9), 62.

Sherman, R. (2013). Building a sense of community on nursing units. *American Nurse Today, 8*(3), 32–34.

Sherwood, G. (1997). Meta-synthesis of qualitative analyses of caring: Defining a therapeutic model of nursing. *Advanced Nursing Practice, 3*(1), 32–42.

Smith, B. (1996). *On the origin of objects.* Cambridge, MA: MIT Press.

Smith, M. (1999). Caring and the science of unitary human beings. *Advances in Nursing Science, 21,* 14–28.

Smith, M. (2011). Philosophical and theoretical perspectives related to complexity science in nursing. In A. Davidson, M. Ray, & M. Turkel (Eds.), *Nursing, caring, and complexity science: For human-environment well-being* (pp. 1–20). New York: Springer Publishing Company.

Smith, M., Turkel, M., & Wolf, Z. (2013). *Caring in nursing classics: An essential resource.* New York: Springer Publishing Company.

Spector, R. (2003). *Cultural diversity in health and illness* (6th ed.). Upper Saddle River, NJ: Prentice Hall Health.

Stace, W. (1955). *The Philosophy of Hegel.* London: Dover Publications, Inc.

Sumner, J. (2006). Concept analysis: The moral construct of caring in nursing as communicative action. *International Journal for Human Caring, 10*(10), 8–16.

Sumner, J. (2010). A critical lens on the instruments of caring in nursing theory. *Advances in Nursing Science, 33*(1), E17–E26.

Sumner, J. (2008). *The moral construct of caring in nursing as communicative action: A theory for nursing practice.* Verlag, Germany: VDM Verlag Dr. Müller Aktiengesellschaft & Co. KG.

Swinderman, T. (2005). *The magnetic appeal of nurse informaticians: Caring attractor for emergence.* Doctor of nursing science dissertation, Florida Atlantic University, Boca Raton, FL.

Swinderman, T. (2011). Technological change in health care electronic documentation as facilitated through the science of complexity. In A. Davidson, M. Ray, & M. Turkel (Eds). *Nursing, caring, and complexity science: For human-environment well-being* (pp. 309–319). New York: Springer Publishing Company.

Tavernise, S. (2008, July 31). Turkish court calls ruling party constitutional. *New York Times.* Retrieved July 31, 2008, from www.nytimes.com/2008/7/31/world/europe/31turkey.html?

Taylor, C. (1989). *Sources of the self: The making of modern identity.* Cambridge, MA: Harvard University Press.

Taylor, C. (1991). *The ethics of authenticity*. Cambridge, MA: Harvard University Press.

Taylor, C. (1994). The politics of recognition. In A. Gutmann (Ed.), *Multiculturalism* (pp. 25–73). Princeton: Princeton University Press.

Teilhard de Chardin, P. (1957). *Le milieu divin*. London: Collins Fontana Books.

Teilhard de Chardin, P. (1959). *The phenomenon of man*. New York: Harper & Row Publishers.

Teilhard de Chardin, P. (1965). *Building the earth*. Denville, NJ: Dimensions Books.

Templeton, J. (1999). *Agape love*. Philadelphia: Templeton Foundation Press.

The New American Bible. (1970). New York: Catholic Book Publishing Co.

Thoma, H. (2003). All at the same time: Holistic science. *Resurgence, 1*(216), 15–17.

Thompson, E. (2006). The problem of "race as a social construct". *Anthropology News, 47*(2), 6–7.

Tiller, W. (2005). Paradigms: The other side. In Arntz, W., Chasse, B., & Vicente, M., *What the bleep do we know!?* (pp. 197–253). Deerfield Beach, FL: Health Communications, Inc.

Tuan, M. (1998). *Forever foreigners or honorary whites?* New Brunswick: Rutgers University Press.

Turkel, M. (2007). Dr. Marilyn Ray's theory of bureaucratic caring. *International Journal for Human Caring, 11*(4), 57–74.

Turkel, M., & Ray, M. (2001). Relational complexity: From grounded theory to instrument development and theoretical testing. *Nursing Science Quarterly, 14*(4), 281–287.

Turkel, M., & Ray, M. (2009). Caring for "not-so-picture-perfect patients:" Ethical caring in the moral community of nursing. In R. Locsin & M. Purnell (Eds.), *A contemporary nursing process: The (un)bearable weight of knowing in nursing* (pp. 225–249). New York: Springer Publishing Company.

United Nations' Educational, Scientific, and Cultural Organization (UNESCO). *Universal declaration on cultural diversity* (UDCD). (2001).

United Nations Millennium Development Goals (MDGs). A global agenda beyond 2015. Retrieved from www.un.org/en/ecosoc/about/mdg.shtml

Vallacher, R., & Nowak, A. (Eds.). (1994). *Dynamical systems in social psychology*. New York: Academic Press, Inc.

Waters, M. (1990). *Ethnic options: Choosing identities in America*. Berkley: University of California Press.

Watson, J. (1979). *Nursing: The philosophy and science of caring*. Boston: Little Brown.

Watson, J. (1988). *Human science, human care*. New York: National League for Nursing.

Watson, J. (2005). *Caring science as sacred science*. Philadelphia: F. A. Davis Company.

Watson, J. (2008). *The philosophy and science of caring* (2nd rev. ed.). Colorado: University of Colorado Press.

Wenger, F. (2006). Culture care and health of Russian and Vietnamese refugee communities. In M. Leininger & M. McFarland (Eds.), *Culture care diversity and universality: A worldwide theory of nursing* (2nd ed., pp. 327–348). Sudbury, MA: Jones and Bartlett Publishers.

Werner, C., & Bell, D. (Eds.). (2004). *Values and valuables*. Walnut Creek, CA: Alta Mira Press.

Winick, C. (1970). *Dictionary of anthropology*. Toto, NJ: Littlefield, Adams & Company.

Wolf, F. (2005). Paradigms: The other side. In Arntz, W., Chasse, B., & Vicente, M., *What the bleep do we know!?* (pp. 197–253). Deerfield Beach, FL: Health Communications, Inc.

Wolin, R. (2006). Jurgen Habermas and post-secular societies. *The Chronicle of Higher Education, Section B*, B16–B17.

Womack, M. (2005). *Symbols and meaning: A concise introduction*. Lanham, MD: Alta Mira Press.

Zimmerman, B., Lindberg, C., & Pisek, P. (2001). *Edgeware: Insights from complexity science for health care leader* (2nd ed.). Irving, TX: VHA Inc.

Select Bibliography

Byrne, D., & Callaghan, G. (2014). *Complexity theory and the social sciences: The state of the art*. New York: Routledge.

Chase, P. (1999). Symbolism as reference and symbolism as culture. In R. Dunbar, C. Knight & C Power (Eds.), *The evolution of culture* (pp. 34–49). New Brunswick, NJ: Rutgers University Press.

Davidson, A., Ray, M., & Turkel, M. (Eds.)(2011). *Nursing, caring, and complexity science: For human-environment well-being*. New York: Springer Publishing Company.

Eriksson, K. (1997). Caring, spirituality and suffering. In M. Roach (Ed.), *Caring from the heart: The convergence of caring and spirituality* (pp. 68–84). New York: Paulist Press.

Hagelin, J. (2005). Science and religion: The great divorce. In W. Arntz, B. Chasse, & M. Vicente, *What the bleep do we know!?* (pp. 131–166). Deerfield Beach, FL: Health Communications, Inc.

McFarland, M. (2006). Madeleine Leininger: Culture care theory of diversity and universality. In A. Marriner Tomey & M. Alligood (Eds.), *Nursing theorists and their work* (pp. 643–662). St. Louis: Mosby-Elsevier.

McFarland, M., & Wehbe-Alamah, H. (Eds.) (2015). *Leininger's culture care diversity and universality: A worldwide theory of nursing* (3rd ed.). Burlington, MA: Jones & Bartlett Learning.

Peat, F. (2002). *From certainty to uncertainty: The story of science and ideas in the twentieth century.* Washington, DC: John Henry Press.

Ray, M., & Turkel, M. (2014). Caring as emancipatory praxis: The theory of Relational Caring Complexity. *Advances in Nursing Science, 37*(2), 132–146).

Roach, M. (Ed.). (1997). *Caring from the heart: The convergence of caring and spirituality.* New York: Paulist Press.

Smith, A., Turkel, M., & Wolf, Z. (Eds.)(2013). *Caring in nursing classics: An essential resource.* New York: Springer Publishing Company.

Toft, M. (2005). *The geography of ethnic violence: Identity, interests, and the indivisibility of territory.* Princeton: Princeton University Press.

Turkel, M., & Ray, M. (2000). Relational complexity: A theory of the nurse-patient relationship within an economic context. *Nursing Science Quarterly, 13*, 307–313.

Wilber, K. (Ed.). (1982). *The holographic paradigm and other paradoxes.* Boulder, CO: New Science Library.

Wolf, Z. (2014). *Exploring rituals in nursing: Joining art and science.* New York: Springer Publishing Company.

Wolfe, A. (2011). *Political evil: How it is and how to combat it.* New York: Vintage Books.

CHAPTER 5

Universal Sources

Examination of the earliest recorded religions reveals three common features: polytheism, animism, and at a slightly later stage a strangely enduring doctrine, the belief in some form of Universal Mind accessible to the individual under suitable circumstances. A great variety of names have described this Universal Mind, among them, Tao, Logos, Brahman, Atman, the Absolute, Mana, Holy Ghost [Spirit], Weltgeist, or simply God. The Universal Mind confers existence on conscious beings in varying degrees, and these beings create, out of the minds bestowed on them and in accordance with principles imposed by the Universal Mind, everything else they call real or existing. (Margenau, 1984, pp. 106 & 129)

Chapter Objectives

1. To appreciate the dynamics of the universal mind and universal sources of religion in culture.
2. To define theology, spirituality, and religion for understanding of transcultural dynamics and caring.
3. To describe spiritual belongingness in religion, science, and nursing.
4. To describe holism, science, and spirituality for nursing.
5. To illuminate spirituality and human caring.
6. To describe transcultural spiritual caring for nursing practice.

Continued

KEY WORDS

Universal Sources • Universal Mind • God • Jesus Christ • Higher power • religion • belongingness • theology • spirituality • religion • holism • complexity science • spiritual nursing • spiritual caring • transcultural spirituality • spiritual suffering

131

Chapter Objectives—cont'd

7. To describe spiritual suffering and spiritual healing for nursing and health-care practice.
8. To identify central precepts of select religions and political and communal theology.
9. To present transcultural caring experiences (case studies) that will illuminate the spiritual in the lifeworld and nursing practice.

KEY WORDS—cont'd
- spiritual healing
- faith-based communities
- diverse religions • Judaism
- Christianity • Islam
- Hinduism • Buddhism
- Shintoism • Confucianism
- Aboriginal and Native Religions • Myth Spirituality
- Integrative Spirituality

Dimension of the Model

Figure 5–1: Dimension of the model: Universal Sources.

This chapter will advance and explore the notion that, when seeking to understand transcultural dynamics in nursing and health, not only caring, ethical, and cultural values play a role but so do things viewed as sacred—the theological, spiritual, and religious. "Religion is a central aspect of any civilization" (Woods, 2005, p. 217) and has been characterized as the Universal Mind and viewed as Universal Sources (see Fig. 5-1) (Margenau, 1984; Ray, 1994, 2010a, 2010b, 2010c, 2011). Thus, the notion of universal as belongingingness can be applied to all cultures in the world. Religions are similar and dissimilar to each other. In the world, "19 major world religions that are subdivided into 270 larger religious groups and an estimated 34,000 separate Christian groups" were identified (Suarez & Lewis, 2005, p. 425). Despite the seeming growth in religion, however, reports show a decline, especially in Christianity in Europe (Eberstadt, 2013). However, the common theme over the course of history is a religious or spiritual inclination toward the discovery of self-in-relation to God (i.e., Higher

Power, Absolute, Almighty, Great Spirit, Source, Creation, and Force) by means of faith and reason (Pope Benedict XVI, 2006). "Faith is the realization of what is hoped for and evidence of things not seen" (Hebrews 11:1, *The New American Bible*, 1987, p. 1534). In essence, faith is trusting in what we do not fully understand. People have felt a religious instinct about the existence of a superior, spiritual reality encompassing our world; but the superior is conceived of in different ways (Heschel, 1954; Joseph, 2002; Leininger, 1991). Universal Sources not only is expressed as a transcendent God or a Higher Power, but also as a mystical force of nature, ancestor worship, myths, or meta-normal experience with or without reference to God (Curtis, 1993; Durkheim & Mauss, 1963; Ray, 1994; Van Iersel, 1973). In the global arena of today, religion or belief is expressed by diverse cultures in complex ways: sometimes through the precepts of monotheistic/God-centered or prophetic religions, such as Judaism, Christianity, or Islam; through the teachings of Eastern, Asian, or indigenous religions, such as Buddhism, Hinduism, Shintoism, and Confucianism; or through New Age spirituality, and spirituality synthesized from diverse views on spirituality, the sciences of complexity and psychology, native spirituality, and even what now are termed political theologies (Arntz, Chasse, & Vincente, 2005; Csikszentmihalyi, 1993; de Vries & Sullivan, 2006; Wiker & Witt, 2006; Wolfe, 2013).

Nursing has long recognized the importance of the concepts of the religious and spiritual in its professional writings and caring practice. Nightingale experienced a spiritual calling, and stated that God spoke to her and called her to his service. Nightingale responded to the call by developing the discipline and profession of modern nursing to meet the needs for health and nursing care (Macrae, 2001).

Subsequently, the spiritual has been honored and exemplified in many nursing philosophies and theories throughout the history of nursing (Alligood, 2014; Smith & Parker, 2015). Nurses are concerned with how their patients construct their reality—how they integrate elements of their spiritual and cultural heritage into the meaning of health and illness (Andrews & Boyle, 2007, 2015; Eriksson, 2006; Leininger, 1991; Ray, 1994, 1997, 1999, 2010a, 2010b, 2010c).

Nursing has been defined as holistic and illuminates caring in the human health experience. Health and illness are holistic processes and correlate neurobiologically, psychologically, culturally, and spiritually. Health and illness involve consciousness and include the dynamics of the human-environment relationship—our personal and cultural histories and relationships, senses, reason, free will, and transcendent nature (Newman, 1986, 1994; Newman, Sime, & Corcoran-Perry, 1991; Newman, Smith, Dexheimer-Pharris, & Jones, 2008; Watson, 2005). Leininger's awareness of cultural illness and health, along with the influence of religion and transcultural caring in her cross-cultural research, culminated in inclusion of religion/spirituality as one of the central dimensions in her theory of Cultural Care Diversity and Universality (1978, 1991, 1997; Leininger & McFarland, 2006; McFarland, 2006; McFarland & Wehbe-Alamah, 2015).

The commitment to holism; harmony of body, mind, and spirit; and transcultural caring as compassion and right action within the dynamics of culture, illuminate the vitality and authenticity of the spiritual in the nurse-patient relationship (Ray, 1989a; 1994, 1997). Scholars and clinicians continue to pursue the relationship between culture, spirituality, and the quality of life by acknowledging caring, compassion, and love (*caritas*) as the foundation of nursing (Eriksson, 2006, 2007; Ray, 1981a, 1981b, 1989a, 1989b, 1997; Watson, 2005, 2008). Understanding human suffering and the need for spiritual healing is a renewed focus for nursing. Palliative care, faith-based transcultural community nursing, and the development of parish nursing (i.e., church-based health promotion and disease prevention) are fulfilling the need (Newlin, Knafl, & Melkus, 2002; Solari-Twadell & McDermott, 2005).

In this chapter, the dimension of the model of Transcultural Caring Dynamics in Nursing and Health Care: Universal Sources illuminate the meaning of the Universal Mind, the Universal God,

and Universal Sources that relates to the idea of the spiritual and religious, and the traditions that shape the moral caring values that all people of diverse cultures hold. By identifying the meaning of Universal Sources (e.g., religious or spiritual traditions) and examining similarities and differences, nurses are more aware of religious beliefs and values and how they influence what emerges and the choices that are made in health and illness. Although the Universal Mind is ubiquitous, Universal Sources—religious and spiritual traditions (e.g., religious holy books, precepts, signs, symbols, rituals, songs, and stories)—of diverse people are specific and vary within and among religions and cultures. As an example, " [t]he United States is the most religious and one of the most diverse and most changing nations in the world' (Suarez & Lewis, 2005, p. 425). Knowledge of religious influences on health and illness is important for nursing. Good cross-cultural comparative evaluation addresses identification of and reflection on similarities and differences between and among religious traditions. Because it is not possible for a nurse to know all elements of the many religions of the world and how specific religious or spiritual beliefs affect a patient's response to illness and health, it is critical to **appreciate, learn about, question,** and **listen** to the accounts of patients and family members' religious and spiritual experiences and compare and contrast them with our own. These actions will help a nurse to understand what is valued in self and others. Active listening or communicative spiritual-ethical caring action will facilitate the provision of comprehensive and competent transcultural spiritual care to patients.

Dynamics of the Universal Mind and Universal Sources

The Universal Mind has shaped man and been shaped by the relationship between God and man or a Higher Power throughout recorded history. The Universal Mind has been illuminated since the earliest times in Western and Eastern philosophies and has been translated into sources of religious or spiritual beliefs and values. Although controversy exists from different *scientific* sources about the idea and nature of God, the *religious* idea suggests that, for example, God as Creator in the monotheistic religions of Judaism, Christianity, and Islam; dharma as the inner lawfulness of being in the Hindu view; and Tao, as the supreme ultimate of heaven in the Confucian view exists (de Vries & Sullivan,

2006; Pope Benedict XVI, 2006a; Pope Francis, 2013; Ray, 1994). "We [human beings] are not some casual andmeaningless product of evolution" (Homily, Pope Benedict XVI, 2008, p. 2). God is personified and considered everywhere, thus universal. The theologian-paleontologist, Teilhard de Chardin described the existence of God and the personification in this way—". . . let the light of your countenance shine upon us in its universality" (1960, p. 132). ". . . [P]eople today have a longing for God, for spirituality, for religion...."(Pope Benedict XVI, 2006b, p. 2). The psychologist, Carl Jung stated that ". . . there has not been one [patient] whose problem in the last resort was not that of finding a religious outlook on life" (Jung 1960, 1964). In this spiritual yearning of the human heart, human beings seek meaning and wisdom, the highest quest of the soul (Smith, 1991). The Biblical scriptures connote that God, the Universal Mind, and humans are relational. The human ability to care and be cared for underscores belongingness to someone or something. As such, God is a living being who cares and loves—a transcendent being outside space and time, yet immanent, within and penetrating the universe. The noted Jewish theologian Buber remarked that ". . . God is the wholly Other; But He is also the wholly Same, the wholly Present" (1958, p. 79). In other words, God, who is Pure Truth, Intelligence, and Love, is *supernatural,* completely transcendent, outside space and time, but revealed on his testimony and authority through sacred books and reason, thus, is immanent, that is wholly the same (never changing) and present by his manifestation to and in the world in "divine light and grace," which surpasses human understanding. "Human or *natural faith* is acceptance of truths on the authority of other men" (Merton, 1951, p. 30). ". . . supernatural grace enters natural faith; the greater one's faith, one's love, through prayer and sacrifice, the more completely one is united to God" (Merton, 1951, p. 256). "There is divine meaning in the life of the world . . . [in this belongingness] we take part in creation, meet the Creator, reach out to Him, helpers and companions" (Buber, 1958, p. 82).

THEOLOGY, SPIRITUALITY, AND RELIGION

It is impossible to divorce true theological and spiritual knowledge from moral conduct or moral improvement in everyday life. *Theology, spirituality, and religion including ethics* are interrelated.

Every religion has some version of the Golden Rule—"do unto others as you would have them do unto you" (Smith, 1991). The foundation of Universal Sources is God or also understood as a Higher Power or the "Good" who reaches out in hospitality and generosity, love and compassion, caring, and justice (Nouwen, 1979; Ray, 1989a). The process of discovering the Universal Mind through the meaning of Universal Sources is understanding the spiritual and religious life, a reaching inward and outward: first to appreciate the soul, our innermost self; second, reaching out to God; and third, reaching out to each other in community (Nouwen, 1975).

Definitions of Theological, Spiritual, and Religious

The theological, spiritual, and religious terms used to explain the transcendent nature of God or a Higher Power often are indistinguishable. For the purposes of this chapter, the following definitions and characteristics of each are *offered.*

Theological refers to the recognition and study of the supernatural or transcendent, God, the creative principle of the universe characterized by an infinite, all-embracing love, completeness, wholeness, and perfection. The finite mind cannot fully grasp the infinite. It is a mystery partially hidden and partially revealed with no definitive human solution (Smith, 1989, 1991). Saint Augustine (1958; Merton, 1961, 1985) acknowledged that there is belief first before understanding. "Originally the term *theology* was applied not to the systematic study of religious dogmas but to the mystical experience" (Capra, Steindl-Rast with Matus, 1991, p. 15). Theology generally is viewed as ". . . the intelligence of God that is the fruit of loving, inquiring, and investigating faith" (Merton, 1985, p. 105). The purpose of theology is to know, love, and serve God. The study and practice of theology is the penetration into the deepest mystery, one's relationship with God by faith, hope, love (i.e., the theological virtues), and through the gifts of grace (i.e., the presence of God), reflection, prayer, reason, and knowledge generation (Spitzer, 2010). There is the endeavor to understand what "religion" as central to Universal Sources implies. By studying the sacred books, such as the *Holy Bible, Qur'an, Vedas, Book of Mormon*; various articles of faith; Catholic Catechism or encyclicals; and principles of Buddha and Confucius, theologians, philosophers, and others interpret, explain, and clarify readings, values, morals, rituals, symbols, and historical traditions.

Spiritual refers to an intelligent and loving presence, an inner communion with someone or thing greater than ourselves. Moreover, spirituality is an inner peace, a realization of the presence of God, Infinite Power, or Creative Force within that flows into or reveals itself in daily life (Goldsmith, 1959). Spirituality is connected with the "soul" (the inner life and the nature of meaning and a meaningful life). Spirituality is connected with diverse cultures and spiritual practices and is not limited to persons who profess a specific religious faith. Spirituality without religion is often interconnected with psychology where there is morality based upon human flourishing, integrated with science and reason (Harris, 2014). As such, spirituality can exist without religion, but authentic religion cannot exist without spirituality (Capra, Steindl-Rast with Matus, 1991). Although we are aware that while seeking the transcendent, God as the highest good and the good as the highest principle in life, we are aware that in life, in culture, even in the history and practice of religion, people suffer and continue to suffer at the hands of evil, by their own bondage to sin or wrongdoing, and by the neglectful and hurtful actions of others, or situations in and of nature. Humans have to deal with the mystery of evil, the "shadow side" of reality, the dark side, or sin (Buber, 1952; De Caussade, 1966; Sanford, 1988; Schwarz, 1995; *The New American Bible*, 1987). Human frailties, vices, and even the supposed good intentions of people have led to abuses and violence against other human beings and animals and the universe itself in all forms, including physical and sexual abuse, persecutions, ethnic prejudices, social and cultural dislocation, wars and "holy" wars based on religious ideologies, and unsustainable practices of the environment (Boulding, 1988; Eriksson, 2006, 2007; Henderson, 2007). Spiritual struggle and distress emerge from pain and suffering. Generally there is a "cry for help" from within to God and others for spiritual healing and transformation, an inner peace that quiets the body, mind, and soul.

Religious refers to the experience of the "holy" (sacred) where the knowledge of God, principles and articles of faith, teachings, and insights from the Holy Books, and religious traditions facilitate the unfolding of the spiritual and religious life—living with others in love and truth. (The noted nursing theorist Watson (2005) refers to caring science as a sacred science.) The root of religion is connectedness to God, and one to the other. "In the beginning was the Word, and the Word was with God, and the Word was God" (John, 1:1, *The New American Bible*, 1987, p. 1322). In this reading from the Bible, the meanings of "was" refer to existence, relationship, and prediction—God's dynamic creative word, preexistent Wisdom, and the ultimate intelligibility of reality (Prologue Interpretation of the Gospel of John, p. 1322). The relationship between God and humans is intrinsically dynamic, manifested by grace (presence and love of God, the seed of wisdom), prayer, meditation, thanksgiving, and good works. Being religious highlights a thirst for meaning—the recovery of wholeness (i.e., body, mind, and spirit)—discovery of a focal point that gives meaning to human existence (Capra, Steindl-Rast with Matus, 1991).

Religion is a call to truth. History shows that there is an overriding conviction in human consciousness that brings people in touch with a truth that transcends a natural law that does not change, (How would the nursing theorist Newman's theory of expanding consciousness relate to this idea of transcendence?) Historical monotheistic (God-centered) religions illuminate the love, mercy, and justice of God for human beings (Merton, 1951, 1985); the mystical religions of the East illuminate purification, mindfulness, righteousness, and human-heartedness (Yu-Lan, 1948). Overall, "truth—wherever it may be found is personal, to be known in personal relationships" (Palmer, 1993, p. 49). "Truth contains the image we are seeking—the image of community in which we were first created, the image of relatedness between the knower and the known that certain philosophies of science now affirm" (Palmer, 1993, p. 31). Being religious generates a sense of belongingness to self, each other, creation, and the Creator. In recent years, there have been accounts of the decline of Christianity, and a decline in the family has been noted at the same time, especially in Europe. Because of these historical facts, Eberstadt (2013) reported that the declines might actually be sparking increased interest in both institutions that have been the cornerstone of civilization and community-building in the West.

Learn More

Names of Select Religions and Philosophies

- Judaism
- Christianity
- Mormonism (Latter-Day Saints [LDS])
- Islam
- Hinduism and Sikhism
- Buddhism
- Confucianism
- Shintoism
- Aboriginal and Native Religion
- Myth Spirituality
- New Age and Integrative Spirituality and Baha'i
- Political and Communal Theologies: Building the Earth

Select Major Religions or Philosophies

Please note: The following presentation of diverse religions or spiritual traditions is not complete but presents central precepts of some of the dominant religions and their symbolism and rituals within select geographical areas of the world. For more in-depth information, readers are encouraged to examine books, journals, and Internet sites dedicated to the study of religion and spirituality, anthropology, nursing and holistic health, parish nursing and faith-based community nursing, transcultural nursing, and spiritual caring. *The International Journal for Human Caring, Journal of Holistic Nursing, Journal of Professional Nursing,* and *Journal of Transcultural Nursing, Spirituality and Health* are examples of excellent sources that integrate the diversity of beliefs, values, and caring into nursing and health care.

Judaism

In Judaism, God is a personal Being wherein a covenant has been established between God and his people as established in the Hebrew scripture (Old Testament) and revealed to the prophets. The covenant is a sacred partnership. As communicated to the prophet Moses, "Thus shall you say to the Israelites: the Lord, the God of your fathers, the God of Abraham, the God of Isaac, the God of Jacob has sent me to you. This is my name forever; this is my title for all generations" (Exodus, 3:1, *The New American Bible*, 1987, p. 60). Judaism

is built on the pillar of the Ten Commandments given to Moses (Exodus, 20:1–17, pp. 77–78, *The New American Bible*, 1987). All the prophets focused on morality in Judaism for the Law. Hebrew Scripture illuminates God as Creator and Lawgiver who guides the faithful in righteous living by giving rules that people as free agents with a free will should obey. Israel was called to be holy as God himself. Moral rightness means commanded by God; moral wrongness means forbidden by God (Rachels, 1986).

In the contemporary world, there are three major movements in Judaism: Orthodox, Conservative, and Reform Judaism (Leffler & Jones, 2005). Orthodoxy maintains Jewish tradition and law as it always was from the Hebrew scripture; conservatism interprets Jewish tradition and biblical literature of human input; and Reform Judaism, which began in Germany, espouses more social action and ethical behavior with less concern for Jewish law (Leffler & Jones, 2005). Another form (the 4th denomination called Reconstructionist) originated in the philosophy of Mordecai Kaplan dating back to 1922 and spoke "more meaningfully to the 20th century world" and focused on building a more civil religion rather than a religion grounded in Biblical tradition in the United States (www.myJewishlearning.com). Kabala is a mystical view in Jewish history, at first passed down to others as an oral tradition highlighting secrets revealed to Adam and spiritual insight through meditative practices into the inner workings of God's creation and the forces of nature. It was initially held as authoritative by most orthodox Jews. Today, Jewish Kabala is a system of oral, written, and meditative belief that is accepted more within the branches of liberal Judaism because of the appeal to the need for a sense of meaning, belongingness, and holiness in life (Wolfson, 2006). Jewish religious practices thus may differ between Israel and other nations, some more orthodox, conservative, or liberal and some secular or political depending upon history and interpretation of Jewish law and ideas (Shapiro, 2007). The center of worship is the synagogue or temple. A major symbol of the Jewish faith is the Star of David.

Christianity

As in Judaism, God is personal, absolutely sovereign, transcendent, and good. God in Christianity is also Trinitarian (Woods, 2005). In Christianity, there is belief in the mystery of the three persons in one: Father, Son, and Holy Spirit. In Christian scriptures, a covenant was established between God and human beings, exemplified through the life and death of Jesus Christ (the second person of the Trinity, known as the Son of God or God incarnate), and reflected in the life of the Christian church through the mystery of the Holy Spirit (the third person of the Trinity) (Pope Benedict, XVI, 2006, 2008). As communicated by the apostle, Saint John, all things came through God, and Jesus was the light of the human race (John, 1:21, *The New American Bible*, 1987, pp. 1321–1357). The Christian life is first and foremost about a person's relationship with God, who is revealed in the life, death, and resurrection of Jesus of Nazareth, the Son of God through the Holy Spirit, hence the Holy Trinity (Pope Benedict XVI, 2006). In Christian thought, theology, as explained by Saint Augustine, is faith; "I believe in order to understand" (cited in Merton, 1985, p. 105). *"Supernatural faith* is the belief in truths revealed by God, on the testimony of God, and because of the authority of God Who reveals these truths to us [in the *Holy Bible*]" (Merton, 1951, p. 30). In other words, *"faith* refers to the positive response of a person who hears God's redemptive Word or who encounters God's redemptive acts in history" (Leffler & Jones, 2005, p. 82). The primary truths revealed by God through Jesus Christ are the theological virtues of faith, hope, and love, and the greatest of these is love (St. Paul, 1 Corinthians, 13). God in Christianity is omniscient, omnipotent, and omnipresent, respectively, knowing everything, all powerful, and present everywhere at the same time (*Catechism of the Catholic Church,* 1994).

Christianity has major faith communities— Catholics, Orthodox (Catholic, Russian, and Greek), Protestants, and Evangelical Christians—who belong to the 34,000 different denominations or churches. Some Christians have mixed feelings about whether or not a person can be an authentic Christian if she is "unchurched" (Leffler & Jones, 2005, p. 20). Each faith community has a common belief in God and in the life and teachings of Jesus Christ through the writings of the New Testament and other holy books and the Holy Spirit (the Trinity). The ways in which the *Holy Bible* and writings are interpreted and lived out in experience (i.e., sacraments, prayers, practices, symbols, and rituals) provide knowledge of the structure and practices of both the oneness and diversity of the Christian religion. Love and mercy are outstanding virtues. For Catholics, the establishment of the Papacy (the church, the succession of Popes, and magisterium) and the pillars of the church in the life of Jesus are central. The mainstays include the Creed, the seven Sacraments, and the Lord's Prayer, and the Ten Commandments and interpretation of the Bible as the Word of God in the liturgy of the Mass, and the prayers of the rosary (*Catechism of the Catholic Church,* 1994). For Christians, the major center of worship is the Church and the symbol of Christianity is the Cross.

There are diverse interpretations of theological and cultural ways of life that guide the faithful in the Protestant communion (Leffler & Jones, 2005), and also the Church of Jesus Christ of Latter-Day Saints (LDS) (or the Mormon Church) founded in the United States around 1830 by Joseph Smith. For many Protestant faiths, the Bible is the ground of all belief and value. For example, most evangelicals invoke the principle of *sola scriptura* (scripture alone) as the canon of the faithful (Leffler & Jones, 2005). For Latter-Day Saints (Mormons) the central foundation for belief is the *Book of Mormon* (Smith, 2005) published in 1830, which illuminates the teachings and revelations of Joseph Smith.

Islam

Allah is known as the God of Islam. Surrendering to Allah is a primary force (Ahmed, 2004; Al-Alwain, 2005). Therefore, "Islam means total submission [of the soul] and surrender to Allah" (Coulson, 1969, p. 1). The *Qur'an* (recitation) is the scripture revealed to the prophet, Mohammed (570-632 CE) in the year 622 in Mecca, present day Saudi Arabia. Chapters of the *Qur'an* are called Surahs (Armstrong, 2002). Traditionally, a Muslim is a person who has *made* submission of his entire being to Allah and Allah's demand is that human beings behave to one another with justice, equity, and compassion. Oneness with God is through knowledge and practice of the five pillars of Islam, which teach people "to walk the straight path" (Smith, 1991, p. 242)—the principles that guide Muslims in their relationship with God.

The five pillars of Islam are related to the path to God. The first pillar is the creed, the confession of faith, the *Shahadah,* ". . . there is no god but God and Muhammad is His Prophet" (Smith, 1991, p. 244). The second is to be constant in prayer (*salat*). The third is charity. The fourth is observance of Ramadan (religious observance to commemorate the beginning revelation of the *Qur'an*), and the fifth pillar is pilgrimage—every Muslim in a position to do so is expected to travel once in a lifetime to Mecca (Smith, 1991, pp. 242–245). The annual pilgrimage to Mecca is known as the Hajj. It is God's will alone that determines the ultimate values and purposes of human life in Muslim thought and Muslim law is the divinely ordained system of God's command (i.e., the Shari'a code of law). This Islamic law is "the whole process of intellectual activity which ascertains and discovers the terms of the divine will and transforms them into a system of legally enforceable rights and duties" (Coulson, 1969, p. 2). The Mosque is the main center of worship. The Crescent is the major symbol of Islam (Armstrong, 2002).

There are two branches of Islam, Sunni (the largest with close to 90% membership [Kurds, a minority population are primarily Sunni Muslims]) and the Shi'a (Shiites). There is a difference in beliefs between the two denominations about who was the legitimate successor to Mohammed. The dominant denomination, the Sunnis, ruled after the time of Mohammed until the end of the World War I. Shi'as (Shiites) were practicing their faith primarily in Persian Iran; they came to more prominence principally during and after the rule of the Iran's Ayatollah Khomeini in 1978. Shi'as also are in some regions in Iraq and Lebanon (Armstrong, 2002). The mystical tradition of Sunni Islam is Sufism, a spiritual practice known in the West by the poetry of Rumi (*The Essential Rumi*, 1995). Sufism focuses on healing love and practicing remembrance, a combination of breath and sound to open the heart to greater love. Islam is diverse and there are different interpretations by scholars and religious leaders of the writings of Mohammed in the *Qur'an*. Muslims live in many different countries of the Middle East and other nations of the world. As one of the fastest growing religions in the modern world, there are different political orientations. Many scholars and religious leaders believe that the difference between Sunnis and Shi'as is mainly political (Armstrong, 2002, p. 206). The rise of the Wahhabi (Wahhabism) reform movement occurred in Saudi Arabia when old nomadic tribal values were subordinated to Islam (The Unity of the Saudi Arabian People, *The Kingdom of Saudi Arabia*, 1993). Wahhabism is a

form of Sunni Islam and is considered orthodox, ultraconservative, and fundamentalist designed to restore "pure monotheistic worship." In Europe, Muslim women are discussing their overlapping Islamic religious and social identities by highlighting their ways of life and mounting counter positions about their differences in interpretation, for example, about the wearing of the veil (*hijab*) and the dress (*abeya* or *burka*), or other generally perceived submissive behaviors. Muslim women are calling for social reform to examine more than one way of perceiving Muslim women in the public arena (Salih, 2007).

Hinduism

Hinduism (from the Hindu meaning, of India) is practiced by 80% of Indians. A religion of more than 1 billion people (one in six people in the world and more than 1.6 million with Hindu foundations in the United States) is practiced by individuals in many nations all over the world (Czerenda, 2006). Hinduism acknowledges an Absolute (also known as Brahman) that is without form, the dharma, which is a universal force, the inner lawfulness of being. The Absolute is never changing, indivisible, but infinitely divisible by reverence of many gods. Thus, "Hinduism is not one codified religion but a compilation of hundreds, perhaps thousands, of smaller belief systems" (Huyler, 1999, p. 31). Emphasis is placed on individual spiritual experience and the realization of the higher self over any religious institution, dogma, or savior. The Absolute, the Brahman, is manifested in different gods and goddesses, the perfect blend of all facets of existence (Huyler, 1999). This polytheism or multiple deities illustrates the many paths to the Absolute. Hence the different branches of Hinduism. One Truth, the Santana Dharma, the eternal law governs everything, the entirety of creation. Hindu principles are expressed through the foundational text, the *Veda* or *Vedas* written more than 6,000 years ago in the ancient form of Sanskrit, called Vedic. To commune with the divine, Hindus may engage in the ceremonial act of the Puja and show reverence to a god or goddess through images using rituals, invocations, prayers, and song (Huyler, 1999). Reincarnation after death is a belief of the Hindu religion (Czerenda, 2006; Huyler, 1999). The temple, as a place of worship, is symbolic of the Hindu religion.

Contemporary Hinduism continues to be influenced by social and cultural traditions, such as the power of the kinship and caste systems, marriage arrangements, the power of women to preserve the family's honor, the wearing of saris by women in many communities, karma, "a person's fate is the outcome of past actions" (Czerenda, 2006, p. 12), and the flawless conduct of women. For example, "a faithful wife is married in each of her rebirths to the same husband, to whom she proves deserving and wins through her virtue" (Czerenda, 2006, p. 13). However, Hindus are changing as the fast-moving environments of contemporary India and Indians around the world are changing. Diverse social and cultural practices, such as a democratic government; a changing or abolishment of the caste system; diverse language structures; improved economic and health conditions; advanced technology (e.g., computers and the World Wide Web); migration; and the changing role of women, family organization and widowhood practices, and tourism are reflective of the new India and multinational Indians. Globalization, cultural change, and migration have prompted increased religious awareness of Hinduism worldwide (Czerenda, 2006).

Sikhism, a religion founded in the 15th century in Punjab, India, by Guru Nanak Dei, Jr. has more than 20 million followers (the 5th largest religion) worldwide. Its principles include devotion to remembrance of God, truthful living, and equality of human beings. Sikhism denounces superstitions, some rituals, and the former Hindu concept of the caste. Ten Gurus are honored in the Sikhism Holy Book, and there is one Living Guru. Symbols of the religion in male members are a turban, beard, steel bracelet, and ceremonial sword worn to represent ideals of honesty, equality, fidelity, meditating on God, and never bowing to tyranny. The symbol of Sikh dress for traditional women is the Salwar Kurta/Punjabi suit, which also is worn by many women in India, Pakistan, and Bangladesh (Retrieved June 18, 2009 from http://www.religioustolerance.org/Sikhism.htm).

Buddhism

Buddhism is a religion based on intelligence, science, and knowledge, whose purpose is the destruction of suffering and the source of suffering based on the teachings of Buddha, the Enlightened One, more than 1,500 years ago (Bhikkhu, 2005). Buddha was first a Hindu and learned from the teachings of Hinduism (*The Vedas*). Buddhism is a religion that is practiced by many people all over the world, especially Asians. It means "the teaching [Tipitaka] of the Enlightened

One . . . who knows the truth about all things, one who knows just 'what is what' (knows things just as they are) and so is capable of behaving appropriately with respect to all things" (Bhikkhu, 2005, p. 2). Buddhists act in accordance with what their own insight reveals, such as how the Laws of Karma are interpreted. Buddhists believe that ". . . a good or bad outcome is a direct result of how they acted" (Hatthakit & Thaniwathananon, 2007, p. 64). There is great respect shown to others in the form of rituals, especially in greetings, the Namasté in India or Wai in Thailand. There is no being in Buddhist faith but through prayers and rituals to the images of Buddha, a deep mystical awareness that leads to "nirvana" can be achieved. The Buddhist comes to the nontheistic realization that all being is "empty" and no "self" is eternal (Alexander, 2006, p. A16). "Buddhists adhere to the doctrine of rebirth after death" (Bhikkhu, 2005, p. 149). The knowledge of the "non-existence of the being, the individual, the self, you and me" [nothing whatsoever is a self or belongs to self] is achieved through knowledge of different spiritual processes, including the eightfold path (i.e., right intent, right speech, right association, right conduct, right livelihood, right effort, right mindfulness, and right concentration), and the four Noble Truths (all things are suffering and desire is the cause of suffering, the drive for fulfillment, hopefulness, and overcoming self-seeking) (Smith, 1991). Reaching Nirvana consists of complete extinguishment of desire by the path, the threefold training of knowledge, morality, and concentration culminating in insight—intuition that is clear and immediate (Bhikkhu, 2005; England et al, 2004).

In the modern world, many people choose Buddhism as a path to compassion and wholeness. Buddhist meditation fosters "serenity, happiness, confidence, and avoidance that provokes anxiety, hopelessness, and fear" (Rinpoche, 2007, p. 50). Buddhism has been influential in modern science and has provided insight into the working of the human mind. The path to the spirit is through the mind, through experiencing it directly by means of qualities of, "wisdom, omniscience, compassion, confidence, and peace" (Rinpoche, 2007, p. 91). The Temple is the place of worship.

Confucianism

Confucianism is a system of thought and moral code based on the teachings of Confucius (551–479 BCE), the Chinese way of life that influences more than 6 million people. Chinese people also have been influenced by Taoism and Buddhism, and other major religions, such as Catholicism and Protestantism. The central precept of Confucianism is living in harmony with human beings and with nature. "In Confucianism, a force in the universe called the Tao (the way) is a unified field that brings together the polarities of the Yin (the negative or feminine element) and the Yang (the positive or masculine element) and is reflected in the Supreme Ultimate, the T'ai Chi (Tzu, 1986). The force focuses on attitude rather than rule to discover who one is and how the physical laws of nature operate in the universe and in the mind. An all-embracing love, or human heartedness (*jen*) and righteousness (*yi*), bring forth the realization that the power continues to flow only when it is passed on to others. "The relationship between mind and matter, between intuition and logic reveals an intricate pattern of compassion and interaction with the balance of nature" (Ray, 1994, p. 260, cited from Tzu, 1986 and Yu-Lan, 1948). To attain these goals, the Golden Rule or "fellow-feeling" is emphasized by a system of interpersonal relationships and good government.

Despite turmoil and conflict in the ancient time of Confucius and in the modern time in China, the moral code of ethics (i.e., humanness and love exemplifying virtues of courtesy, magnanimity, good faith, diligence, and kindness) was and is promoted. The strongest moral center for ethical relationships is the family with father and son having the strongest relationship; a woman enters into the family of her husband after marriage in traditional Chinese culture. In modern China, population is restricted and numbers of children are limited mainly to one child per couple or family, although this policy is beginning to change. Relationships primarily are hierarchical except those between friend and friend. For followers, Confucianism is a form of education with no priests, no sects, and no creed; however, there is sacrifice to the spirits and prayers, rituals, and rites directed to "heaven." Thus, heaven is viewed as a force in human affairs, and ancestor worship is practiced. "Outside China, Chinese peoples and the civilizations influenced by China still revere Confucius in various ways. In modern Hong Kong (now a part of China), Taiwan, and Singapore, with primarily Chinese populations, Confucius is held in high regard. In Vietnam, Korea, and Japan, Confucian ethics and ideals remain part of the

cultural values" (Hoobler & Hoobler, 2004, p. 16). However, in these cultures, especially South Korea and Vietnam, there also has been a strong focus on the Christian faith.

Shintoism

Shinto is the native religion in Japan with its roots dating back to 500 BCE. Shintoism is animistic, venerating almost any natural objects, including leaders, scholars, and warriors. The principal deity of Shintoism is the Sun Goddess (the nation of Japan is called Nippon, which denotes "the Origin of the Sun" and the flag's red dot symbolizes the sun). Ancient mythology highlights Amaterasu, the Goddess of the Sun, the ruler of heaven, and the legendary ancestor of the Imperial Family. Other religions are practiced in Japan, one being Buddhism, which dates back to the 6th century. For a period, Buddhism was considered the religion of Japan until Shintoism was reinstated as the state religion in 1868. Many of the Shinto deities came to be recognized as the Buddha himself, but tradition says that Buddha was a manifestation of Shinto deities. There is no doctrine in Shintoism, but prayer (*norito*) is used to address the deity. Prayers also are chanted by Shrine priests. More than 80,000 shrines, the central places of worship, have been erected in sacred spots throughout Japan and have been consecrated to the Shinto pantheon. Four are dominant: Hachimangu (the 15th Emperor Ojin, the god); Tenjin, heaven's god, the deity of learning; Inari, the god of the harvest and foxes (placed at the entrance to Torii gates in front of shrines); and Jingu, which is associated with the Imperial Family. Purification is essential for Shintos, where before approaching the deity, there is a ceremonial cleaning of the mouth and hands with water using a stone-wash basin at the entrance to a shrine. Shrines have two-part structures that represent the oratory, called Haiden, and the Honden, the main dwelling or inner sanctum of the deity that houses mirrors (the symbol of the Sun Goddess), swords, and jewels, serving as spirit substitutes. Prayers are uttered after first clapping hands twice to make sure the god is listening, bowing once, placing coins into a wooden offertory box, and praying. Different rituals for good health and happiness mark the stages of the Japanese throughout their lives (Ruparell, 2000; Sivananda, 2005).

Aboriginal and Native Religions

Aboriginals or indigenous peoples of the world manifest oneness with nature. At the same time, indigenous people, often referred to as tribal or First Nations' people in the Americas, and Aboriginals in Australia have different cultural backgrounds, languages, and religions. The Great Spirit or God is recognized as present in all creation and is the foundation of native religion (Kinast, 2006, p. A16). The fundamental values of Native peoples illuminate a delicate balance among the indigenous groups themselves, other people, and the environment or earth. In Australia, the Aboriginal way of life was initially nomadic and rooted in kin relationships; personal possessions were limited to what the person could carry and what was necessary for hunting and food gathering (Baglin & Mullins, 1969). Now the Aboriginal (Koorie culture and others, such as the Torres Strait Islander people) mostly are rooted in the major cities and outback regions of Australia (Ray, 2001). In the Americas, the land is important to the Native people who number more than 2.5 million American Indians and Alaska Natives, and 1.6 million who consider themselves of Native/First Nations' ancestry (Hill, 2002; *Statistics Canada*, Canada 2001 Census, May 15, 2001; First Nations Statistics, 2001/2002, *United States Census Bureau*, 2000). The land was considered given to Native people by the Great Spirit because he put them on the land to come and go and live in their own way. The land continues to be important despite losses to "new world" conquerors (McMaster & Trafzer, 2004; Curtis, 1993). The people of the land could not come and go as freely but were confined to reservations. Mindfulness and compassion for the land and all beings continue as central beliefs (Lowe & Nichols, 2013; Ywahoo, 1987). In 1999 in Canada, the new territory set aside for the Inuits (formerly Eskimos) is named Nunavut, which means "Our Land" (Hill, 2002, p. 66). Oral traditions and other writings teach the maintenance of harmony of mind and antidotes to disharmony. Right relationship to self, family, tribe, clan, nation, and the planet is important to maintain harmony, although modern spiritual and mental health problems, as in the general world culture, have emerged. Each voice and opinion is part of a circle, a unity that highlights the energy in all, and is seen as an ever-present essence (Great Mystery) burning in the heart of every being (Ywahoo, 1987). Diverse tribes also have accepted Christian religious traditions. Long-houses are places of worship but they also are the gathering place for sharing food and community for Indian people. Each year at the annual powwow(s) (the term refers to the sacred) in North America, Native Indians with their Medicine people gather together to celebrate their history and culture(s) with traditional ceremonies that honor the Great Spirit, the land, and each other. The ancient and enduring wisdom of the holy people is passed along through prayers, songs, rituals, and stories (McMaster & Trafzer, 2004).

Myth Spirituality

In the history of mythology, contrary to the common use of the term as legend or illusion, the world is expressed through stories and artistic symbols and the oral traditions of different eras and cultures. Myths are passed on from one generation to the other and are an attempt to explain the meaning of the world in story form, primarily through oral tradition but also through literature and art (Ions, 1999). Myths can be embedded in religious traditions, for example, in the Bible, or also stand on their own in many cultures. Anthropological references illuminate the fact that mythologies are living forces, not just stories related to cultural heritage. They are captured in carvings and paintings in tombs and symbolized in pottery, paintings, and sculpture. The myth stories of ancient Egypt, Greece, Rome, and India; the Celtic and Norse mythologies; and the stories of the Americas, Persia, Africa, China, and Japan try to explain life and death, creation, day and night, the afterlife, and the fight against darkness, demons, and the underworld. The Mesoamerican calendar systems of the Aztecs and Mayans; the ancient astrology of the moon, sun, and stars; and the feats of great heroes and heroines are vivid examples of the creative expression in mythology (Ions, 1999). From the viewpoint of health and illness, cold-and-hot theories or yin-and-yang philosophies, the evil eye ritual and other rituals used to understand life, expel or chase away evil spirits and explain the mysteries of life. "In a sense, a myth is a sacred narrative with a moral message . . ." (Ions, 1999, p. 6).

New Age or Integrative Spirituality

In New Age spirituality or what is viewed as an integrative spirituality (Burnham, 1989; Wilber, 2006), the ideas of power, force, creativity, and spiritual healing are embraced. The philosophy carries with it the ideas of belongingness, belonging to the universe, and self-in-relation (Capra et al, 1991; Wilber, 2006). New Age spirituality honors the spiritual as a creative force and recognizes our common humanity and our responsibility to the universe. The integrative movement may espouse one religion, and often one government, or appreciation of many religions or beliefs. A contemporary and important faith, the Baha'i teaches that all creatures are of one God, as creations of one God, and are part of one family. God has revealed himself to humanity through Divine Messengers, such as Abraham, Krishna, Buddha, Jesus, and Muhammad, which for the Baha'i make up the oneness of God, and oneness of the human family, and the oneness of religion (http://www.bahai.org, retrieved August 2, 2008).

Integrative spirituality applies in-depth approaches to understanding the self, such as mindfulness, meditation, and yoga; select principles especially from Native spirituality and Buddhism; and other truths of Judaism and Christianity, such as respect and love. Thus, this approach promotes ethics, the idea of serving and seeking the good of the other and the earth (Wilber, 1982, 2006).

Diversity is honored with a commitment to people of all races and cultures. Responding to the need to care for the universe and the more than 6 billion people who inhabit it, the spiritual movement is propelling people to examine lifeworld problems and issues that potentially may harm or are harming the planet and the people in it, no matter what culture or religion. There is a call from messengers with diverse political, religious, and secular views to take individual and collective responsibility. A concept called the "love economy," embracing social, environmental, and ethical auditing that reflects the triple bottom line (i.e., people, planet, and profit) is influencing different groups, nations, and corporations to increase accountability for the following ideas: sustainability, low-environmental–effect decisions and environmental rights, workplace safety, fair labor standards, improved education and health care, nutrition, slow-food movement (e.g., sustaining small farms), clean technology, and human rights (Henderson, 2007).

As societies are becoming informed about global issues, the reality of the human family as a network of relationships is unfolding. In science and spirituality, complexity science teaches about interconnectedness and "emergent" systems (Peat, 2002). New Age spirituality teaches about the oneness of all, the inseparability of mind, body, and spirit, and ". . . the need [for] a new kind of rationality that includes not only our powers of analysis and logical deduction, but also our empathy and aesthetic response to the natural world" (Briggs & Peat, 1999, p.122).

POLITICAL AND COMMUNAL THEOLOGIES: BUILDING THE EARTH

Aspirations for appreciating a common humanity, common hope, and spiritual integration in the wake of historical geopolitical struggles has raised concerns about how a world community can move toward cooperation and peace. In 2006, de Vries and Sullivan published a book, *Political Theologies,* with numerous secular (concerned with things of the world) and religious authors who shared essays that critiqued the past, examined the present, and proposed ways to build the earth in the age of interculturality and globalization. The rediscovery of the universal religious principles of faith, hope, and love were illuminated. By revisiting and questioning the historical integration of spirituality and secularism, scholars began to see, value, and even anticipate the visibility of religion in the public sphere. The period of the Enlightenment of the 17th and 18th centuries in Western history highlighted the replacement of the theological virtues of faith, hope, and love with the secular merits of liberty, equality, and fraternity (De Duve, 2006, p. 654). Religion (as a universal concept) was relegated to the private sphere (de Vries & Sullivan, 2006). However, in what is now called the "postsecular" world (i.e., where the spiritual and material are integrated), there is a changed attitude in the print and electronic media, and local and global communities that examines religion and its abiding tenets. Scholars and politicians are recognizing the persistent role of religion, primarily virtues of patience, tolerance, and even love of enemies in conjunction with moral principles and open communication in civic life especially when investigated against the background of intercultural dissension, prolonged conflict, and war. A leading social philosopher, Habermas, (2006) stated that "liberal political culture may even expect its secularized citizens to participate in efforts to translate relevant contributions from a religious language [theological virtues] into a publically accessible one" (p. 260). Comparing and contrasting secular principles of liberty, equality, and fraternity with cultural beliefs and the religious principles of faith, hope, and love are emerging (De Duve, 2006). Translating references to the virtues set forth in the Scriptures that illuminate the religious meaning in the forms of compassion, love, morality, and justice are beginning to appear in public discourse and policies. In Europe, where postmodern philosophy embraced relativism and rejected universal values associated with religious morality, and highlighted the idea that "God is dead," there is a transformation. In the United States, despite its adherence to the rule of the separation of church and state, references to God have been sustained because of the history and constitutional foundation of its principles of democracy. In the past decade, the idea of God is becoming more visible in the public square and supported by the majority of the citizens. After the tragic events of September 11, 2001 in the United States, the universal principles of "good *and* evil" were once again elucidated in private and public domains (Berman, 2004; Wolfe, 2012). Subsequently, in theology, ethics, and government, the prevailing postmodern philosophy of moral relativism with its focus on moral particulars or individual moral decisions were viewed and studied in relation to *universal* ethical principles of good and its opposite, evil. The unfolding of the new paradigm in science as interconnectedness, and the raising of spirituality to a public realm to accommodate concerns for human and environmental rights, justice, and care of the poor, immigrants, and the vulnerable brought forth increasing respect for universal moral principles. At the same time in trying to understand how to benefit all people and things of the universe, a renewed interest in the foundations of religion as agape love was articulated (Ray, 2010a, 2010c). The basic principle of God's love for his people as unconditional and human beings' love for God and love of neighbor even the principle of loving one's enemy came to light (Templeton, 1999). Love in this sense, is communicated in the daily prayer of the Shema for Jews that addresses the love for God and neighbor (Deuteronomy 6:4–5 and Leviticus 19:18, respectively), and articulated in the excerpts from *New Testament Scripture*, such as the *First Letter of John* in the New Testament that God is love and we are to love our neighbor as ourselves (1 John 4:16 and Mark 12:29–31 respectively) (from Pope Benedict XVI, *Encyclical Letter* 2005, "*Deus Caritas Est*" [God is Love]) and taught in the writings of the *Qur'an*, which reminds followers of Islam that true charity is given to those in need and also anticipated in those who cannot ask for help, who are ashamed or unaware of their need or of others' capacity to help (from the *Qur'an, Sura [Chapter]* 51:19 in Templeton, 1999, p. 39). Love thus is considered *agape* or unconditional love. It recognizes that enemies exist but it means that we are to love our enemies without selfish motives because love is from God

(1 John 4:7, *The New American Bible*, 1987). As we have learned, the spiritual refers to an intelligent and loving presence, an inner communion with someone or thing greater than ourselves, a realization of the presence of God, an Infinite Power or Creative Force that flows into or reveals itself in daily life (Goldsmith, 1959). The quest for God is a quest for wholeness and unity in daily life. New approaches to the study of physics, health sciences, political and economic sciences, technology, and art are prompting an investigation into the human-spiritual-science relationship (Arntz et al, 2005; Capra et al, 1991; Vaught, 1982). The changes in views of science and the force of technology now seen as coexistent with humanity, or that technology may transcend biology, or the idea of an age of spiritual machines (Kurzweil, 2005) are challenging researchers and scholars to contemplate the meaning of an intelligent universe, creative force, and the concepts of the whole, unity, and endless possibilities (Artnz et al, 2005). What truly is the relationship between the human and the universe? What is the relationship between the unity of cultures and the diversity of beliefs? Religious virtues of faith, hope, and love, the truth of the Scriptures and other Holy Books are stimulating awareness and encouraging the search for understanding. "Socially, the fusion and intermingling of races [cultures] are leading directly to the establishment of an equally common form, not merely of language, but of morality and ideals" (Teilhard de Chardin, 1965, p. 78). Humans are integral, body, mind, and spirit (soul). Historical and formal religions present God as universal love. Religion is connected with the "soul" (the inner life) and through contemplation and prayer gives purpose and meaning to life with the goal of sparking moral action. In the restored political and communal theologies and changing postsecular world of today, the call is to build the earth—a civilization of love, respect, and justice for diverse cultures and spiritual practices. Habermas (in Wolin, 2006) recognized that a new postsecular (postmaterial) moral, political, and economic world that integrates ethical, religious, and spiritual views always must be examined within a context of openness and suspension of anyone's *particular* religious or spiritual conviction as the path to truth. The intrinsic worth of each person and the diversity of meaning of *all* views need to be respected and honored. By honoring the virtues of faith, hope, and love in both private and public life in relation to the

civic standards of freedom, equality, and fraternity, the call will be answered through transcultural communicative spiritual-ethical caring (Boulding, 1988; Delio, 2014; Pope Benedict XVI, 2005; Ray, 1997, 2005, 2010a, 2010b, 2010c; Ray & Turkel, 2014; Teilhard de Chardin, 1965; Watson, 2005).

The Dynamics of the Universal Mind: The Religious Person

Religion comes from the Latin word *religio*, a rebinding to, connecting to, or in contemporary terms, belonging to the universe (Capra et al, 1991). The notion of *homo religiosus* (religious man) beckons the inner soul to confront reality, to discover ". . . everything that is true and beautiful in creation" (Teilhard de Chardin, 1960, p. 97). From an anthropological viewpoint, this binding to the universe was the foundation of primal religion where, first and foremost, tribes were bound to each other, to animals, plants—to nature itself. "Human beings and nature belong to each other" (Smith, 1991, p. 375). No line separated the sacred and the secular, the holy and worldly. Division between the sacred and the secular emerged throughout the centuries in the historical religions; however, as the light of understanding has been deepening in science, culture, and religion, the dynamics of *unity* between the sacred and secular again is becoming more apparent (Capra et al, 1991; Delio, 2014; Peat, 2002; Spitzer, 2010; Thoma, 2003). Paradoxically, as the dialogue between science and religion is becoming more apparent, many people of different cultures of the world continue to live out their lives to a large extent within contexts of social, political, and religious strife, conflict, and war with a general fear of living together (Ray, 2010c; Sanford, 1988; Valenta, 2006; Wolfe, 2013). In the wake of severe political and religious unrest in pluralistic societies, leading social philosophers and theologians note that dialogue and communicative action must be the core. People in politics must deal with nation-states and ethical and spiritual responsibility to the public good; people in theology must deal with covenants of faith, hope, and love in the context of political movements involving religion and violence (de Vries & Sullivan, 2006; Schmitt, 1985; Wolfe, 2013).

APPROACHES TO GOD

Five basic approaches to God have been identified—theist, pantheist, panentheist, agnostic, and atheist (Shapiro, 2007). Each offers views of God and nature. Theists recognize God as one who is a transcendent supernatural who created the world and who loves, rewards, judges, and punishes (Buber, 1952, 1958) and also one who is immanent, wholly present as love *in* the universe (Delio, 2014; Merton, 1951; Saint Thomas Aquinas, 1967). Both Judaism, the first faith community to whom the God of the Bible revealed himself, and Christianity recognize the transcendent authority and love of God; in Christianity God also is manifest in Jesus Christ, the Son of God. Pantheists recognize that God *is* all; this is recognized in the Hindu faith; panentheists recognize God *in* all, such as "New Age" spiritualists. Atheists say God does *not* exist and agnostics are not sure (Shapiro, 2007).

In contemporary world culture, people of faith choose many paths to God. They hold different meanings of God in response to history and tradition, culture, knowledge, understanding, grace, and insight of the concept of God and the search for the good in self and others. Diverse cultures use the name God and other names, such as Jesus, Great Spirit, Higher Power, the Word, Holy Spirit, Absolute, Deity, Sun, Force, and so forth. In the Christian sense, God is also known as the Trinity, the mystery of three persons in One God (Father, Son [Jesus Christ] and Holy Spirit) (Merton, 1951; Pope Benedict XVI, 2005, 2006; Ratzinger, 2007). The Jewish theologian, Heschel (1954) acknowledged God as a stillness that surrounds and hovers over the restlessness of the world, the secret stillness that precedes our birth and succeeds our death.

UNIVERSALITY AND DIVERSITY OF SPIRITUAL BELIEFS AND VALUES

Communities from ancient times to the present have shared common cultural yet diverse spiritual beliefs and values (Van Iersel, 1973). Universality or commonality derives naturally from shared human experience and education. "A feeling of belonging and moral agency flows from unity among relationships" (Koerner, 1997, p. 63). Universality also means the universal love of God; thus experience is guided by this objective truth and expressed diversely (Pope Benedict, XVI, 2008, p. 6). Diversity derives from specific values and beliefs that have been generated and transmitted by people of different cultures over time (Leininger, 1970, 1978, 1991; Leininger & McFarland, 2006). The focus of diversity is the actual lived experience, values, and beliefs and the choices that are made by different culture groups. The search for discovery of the self-in-relationship produces cooperation and competition. The complexities of living often generate misunderstanding and manifest as political and economic chaos, competition for power and resources, religious and ideological friction, cultural humiliation, dissension, terrorism, and even war by one culture group or another. Education and continuous communication will be the keys to appreciating a diverse universe and to transcending distinctions of race, color, nationality, religion, and ideology (Ho, 2003). "An education in transcendence prepares us to see beyond appearances into the hidden realities of life—beyond facts into truths, beyond self-interest into compassion, beyond our flagging energies and nagging despairs into *love,* required to renew the community of creation" (Palmer, 1993, p. 13).

Spiritual Belongingness

Spiritual belongingness relates to Universal Sources and Universal Mind in the sense that belongingness refers to how the wisdom of spirituality (theology) shares parallel insights into the reality of the nature of the universe (cosmology and history). These insights have been generated by the new sciences of the complexity, the quantum, and beyond (Capra et al, 1991; Peat, 2002). The new sciences highlight interconnectedness or belongingness; there are no separate or isolated objects in the universe; however, God as the Universal Mind reveals the paradox and mystery of integrality, both as object in the sense of the supernatural, and subject in presence in the universe. The Hebrew and Christian Scriptures reveal the interrelationship between God and man. In the new sciences, the observer of phenomena in the universe is not separate from what is observed; this is considered oneness, unity; the observer and the observed belong to each other. Thus, the belongingness that is articulated in theology is also central to science. "Theology looks at reality under the aspect of our relationship to God, the Horizon, while science narrows its focus to what is contained within the horizon" (Capra et al, 1991, p. 159). Although the following examples show distinct notions of spiritual belongingness in the three monotheistic religions, most religions or spiritual and principle-based foundations of thought illuminate beliefs and values that pertain to a set of precepts that help a person or culture group find belongingness. The moral frameworks, such as the Ten Commandments, guide people in their relationship to self, others, and their ultimate reality (Suarez & Lewis, 2005). In the major monotheistic religious traditions of Judaism, Christianity, and Islam, the reference point of belonging and unity is God. "God is the center toward which all forces tend" (Heschel, 1954, p. 7).

In Jewish theology, the covenantal relationship between God and his people is primary. Heschel (1954) remarked that "[f]aith is the beginning of intense craving to enter an relationship with Him who is beyond mystery, to bring together all the might that is within us with all that is spiritual beyond us" (pp. 109–110). The covenant is a sacred partnership. God announced himself to Moses, "I am the God of your father, ...the God of Abraham, the God of Isaac, the God of Jacob" (Exodus, 3:6, *The New American Bible*, 1987, p. 60). In Jewish scripture the reciprocal relationship of God and human beings is revealed in Deuteronomy (30:19–20, *The New American Bible*, 1987), "I have set before you life and death, the blessing and curse. Choose life, then, that you and your descendants may live by loving the Lord, your God, heeding his voice and holding fast to him...." (p. 209). Israel was called to be holy as God Himself. In scripture, "The Lord said to Moses, 'Speak to the whole Israelite community and tell them: Be holy, for I, the LORD, am your God, am holy'" (Leviticus, 19:1–3, *The New American Bible*, p. 120). The Divine Command and rules of conduct including the Ten Commandments were given to the people of Israel and reinforce how God and his people are interconnected.

Within the many expressions of Christianity, Catholicism, and the various denominations and nondenominations of Protestantism, the ultimate perfection of an informed Christian conscience, despite evil, sin, or the frailties of the will, is *love* (Merton, 1951; Pope Benedict XVI, 2005). Nouwen exclaimed that "[t]he perfect love that drives out all fear is divine love in which we are invited to participate" (1986, p. 36). God looks for us before we look for him (Chester, 2005). In the Christian scripture, Jesus Christ, love manifest on earth and in heaven, states, "Make your home in me as I make mine in you" (John, 15:4, *The New American Bible*, 1987, p. 1347). The New Testament scriptures illuminate how Jesus taught about love and a relationship with God and neighbor. For example, in the *Sermon on the Mount,* Jesus gave the people the Beatitudes, a guide to living and loving God and their neighbor, and loving their enemy, and the spiritual rewards that they would reap (Matthew, 5:3–10, *The New American Bible*, 1987, pp. 1191–1192).

Jesus also taught the people how to pray and seek forgiveness with the recitation of *the Lord's Prayer* (Matthew, 6:9–13, *The New American Bible*, 1987, p. 1195). Steindl-Rast stated that "[t]he moral dimension of Christianity is always consequent on the inner transformation experienced as a free gift from God" (Capra et al, 1991, p. 50). Humans are made in the image and likeness of God. Therefore, the Christian faith is considered a supernatural vocation—human beings are called to a fullness of life that far exceeds the dimensions of earthly existence; it consists in sharing the very life of God, the unification of the soul of a human being to God in this life and in eternity (Pope John Paul II, 2006). Four pillars sustain and guide the faithful—the creed, the confession of faith; the sacraments (baptism, penance, communion, confirmation, marriage, holy orders, anointing of the sick in the Catholic tradition, and baptism and marriage in the Protestant traditions); the Ten Commandments; and the *Lord's Prayer*, the scriptural Word of God. Faith in God through ritual practices of the Christian religious faiths facilitate closer union with God, thus, a true sense of belongingness to the "mystery" that is continually unfolding in the lives of people and the lifeworld.

In the Islamic tradition, the message of the *Qur'an* (1980) illustrates a relationship to God (Yassine, 2004). "Allah brought you out of your mothers' wombs devoid of all knowledge, and gave you ears and eyes and hearts, so that you may give thanks" (The *Qur'an*, 1980, *Sura*, 16:77). Oneness with Allah is through knowledge and practice of the five pillars of Islam, which teach people "to walk the straight path" (Smith, 1991, p. 242)—the principles that guide Muslims in their relationship with God. The first pillar is the creed, the confession of faith, the *Shahadah*, "*. . . there is no god but God and Muhammad is His Prophet*" (Smith, 1991, p. 244). The second is to be constant in prayer. The third is charity. The forth is observance of Ramadan and the fifth pillar is pilgrimage—once during a lifetime, every Muslim in a position to do so is expected to travel to Mecca (Saudi Arabia) where God's revelation to Muhammad was first disclosed (pp. 242–245).

The *mystery* of God is expressed as belonging to Creation, the Great Spirit, the Infinite, or the Absolute in many other religious traditions. In the Eastern traditions, for example, in Buddhist philosophy, belonging to truth is understood through contemplating the nature of things. Oneness is the ultimate reality discovered through disciplined mindfulness and infinite compassion and results in enlightenment (Capra et al, 1991). As an animistic religion (attribution of a living soul to inanimate objects and natural phenomena), Shintoism focuses on the Deity, the central Deity being the sun and ways to purification through worship and prayer rituals (Ruparell, 2000). The foundational texts of Hinduism, the *Vedas*, and the Upanishads (genealogies, correspondences, and the significance of the Vedic rites) and the Laws of Manu also support the notion of oneness with the divine reality, called the Absolute among Hindus (Czerenda, 2006).

The religious culture of diverse indigenous, native, Indian, or First Nations' peoples illuminates the strength of belongingness to the universe and relationships to each other. In traditional Native or Aboriginal culture, people belong to the Great Spirit, Creator Being, and all of nature, water, and earth including the heavens and clan(s), tribes, or first nations through the rituals and symbols that represent native beliefs of more than 1,000 indigenous cultures in the Americas and Oceania. Aboriginal/native people have traditionally held the view of oneness with the universe. Native religion teaches becoming the best human being one can be to fulfill one's potential of peacekeeper, calling forth harmony and joy in all relations (Ywahoo, 1987; McMaster & Trafzer, 2004). Joseph, Nez Perce Chief stated that "[w]e were taught to believe that the Great Spirit sees and hears everything, and that he never forgets; that hereafter he will give every man a spirit-home according to his deserts. . . . This I believe, and all my people believe the same" (Curtis, 1993, p. 22). Through dialogue and observation of indigenous peoples and their religions, medicine people, rituals and symbols, contemporary scientists and theologians are becoming more informed about the meaning of belonging to the universe (Capra et al, 1991; McMaster & Trafzer, 2004; Peat, 2002, 2003; Watson, 1987).

SPIRITUAL BELONGINGNESS AND COMPLEXITY SCIENCE

Belongingness is central to cultures and subsequently science as a part of culture. Belongingness between and among individuals and their tribes, clans, and social group(s) is manifested in ancestral wisdom. As part of the history of human culture throughout the ages, the formulation of principles of creation, laws or divine commands and then the physical, social, and human science gave order to people's lives (Davidhizar & Giger, 2003; Durkheim & Mauss, 1963; Evans-Pritchard, 1965; Giger, & Davidhizar, 1998; McMaster & Trafzer, 2004; van Manen, 1990, 2014). As we have learned, the new sciences of complexity (quantum physics, chaos theory, holography and holistic science, emergent complexity) provide some understanding of the notion of belongingness or interconnectedness that is advancing in science today (Battista, 1982; Briggs & Peat, 1984; Capra et al, 1991; Goodwin, 1994, 2003; Kurzweil, 2005; Peat, 2002, 2003; Spitzer, 2010; Tudge, 2003). The science of "emergent complexity" acknowledges that everything in the universe is whole, more than the sum of its parts, and is continually emerging (Bar Yam, 2004). The universe as a web of relationships is mysterious yet self-organizes into structured patterns. An order that we might not expect to see emerges. Quantum theorists and researchers attempt to investigate and interpret patterns of wholeness primarily through mathematics and mathematical modeling. They seek to discover knowledge of patterns of energy, the intertwined unity and ultimate oneness in the universe. Western philosophers and scientists are looking to eastern and aboriginal philosophies to deal with the way in which principles of "reality" can be better understood. In the past, Western scientific thought espoused rules for reality that highlighted materialism, determinism, reductionism, and objectivity and breaking the universe into parts—the traditional Cartesian notion that the *dynamics* of the world can be understood primarily from the properties of the parts. In this view, there is no other reality but material. Everything can be reduced to elements of physics and chemistry (Wiker & Witt, 2006).

In the new view of the sciences of complexity, the *dynamics* of the world are understood as networks of relationships where "the units of matter and those exploring them are entangled in a unity [oneness] not separated in lonely isolation from one another" (Goodwin, 2003, p. 15). In essence, the knower (the seeker of knowledge) and the known (the subject to be known) are interconnected, are one. The universe is intersubjective and relational, not objective and materialistic. Quantum scientists are learning about and weaving together knowledge of the patterns of the unbroken wholeness of existence (Briggs & Peat, 1984; Byrne & Callaghan,

2014; Capra et al, 1991; D'Aquili & Newberg, 1999; Holmes, 2007; Kurzweil, 2005; Lemkow, 1990; Peat, 2003; Thoma, 2003). As the new sciences are a complex living reality, patterns of interconnected energy are just like human beings (Arntz et al, 2005; Rogers, 1970, 1994; Wiker & Witt, 2006). The world is meaningful, purposeful, elegant, beautiful, and intelligent; someone cares (Wiker & Witt, 2006). The complex scientific knowledge corresponds, in part, to the *ways of thinking* from passages, for example, the *Book of Psalms* [of the *Holy Bible*] (1993), and of vanishing ways of life of aboriginal or native peoples who had insights into a more intelligible understanding of the universe and the whole (Peat, 2002, 2003).

Among scientists, nursing is leading the way in understanding the complexity of relationships because of its focus on relationships, holism, culture, and relational caring, including understanding how nature and the environment play a significant role in human health and well-being (Davidson & Ray, 1991; Davidson, Ray, & Turkel, 2011; Newman, 1986; Nightingale, 1860/1969; Ray, 1998, 2010a, 2010b, 2010c; Ray & Turkel, 2014; Turkel & Ray, 2000, 2001). Choice (reasoned, ethical, and intuitive thought) is identified as the "conductor of the symphony" (Davidson & Ray, 1991; Davidson, Ray, & Turkel, 2011).

Consciousness, Science, and Spirituality

Supernaturally, there is a relationship between God as the source of creation and humans, the creative experience that guides truth. Within *human* nature, the mind and the brain are responsible for all experience (d'Aquili & Newberg, 1999). Thoughts matter. They are the constructs of reality, "a structure in which reality is patterned" (Arntz et al, 2005, p. 247). Patterns of reality show interconnectedness. In science, the "connectivity hypothesis" is being advanced; biology, physics, and sociology, for example, are for the first time exchanging ideas that move each of those sciences ahead. A new synthesis called neurotheology that integrates knowledge of the brain, science, spirituality, and religious experience is taking shape (Joseph, 2002). The connectivity hypothesis is the feedback of active information that shows and creates coherence among electrons, photons, molecules or cells, humans, societies, cultures, and civilizations (Arntz et al, 2005). The most complex of all information systems, the mind, a collection of tens of billions of neurons connected through trillions of neurotransmitters that result in conscious and unconscious activities is ". . . a perpetually evolving [neurobiological and electro-chemical] *event* rather than a distinct entity" (Rinpoche, 2007, p. 52). Thus, as Jung concluded "[c]onsciousness is not an entity, nor just a perspective, but a process that always implies a consciousness of something [self, others, God, things, thoughts, feelings and so forth]" (Cope, 2006, p. 5). In nursing, we see this notion of expanding consciousness expressed by nursing theorist Margaret Newman (Brown & Alligood, 2014; Newman et al, 2008). The idea of event or process is illuminated even more when genetics, spirituality, and technology are added to the picture. In the relationship among the human mind, genes, and technology, researchers state that ". . . the speed and learning capacity of the human mind is reaching its limits" (Holmes, 2007, p. 42) through traditional and formal educational means. Kurzweil, a futurist, wrote that the future will integrate the human and machine in which "information-based technologies will encompass all human knowledge and proficiency, ultimately including the pattern-recognition powers, problem-solving skills, and emotional and moral intelligence of the human brain itself" (2005, p. 8) including neurotheology—how the mind mediates our experience with God (D'Aquili & Newberg, 1999; Delio, 2014; Joseph, 2002). Technology and its powers are expanding so rapidly that it is constantly changing the human perception of reality. As humans in fact "merge" with machines, as in what has been happening over the past 40 years regarding humans and computer technology, humans and technology are considered "one" (Smith, 1998). A new dialogue about the nature of science, technology and the moral responsibility of what it means to be human and spiritual is beginning (Capra et al, 1991; Ess, 2014; Wiker & Witt, 2006). No longer can the scientist claim objectivity or neutrality. The idea of nature as an entangled web of relationships challenges scientists, technologists, philosophers, theologians, and health-care personnel to discuss the meaning of the human being in the new world of the interconnectedness between science and technology, science and theology, the belongingness that gives us a new vision of reality (Capra et al, 1991; O'Murchu, 1997; Smith, 1998; Wiker & Witt, 2006). Now, the challenge relates to the question of teleology, the question of the overall design and purpose of the universe and nature, and how humans should participate in the world and the universe as a whole.

SPIRITUAL BELONGINGNESS AND THE WORLD COMMUNITY

Awareness of the universality of spiritual meaning and the multiple and diverse ways of expressing spirituality facilitate understanding of transcultural spirituality and caring. Knowledge of transcultural spirituality not only is important to individuals in transcultural nursing and health-care situations but also to the meaning of "multicultural" understanding within nations. The new concepts of multiculturalism, interculturality, postmulticulturalism, or "postnational allegiance" that are emerging as culture groups migrate all over the world identify the need to understand multicultural spiritual beliefs and values. Increased spiritual suffering because of old and new injustices has been highlighted. Old injustices continue: racial and intercultural social and health-care issues persist even though there is more education; terrorism and war continue to emerge even though there is more diplomacy; poverty is pervasive even though there are adequate resources to share. New injustices abound and stem from the exploitation of the human heart through Internet pornography, and worldwide sex trafficking. There is more manipulation of the minds of people with the promise of excitement and freedom through unrestrained Internet sites, and the use of drugs and alcohol. "Even our common habitat, the earth itself, groans under the weight of consumerism, greed, and irresponsible exploitation" (Pope Benedict XVI, 2008, p. 6). "Wasteful" energy consumption, abuses of the land, and man-made contributions to climate change and global warming (Henderson, 2007) increase suffering. A loss of hope in the present and future, however, has enhanced the reemergence of religion in the realm of politics and public policies (Delio, 2014; de Vries & Sullivan, 2006; Postero, 2007; Salih, 2007; Taylor, 1994).

SPIRITUAL BELONGINGNESS AND NURSING

All her life, Florence Nightingale, the mother of modern nursing, was drawn to the life of mystics—prophets, saints, and people who experienced reality from a transcendent perspective (Calabria, 1990). Macrae (2001) pointed out that "[c]ross-cultural studies of the mystical perspective reveal experiences of timelessness, of creative power, of profound love and compassion, of touching upon truth, and of union with God or a *transcendent reality*" (p. 5). According to Nightingale, mystical experience was a source of wisdom and strength to fulfill one's purpose in the world (Dossey, 2000; Macrae, 2001). And her purpose was nursing, a call from God to help the sick and poor. Nightingale (1860/1969) believed that "nature [i.e., the manifestation of God] alone cures . . . and what nursing has to do is put the patient in the best condition for nature to act upon him" (p. 133). In her experiences in Egypt, Nightingale understood that the ancient view of good and evil were complementary processes in a dynamic universe (Calabria, 1990). From her experiences in the Crimea, Nightingale also understood that religious divisiveness can impede a spiritual cause. In her study of comparative religions and mystical elements, she concluded that "spirituality is not the property of any one religious tradition; it is a part of human nature, the highest level of human consciousness" (Macrae, 2001, p. 27). Nightingale and other religious sisters and deaconesses before her led the way in establishing the "spiritual" in nursing and made it possible for nurses of different religious commitments to relate to one another, not from a basis of stereotypical mistrust or misunderstanding but in a completely open and caring approach. Throughout the history of nursing, many nursing theorists who followed Nightingale integrated spirituality into their theories and their theories are used to guide the practice of nursing (Alligood, 2014; Parker, 2006; Marriner, Tomey, & Alligood, 2006; Smith, 2015). Nursing is holistic, more than the sum of its parts, the integration of body, mind and spirit: nurses first ". . . meet others as human beings who have so much in common: a heart, a face, a voice, the presence of a soul, fears, hope, the ability to trust, a capacity for compassion and understanding, the kinship of being human" (Heschel, 1954).

Holism, Nursing Science, and Spirituality

The holistic science of nursing has provided nursing with understanding of the complexity of human relationships and the complexity of the meaning of the integral relationship of the human and environment. Holism, first introduced to nursing by Rogers (1970, 1994) more than 40 years ago is characterized as the science of unitary human beings (SUHB). Rogers' theory influenced other nursing scientists of the holistic nature of nursing by illuminating the meaning of wholeness as the integral nature of the human and environment, multidimensionality, dynamism, and energy flow, in essence integration of the body, mind, spirit, and the environment. Other

theorists who followed in Rogers' footsteps characterized nursing as caring and the nature of health as expanded consciousness (Newman, 1986; Newman et al, 1991, 2008). Nursing as holistic, nursing as a human science and a science of human becoming (Parse, 1981, 1995), nursing as human-environment well-being (Davidson & Ray, 1991; Davidson, Ray, & Turkel, 2011; Ray & Turkel, 2014), nursing as the essence of caring and culture (Leininger, 1981, 1991; Leininger & McFarland, 2006; Swanson, 1999), and nursing as relational caring dynamics (Coffman, 2006, 2014; Ray, 1994, 1998; Ray & Turkel, 2014; Turkel, 2007; Turkel & Ray, 2000, 2001) highlight the complexity of nursing. Nursing scientists understand the process of human-environment interconnectedness, and information systems as systems of energetic caring transformation. Accordingly, and in conjunction with the new science of complexity, nursing is a dynamic process of thought and action, a structure of reality that is holistic and moral and patterned toward meaning. As a process of caring in the human health experience, the nurse and patient are in relationship and are continually emerging; they belong to each other and are seeking well-being and transformation, body, mind, and spirit. In today's complex healthcare environment, a person may continue to be objectified and viewed in parts rather than a whole. From a nursing science viewpoint, however, the patient can be considered holographic; the whole is in the part and the part in the whole. If a nurse is caring for a specific part of the body at one point in time, for example, the heart, the nurse is still caring for the whole, body, mind, and spirit. A holistic science acknowledges an unbroken circle of existence. We are aware and conscious of our belongingness to God, each other and the environment, the integration of body, mind and spirit. Holism provides the insight toward foresight—how human, spiritual, scientific, and technological knowledge coalesce and cocreates a wiser future for the discipline and profession of nursing (Davidson, Ray, & Turkel, 2011; Watson, 2005).

SPIRITUAL CARING IN NURSING

Spiritual caring in nursing speaks of relationship, human dignity, compassion (love and mercy), and justice (human rights) for another in his suffering and need (Ray, 1989a, 1997, 1999, 2010a, 2010b, 2010c; Watson, 2005; Yuan & Porr, 2014). It is a spiritual and ethical way of being. The need for health and nursing care is universal and the *Code of Ethics for Nurses* (2001) states that "[n]ursing care aims to maximize the values that the patient has treasured in life and extends supportive care to the family and significant others" (p. 7). Nurse caring incorporates first and foremost the ethical imperative of respect for persons (*Code of Ethics for Nurses with Interpretive Statements*, 2001, www.nursingworld.org/code-ofethics; Rachels, 1986). Respect for persons presumes that there must be equal value given to all people. Leininger, as one of the first nurses to acknowledge the notion of cultural universality and cultural diversity, understood the depth of meaning that cultural identities and culture-specific beliefs and values have to patients and families (Leininger, 1978, 1991, 1997; Leininger & McFarland, 2006; McFarland & Wehbe-Alamah, 2015). From the spiritual caring perspective, many theorists described the nature of human caring as a transpersonal and sacred philosophy, science, and practice (Boykin & Schoenhofer, 2001; Leininger, 1978; 1991; Leininger & McFarland, 2006; McFarland, 2006; Ray, 1981a, 1981b; 1997, 2007, 2010a, 2010b, 2010c; Roach, 1987/2002, 1997; Watson, 1979, 1988, 2005). Transcultural nursing, advanced first by Leininger (1991, 1997; Leininger & McFarland, 2006; McFarland & Wehbe-Alamah, 2015), reinforces how transcultural care/caring as ethical and spiritual play a role in the practice of nursing. Watson (1979, 1988, 2005, 2008) illuminated the nature of human caring and spirituality that makes healing possible. When a nurse engages himself in the caring moment of a transpersonal relationship with a patient or significant other, the potential for healing of body, mind, and spirit of both the patient and the nurse unfolds. The essence of the caring moment in the caring/healing relationship is the preservation, enhancement and protection of human dignity, wholeness, and integrity or harmony of body, mind, and spirit (Watson, 1997, 2005, 2008). Swanson (1999) detailed Watson's (2005) caring moment by the following actions: *knowing* or striving to understand an event and its meaning for the other; *being with* or being emotionally present; *doing for* the other; *enabling* or facilitating the other's movement through life events; and *maintaining belief* or sustaining faith in the other to face a future with meaning. Ray (1981b) illuminated that love and caring were synonymous—that the copresent and loving relationship of one with the other in nursing facilitated the well-being of the other. Ray (1981b, 1997) discussed the idea of divine love as the foundation for nursing. As

caring became a significant force in contemporary nursing, articulation of the spiritual became stronger, such as in Leininger's (1978, 1991, 1997) integration of culture and spirituality, Ray's (1981a, 1981b, 1997, 2006, 2010a, 2010b, 2010c) integration of spiritual-ethical caring and complex organizations, Roach's (1987/2002) philosophical and theological analysis of caring in nursing practice, Eriksson's (1997, 2006, 2007) philosophy of suffering and caritas (love), and Smith's (1999) transtheoretical synthesis of caring in Watson's theory, and love in Rogers' SUHB. Watson (2005) elaborated further on the nature of spirituality and the universality of love by referring to Teilhard de Chardin and stating that love is not just characteristic to human beings but is coextensive with the universe, is cosmic, the general property of all life. Furthermore, Watson (2005) remarked that the transpersonal connection ". . . goes beyond the personal, physical ego self and connects with the deeper, more spiritual, transcendent, even cosmic connections in the universe" (p. 203). To address some of these problems, in the past decade, spiritual caring has been introduced into some nursing school curricula. Research is taking place to reveal the meaning of caring and spirituality by many new nursing scholars, such as Touhy's research of nurse caring, spirituality and the elderly (Touhy, 2002; Touhy, Strews, & Brown, 2005). Some hospitals have engaged the services of chaplains, priests, ministers and rabbis, and other professionals with knowledge of spirituality and patient care needs. Also, other faith-based communities have evolved, generating new roles, such as faith-based community nursing and parish nursing (Dyess, 2011; Dyess & Chase, 2012; Smith, 2004; Solari-Twadell & McDermott, 2005). Parish nursing, a specialized practice of professional nursing in churches, embraces the spiritual dimension as central to practice when providing physical and cultural care to parishioners.

TRANSCULTURAL CARING SPIRITUALITY

The ideal of caring as love and the universal energy of the universe as whole, presents the foundation for a blueprint for cocreating harmony in the world and culturally specific choice for health and well-being (Eriksson, 2006; Ray, 1997, 2010a, 2010b, 2010c; Watson, 2005). In a copresent transcultural spiritual relationship, nurses hold others in their hands. "It is in the Other that we see ourselves and the infinity and mystery of our own soul, reflected back to us through Other" (Watson, 2005, p. 81). By virtue of nurses' caring mandate, nurses are coresponsible to identify patterns of suffering and loss of meaning for patients. Patterns of suffering are complex and divergent, from physical to mental, and cultural to spiritual health problems. Many professionals, such as nurses, psychiatrists, psychologists, physicians, social workers, and chaplains are called upon to use spiritual healing by understanding religious and cultural values and beliefs and integrating holistic spiritual/religious care practices for patients. In transcultural nursing, trying to understand not only the spiritual nature and religions of persons but also the idea of our own spiritual self-awareness can assist nurses in providing more culturally relevant and competent care to patients of all cultures.

SPIRITUAL SUFFERING AND HEALING

Upholding and preserving cultural diversity and patients' identity within a unity of purpose manifest spiritual-ethical caring. By being aware of and knowledgeable about specific religions and spiritual values of diverse cultural groups, nurses have an appreciation for the way in which spiritual suffering emerges. Subsequently they can facilitate how culturally and spiritually centered health-care choices are made (Ray, 1994, 2010a, 2010b, 2010c). It is important to understand spiritual suffering and spiritual healing.

Spiritual suffering emerges under the following circumstances: not having a sense of belonging, not feeling safe, cared for, protected, and loved (Nouwen, 1986). Spiritual suffering reveals violations of human dignity (Eriksson, 2006; Purnell & Mead, 2007). When personal, spiritual, or religious beliefs and values conflict, inner anguish, pain and suffering, illness, disease, distress, and struggle become visible. Often, spiritual struggle occurs intentionally or unintentionally, for example, when people suffer loss: when natural and planned disasters occur wherein people are displaced or driven from their homes; when people are placed in refugee camps or try to escape violence in their own countries; when people have no health care or no one to care for them; when people are hidden away or homeless because of drug use, alcohol use, or mental illness; and in general when people have no shelter from the "storms" of life (Nouwen, 1979).

Overall, many factors contribute to spiritual suffering and may come to light:

- When values and beliefs collide
- When the ethical self or conscience is troubled
- When there are feelings of absence of not belonging to God, to family and friends, or to the community
- When there is a feeling of anger or alienation from God, family, and friends
- When physical, emotional, or sexual abuse is experienced
- When suffering or pain overwhelm
- When physical, emotional, and spiritual survival is at stake
- When identity is threatened
- When feelings of love, peace, and harmony may be challenged
- When illness is overpowering
- When death looms

Consequently people often become confused, troubled, depressed, suicidal, or even homicidal. As spiritual struggle increases, faith and hope can increase or decrease. Generally, in the case of so much pain and suffering, loss and grief are experienced (see the Stages of Grief by Kübler-Ross, 1997). Either spiritual struggle can be reconciled, or spiritual "illness" may be identified. In 2000, with the increase in spiritual suffering, the American Psychiatric Association identified any reference to the religious or spiritual as a "problem, an illness, a disease entity" (rather than ignoring it) with the classification category of Religious or Spiritual Problem in the DSM-IV (2000), *Diagnostic and Statistical Manual of Mental Disorders of the American Psychiatric Association* (p. 741).

Even though spirituality has been identified in mental health care, the holistic image of the integration of body, mind, and spirit and understanding of the cultural context of the meaning of suffering may be overlooked. In her book, *The Suffering Human Being*, the nursing scholar Eriksson (2006, 2007) believes that "[w]e must return to the question of what caring actually means and what should constitute the fundamental interests of caring and caring science" (Eriksson, 2006, p. 93). Eriksson's worldview for the health professions highlights the question of meaning. The primary focus of the professionals' responsibility is to link the person's suffering to relationships, to health, to one's whole life. Spiritual difficulty or illness needs spiritual healing, caring, love, understanding, and sometimes professional counseling and medication if appropriate.

Spiritual healing is nurturing the soul and cultivating depth and sacredness in everyday life by reaching out to an Infinite Source (Moore, 1992; *The Book of*

Psalms, 1993; *The New American Bible*, 1987). Spiritual healing is *trust*—trust in God and others to come to our rescue, to be there for us in suffering and need. Helping to restore a person's dignity and self-esteem through compassion and moral action is the role of caring professionals. This role becomes especially important with persons who have served in the military and suffer the wounds of war. Spiritual healing encompasses the search for authenticity and truth, search for belongingness to God and others, and fostering holiness (Eriksson, 2006; Moore, 1992; Palmer, 1993; Wilber, 2006). When acknowledging the meaning of suffering and the need to belong, we, at the same time, acknowledge the pain or the "dark side of the soul." Authenticity is revealed—the limited and brokenness of love and the unlimited and unbrokenness of God (Nouwen, 1986). People in general believe that spiritual responsiveness and forgiveness make the struggle or suffering in life and illness worthwhile (Eriksson, 2006; Morse, 2001). Care of or nurturing the soul is made possible by personal, interpersonal, and professional communication (i.e., prayer, sharing, caring, and counseling). The anguish initiated by suffering calls for relief. For *some* religious persons, suffering can be a cause of joy. Many people offer up their sufferings (redemptive suffering) for a life of love and peace and for eternal life, for "a new life of resurrection" (Dear, 2007, p. 73).

Caring itself is coexistent with suffering. Consider the meaning of the word compassion. In times of illness, dying, and death, professional and lay caregivers feel, through compassion, the pain of the other (De La Rosa & Goke, 2007; Purnell & Mead, 2007). Compassion, as suffering with the other, illuminates the spiritual in all of us. As nurses, we are "wounded healers" (Nouwen, 1979; Ray, 2008). We are called upon to transcend sadness. Through genuine love and reaching out to others through spiritual healing, nurses facilitate and assist patients (or other caregivers) to finding meaning in suffering and pain. As a wounded healer, nurses also find healing for themselves (Nouwen, 1979, 1986; Hatthakit & Thaniwathananon, 2007; Lange, 2007).

The Unique Role of Nurses in Spiritual Healing
Nurses in particular have a unique responsibility to care for the soul of the other because of their commitment to holism (harmony of body, mind, and spirit), culture, and human caring. Nightingale (1860/1969) remarked that nursing is putting people in the right condition so that nature can act

on them (referring to nature as the manifestation of God). Spiritual caring is the mandate and nursing is the art of spiritual caring (O'Brien, 2002). One of the most important arenas of patient care that is entrusted to the nurse is the responsibility for the alleviation of pain (i.e., physical, emotional, or spiritual). When in the presence of a nurse, patients request relief from pain and suffering, generally by means of medication. The nursing theorist Eriksson (2006) remarked that "[t]he history of suffering belongs together with the history of compassion and the responsibility we are prepared to assume to [and for] each other" (p. 31). Moreover, Eriksson stated that "[t]o cause suffering for the other is simultaneously to violate one's own dignity and to deny one's own holiness" (p. 31). Nurses should not be engaged in the cause of suffering for any reason to a patient with the exception of and when necessary, treatment protocols, which may inflict bodily pain or emotional hurt. Caring deeply involves nurturing, comforting, and compassionately communicating with the patient to gain knowledge and insight into the struggle with physical, emotional, or spiritual distress.

At the same time, attention to the use or abuse of technology in the care of the patient, and dying and pending death requires diligence by the nurse (Ray, 2007). Patients often cannot express their suffering in tangible and easily describable terms, so nurses as trusted caregivers are called upon to translate its meaning. If the patient is an infant, child, or is not conscious, the nurse needs to be able to intuit the energy level and need, and respond accordingly.

Ways to Spiritual Healing
The ways to spiritual healing are many and varied, such as communicating with God or a Higher Power through personal prayer and the prayers of others, sacred services, communicating with family and friends, and seeking help from other professionals. Seeking spiritual direction and communicating with religious leaders help people to heal from suffering and loss. Other spiritual practices, such asreflection and meditation, visualization, art and music therapy, and ancient rituals, open consciousness to divine energy (Goldsmith, 1959). A transcultural caring science enfolds transcultural spirituality including theology, religion, and ethics into knowledge of culture care diversity (recognition of differences in) and

universality (commonalities) for the purposes of the preservation and maintenance of cultural beliefs and values, accommodation and negotiation, and repatterning or restructuring of cultural choice for health and well-being (Leininger, 1991; Leininger & McFarland, 2006; McFarland & Wehbe-Alamah, 2015). Appreciation, understanding and choice are strengths of the coparticipative spiritual and ethical caring relationship. Transcultural spiritual-ethical caring thus includes:

- Respecting all people
- Being open to cultural/multicultural beliefs and values
- Embracing understanding of the meaning of moral and spiritual development in self and others
- Being accountable to and responsible for the other no matter what the religious beliefs are
- Attempting to secure human rights
- Mediating care
- Designing nursing care plans within hospitals and communities that facilitate choices and improve the lifeworld of patients from all cultures

By appreciating, listening, consoling, comforting, praying for, guiding, and energizing patients (and family members or significant others) to find meaning in suffering and pain, the art of spiritual healing is enacted. Nurse caring is thus significant and transforming. It fulfills the mandate of Nightingale. Through the self or with the assistance of professional religious leaders, the nurse as a spiritual healer fulfills the quest for wholeness, for belongingness, for overcoming fragmentation and loss, and, when necessary, sets in motion the right spiritual action for healing, health or a peaceful death.

A profound way to spiritual healing for the nurse is captured in the following poem of loss, love, and *Infinite Love* by Sandra Lynch in *The Heart of Nursing* (Wendler, 2005, p. 95).

Song for a Baby, Lost

Elijah, you may have been just one
Tiny drop
Upon this earth
But you touched the heart
Deep within . . .
Your deep brown eyes.
You touched me
Pools of gentle, sweet softness,
With a blessing.

Sweet, pure Elijah
You are God's holy baby
You dance with angels
And your laughter rings through the heavens
I hear your voice
Mingling with the sound of a
Bird song.
Thank you, Elijah.
Sweet baby Elijah, you are forever
A song in my heart.
(Used with permission by Sigma Theta Tau
International, 2009)

Summary

Universal Sources and Universal Mind as the theological, spiritual, and religious dimensions of culture give meaning to human beings of all cultures. The spiritual life is the journey of the soul—a light of conscience or moral knowledge of reaching out to a Universal Source and of addressing issues of good and evil and how to live in right relationship with self and others. This chapter highlighted the following:

- The Universal Mind captures the notion of deep beliefs about Universal Source(s) that shape values of diverse cultures and morality and ultimately form the basis of transcultural spirituality.
- The integration of theology and science is bringing us to a new understanding of the meaning of belongingness—to the God in and of the universe, the Universal Source(s), the Universal Mind (O'Murchu, 1997).
- The person is elevated in the spiritual life through faith, grace, prayer, meditation, and the gift of right reason by his or her relationship to God, defined also as the Divine, Infinite, Absolute, Jesus Christ, Allah, Creative Spirit, Higher Power, force, nature, creativity, healing, aboriginal myths, and stories.
- People express diverse religious beliefs and values, for example, Judaism, Christianity, Islam, Hinduism, Buddhism, Confucianism, Shintoism, Native Spirituality, and Integrative Spirituality by virtue of what is learned and transmitted within their historical cultures and/or transmitted by contact with people from different religions.
- For people whose beliefs do not correspond to beliefs about a God as a Universal Source, most hold universal virtues of charity and respect for persons, justice, and human rights that give hope and meaning to existence (Wielenberg, 2005).

- Science, theology, and social and health sciences, and even political and economic sciences, are beginning to come together to dialogue about the purpose and nature of the universe as we are discovering the interconnectedness of all things.
- Science has brought us to a new understanding about the sphere of belongingness (Capra et al, 1991).
- Belonging to the universe is the new hymn of science and theology (Delio, 2014).
- "The pivotal shift in spirituality's meaning for the twentieth [twenty-first] century resides in the birth of a worldview of interdependence or relationality. In its broadest sense . . . spirituality is the relational component of lived experience" (O'Murchu, 1997, p. 65) and religious virtues of faith, hope, and love are the foundation to lived experience (Pope Benedict XVI, 2005).
- Scientists and theologians see the universe as beautiful and intelligent.
- Transcultural spirituality is universal and points the way to understanding the cultural and religious forces that facilitate health and healing.
- The forces of compassion and justice light the way of the soul toward holistic health and harmony of body, mind, and spirit.
- Compassion and justice point the direction for authentic dialogue and peaceful coexistence.
- Cycles of fear, hatred, evil, war, and retaliation that impact health and well-being can be changed by appreciation of our belongingness to a Creator who cares, and our common humanity, and the responsibility we have for each other.
- Changing our internal image of reality can change the world (Harman, 1998).
- Dialogue increases understanding about differences and similarities in the quest for wholeness, compassion, and love.
- Transcultural spiritual-ethical caring is knowledge of a shared perception of the good and a desired form of life that is authentic.
- Cultures survive and grow only if they can draw their strength from compassion and love, recognition, appreciation, protection, justice, human rights, and mutual constructive criticism. Diversity within a unity of purpose then becomes a reality.

- Nursing has theological/spiritual roots (See Jeanne Mance, 2009, first lay nurse to practice in North America, Nightingale [1860/1969], mother of professional nursing, and religious sisters and others who advanced nursing over the years).
- Each nurse as a holistic caring scientist and artist is a part of the spiritual oneness of the mystery of the universe. As nurses engage in caring practices in general and spiritual caring practices in particular, the bonds of our common humanity are strengthened.
- All nurses are transcultural nurses by understanding the diversity of human culture and the diversity of beliefs and values.
- As a dynamic, holistic, multidimensional, and transcultural caring science, the sacred science of nursing involves love as the highest form of consciousness (Eriksson, 2006; Ray, 1981a, 1981b, 1997, 2010a, 2010b, 2010c Smith, 1999; Watson, 2005).
- Spiritual suffering and healing can be enhanced by empathy, spirituality, and transcultural communicative spiritual-ethical caring action in nursing practice around the globe.
- Transcultural nurses have the ability to facilitate choices for healing, health, and well-being.
- The Universal Mind as theological, spiritual, and religious consciousness gives meaning to nursing's declaration of health for all humanity, all cultures.
- Transcultural nursing's local and global responsibility is to unite in programs of action, such as parish nursing, faith-based community nursing, and organizations that attempt to achieve health for all humanity (Miller et al., Transcultural Nursing Society Position Statement on Human Rights, 2008; *Nightingale Declaration for a Healthy World*, American Holistic Nurses Association, 2007).
- The commitment to faith in all people, and love and transcultural caring is hope for the world.

*In this chapter on Universal Sources, the author is aware of her limitations in discussing this subject matter. The content presented is an invitation to study the area of religion and spirituality further within and across the sacred books and literature of all religions to provide competent transcultural nursing and health care.

Transcultural Caring Experiences

When reviewing the following transcultural caring experiences (stories/case studies), please refer to your own experience, religion, spiritual understanding, Biblical history, and other "holy" books and literature to pursue knowledge of world religions in a pluralist world. Refer to different literature and Web sites to assist with your search to compare and contrast central tenets of different religions.

Carol's Story*

Based upon the book: *The Life of Illness* (1993) by Carol T. Olson

*Carol was one of my Doctor of Philosophy students from whom I learned much about suffering, pain, persistence, endurance, courage, and faith in God.

Carol T. Olson, a Canadian woman of Scandinavian descent, had four siblings—two brothers and two sisters. Her mother was deeply religious and devoted to her children. She had been a high school teacher and principal before marriage. Carol's father was a Lutheran minister and part of a large faith community in Western Canada. He was the first director of the Canadian Lutheran Evangelistic Movement and the World Mission Prayer League. He also was a radio pastor for many years, serving the needs of people in Alberta, Saskatchewan and British Columbia. The family had an uncompromising faith in God, trusting that God would provide a way for each member of the family. Each day, the family was committed to devotion to God—saying morning prayers followed by family singing of the Lord's Prayer and other hymns and evening devotions, praying while kneeling at the bedside with their mother. Each of the children in the family suffered from severe polycystic kidney disease, including Carol. Two of the children, a boy and girl, died early in life from kidney failure. During Carol's teenage years, two more of her siblings died from kidney failure after suffering great physical difficulties and pain and experiencing both the hope and trauma of dialysis machines at a time when they were in their infancy and pharmacological research in immunology was developing slowly. Also, during this period of the illness and death of her siblings, Carol's father died suddenly of a heart attack.

Despite the pain that Carol felt from all the loss, she wondered how her father and her siblings could have accomplished so much in their lifetimes. Carol answered her own question. Their secret belonged to God. Carol was a very religious woman. She coped with her kidney disease with patience and grace. She was a pioneer to the many advances in kidney disease as well as to technological and therapeutic developments. Carol's questioning continued as she pursued her education, and underwent the many challenges to sustain life. She explained that medical technology gave her life. But medical technology has no life, no soul that suffers pain and thrives in hope. Carol stated, "What is life that technology is not sufficient for life?" By her research questions, reflection, and writing, Carol wanted to help herself, the rest of the world, especially doctors, nurses, and technicians, "live in understanding." She concluded, with help from the contributors to her research (i.e., nurse, teacher, doctor, minister, and mother) who read literature such as Tolstoy's *The Death of Ivan Ilyitch*; Erickson's *With all my Heart*; Camus' *The Plague*; Florence Nightingale's *Notes on Nursing*; and Lord Tennyson's *In Memoriam* that the good of illness is love. In a life of illness, there is no life in us other than the love of God, family, friends, and community (Olson, 1993, pp. 1–5).

Questions for Analysis of Carol's Transcultural Caring Experience: The Life of Illness

You, as a nurse, are assigned to care for Carol in the Dialysis Center of the hospital. She has come to the hospital after a severe bout with fatigue after classes at the university (she is taking postdoctoral studies in secondary education). Her hemoglobin, potassium, and sodium levels are out of control. Because of her general weight loss from the many years of polycystic kidney disease, continuous dialysis, and nutritional challenges, Carol is feeling very exhausted. She also is exhibiting signs of deep sadness. Right now, Carol's skin is dry and itchy and she is uncomfortable. You have been Carol's nurse in dialysis for many years and know the history of her suffering and endurance with the disease and the technology and the experiences of her family who encountered "lives of illness." You are familiar with the fact that Carol has been involved in research and had opportunities to experience some of the new advances in dialysis treatment and pharmacology.

You also have learned more about the general care of the patient with kidney disease, including the potentialities for renal transplant surgery and care. Lately, you have taken a hospital ethics course where end-of-life decisions and advance directives (patient wishes and decisions) were discussed. You also took courses in holistic and alternative health care at the local university school of nursing. As a nurse, you always marveled at how Carol and her mother dealt with everyday struggles of human existence. Through your discussions with Carol (and her mother), you know that she has a deep Christian faith and lives a "life of prayer" and dedication to the Christian life. You are aware from sharing with Carol that she and her mother believe that the family will be together again in eternity.

Reading Olson's book, *The Life of Illness,* will assist with these questions and your answers.

Reflective Nursing Practice: Transcultural Caring Spirituality

- How does Carol's life story make you feel? What does suffering mean to you as you contemplate Carol's story?

- What do you think about the role of spirituality in nursing and health care? How does faith enter into your call to care, not only for Carol but also for other patients?

- What is transcultural spirituality? How do you see spirituality viewed as transcultural, for example, when a nurse has a different spiritual belief than his or her patient?

- Does Carol's story conjure up feelings about the meaning of faith, hope, and love and mercy?

- Are there differences in the Christian faith, in general, or in particular Christian religions? Could you introduce any holistic care practices given that nursing addresses health as the harmony of body, mind, and spirit (soul)? Would there be any conflicts with Christianity or any other religion?

- Compare and contrast the different health-care systems of physical, technological, pharmacological, and spiritual care. What responsibility do you as a nurse have to take into account regarding the faith and moral foundation of patients in facilitating the making of decisions/choices about nursing care or patient self-care as they live out the life of illness? Does it make a difference if the patient is living in Canada where Carol and her family are from?

- What does chronic illness and pain mean to you? What are the signs and symptoms of chronic renal disease?

- What does technology and pharmacology mean in the life of a patient with kidney disease?

- How would the team of physicians, researchers, nurses, and nutritionists, and social workers care for and play a role in chronic illness?

- Do you feel any signs of spiritual distress that might be coextensive with Carol's life of illness? Do you think Carol might feel spiritual distress even though she has a strong faith?

- Do you have feelings about injustice in the life of Carol?

- What do end-of-life decision and advance directives mean to you?

- How would you introduce the notion of spiritual (pastoral) care to the team of caregivers if it is not a foundation for care in your hospital or care experience? Should a chaplain be on the team given the strength of faith in many patients' lives? What if the chaplain is a different faith than a patient? How would you handle that challenge?

Further Reflection on Spirituality

When you contemplate the life of illness of Carol and the trauma that she and her mother encountered when each of her siblings died of kidney disease and her father died suddenly of a heart attack, reflect upon concepts, such as *health-care theology* and *social justice.*

- Do you feel any signs of spiritual distress that might be coextensive with Carol's life of illness?

- Do you think Carol might feel spiritual distress even though she has a strong faith?

- What do you think about social justice? Is there a relationship among religion, spirituality, culture, health care, and health-care policy from your viewpoint?

- What do you think about programs of study for faith-based community or parish nursing? Should they be adopted by more churches and synagogues?

- Where are they located in your community?

Jim's Story

The Owl: The End Is Nigh

My husband Jim was dying of lung cancer, a disease for which no primary care physician or oncologist had an answer because Jim had no risk factors. He had never smoked cigarettes or been around toxic substances in his job as an accountant with a telephone company. He had been a Marine though during the Vietnam conflict more than 30 years earlier and there was some discussion that maybe he had exposure to Agent Orange, a substance used for defoliation of brush in the jungle.

Jim survived with metastatic lung cancer beyond the 5-year mark, after first having surgery, then radiation, and then many years of chemotherapy with participation in new and different research protocols. Jim survived because of his deep religious faith and spiritual nature. Jim lived his life as a Catholic, a man of principle, always praying and responding to the call of the Lord. He was deeply devoted to his family, nursing, and me, his wife. He loved nature and everything in it, especially rabbits, ducks, birds, even spiders. Jim always believed in the value of nurses because, as Jim said, "they care." His doctor loved him like a brother. Family and friends of all religious faiths prayed for him. Fran and Eleanor, his special nurse friends, performed "therapeutic touch" (i.e., healing touch and Reiki). Good friends, Carolyn and Tom were always there for him. The university faculty bestowed upon him an Honorary Professorship, which was one highlight of his life. As Jim's caregiver, I was very afraid; I think Jim was too, but he had dealt with the fear of death as a combat Marine so perhaps he had a better understanding of the "shortness of life." I tried to give Jim all the love, support, and prayers I could and find and fight for the best cancer care and healing modalities available. Often, the insurance system in the United States provided barriers to the best care available.

Five and one-half years into Jim's battle with cancer, his body was failing but his mind was clear and his spirit strong. As time went on, one night Jim woke me and asked, "Do you hear the owl?" I did. The owl was hooting softly in the distance—but just for a moment or two. (We lived a little outside of Denver near the foothills of the Rocky Mountains. We had never heard the hooting of the owl before.) Jim pondered and said, "God is calling me home." I listened in silence, finally reassuring him, knowing in my heart what that meant.

A few nights later, Jim woke me again. He said, "Do you hear the owl?" I said, "Yes." Jim's voice was so strong when he responded, "God is calling me home." Though it was so hard for me to say, I agreed, "God IS calling you home." We never heard the owl again.

In less than a week, after a surprise Thanksgiving Day visit from his sister and children from Utah, a visit from our priest who gave him the Sacrament of the Sick in preparation for his journey to God, and less than a day in hospice with two very caring nurses, Jim died encircled by friends and me, his loving wife. Through the prayers and care by his human family who surrounded him after a difficult night and day of suffering, Jim died—he faded away to a life with God in eternity. In the room, I was aware of the "presence of God and his spiritual family, the Communion of Saints" (a central precept of the Catholic faith from Hebrews 12:1–2, *The New American Bible*, 1987, p. 1536). Jim had a Catholic funeral mass, buried with full military honors, and laid to rest beside his parents.

Questions for Spiritual Caring Analysis of Jim
Reflective Practice

- How does the transcultural caring experience of Jim call forth in you an understanding of spirituality in Jim and his family? Compare and contrast your own spiritual faith with that of Jim's (transcultural spirituality). What is the relationship among religion, spirituality, and health care from your view point? Does Jim's story conjure up feelings about the meaning of faith, hope, and love that is reappearing in nursing as caring and in the public sphere?
- Contemplate the meaning of suffering with cancer for more than 5 years and its effect on the patient and family. For reflections: What is the meaning of an overwhelmed patient from your understanding, for example, are they getting the right care or treatment—are there too many suggestions for treatment or care or wellness care now that it is becoming a part of cancer care, too many or too few caregivers, too many appointments or not enough home visits, and so forth? Should and how can caring nurses become the primary coordinators of care for patients?

- What does the dying process in Jim's story mean, and what does the dying process mean to you? What do suffering, courage, and hope mean to you as you contemplate Jim's story?
- What is the meaning of spiritual care and a faith-based foundation to care and treatment? Why is spiritual care so important to patients and patients with cancer?
- What is holistic nursing and caring in Jim's story? What emotional fears are present in Jim's story? Is there such a thing as the theology of the body, mind, and spirit (soul) for nursing and health care?
- What are the signs and symptoms of lung cancer and of metastatic lung cancer? Ponder treatments, such as radiation and pharmacological chemotherapies, as you as a nurse of care for a cancer patient over time.
- How does transcultural nursing (i.e., values, faith traditions, signs, symbols, and rituals) enter into the portrait of Jim's story? What cultural and faith rituals are present in Jim's story? What significance do signs and symbols and rituals have for you as a person, professional nurse, or nursing student? What do you think about the sign and symbol of the owl in Jim's story? How did the symbol of the owl affect you? What is the importance of signs, symbols, and ritual in culture in Jim's story? Do you know the meaning of the symbol of the owl in native spirituality? Can you see that spirituality can be viewed as transcultural, for example, if you have a different spiritual or religious belief or set of values than Jim? What about other ceremonial cultural rituals, such as military honors for a veteran of the U.S. Marine Corps? Can you think of rituals in your own faith or in nursing that are significant?
- What signs of the end of life were present in Jim's story? What does end-of-life care mean to you? How are physical, emotional, and spiritual qualities integrated? What responsibility do you as a nurse have to take into account in relation to the faith and moral foundation of patients in facilitating the making of end-of-life decisions/choices about their care or patient self-care as they live out the life of suffering, pain, hope, and courage in the dying process at the end of life? What care should be given a wife as caregiver and who also is a nurse? What care should be given to any family member with a patient who is suffering from cancer? How would you introduce the notion of spiritual care and end-of-life care to your team of caregivers if they do not have a holistic focus?

Further Reflection on Transcultural Spirituality and Holistic Nursing

- Do you have feelings about injustice in the life of Jim or any other patients because you think they may not have deserved what happened to them?
- Do you feel any signs of spiritual distress, especially contemplating military service and war, injury, trauma, especially when wars may not be unanimously supported in one country or another? What do you think about post-traumatic stress disorder (PTSD) or spiritual distress in military personnel, veterans, or their families?
- Contemplate the use of chemotherapy in conjunction with alternative nursing practices, such as therapeutic touch, healing touch, and Reiki. Do you think these practices should be integrated into professional nursing practice?
- Do you think that alternative practices are forms of spiritual care or are they, as some theological scholars, think, antitheological or anti-Christian? Could you introduce any holistic care practices given that nursing addresses health as the harmony of body, mind, and soul? How would you, as a nurse, discuss different therapeutic practices?
- What do you think of pastoral care for the sick and dying? What is your view of healing? Would you or how would you as a team leader in professional situations, whether in the hospital or hospice care, raise a discussion of the integration of scientific medicine with alternative health care and holistic nursing practices with your team of physicians, researchers, nurses, nutritionists, social workers, and chaplains or pastoral care practitioners?
- If your hospital or hospice care unit did not have a pastoral care team, would you raise the subject?
- Contemplate differences, review this chapter, and search the literature or Web sites to understand more about different faiths: Christian, Jewish, Native, Muslim, Buddhist, Hindu, or other religions.

Do you think that diverse religious or spiritual practices of different ethnic groups are or should be an integral part of care in any professional setting? How would you approach patients about their religious practices and rituals to develop a plan of cultural care and provide culturally relevant and competent care? How would you integrate traditional practices of a specific culture group with scientific and professional Western care practices? Think about your own cultural background or that of your relationship with a close relative or friend, how would you support the patient and the patient's family?
- How would you provide caring, concern, and kindness for a patient who was not religious or spiritual during illness and at the end of life?

References

Ahmed, A. (2004). *Postmodernism and Islam: Predicament and promise*. London: Routledge.

Al-Alwain, T. (2005). *Issues in contemporary Islamic thought*. Cairo: International Institute of Islamic Thought.

Alexander, S. (2006). How religions are similar and how they are not. *Florida Catholic*, October 2006, p. A 16.

American Nurses Association. Http://www/nursing-world.org/codeofnursingethics

American Psychiatric Association (2000). *Diagnostic and statistical manual of mental disorders* (4th ed). Washington, DC: American Psychiatric Association.

Andrews, M., & Boyle, J. (2007). *Transcultural concepts in nursing care* (5th ed.). Philadelphia: Lippincott Williams & Wilkins.

Andrews, M. & Boyle, J. (2015). *Transcultural concepts in nursing care* (7th ed.). Wolters Kluwer Health.

Armstrong, K. (2002). *Islam*. New York: The Modern Library.

Arntz, W., Chase, B., & Vincente, M. (2005). *What the bleep do we know!?* Deerfield Beach, FL: Health Communications, Inc.

Baglin, D., & Mullins, B. (1969). *Aboriginals of Australia*. New South Wales: Shepp Books.

Bahia religion. Retrieved August 2, 2008 from http://www.bahai.org.

Bar-Yam, Y. (2004). *Making things work: Solving complex problems in a complex world*. Boston: NECSI, Knowledge Press.

Battista, J. (1982). The holographic model, holistic paradigm, information theory and consciousness. *The Holographic Paradigm and other Paradoxes*. Boulder: New Science Library.

Berman, P. (2004). *Terror and liberalism*. New York: W. W. Norton & Company.

Bhikkhu, B. (2005). *Handbook for mankind (Buddhism)*. Thailand: National Buddhism Center.

Boulding, E. (1988). *Building the global civic culture*. New York: Teachers' College Press.

Boykin, A., & Schoenhofer, S. (2001). *Nursing as caring: A model for transforming practice*. Sudbury, MA: Jones & Bartlett.

Briggs, D., & Peat, F. (1984). *The turbulent mirror*. New York: Harper & Row, Publishers.

Briggs, J., & Peat F. (1999). *Seven life lessons of chaos*. New York: Harper Collins Publishers.

Brown, J., & Alligood, M. (2014). *Margaret Newman, Health as expanding consciousness* (8th ed.). St. Louis: Elsevier.

Buber, M. (1952). *Good and evil*. New York: Charles Scribner's Sons.

Buber, M. (1958). *I and thou*. New York: McMillan.

Burnham, F. (Ed.). (1989). *Postmodern theology: Christian faith in a pluralist world*. San Francisco: HarperSanFrancisco.

Byrne, D., & Callaghan, G. (2014). *Complexity theory and the social sciences*. New York: Routledge.

Calabria, M. (1990). Spiritual insights of Florence Nightingale, *Quest 3*, 66–74.

Capra, F., Steindl-Rast, D., with Matus, T. (1991). *Belonging to the universe*. SanFrancisco: HarperSan Francisco.

Catechism of the Catholic Church. (1994). (Liberia Editrice Vaticana). The Vatican: Liguori Publications.

Chester, M. (2005). *Divine pathos and human being: The theology of Abraham Joshua Heschel*. London: Valentine Mitchell.

Chinn, P. (2013). *Peace and power: New directions for building community* (8th ed.). Burlington, MA: Jones & Bartlett Learning.

Code of ethics for nurses with interpretive statements. (2001). Washington, DC: American Nurses Association.

Coffman, S. (2006). Marilyn Anne Ray: Theory of bureaucratic caring. In A. Marriner Tomey & M. Alligood (Eds.), *Nursing theorists and their work* (pp. 116–139). St. Louis: Mosby-Elsevier.

Cope, T. (2006). *Fear of Jung.* London: Karnac.

Coulson, N. (1969). *Conflicts and tensions in Islamic jurisprudence.* Chicago: The University of Chicago Press.

Csikszentmihalyi, M. (1993). *The evolving self.* New York: Harper Collins Publisher.

Curtis, E. (1993). *Native American wisdom.* Philadelphia: Running Press.

Czerenda, A. (2006). *"The show must go on": A caring inquiry into the meaning of widowhood and health for older Indian widows.* Doctor of Nursing Science Dissertation, Florida Atlantic University (Publication Number: ATT 3222085. Proquest Document ID #: 1176546131), Boca Raton, FL.

D'Aquili, E., & Newberg, A. (1999). *The mystical mind: Probing the biology of religious experience.* Minneapolis, MN: Augsburg Fortress Publishers.

Davidhizar, R., & Giger, J. (2003). *Transcultural nursing: Assessment & intervention.* St. Louis: Mosby.

Davidson, A., & Ray, M. (1991). Studying the human-environment phenomenon using the science of complexity. *Advances in Nursing Science, 13*(2), 73–87.

Davidson, A. Ray, M., & Turkel, M. (Eds.) (2011). *Nursing, caring and complexity: For human-environment well-being.* New York: Springer Publishing Company.

Dear, J. (2007). Transfiguration: A meditation on transforming ourselves and our world. *Spirituality and health, March–April,* 72–73.

De Caussade, J. (1966). *The sacrament of the present moment.* San Francisco: HarperSanFrancisco.

De Duve, T. (2006). Come on, humans, one more effort if you want to be post-Christians! In H. De Vries & L. Sullivan (Eds.), *Political theologies: Public religion in a post-secular world* (pp. 652–690). New York: Fordham University Press.

De La Rosa, R., & Goke, K. (2007). Reflections on suffering and culture in Iraq: An army nurse perspective. *International Journal for Human Caring, 2*(2), 53–58.

Delio, I. (Ed.) (2014). *From Teilhard to Omega.* Maryknoll, NY: Orbis Books.

De Vries, H., & Sullivan, L. (Eds.). (2006). *Political theologies: Public religions in a post-secular world.* New York: Fordham University Press.

Dossey, B. (2000). *Florence Nightingale: Mystic, visionary, healer.* Philadelphia: Lippincott, Williams & Wilkins.

Douglas, M., Uhl-Pierce, J., Rosenkoetter, M., et al. *Standards of practice for culturally competent care: 2011 update.* Journal of Transcultural Nursing, 22(4), 317–333.

Durkheim, E., & Mauss, M. (1963). *Primitive classification* (R. Needham, Trans.). Chicago, IL: The University of Chicago Press.

Dyess, S. (2011). *Faith: A concept analysis.* Journal of Advanced Nursing, 67(12), 2723–2731.

Dyess, S., & Chase, S. (2012). *Sustaining health in faith community nursing practice: Emerging processes that support the development of a middle-range theory.* Holistic Nursing Practice, 26(4), 221–227.

Eberstadt, M. (2013). *How the West really lost God: A new theory of secularization.* West Conshohocken, PA: Templeton Press.

England, J., Kuttianimattathil, J., Prior, J., Quintos, L., Kwang-Sun, D., & Wickeri, J. (Eds.). (2004). *Asian and Christian theologies.* Delhi, India: Orbis Books.

Eriksson, K. (1997). Caring, spirituality and suffering. In M. Roach (Ed.), *Caring from the heart: The convergence of caring and spirituality* (pp. 68–84). New York: Paulist Press.

Eriksson, K. (2006). *The suffering human being.* (C. Peterson & J. Zetterlund [Eds.]). Chicago: Nordic Studies Press.

Eriksson, K. (2007). Becoming through suffering-The path to health and holiness. *International Journal for Human Caring, 2*(2), 8–16.

Ess, C. (2014). *Digital media ethics.* Cambridge, UK: Polity Press.

Evans-Pritchard, E. (1965). *Theories of primitive religion.* Oxford: Oxford University Press.

Giger, J., & Davidhizar, R. (1998). *Canadian transcultural nursing: Assessment and intervention.* St. Louis: Mosby.

Goldsmith, J. (1959). *The art of spiritual healing.* San Francisco: HarperSanFrancisco.

Goodwin, B. (1994). *How the leopard changed its spots: The evolution of complexity.* New York: Simon & Schuster.

Goodwin, B. (2003). Patterns of wholeness. *Resurgence, 1*(21), 12–14.

Habermas, J. (2006). On the relations between the secular liberal state and religion. In H. DeVries & L. Sullivan (Eds.), *Political theologies: Public religion in a post-secular world* (pp. 251–260). New York: Fordham University Press.

Harman, W. (1998). *Global mind change* (2nd ed.). San Francisco: Berrett-Koehler Publishers, Inc.

Harris, S. (2014). *Waking up: A guide to spirituality without religion.* New York: Simon & Schuster.

Hatthakit, U., & Thaniwathananon, P. (2007). The suffering experiences of Buddhist Tsunami survivors. *International Journal for Human Caring, 2*(2), 59–66.

Henderson, H. (2007). Alternative future/s. *Spirituality and Health. March-April,* 69–71 & 92–93.

Heschel, A. (1954). *Man's quest for God.* New York: Charles Scribner's Sons.

Hill, L. (2002). *American Indians.* New York: Workman Publishing Company, Inc.

Ho, M. (2003). Dance of life. *Resurgence, 1*(216), 18–19.

Holmes, W. (2007). Expanding the human mind: The future of the brain. *The Futurist, 41*(4), 41–46.

Hoobler, T., & Hoobler, D. (2004). *Confucianism.* New York: World Religions, Facts on File, Inc.

Huyler, S. (1999). *Meeting God: Elements of Hindu devotion.* New Haven: Yale University Press.

Ions, V. (1999). *The history of mythology.* New York: Quadrillion Publishing, Inc.

Joseph, R. (Ed.). (2002). *Neurotheology: Brain, science, spirituality, religious experience.* San Jose, CA: University Press.

Jung, C. (1960). *Psychology and religion* (The Terry Lecture Series)(Original Publication 1938 by Yale University Press). Binghamton, NY: The Vail-Ballow Press, Inc.

Jung, C. (1964). *Man and his symbols.* Garden City, New York: Doubleday & Company, Inc.

Kinast, R. (2006). Different religions can resemble each other. *Florida Catholic,* October 2006, p. A16.

Koerner, J. (1997). Cocreation of culture through choice. In J. Dienemann (Ed.), *Cultural Diversity in Nursing* (pp. 63–69). Washington, DC: American Academy of Nursing.

Kübler-Ross, E. (1997). *On death and dying.* New York: Scribner.

Kurzweil, R. (2005). *The singularity is near.* New York: Viking.

Lange, B. (2007). The prescriptive power of caring for self: Women in recovery from substance use disorders. *International Journal for Human Caring, 2*(2), 74–80.

Leffler, W., & Jones, P. (2005). *The structure of religion: Judaism and Christianity.* Lanham: University Press of America, Inc.

Leininger, M. (1970). *Anthropology and nursing: Two worlds to blend.* New York: John Wiley & Sons.

Leininger, M. (1978). *Transcultural nursing: Concepts, theory and practices.* New York: John Wiley & Sons.

Leininger, M. (Ed.)(1981). *Caring: An essential human need.* Thorofare, NJ: Charles B. Slack, Inc.

Leininger, M. (1991). *Culture care diversity and univer-sality: A theory of nursing.* New York: National League for Nursing Press.

Leininger, M. (1997). Transcultural spirituality: A comparative care and health focus. In M. Roach (Ed.), *Caring from the Heart: The Convergence of Caring and Spirituality.* New York: Paulist Press.

Leininger, M., & McFarland, M. (2006). (Eds.). *Culture diversity & universality: A worldwide nursing theory* (2nd ed.). Sudbury, MA: Jones & Bartlett.

Lemkow, A. (1990). *The wholeness principle: Dynamics of unity within science, religion & society.* Wheaton, IL: Quest Books.

Lowe, J., & Nichols, L. (2014). *Utilisation of a Native American nursing conceptual framework: Implications for practice and research.* Australian Journal of Advanced Nursing, 31(2), 13–22.

Macrae, J. (2001). *Nursing as a spiritual practice.* New York: Springer Publishing Company. Margenau, H. (1984). *The miracle of existence.* Woodbridge, CT: Ox Bow Press.

Mance, J. (2009). *Celebrating women's achievements-Canadian Women in Science-Jeanne Mance.* Library and Archives of Canada/Bibliothèque et Archives Canada. Retrieved June 18, 2009, from http://www.collectionsCanada.gc.ca/women/002026-410-e.html

Margenau, H. (1984). *The miracle of existence.* Woodbridge, CT: Ox Bow Press.

Marriner Tomey, A., & Alligood, M. (Eds.). (2006). *Nursing theorists and their work.* St. Louis: Mosby-Elsevier.

Martin, M. (2013). *Perceived discrimination of Muslims in health care in the United States.* (Order No. 3585040, Florida Atlantic University, Proquest

Dissertations and Theses, 209.) Retrieved from http://search.proquest.com/docview/1508821207?accountid=131239. (1508821207).

Martin, M. & Ray, M. (2015). *Gender equality and the empowerment of women in Arab countries: A transcultural caring perspective.* International Journal for Human Caring. 19(1), 13-18.

Martin, M. (in press). A model for understanding the Muslim patient: Using Ray's Transcultural Caring Dynamics in Nursing and Health Care. Research and Theory for Nursing Practice.

McFarland, M. (2006). Madeleine Leininger: Culture care theory of diversity and universality. In A. Marriner Tomey & M. Alligood (Eds.), *Nursing theorists and their work* (pp. 643–662). St. Louis: Mosby-Elsevier.

McFarland, M., & Wehbe-Alamah, H. (2015). *Leininger's culture care diversity and universality: A worldwide theory of nursing* (3rd ed.). Burlington, MA: Jones & Bartlett Learning.

McMaster, G., & Trafzer, C. (Eds.). (2004). *Native universe.* Washington, DC: Smithsonian Institution.

Merton, T. (1951). *The ascent to truth.* New York: Harcourt Brace Jovanovich Publishers.

Merton, T. (1961). *New seeds of contemplation.* New York: New Directions Books.

Merton, T. (1985). *Love and living* (N. Stone & P. Hart [Eds.]). New York: Harcourt Brace Jovanovich.

Miller, J., Leininger, M., Leuing, C., Pacquia, D., Andrews, M., Ludwig-Beymer, P., & Papadopoulos, I. (2008). Transcultural nursing society statement of human rights. *Journal of Transcultural Nursing, 18*(1), 5–7.

Moore, T. (1992). *Care of the soul.* New York: Harper-Collins Publishers.

Morse, J. (2001). Toward a praxis theory of suffering. *Advances in Nursing Science, 24*(1), 47–59.

Newlin, K., Knafl, K., & Melkus, G. (2002). *African-American spirituality: A concept analysis.* Advances in Nursing Science, 25(2), 57–70.

Newman, M. (1986). *Health as expanding consciousness.* St. Louis: Mosby.

Newman, M. (1994). *Health as expanding consciousness* (2nd Ed.). New York: National League for Nursing Press.

Newman, M., Sime, M., & Corcoran-Perry, S. (1991). The focus of the discipline of nursing. *Advances in Nursing Science, 14*, 1–6.

Nightingale, F. (1969). *Notes on nursing: What it is and what it is not.* New York: Dover. (Original work published 1860)

Nightingale Declaration for a Healthy World. (2007). American Holistic Nurses Association (AHNA), Flagstaff, Arizona.

Nouwen, H. (1975). *Reaching out: The three movements of the spiritual life.* New York: Doubleday.

Nouwen, H. (1979). *The wounded healer.* New York: Doubleday & Co., Image Books.

Nouwen, H. (1986). *Lifesigns.* New York: Doubleday.

Nouwen, H., McNeil, D., & Morrison, D. (1982). *Compassion.* New York: Doubleday.

O'Brien, M. (2002). *Spirituality in nursing* (2nd ed.). Sudbury, MA: Jones and Bartlett Publishers.

O'Brien, M. (2013). *Spirituality in nursing* (5th ed.). Burlington, MA: Jones & Bartlett Learning.

Olson, C. (1993). *The life of illness.* Albany, NY: State University of New York Press.

O'Murchu, D. (1997). *Quantum theology: Spiritual implications of the new physics.* New York: The Crossword Publishing Company.

Palmer, P. (1993). *To know as we are known.* San Francisco: HarperSanFrancisco.

Parker, M. (Ed.). (2006). *Nursing theories, nursing practice* (2nd ed.). Philadelphia: F. A. Davis Company.

Parse, R. (1981). *Man-living-health: A theory of nursing.* New York: Wiley.

Parse, R. (1995). *Illuminations: The human becoming theory in practice and research.* New York: National League for Nursing Press.

Peat, F. (2002). *From certainty to uncertainty.* Washington, DC: Joseph Henry Press.

Peat, F. (2003). From physics to Pari: A continuing search for answers. *Resurgence, 1*(216), 24–26.

Pope Benedict XVI. (2005). Encyclical Letter *"Deus Caritas Est" (God is love),* Retrieved June 18, 2009, from http:www.vatican.va/holy-father/benedict_xvi_enc-2005/225_deuscaritasest_en.html

Pope Benedict XVI. (2006a). Prepolitical moral foundations of a free republic. In H. de Vries & L. Sullivan (Eds.), *Political theologies: Public religion in a post-secular world* (pp. 261–268). New York: Fordham University Press.

Pope Benedict XVI. (2006b). The split in modern morality. *Restoration, 60*(5), 2, 8.

Pope Benedict XVI. (2008). Our relationship with God. *Restoration, 61*(6), 6.

Pope Francis. (2013). Lumen fidei (the Light of Faith–Encyclical Letter. Retrieved from www. m.vatican. va./context/encyclicals.documents/papa-francesco-20130629-enciclia-lumen-fidei.html

Pope John Paul II. (2006). You are of inestimable worth. *Restoration, 59*(2), 2.

Postero, N. (2007). *Now we are citizens.* Stanford, CA: Stanford University Press.

Purnell, M. & Mead, L. (2007). When nurses mourn: Layered suffering. *International Journal for Human Caring, 2*(2), 47–52.

Rachels, J. (1986*). The elements of moral philosophy.* New York: Random House.

Ratzinger, J. (Pope Benedict XVI). (2007). *Jesus of Nazareth* (A. Walker, Trans.). New York: Doubleday.

Ray, M. (1981a). A study of caring within an institutional culture. *Dissertation Abstracts International, 42*(06) (University Microfilms No. 8127787).

Ray, M. (1981b). A philosophical analysis of caring within nursing. In M. Leininger (Ed.), *Caring: An essential human need.* (pp. 25–36). Thorofare, NJ: Charles B. Slack, Inc.

Ray, M. (1989a). Transcultural caring: Political and economic visions. *Journal of Transcultural Nursing, 1*(1), 17–21.

Ray, M. (1989b). The theory of bureaucratic caring for nursing practice in the organizational culture. *Nursing Administration Quarterly, 13*(2), 31–42.

Ray, M. (1994). Transcultural nursing ethics: A framework and model for transcultural ethical analysis. *Journal of Holistic Nursing, 12*(3), 251–264.

Ray, M. (1997). Illuminating the meaning of caring: Unfolding the sacred art of divine love. In M. Roach (Ed.), *Caring from the heart: The convergence of caring and spirituality.* New York: Paulist Press.

Ray, M. (1998). Complexity and nursing science. *Nursing Science Quarterly, 11*, 91–93.

Ray, M. (1999). Transcultural caring in primary health care. *National Academies of Practice Forum, 1*(3), 177–182.

Ray, M. (2001). Transcultural assessment. In S. Koch & S. Garratt (Eds.), *Assessing older people.* New South Wales, AU: Maclennan & Petty.

Ray, M. (2006). Marilyn Anne Ray's theory of bureaucratic caring. In M. Parker (Ed.), *Nursing theories &*

nursing practice (2nd ed., pp. 360–368). Philadelphia: F.A. Davis Company.

Ray, M. (2007). Technological caring as a dynamic of complexity in nursing practice. In A. Barnard & R. Locsin (Eds.), *Perspectives on technology and nursing practice.* United Kingdom: Palgrave.

Ray, M. (2008). Caring scholar response to "Achieving compassionate excellence: A cooperative accelerated BSN program". *International Journal for Human Caring, 12*(2), 39–41.

Ray, M. (2010a). *Transcultural caring dynamics in nursing and health care.* Philadelphia: F. A. Davis Company.

Ray, M. (2010b). *A study of caring within an institutional culture: The discovery of the Theory of Bureaucratic Caring.* Germany: Lambert Academic Publishing.

Ray, M. (2011). Complex caring dynamics: A unifying model for nursing inquiry. in Davidson, A., Ray, M., & Turkel, M. (2011). *Nursing, caring, and complexity science: For human-environment well-being* (pp. 31-52). New York: Springer Publishing Company. (Reprinted with revisions from original article published in Theoretic and Applied Chaos in Nursing, 1994).

Ray, M., & Turkel, M. (2012). *The transtheoretical evolution of caring science in complex systems.* International Journal for Human Caring, 16(2), 28–49.

Ray, M., & Turkel, M. (2014). *Caring as emancipatory nursing praxis: The theory of Relational Caring Complexity.* Advances in Nursing Science, 37(2), 132–146.

Rinpoche, Y. (2007). Destined for joy. *Spirituality and Health, March-April,* 48–53.

Roach, M. (Ed.). (1997). *Caring from the heart: The convergence of caring and spirituality.* New York: Paulist Press.

Roach, M. (2002). *The human act of caring* (rev. ed.). Ottawa: Canadian Hospital Association. (Original work published 1987)

Rogers, M. (1970). *An introduction to the theoretical basis of nursing.* Philadelphia: F. A. Davis Company.

Rogers, M. (1994). The science of unitary human beings: Current perspectives. *Nursing Science Quarterly, 2,* 33–35.

Ruparell, T. (2000). Shintoism. In Ian S. Markham (Ed.), *Encountering religion: An introduction to the religions of the world.* London: Blackwell Publishing Ltd.

Saint Augustine. (1958). *City of God* (G. Walsh, D. Zema, G. Monahan, & D. Honan, Trans.). New York: Doubleday.

Saint Thomas Aquinas. (1967). *Summa theologiae. The emotions* (Vol. 19). New York: McGraw-Hill Book Company.

Salih, R. (2007). Muslim women and the public sphere in Europe. *Anthropology News, 48*(5), 14–15.

Sanford, J. (1988). *Evil: The shadow side of reality.* New York: Crossroad.

Schmitt, C. (1985). Political theology (G. Schwab, Trans. & Intro.). Chicago: The University of Chicago Press.

Schwarz, H. (1995). *Evil: A historical and theological perspective.* Minneapolis: Fortress Press.

Shapiro, R. (2007). Why aren't you an atheist?..Why connect spirituality and Health? *Spirituality and Health, 10*(2), 16–17.

Singer, P. (Ed.). (1993). *A companion to ethics.* Oxford: Blackwell Publishing.

Sivananda, S. (2005). Shintoism. Retrieved June 18, 2009, from http://www.dishq.org/religions/shintoism.htm

Smith, H. (1989). *Beyond the post-modern mind* (rev.). Wheaton, IL: The Theosophical Publishing House.

Smith, H. (1991). *The world's religions.* San Francisco: HaperSanFrancisco.

Smith, J. (1998). *On the origin of objects.* Cambridge, MA: The MIT Press.

Smith, J. (2005). *The book of Mormon: The original 1830 edition.* Berkeley, CA: Apocryphile Press.

Smith, M. & Parker, M. (Eds.). (1999). Caring and the science of unitary human beings. *Advances in Nursing Science, 21,*14–28.

Smith, M. (Ed.) (2015). *Nursing theories and nursing practice* (4th ed.). Philadelphia: F. A. Davis Company.

Smith, M., Turkel, M., & Wolf, Z. (2013). *Caring in nursing classics: An essential resource.* New York: Springer Publishing Company.

Smith, M. J., & Liehr, P. (2014). Story theory. In M. J. Smith & P. Liehr (Eds). *Middle range theory for nursing* (3rd ed.) (pp. 224–257). New York: Springer Publishing Company.

Smith, S. (2004). *Parish nursing: A handbook for the new millennium.* New York: Howorth Pastoral Press.

Solari-Twadell, P., & McDermott, M. (2005). *Parish nursing: Development, education and administration.* St. Louis: Mosby.

Spitzer, R. (2010). *New proofs for the existence of God: Contributions of contemporary physics and philosophy.* Cambridge, U.K.: William B. Eerdmans Publishing Company.

Statistics Canada. Canada 2001 Census, May 15, 2001. First Nations Statistics, Statistics Canada, *Winter 2001/2002,* Aboriginal Peoples Survey. Retrieved July 24, 2007, from http://www.library.ubc.ca/xwa/stats.htm.

Suarez, Z. & Lewis, E. (2005). Spirituality and culturally diverse families: The intersection of culture, religion, and spirituality. In E. Congress & M. Gonzalez (Eds.), *Multicultural perspectives in working with families* (2nd ed., pp. 425–441). New York: Springer Publishing Company.

Swanson, K. (1999). What is known about caring in nursing science? In A. S. Hinshaw, Fleetham, S., & Shaver, J. (Eds.). *Handbook of clinical nursing research* (pp. 31–60). Thousand Oaks, CA: Sage.

Taylor, C. (1994). The politics of recognition. In A. Gutmann (Ed.), *Multiculturalism* (pp. 25–73). Princeton: Princeton University Press.

Teilhard de Chardin, P. (1960). *Le divine milieu.* New York: Harper & Row, Publishers.

Teilhard de Chardin, P. (1965). *Building the earth.* New Jersey: Dimension Books.

Templeton, J. (1999). *Agape love: A tradition found in eight world religions.* Philadelphia: Templeton Foundation Press.

The Book of Psalms. (1993). New York: Dover Publications Incorporated.

The Essential Rumi (C. Bark with J. Moyne, Trans.). (1995). San Francisco: HarperSanFrancisco.

The Kingdom of Saudi Arabia (9th ed.). London: Stacey International.

The New American Bible. (1987). Nashville: Thomas Nelson Publishers.

The Qur'an (1980). (Checked and revised by Mahmud Zayid). Beirut: Dar El-Choura.

Thoma, H. (2003). All at the same time. Holistic science. *Resurgence, 1,* 15–17.

Touhy, T. (2002). Touching the spirit of elders in nursing homes. *International Journal for Human Caring, 6*(1), 12–17.

Touhy, T., Strews, W., & Brown, C. (2005). Expressions of caring as lived by nursing home staff, residents, and families. *International Journal for Human Caring, 9*(3), 31–37.

Tudge, C. (2003). Set thine house in order: Science and religion. *Resurgence, 1*(216), 27–31.

Turkel, M. (2007). Marilyn A. Ray's theory of bureaucratic caring. *International Journal for Human Caring, 11*(4), 57–70.

Turkel, M., & Ray, M. (2000). Relational complexity: A theory of the nurse-patient relationship within an economic context. *Nursing Science Quarterly, 13*(4), 307–313.

Turkel, M., & Ray, M. (2001). Relational complexity: From grounded theory to instrument development and theoretical testing. *Nursing Science Quarterly, 14*(4), 281–287.

Tzu, L. (1986). *The Tao of power* (R. Wing, Trans.). New York: Doubleday.

United States Census Bureau. (2000). American Indian and Alaska Native Data and Links, 2000. Retrieved July 24, 2007, from http://factfinder.census.gov/home/aian/index/html

Valenta, M. (2006). How to recognize a Muslim when you see one: Western secularism and the politics of conversion. In H. DeVries & L. Sullivan (Eds.), *Political theologies: Public religions in a post-secular world.* New York: Fordham University Press.

Van Iersel, B. (1973). The alternation of secularizing and sacralizing tendencies in scripture. In A. Greeley & B. Baum (Eds.), *The persistence of religion.* New York: Herder and Herder.

van Manen, M. (1990). *Researching lived experience.* Albany, NY: State University of New York Press.

van Manen, M. (2014). *Phenomenology of practice.* Walnut Creek, CA: Left Coast Press.

Vaught, C. (1982). *The quest for wholeness.* Albany, NY: State University of New York Press.

Watson, J. (1979). *Nursing: The philosophy and science of caring.* Boston: Little Brown.

Watson, J. (1988). *Human science, human care.* New York: National League for Nursing.

Watson, J. (2005). *Caring science as sacred science.* Philadelphia: F. A. Davis Company.

Watson, J. (2008). *Nursing: The philosophy and science of caring* (rev..ed.). Boulder, CO: University Press of Colorado.

Wendler, M. (Ed.). (2005). *The heart of nursing.* Indianapolis, IN: Sigma Theta Tau International.

Wielenberg, E. (2005). *Value and virtue in a Godless universe.* Cambridge: Cambridge University Press.

Wiker, B., & Witt, J. (2006). *A meaningful world: How the arts and sciences reveal the genius of nature.* Madison, WI: Intervarsity Press.

Wilber, K. (Ed.). (1982). *The holographic paradigm and other paradoxes.* Boulder, CO: New Science Library.

Wilber, K. (2006). *Integral spirituality: A startling new role for religion in the modern and postmodern world.* Boulder, CO: Shambhala.

Wolfe, A. (2011). *Political evil: What it is and how to combat it.* New York: Vintage Books.

Wolfson, E. (2006). *Venturing beyond: Law and morality in Kabbalistic mysticism.* Oxford: Oxford University Press.

Wolin, R. (2006). Jürgen Habermas and post-secular societies. *The Chronicle of Higher Education, Section B,* B16–B17.

Woods, T. (2005). *How the Catholic church built western civilization.* Washington, DC: Regnery Publishing, Inc. www.myJewishlearning.com

Yassine, A. (2004). *Winning the modern world for Islam.* Iowa City, IA: Justice and Spirituality Publishing, Inc.

Yuan, H., & Porr, C. (2014). *Integrating spiritual care into a baccalaureate nursing program in Mainland China.* Journal of Holistic Nursing, 32(3), 240–243.

Yu-Lan, F. (1948). *A short history of Chinese philosophy* (D. Bodde, Ed.). New York: Free Press.

Ywahoo, D. (1987). *Voices of our ancestors: Cherokee teachings from the wisdom fire.* Boston: Shambhala.

CHAPTER 6

Transcultural Caring Inquiry: Awareness, Understanding, and Choice

*Deep within us, emergent when the noise of other appetites is
stilled, there is a drive to know, to understand, to see why, to
discover the reason, to find the cause, to explain.*
(Lonergan, 1978, p. 4)

Chapter Objectives

1. To illuminate transcultural caring inquiry in nursing.
2. To describe transcultural caring art.
3. To define **awareness, understanding,** and **choice** as
   knowledge-in-process and the principles of transcultural
   communicative spiritual-ethical caring in nursing and
   health care.
4. To discuss the nature of transcultural caring evidence.

KEY WORDS
Transcultural caring inquiry
• nursing art • evidence
• knowledge-in-process
• reflective action
• communicative spiritual-
ethical caring • awareness
• understanding • choice
• moral accountability
and responsibility • culture
broker

Chapter Objectives—cont'd

5. To review the Transcultural Caring Dynamics in Nursing and Health-Care Theoretical Model as the foundation for knowledge-in-process for transcultural nursing practice.

   5.1 To appreciate the concept of transcultural spiritual-ethical caring as the ground of transcultural caring dynamics in nursing and health care.

   5.2 To discuss the intimate art of transcultural spiritual-ethical caring.

   5.3 To discuss transcultural context: culture, conflict, and cultural transformation.

6. To discuss a process for transcultural caring competency (personal accountability and professional responsibility) in nursing practice.

7. To discuss transcultural communicative spiritual-ethical caring.

   7.1 Unfolding the art of transcultural communicative spiritual-ethical caring.

   7.2 The practice of transcultural spiritual-ethical caring.

8. To present tools for transcultural caring inquiry and assessment.

   8.1 Transcultural Caring Dynamics Assessment Tool.

   8.2 Ray's Transcultural Communicative Spiritual-Ethical CARING Tool for Transcultural Caring Competency.

   8.3. Culture-Value Conflict Assessment Tool.

   8.4 Dynamics of Transcultural Caring for Choice Tool.

   8.5 Transcultural Caring Negotiation Tool.

9. To present three transcultural caring experiences to illustrate transcultural caring assessment and evaluation.

Center of the Transcultural Caring Dynamics Model for Nursing and Health Care

Figure 6-1: *Center* of the transcultural caring dynamics (awareness, understanding, and choice) model for nursing and health care.

Introduction

Nursing practice is a human science and an art. Human science is interpretation of the meaning of lifeworld experiences for the purposes of understanding. It is similar to art. Art is the visionary eye through which we see *in* the other, facets of ourselves (Bronowski, 1978). Human science and art is a relationship, the mirror of ourselves, which sees its own humanism. We attach value to the vision cocreated in relationship in the forms of: insight and awareness, love, commitment, fairness, loyalty, thought, skill, and efficiency (Bronowski, 1978). Nightingale (1860/1969; 1992) considered nursing as the highest form of art because all of nursing's thoughts and actions are directed toward the art of understanding. Nurses constantly seek insight and understanding through reflective consciousness and spiritual-ethical understanding of the meaning of relationship in the forms of respect, compassion, and communication. This insight uses all forms of evidence (empirical and human science) to become aware and to understand patterns of meaning of human caring, ethics, culture(s), and spirituality of patients, families, and professionals for the purposes of facilitating choices (Boykin & Schoenhofer, 2001; Carper, 1978; Chase, 2004; Ray, 1994a, 1994b, 1998a, b; 1998a, 1998b, 2010a, 2010b, 2010c; Ray & Turkel, 2014; Turkel, 2006a, 2006b). Transcultural caring inquiry is knowledge-in-process, communicative spiritual-ethical caring. The action is dynamic and cocreates choices. This chapter will present ways of knowing for transcultural caring inquiry to illuminate awareness, understanding, and choice in relation to the Transcultural Caring Dynamics in Nursing and Health-Care Theory and Model (narrative presented in Chapters 2–5) and various tools/models for transculturological assessment. The tools for assessment and analysis include transcultural caring assessment tools, a tool for evaluation of the potential for culture-value conflict, and tools to address a nurse's accountability and responsibility in transcultural caring negotiation to facilitate choice(s) for health, healing, well-being, and a peaceful death.

Transcultural Caring Inquiry

Transcultural caring inquiry as insightful evidence is a critical and comprehensive methodology. This method is a relational approach, a process to assess, discern, interpret, understand, and judge the meaning of ways of life. In this book and presentation, *evidence* is integral; it is insight and knowledge-in-process gleaned from the Transcultural Caring Dynamics in Nursing and Health-Care Theory and Model, that is, communication, using information and applying caring, knowledge, transcultural ethical caring principles, transcultural context, and the universal sources in conjunction with the tools of assessment for awareness, understanding, and choice in nursing situations (i.e., transcultural caring experiences or real world nursing practice experiences). The elements of transcultural caring evidence are pictured in Figure 6-1 and defined as follows (Davidson & Ray, 1991; Davidson, Ray, & Turkel, 2011; Gadamer, 1986; 1990; Lonergan, 1958, 1972; Ray 1998b):

Awareness is insight and reflection into the relational self; the self and others as multicultural beings. Awareness is an awakening and openness to the spiritual-ethical caring way of life that integrates feeling and intellect, emotion and knowledge, and insight and understanding. Awareness symbolizes caring as the essence of nursing, ethical principles, transcultural context, and universal sources, the foundation for appreciation, responsiveness, discernment, and emerging competency in transcultural communicative spiritual-ethical caring action for nurses in practice, education, administration, and research.

Understanding is participation in the cocreative and emergent present moment that reflects and captures possibilities of meaning involving recollection of past knowledge (one's past experience and scientific and artistic knowledge), an anticipated future (hope in what may emerge), and intuitive knowing (direct apprehension of an encounter) for the self-in-relation. The encounter of the present moment is knowledge-in-process where transcultural, communicative spiritual-ethical caring action (reflective action) is evoked. Knowledge-in-process emerges as both reflective and unlimited or unfolding evidence (the meaning of the "living present") as individuals relate to and learn from each other. Thus, understanding symbolizes participation in an ongoing, cocreative, or aesthetic, communicative process of knowledge seeking with self and others (i.e., patients, significant others, and professionals) that captures *within* the emerging present moment, the possibilities of meaning involving "listening to and hearing" evidence from patients' histories and experience, scientific inquiry, and research. As such, understanding is intentional consciousness that is, *at once*, past, and future lived out in the emerging present moment. The context of virtual relationships in the present moment is also an evolving consideration (Grumime, Barry, Gordon & Ray, in press; Wu & Ray, in press). In transcultural nursing, professionals are seeking understanding of patients' patterns of cultural/multicultural meaning and the human processes associated with health, suffering, distress, illness, dying, and death.

Choice is complex; it is a dynamic that is *continually emerging* through awareness, discernment, understanding, interpretation, intuition, and respect for and judgment of patterns of meaning as people progress through different moments and encounters in the journey of life. Choice symbolizes continuous discernment of the patterns of meaning in the pursuit of right action as people participate in the art of choosing. Choice unifies, organizes, and transforms body, mind, and spirit. In transcultural nursing, transformative choice integrates awareness and understanding of multicultural lifeways that affect a person's health, healing, well-being, dying, or death in the context of family, institutions, and local and global communities including virtual communities.

THE NATURE OF CARING EVIDENCE

From the definitions of awareness, understanding, and choice, we see that the nature of transcultural caring insight and thus, transcultural evidence is dynamic, complex, and unlimited. Evidence is all that is known and what is continually unfolding in experience; evidence is continually emerging and is always being revealed (Heidegger, 1962, 1972, 1977). Evidence as knowledge-in-process, reflection-in-action, and as a comprehensive *relational* method illuminates transcultural, communicative spiritual-ethical caring (CARING—compassion, advocacy,

respect, interaction, negotiation, and guidance; see the related tool to follow). As such, evidence is much more complex than what is captured in books or journals or what may be stored in a computer. In essence, evidence is not only empirical science, but also, human science. It includes not only scientific information that is condensed into the computer but also what can be imagined, visualized, remembered, judged, or intuited. Evidence also is composed of how it is understood *in* lifeworld experience, such as health as desired by patients and health-care professionals, suffering as sensed by nurses, pain as felt by patients, diverse cultural rituals as practiced, prejudice as learned, actions as communicated (Reeder, 1984, 1992, 2007). Transcultural evidence recognizes and captures the dynamic of patterns of culture: values, beliefs, attitudes, symbols, rituals, and behaviors of people of diverse ethnicities and culture groups. Transcultural evidence is cross-cultural knowledge-in-process (the intimate art of caring)

Learn More

Examples of Illuminating Awareness, Understanding, and Choice to Enhance the Theory of Transcultural Caring Dynamics in Nursing and Health Care

1. **Awareness** of transcultural spiritual-ethical caring as a way of being
   * **Awareness** illuminates personal and professional reflection, attentiveness, and responsiveness of the nurse-patient relationship as knowledge-in-process unfolding (transcultural communicative spiritual-ethical caring). Awareness highlights the foundation of transcultural caring as a spiritual and ethical way of being.
2. **Understanding** of knowledge-in-process
   * **Understanding** illuminates knowledge-in-process of categories of complex cultural information—individual cultures or ethnic histories, society and models of community, communication and technological systems, political structures and networks of relationships, economic structures and allocation of resources, social policy and policy brokering. These categories are the foundation of the theory developed in this book, the Essence of Caring, Transcultural Caring Ethics, Transcultural Context, and Universal Sources.
   * **Understanding** also encompasses potentialities for culture-value conflict for discernment in seeking understanding of self and others in relationship.
3. **Choice** illuminates transcultural communicative spiritual-ethical caring dynamics
   * **Choice is dynamic complexity**—a metaphor that encapsulates cocreative patterns of meaning as diverse people interact.
   * **Choice is a process** of recognizing, witnessing, discernment of cocreative patterns of meaning, and negotiation for decision and change.
   * **Choice cocreates** unity and organization (i.e., agreement, understanding, respect, appreciation, compromise, and reconciliation) and transformation to health, healing, well-being, dying, or death.
   * **Choice embodies** continual discernment and practical wisdom.
   * **Choice** as spiritual-ethical ways of caring, the ethics of accountability and responsibility, understanding, agreement, compromise, and reconciliation complete the circle of transcultural caring.

that is continually being revealed and interpreted through communicative spiritual-ethical caring action as people relate and interact.

Transcultural caring inquiry in nursing is a journey of compassion that involves the "speaking together" between the one caring and the one cared for. This immersion into the human encounter reveals the holistic nature (i.e., body, mind, and spirit) that is nursing (Ray, 1991, 1997a, 2010a, 2010b, 2010c; Watson, 1979, 1988, 2005, 2008). There is shift from a focus on I, you, or they to a "compassionate we" in the interaction. The artistic (aesthetic) power of compassion comes from a "wounding of the heart" by the other where the other enters into us and makes us other, a felt realness or authenticity, a depth of the sharing of being (Buber, 1965; Ray, 1991, 2010c). From this sharing, knowledge and understanding of what it means to be human and in need or suffering is felt and unfolds.

THE THEORY AND MODEL OF TRANSCULTURAL CARING DYNAMICS IN NURSING AND HEALTH CARE: A REVIEW

Evaluation of the theory and model that guides this book (see Chapters 2–5) shows that transcultural caring represents knowledge-in-process, the interface among caring as the essence of nursing, transcultural caring ethics, the transcultural context (person as the multicultural self, and person in family, institutional, local, and global communities), and universal sources (the spiritual). Transcultural caring knowledge-in-process (the intimate art of caring) gives us a source of awareness and understanding of self and other by uniting in relationship "the knower and the known" (Reeder, 1984, 1992, 2007). Although different, both self and other are seeking understanding of how we ought to live as we share a common world (spiritual-ethical caring). "The shape of our knowledge becomes the shape of our living [our art or practice]; the relation of the knower to the known becomes the relation of the living self to the larger world. . . . We are part of nature and history" (Palmer, 1993, pp. 21, 34).

SPIRITUAL-ETHICAL TRANSCULTURAL CARING

Spiritual-ethical caring is the *ground* of transcultural caring in nursing. The concepts of the spiritual and ethical help us to understand how we ought to live as we interact with each other for the good of others. Spiritual-ethical values are a plan for life, a code of conduct that unfolds in the art or practice of nursing. The spiritual opens us to the unfolding of the mystery of and seeking the higher good of human life and relationships. The "good" is both a spiritual good instilled in conscience through the I-Thou relationship (Buber, 1958; Ratzinger, 2007), and a social good that fosters distinguishing or judging what is good from what is bad in the lifeworld (Palmer, 1993). Spiritual-ethical caring is spiritual, philosophical, emotional, interactive, and practical. It encompasses spiritual virtues, such as faith and hope; relational human virtues, such as being copresent with others, compassion (sympathy and empathy), and love; ethical virtues, such as doing good (beneficence), doing no harm (nonmaleficence) truth telling, and being responsible and just; and practical virtues, such as communication, transcultural mediation, and facilitation of choice. Caring as spiritual and ethical is a human science and an art (Eriksson, 1997; Ray, 1981a, 1981b, 1991, 1997a, 1997b; Watson, 2005). *Transcultural caring* as a complex phenomenon incorporates compassion through love in response to suffering and need with right action or justice and fairness within an understanding of cultural dynamics (Ray, 1989a, 1989b, 1999a, 1999b). Love is a spiritual and human energy, that surrenders to the "compassionate we"—the unfolding art of caring for another. Rather than being educated away, love is integral as we become coparticipants and cocreators in a community of authentic relationships with other persons and things of the universe (see Figs. 2-2, 2-3, and 2-4).

The Intimate Art of Transcultural Spiritual-Ethical Caring

To address the processes of transcultural caring art as the "compassionate we," the following will illuminate the intimate art of nursing. Often, the intimate caring art is invisible to others or taken for granted. Generally what is known about the art of nursing is translated into external forms (competencies, skills, or tasks). Watson (1992), referencing Nightingale, declared that "the need to reiterate the interconnection between person and environment, between person and nature, between the inner and outer worlds, between the private and the public, between the physical and the spiritual as part of the natural healing responses of people and civilizations; [there is] the need to systematically develop nursing practice. . . . Even the roots of nursing throughout time have been based on a philosophy and commitment to caring and healing" (pp. 80–81). The following is a presentation of the "art of awareness, understanding, and choice," transcultural nurses' commitment to the intimate art of the caring relationship, a spiritual-ethical call initiated first by Nightingale, kept alive by professional nurses, and continuing as knowledge-in-process (reflective action) illuminated through transcultural communicative spiritual-ethical caring.

The intimate art of professional nursing is a portrait of the meaning of the "living present," knowledge-in-process. This process of nursing is compassion and transcultural advocacy to facilitate right action, the ethic of reconciliation. Gadow's (1980) philosophy of existential advocacy contributes to understanding the living present. Within this philosophical foundation, the patient and the nurse can freely decide or choose through awareness and understanding how the relationship and patterns of meaning will unfold. In the situation of potential language or cultural differences, the meanings of situations may seem more complex but "looking for" and "connecting with" the simple, the human and humane is what is called for. Gadow adopted the belief that "the nurse [more than any other health care professional] attends to the patient as a whole, not just as a single problem or system" (1980, p. 81). While honoring her own professional and scientific knowledge and her own strengths and weaknesses, the nurse attends first to the ordinary intimacies of everyday life, experiencing the person as a unique individual in his or her cultural/multicultural complexities with his or her own strengths and weaknesses, and ability to make choices. Advocacy in Gadow's view is based upon the assumption of self-determinism—about what individuals want to do or how they choose. Often nurses can become paternalistic because of the "power elitism" or what is vested in the nurse as a professional who can limit the freedom or rights of individuals. Paternalism is a violation of the right of authentic self-determination or freedom of choice, which is the most fundamental and valuable human right (Gadow, 1980). Thus, authentic self-determinism facilitated in relationships is to help persons become clear about what they want to do by helping them discern and clarify their values and beliefs in a situation to reach decisions that express their complexity of values. These values are cultural and include religious and ethical values. As Gadow pointed out, often in the education of nurses, a dichotomy between the personal and the professional is articulated. She remarked that nurses are taught or they choose to

help patients make decisions, but at the same time they may feel that they must be wary of becoming too personal in interactions, that is, revealing too many personal feelings, values, or peculiarities. Often nurses believe that it is right and good to be caring but sharing emotions or feelings is to be avoided. The scientific, technical, or managerial ways of behaving seem to be more encouraged in many educational programs or health-care institutions. Interestingly, Gadow expressed the value of nursing as holistic, and remarked that "regarding the *patient* as a 'whole' [integrated body, mind and spirit], would seem to require nothing less than the *nurse* acting as a 'whole' person" (1980, p. 87).

How does the nurse act holistically—personally and professionally? The nurse is also a multicultural self (the ethic of accountability). In the professional relationship, the nurse must be interested in the other's *good* in that "living present" more than in his or her own. In a sense, it can be understood as making a sacrifice. The patient, on the other hand, by virtue of the fact that his or her health is at stake, he or she will be concerned about his or her own good and relate specifically to his or her body in pain or suffering. Only the patient can experience his or her own interiority, center, or heart, in what he or she is experiencing in his or her own lived nature. In contrast, the nurse, while recognizing the person as person, experiences the patient's body also as a technical object, a thing to be regarded scientifically or technically. The nurse and the patient experience modes of access to the patient's body *differently* and thus their understanding is different. The patient is oriented and aware primarily of his or her own uniqueness while the professional is oriented toward the patients not only as a unique person to be cared for but also, with different types of scientific, technical, and sociocultural representations (for example, diagnoses, cultural desires, pharmacological needs, and so forth). Sometimes the business of organizations (economics of time) interferes with involvement and contributes to avoidance of honoring the cultural uniqueness, the aesthetic, and the spiritual in patient care. Prioritization of the scientific or technical realms can take precedence over human and spiritual needs and blur the quality of the interrelationship.

Ray (1981a, 1989a, 1989b, 1994a, 1994b, 1997a, 1997b, 1998a, 1998b, 2001a, 2001b, 2007a, 2007b; Ray & Turkel, 2012, 2014; Ray, Turkel, & Marino, 2001; Turkel & Ray, 2009), however, found that nurses do integrate the complex context into the meaning of caring relationships, however silent. The sociocultural as technical, economic, political, and legal emerge as a synthesis with the spiritual-ethical caring of the patient. Questions arise as to the *meaning* of the synthesis of the personal, professional, and contextual. What intentions prevail? If intentionality is a philosophy of presence (Heidegger, 1977; Reeder, 1984, 2007; Smith, 1998), participation of the entire self integrates every resource of persons and the context. Gadow (1980) reinforced the belief that advocacy implies that patients can be assisted in reaching decisions that express their complex totality as individuals *only* by nurses who themselves act out of the same explicit self-unity (the holism of body, mind, and spirit), allowing no dimension of themselves to be exempt from the professional relationship. Because of the immediate, sustained, and often intimate nature, and its scientific, technical, and ethical complexity of nursing care, the relationship offers avenues for every dimension of the professional to be engaged. The nurse expresses the emotional, rational, esthetic, intuitive, physical and philosophical (Gadow, 1980) with compassion, which is the motivator for "the wounding" of the self by the other to form the "compassionate we" (Ray, 1991, 2007a, 2007b; Turkel & Ray, 2009). To capture the meaning, we enact the power of love to suffer with the other, feel the other's pain, imagine what it is like to be the other, in essence become the other (Eriksson, 1997; Frankl, 1984). The direction of feelings toward the other's suffering and joy facilitates the integration of human and complex systems (the living present or cocreative emergence). Nursing is one of the few professions that finds its soul in the living present and in cultivating practical wisdom (Ray, 1994a)— synthesizing the dynamics of caring, the ethics of principles as moral experience, the sociocultural including the technological and socioeconomic contexts, and the spiritual to facilitate further understanding of what it means be human. As Gadow (1980) reported, the nurse is an advocate who participates *with* the patient in determining the personal meaning that the experience of illness, suffering, or dying has for that individual. At the same time, the nurse is determining the meaning of the nursing situation for herself.

TRANSCULTURAL CONTEXT: CULTURE, CONFLICT, AND CULTURAL TRANSFORMATION

In the unfolding of the intimate art or practice of transcultural caring, culture, conflict, and competency

emerge within the knowledge-in-process, transcultural caring competency challenges nurses to address the meaning of evidence as unlimited, concepts that are developed in this book, transcultural caring, transcultural caring ethics, the transcultural context and universal sources and their relationship to awareness, understanding, and choice. The Transcultural Caring Dynamics in Nursing and Health-Care Theory and Model reveals how transcultural caring competency may be achieved.

Culture is dynamic complexity and choice. Yet more than 300 definitions of culture have prevailed across a variety of disciplines ranging from all life-world phenomena to creativity (Baldwin, Faulkner, Hecht, & Lindsley, 2006, p. xvi). Often culture and ethnicity become blurred, especially in the contemporary global community of today. Because ethnic boundaries in the past have gone through rapid transformation as the world has shrunk through mass communication and transportation, many people think of themselves as multicultural (Rockefeller, 1994; Taylor, 1989, 1991; Waters, 1990). "To identify ethnically, to make it a prominent feature of one's identity [especially in the West], requires a conscious choice" (Tuan 1998, p. 25). Therefore, transcultural competency in the traditional sense of the term as culture-specificity is forever more challenging.

Forms of diversity, such as panethnicity, multiculturalism, and interculturality/transculturality have become the order of the day (Gutmann, 1994). But has panethnicity truly superseded previous forms of discourse? What new patterns of meaning contribute to our understanding of cultural diversity? Is there any one culture that triumphs over others? We can see that, because of the complexity of culture especially in the developed world, terms, such as acculturation, assimilation, and adaptation that historically have been used to demonstrate cultural integration could be in question. We often see these words still used to describe how one group should adapt or integrate into a community or nation. For purposes of clarification, *acculturation* usually deals with the <u>evaluation</u> of cultural changes when there is long-term contact between any <u>two</u> cultures (Kim, 1989); *assimilation* often is used interchangeably with acculturation but generally refers to achieving <u>cultural homogeneity;</u> and *adaptation* often means <u>psychological adjustment or personal development</u> as a result of response to cultural assimilation and cultural change (Yapple & Korzenny, 1989). The acceptance of multiple identities (panethnicity) in contemporary life gives us pause to reflect upon whether or not terms, such as acculturation and assimilation are as relevant as they once were, especially as we recognize and accept more cultural diversity within nations or the world at large.

Culture, although thought of as integral and binding, is more often than not, a choice to accept or decline certain rituals, meaning systems or symbols of one's time-honored heritage. Although the view of culture as dynamic complexity and choice gives more freedom to decide one's identity in the new world of multiculturalism or interculturality, there continues to be extensive disagreement. Often we see that decisions made in accepting multiple identities and supporting cultural diversity and immigration in some Western countries result in what citizens call cultural fatigue. Tolerance and open-mindedness give way to *cultural fatigue* that gives birth to new prejudices or reinforces old ones. We can see this result with the influx of immigration (especially illegal) to Westernized nations from nations where poverty and political instability have existed.

Because the concept of culture is so complex, it is paradoxical. It can be thought of as conflictual or freeing, prejudicial or flexible, closed or open, power-based or cocreative. On the one hand, many nation-states are struggling to achieve national identity and recognition (Lestig & Koesler, 2000). On the other hand, many nation-states are struggling with the changes brought about by increasing multiculturalism and open borders, for example, the current member states of the European Union. There has been a movement from ethnic pride to ethnic terrorism (Volkan, 1998). Wars related to the culture of power and sectarianism are looming all over the world. Volkan (1998) stated that "[w]hen ethnic groups define and differentiate themselves, they almost invariably develop some prejudices for their own group against the others' group. . . . Ethnicity has no existence apart from interethnic relations" [from the Committee of International Relations of the Group for the Advancement of Psychiatry, (p. 22)]. In a digitalized world, the media capture the many meanings associated with panethnicity and/or multiple identities. "It has been noted that a vast majority of nations today are no longer (if they ever were) ethnically homogeneous (see Kymlicka, 1995)" (Kalifon & Mollov, 2006, p. 4).

The complexity of cultural diversity or multiculturalism has stirred up emotions that range from love to hatred, understanding to misunderstanding, confidence in the future to confusion about the future. The construction and deconstruction of cultural identity paints a not-so-picture-perfect portrait of multiculturalism. To look more deeply into the issue, we can learn much from what the new sciences of complexity or quantum sciences and quantum theology tell us. Science and theology state that the future is open, approximate, uncertain, unfolding, and inexhaustible (O'Murchu, 1997; Peat, 2002); the new epistemology (knowledge-in-process) highlights knowledge unfolding in a network of relationships (Capra, Steindl-Rast, with Matus, 1991). What is the universal cultural language that is capable of expressing human realities and spiritual values? The language is *compassion and choice*; compassion for others and choice as to how we want to be, how we want to live in this age of communication, interconnectedness, and belongingness. Because of historical circumstances, economic, political, or military power and in some cases religious zeal, one nation or a group of nations may be designated as a superpower or dominant power. Sociocultural ramifications emerge. Conflict, hostility, violence, and even war, often ensue. Competition rather than equitable cooperation takes over. What is next? Important ideas are emerging despite injustices, violence, terrorism, and war. In response to global systemic crises, transformation, and redefinitions of culture are emerging that address culture as dynamic complexity and choice—culture as creation and cocreation (Baldwin, et al, 2006; Pollock, 2006; Stoll, 2006). To illustrate this idea of creation or cocreation and choice, in the European Union, where there is the movement of unity among nations with no defined borders and a common currency, a concept of "newropean" is emerging with publications, such as the *Newropeans Magazine* identifying global Europe (Retrieved August 2006, from *Newropeans Magazine,* http://www.newropeans-magazine.org/). Intranational and international discourse is beginning to revolve around issues of consociationalism (Kalifon & Mollov, 2006) and sociality with a new view from the expansion of social media called Generation F (Behar, 2013), which speaks to the character of how human beings who are different should live and communicate together and to the quality of their human and human-technological relationships (Boulding, 1988; Dewey in Bernstein, 1986; Kalifon & Mollov, 2006; Ray, 1989a, 2010a, 2010b, 2010c; Ray & Turkel, 2014). This concept of community has been advanced in Northern Ireland and is emerging in Israel and Palestine and is being evaluated in the digital world.

Demands revolve around new approaches to issues of transcultural interaction and dialogue, human and land rights, immigration, participatory democracy, liberty, freedom, resources, economic justice, and rules of law (Arrien, 1993; de Vries & Sullivan, 2006; Economy & Levi, 2014; Hahnel, 2005). The ways of the teacher, healer, and visionary recognize the richness of diversity and the common human family—the unfolding of spiritual democracy and spiritual technology: the realignment of the domains of the political and religious and the social and spiritual effect of technology for the future of humankind (de Vries & Sullivan, 2006; Kurzweil, 2005). The intelligent man [woman] is always open to new ideas. In fact, the idea is stated in an ancient Biblical saying from Proverbs (18:15), "The mind of the intelligent gains knowledge, and the ear of the wise seeks knowledge" (*The New American Bible,* 1970, p. 719).

TRANSCULTURAL CARING COMPETENCE IN NURSING PRACTICE

Looking for new ideas has never been lacking in nursing. Understanding the importance of the multiple meanings of culture and providing culturally congruent care is one of the creative aspects and challenges of nursing education, research, and practice. Integration of guidelines for cultural competency is beginning to appear in nursing education and practice (Leininger, 1970, 1978, 1991, 1995, 1997; Leininger & McFarland, 2006; McFarland, 2006; McFarland & Wehbe-Alamah, 2015; Lipson & DeSantis, 2007; Purnell & Paulanka, 2008; Ray, 2010a, 2010b, 2010c; Ray & Turkel, 2014). Cultural competence addresses the critical nature of cultural illness and health and cultural care diversity in health and illness (Jeffreys, 2006; Spector, 2008). Transcultural caring competence in nursing practice calls forth presence and moral accountability and ethical responsibility—illuminating the moral voice of nurses to serve the good of humankind through compassion and justice. By learning, listening to, reflecting upon, and seeking understanding of what is needed to engage in trans-cultural communicative spiritual-ethical caring action, nurses can positively affect not only patients and their families but also, the future of health care in local and global arenas. To reiterate, *transcultural caring competency* illuminates how we *ought* to live and practice nursing when we relate to others who may be different from ourselves yet share a common world, common resources, and common opportunities in an interdependent universe. The concept of "the

moral is slowly regaining a place of honor . . . . it is becoming ever more clear that we should not do everything that we can do [for example, abuse humans through biotechnologies, destroy people and nations through the use of bombs, or harm the environment through wanton greed]" (Ratzinger, 2007, p. 43). It is becoming more evident that there is a call for serious and continuous dialogue to address the great concerns of today. In nursing, it is not easy to be responsive to all the challenges facing human caring for people who may have perpetrated the creation of evil against other humans and the environment, even history, but nurses through their spiritual-ethical caring are "asked" to rise above the pain to heal the pain of the perpetrators. Thus, transcultural human caring practice as a distinctive form of human spiritual-ethical activity that conveys the *moral character of participatory life itself* and thus contributes to the understanding of the ethical and spiritual in human life, the ability to distinguish the good from the bad, and to share in the rich experiences of diversity and commonality of community life.

TRANSCULTURAL COMMUNICATIVE SPIRITUAL-ETHICAL CARING

Transcultural communication encompasses interpersonal communication between or among members of diverse culture groups (including ethnic and racial); comparing and contrasting of intercultural and cross-cultural communicative patterns; channels of communication through different forms of media (i.e., radio, television, Internet); and comparative mass communication (Asante & Gudykunst, 1989; Gudykunst 2001, 2005). Transcultural communicative spiritual-ethical caring involves awareness, understanding a person in the context of caring, the spiritual and ethical and the sociocultural as a universal, and the capacity to facilitate choice. The person in context reflects spiritual, ethical, social, cultural, ethnic, and racial integration. At the same time, the person in context reflects the social structures that

❖ *Nursing Reflection*

Transcultural caring competence in nursing practice calls forth presence and moral accountability and ethical responsibility—illuminating the moral voice of nurses to serve the good of humankind through compassion and justice.

make up the context, the patterns of meaning in the sociocultural or institutional cultures, communities, nation-states, and the globe: the political, economic, legal, technological, and humanistic, including the spiritual and ethical dimensions that are complex and dynamic, and as advanced by Ray as the Theory of Bureaucratic Caring (Coffman, 2006, 2014; Ray, 2005; Ray & Turkel, 2014, 2015; Turkel, 2007). Health and illness do not only involve physical and mental elements of what it means to be human, but also what a society at large believes about health, illness, and care. Such an understanding develops through thoughtful insight, knowledge, ethical responsibility, and open communication. The present age of communication demands that communication in context must include attention to the *needs* of the other permitting and facilitating reasonable communication of participants in community life and social media. Habermas (1986, 1987, 1995; Ray, 1991, 1999a, 1999b; Sumner, 2006, 2008), the leading philosopher and theorist of communicative action, claimed that every person or group fostering inquiry is located in a context (social and historical), which influences not only the inquiry but also the knowledge produced. For Habermas, the distinctive form of human interaction is the dialectic of the moral life, where claims to right and wrong are inherent and emergent in all forms of communication and rely upon rationality and wisdom (Ray, 1992, 1999a; Sumner, 2008). Through communication, persons reveal patterns of cultures to which they are connected, thus, communication is complex and dynamic. Sometimes serious questions of communication arise at a global level. People question whether or not the average citizen is heard. Diverse views are usually reconciled in political discourse within or between governments; however, within or between culture groups there emerges different "takes" on the meaning, often illuminating the need for mediators to resolve or broker serious interrelational communicative issues (Huyssen, 2003).

With the escalation of social media, more ethical questions continue to arise from interrelational technological communication (Ess, 2014).

In transcultural communicative spiritual-ethical caring, the focus is on the patient and family or significant other and the moral accountability and ethical responsibility of the nurse. Listening to and hearing the needs of patients and especially patients and families with diverse views of healthand healing requires authentic communication—communion with and participation in cocreating meaning that illuminates awareness, understanding, and the ability to facilitate choice. *Awareness, understanding, and choice for the patient engender compassion through love, fairness, and justice toward right action* (Ray, 1989a). Transcultural caring generally is caring between equals but at the same time, in the nurse-patient relationship, we may not always have sustained equality. In a professional relationship, the nurse has a specific body of nursing knowledge and skill that the patient is seeking, which can be viewed as having power and can be used to overpower the patient. Sumner (2006) reminds us that "[i]f the interaction is unidirectional (nurse directed towards patient, there is no reciprocity in meeting the innate human needs and unity of purpose), then it is hypothesized that this is not caring in nursing" (p. 14). The process in transcultural communicative spiritual-ethical caring action must be empowering and holistic—ethical, spiritual, and respectful of culture(s) in the nursing situation. This nursing situation today can also be a technological caring relationship mediated through diverse social media outlets. Transcultural communicative spiritual-ethical caring action is the means of using caring knowledge and skill to assist in freeing the patient from fear, suffering, grieving, and pain and pursuing a unity of purpose toward the goals of health, healing, or a peaceful death. There is a transformation for both the patient and nurse (see Fig. 6-2).

Figure 6-2: Transcultural spiritual-ethical caring action of nursing. *Adapted in part from Gadow, S. (1980). Existential advocacy: Philosphical foundation of nursing. In S. E. Spicer and S. Gadow (Eds.), Nursing images and ideals. New York: Springer & Co.*

Transcultural Spiritual-Ethical CARING Action of Nursing

Spiritual-ethical caring encompasses existential advocacy: the effort to help persons become clear about what choices they want to make by helping them understand, discern, and clarify their values in the transcultural nursing situation, and on the basis of that self-examination make choices for health, healing, or a peaceful death.

Tools for Transcultural Caring Inquiry and Assessment

The following are assessment TOOLS, which help to explain the process of transcultural knowledge-in-process and transcultural caring competency. These tools provide assistance and a guide with transcultural assessment and awareness, understanding, and choice for transcultural caring in nursing practice situations. The tools can be used individually or collectively when applied to a transcultural caring situation. The specific tools to be addressed include:

- Transcultural Caring Dynamics Tool (for Patient and Family Assessment)
- Ray's Transcultural Communicative Spiritual-Ethical CARING Tool for Culturally Competent Practice
- Transcultural Culture-Value Conflict Assessment Tool
- Negotiation Tools
  - Dynamics of Transcultural Caring for Choice Tool
  - Transcultural Caring Negotiation Tool

For Your Reflection

Contemplate the following points when using any of the *tools* in the transcultural caring relationship:

- Determine the language or interpreter needs.
- Act compassionately with patient, family members, or significant others.
- Determine the nature of evidence in transcultural caring (empirical scientific quantitative) and human scientific (qualitative) evidence.
- Interact in a mutually collaborative manner to develop a trusting relationship.
- Communicate spiritual-ethical caring by ethical interaction, showing respect, and serving the good of the patient, family members, or significant others.
- Determine how best to interact ethically when technology is employed.
- Identify with the patient and family, the cultural/multicultural values, beliefs, attitudes, and opinions.
- Ask about traditional cultural practices that influence health and healing.
- Identify the religious or spiritual system of the patient and family.
- Ask about religious or spiritual practices and their influence in health and healing.
- If appropriate, ask about the patient's, family's, and significant others' needs about dying and

death rituals practiced within a particular religion or spiritual relationship.
- Determine how much information can be absorbed by all members of the interaction by attentively listening.

Transcultural Caring Dynamics Tool

An explanation of the Transcultural Caring Dynamics Tool (see Fig. 6–3) (an adaptation of Ray's Theory of Bureaucratic Caring (Coffman, 2014; Ray, 2010b; Ray & Turkel, 2015) for patient and family assessment follows.

SOCIOCULTURAL

- Determine how the universal environment, including the environment of a hospital, clinic, outpatient center, family, or community influences the patient in health or illness.
- Be aware of the symbolic behavior (i.e., nonverbal gestures or behavior) of the patient, family members, or significant others.
- Identify the ethnic foundation of the patient, family, or significant others.
- Identify the kinship structure (i.e., patient and family relationships).
- Identify patient's support system by determining the current living arrangements and social

Transcultural Caring Dynamics

The Universal Environment

Figure 6-3: Transcultural caring dynamics: The universal environment.

networks (if possible, sketch out a kinship structure or genealogy of the patient and illnesses).

- Discover intergenerational relationships (i.e., harmonious or conflictual).
- Identify the decision makers (for health care and living) in the family or significant others.
- Assess the environment of the patient and family and significant others.

PHYSICAL

- Identify with the patient, family members, or significant others, the patient's physical needs.
- Identify patterns of culture and health and scientific and ethnopharmacological needs.
- Determine, with sensitivity, the patient's meaning and perceptions of health, health problems, diagnosis, causes, symptoms, suffering and grief, pain, and prognosis.
- Determine if the patient (or a family member) has served in the military or is a veteran.
- Discover if there are physical, mental, or spiritual challenges to well-being.
- Identify the activities of daily living and any limitations.
- Determine the medications or other traditional folk preparations used.
- Determine if there are health practitioners or traditional healers serving patient needs or if there is a desire for a healer to serve the needs of the patient.
- Ask if there is anything that makes the patient feel better or worse.
- Request information about nutritional needs and food preferences of the patient.
- Identify whether or not traditional cultural foods are desired.
- Determine if the hot-and-cold system of food intake is adhered to.

ECONOMIC

- Determine sensitively with the patient, family, or significant others, the socioeconomic status of the patient.
- Determine the short- and long-term care: economic, social support, and living arrangements, and needs of the patient.
- Determine whether or not the patient can afford the prescription medication(s).
- If or when appropriate, arrange with the social worker for economic support of the patient and family (this notion is also under Political).

TECHNOLOGICAL

- Determine if there are or will be technological equipment needed for patient support, home care, or rehabilitation, and technical assistance with daily living activities for the patient and family.
- Determine if the patient has a computer and Internet service and telephone for continual communication of needed information.
- Determine how family is communicating with the patient (e.g., via Facebook, Twitter, Skype, etc.).
- Arrange for a tele-interpretation if necessary for the patient and family or significant other(s).
- Ask about the driving patterns of the patient especially for the elderly.

POLITICAL

- Determine power relationships between professional and patient and family or significant others. (Power is using knowledge, skill, and cocreative participation in the service of the good of the other [Brown, 2002].)
- Be aware of and seek understanding of the complex processes of negotiation within transcultural communicative caring action.
- Determine the insurance system (i.e., private or public) of the patient, if appropriate.
- Determine (with the social worker if available) whether or not there should be local or national governmental intervention or Veterans' Administration assistance with care needs.

LEGAL

- Determine what policies and regulations, if any, facilitate the provision of culturally sensitive spiritual-ethical caring.
- Be aware of the legal ramifications of boards of nursing for licensure to practice, patient safety issues, and sensitivity to transcultural nursing.
- Understand the regulatory bodies of the institutional, international community and ethical and legal statements in relation to the practice of nursing.
- Determine what the legal needs of the patient are in relation to culturally sensitive health care, especially for the elderly.
- Facilitate the naming of a health-care surrogate or advocate for the patient—someone who can speak on behalf of and who understands the patient in ethnocultural health-care matters.

- Ask if (primarily in the United States and some other Western nations), the patient has a living will and a durable power and durable medical power of attorney for health care so that a family member or significant others can speak on behalf of the patient.
- If in the United States, make sure that Health Insurance Portability and Accountability Act of 1996 (HIPAA [Public Law 104-191, 104th Congress]) privacy requirements are followed.

EDUCATIONAL

- Mutually identify and develop a process of open, mutual communication and guidance for the provision of culturally relevant care.
- Determine the education and educational needs of the patient, family, or significant others.
- Provide assistance with diagnosis, symptoms, and health-care needs based upon mutual understanding of needs and desires and patterns of culture.
- Identify expectations for ongoing nurse and physician and/or traditional healer care, home care, assisted living (i.e., short- or long-term care), nursing home (i.e., long-term care), further hospitalization, and family and community support.
- Cocreate a culturally relevant plan of care for the diagnosis, and treatment plan with the patient, family, or significant others for immediate and further care.
- Determine what type of social media for communication and education purposes will be used.

UNIVERSAL ENVIRONMENT

- Identify the health-care system as a living system and as a structure.
- Identify the organization of traditional or "folk" health care in nongovernment organizations, such as small and large group ethnic or religious identities.
- Understand *alternative* healing systems in non-Western and Western nations that may have an effect on the health and healing processes of the patient and family or significant others.
- Consider how the health-care system as a *living* system is involved in the understanding of transcultural nursing leadership and management and the spiritual-ethical caring practice of nursing and health care.
- Recognize how the organizational and community *context* plays a significant role in beliefs, values, attitudes, and behaviors of all people

(patients and families and "families of choice" [in a culturally dynamic world where genealogical families or kin are dispersed, some people chose "a family" and it becomes their family], and professionals engaged in cocreating life patterns of culture and meaning).

- Evaluate organizations as social structures with bureaucratic systems, economic, political, legal, technological, sociocultural, spiritual, ethical, and humanistic dimensions, and how the organizational processes are integrated into health-care decisions.
- Understand the relationship between complex organizational values and leadership in nursing and health-care systems.
- Understand the ecosystems and bionetworks that make up our environments and influence patient's and professional's health.
- Examine how organizations within and outside an institution and other regulatory bodies affect quality and safety of the provision of transcultural nursing to patients (Coffman, 2006, 2014; Davidson, Ray, & Turkel, 2011; Ray, 1989b, 2001a, 2001b, 2001c; Ray, 2005, 2007, 2010a, 2010b, 2010c; Ray & Turkel, 2014).

Ray's Transcultural Communicative Spiritual-Ethical CARING Tool for Cultural Competency

This tool can be used for guidance in transcultural communicative spiritual-ethical caring action. It uses the acronym of CARING to outline the process of transcultural caring communication for patient care: Caring, Advocacy, Respect, Interaction, Negotiation, and Guidance (see Fig. 6-4). It can be used when communicating transculturally with a patient. The CARING acronym is central to the tool and the word itself guides the transaction to understand the meaning of health and illness for the patient and significant others. The concepts representing, the acronym CARING outlined in the tool have been interwoven throughout the narrative texts of previous chapters.

Culture-Value Conflict Assessment Tool

EVALUATION OF POTENTIAL FOR CULTURE-VALUE CONFLICT FOR TRANSCULTURAL ASSESSMENT

To make possible transcultural assessment, transcultural communicative caring action, and cocreative

Ray's Transcultural Communicative Spiritual-Ethical CARING Tool for Cultural Competency

Transcultural communicative caring is a multidirectional way of caring in professional life that encourages transcultural communication (symbolic interaction, oral or linguistic interaction [or through an interpreter or video-conferencing]) to mutually understand the needs, suffering, problems, and questions of people that arise in culturally dynamic situations.

C: Compassion
- Respond lovingly in authentic presence in person or via electronic communication by opening one's mind and heart to the other.
- Act ethically by doing good, being fair, and facilitating choice.

A: Advocacy
- Discern by discovering, ascertaining, distinguishing the vision of reality (worldview) of the other, and the contributions to the situation of the patient, family or significant other to facilitate mutual understanding and transformation.

R: Respect
- Respect the culture (including the traditional or folk culture) of the patient and family, and the dynamics of the transcultural relationship of the patient, family, and community.

I: Interaction
- Act competently by interviewing, listening, and manifesting transcultural knowledge and skill.
- Ask questions to enhance the history and physical examination:
  - What do you think is causing your suffering/pain/problem?
  - How are you affected by the suffering/pain/problem?
  - What do you think may help or benefit you?

N: Negotiation
- Mediate relationships and codevelop a plan of care by transcultural caring: allowing, recognizing, acknowledging, encouraging, affirming, confirming, and transforming the transcultural encounter.
- Cocreate transforming self/life patterns by understanding the power within and the life-world patterns that promote connection of one to the other in community.
- Mutually shape and devise a plan of care from the shared alliance (ethics of caring and responsibility [agreement, compromise, and understanding]) in choice-making with patients and family/significant others.

G: Guidance
- Coeducate, codirect, advise, counsel, and inspire hope.

Figure 6-4: Ray's transcultural communicative spiritual-ethical CARING tool for cultural competency. *Adapted from Ray's Transcultural CARING tool in Ray, M, & Turkel, M. (2001). Culturally based caring. In L. Dunphy & J. Winland-Brown (Eds.), Primary care: The art and science of advanced practice nursing. Philadelphia: F. A. Davis Company.)*

choice making in nursing practice, consider some issues that may occur between the lifeworld and the system. Because of global interconnections and the electronic media, the reality of conflict, violence, suffering, and war often seems stronger than the reality of belongingness, interdependence, human caring interaction, and relationship, and nation building. Huyssen (2003) highlighted the difficult issues of conflict as a way of life—what happens to individuals and groups as they are exposed to long-term conflict—the politics of public memory in relation to cultural memory. This reality has affected the health of many culturally diverse groups/nations, such as First Nations' people (Native Americans), aboriginals of Australia, and the Maori of New Zealand (Lowe, 2002; Lowe & Crow, 2009; Mason, 1998) and, in the conflict of today, many European, Middle Eastern, and African nations (Eril, Nunning, & Young, 2014). Huyssen remarked that there is a quest for the politics of forgetting—the process of moving forward in reconciliation and peace development in the global community. " . . . [T]he intense focus on memories of the past may block our imagination of the future and create a new blindness in the present. At that stage we may want to bracket the future of memory in order to remember the future" (Huyssen, 2003, pp. 182–183). Lederach (1999) and Appleton (2005) wrote of how to remember the future in the process of reconciling conflict and violence by understanding its progression.

The "visual grammar" (i.e., television and Internet media) communication as much of the media is called today, presents a way of seeing that is fast-paced and action-oriented, now seemingly substituting shock and fear for reflection on the essence of what people can do to make things more harmonious and beautiful (Yapple & Korzenny, 1989, p. 300). Questions arise as to whether or not the products and structures of cultures are being replaced by modes of thought influenced primarily by elements of mass communication. Is conflict enflamed by the rhetoric of "visual grammar"? Can new ways of communicating be nurtured? A philosopher of our time, Habermas (2006), saw an answer in an engaged citizenry in secular and religious approaches to life through the nurturing element of communicative action in the world community. Tolerance and assuming the standpoint of the other (compassion from the nursing viewpoint), the hallmarks of Habermas' (1986, 1987, 1995) theory of communicative action, assist in understanding the meaning of a seeking the good for a common humanity.

As the philosopher Hegel reminds us, conflict is what creates the conditions for change. Hegel noted that progress unfolds *only* through the conflict generated by contradictions, the dynamic of the dialectic: thesis, antithesis, and synthesis. "Every sociocultural system, considered a thesis, view, or argument tends to generate its own internal contradictions (antithesis or opposite); this leads to conflict, which can only be resolved by the transformative process, an alteration of the given system toward a new order, integration, or synthesis. The new system or synthesis then becomes the thesis, and the process begins again" (Hegel, in Bee, 1974, p. 31). Cultural change or change in illness from crisis to healing illuminates this process. Cultural change is a cocreative expression as people interface, and beliefs, values, and attitudes and historical traditions are valued and challenged.

Dimensions of the Culture-Value Conflict Assessment Tool

This tool signifies a journey into understanding the conflicts that may affect nurses as they engage in transcultural interactions and communication,

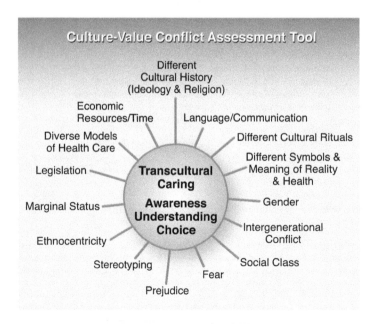

Figure 6-5: Culture-value conflict assessment tool.

including virtual communication. Transcultural caring practice as a distinctive form of human spiritual-ethical activity conveys the moral character of participatory life. The Culture-Value Conflict Assessment Tool reveals what potentially may be cocreated or what emerges when a person or people of diverse groups interact together to cocreate an ethic of accountability and responsibility. Review the detailed description that follows.

DIFFERENT CULTURAL HISTORY (IDEOLOGY AND RELIGION)

Different cultural histories, ideologies, and religions have the potential for increasing conflict in human relationships. In medicine, medical anthropology, and the health-care arena in general, there are differences in the ways in which nature or the physical and the cultural are understood and thus are differentiated (Brown, 1998; Kehoe, 1998; Peacock, 1986). Beliefs, values, attitudes, and behaviors are formulated by the way in which people construct reality and give and find meaning. These units of experience or cultural patterns, expressions, memories, and occurrences are not mere reflections of society, but are commentaries on or illuminate meanings *in* society itself (Eril, Nunning, & Young, 2014; Turner & Bruner, 1986). As we have learned, every person is an energy pattern that encompasses meanings influenced by our biology, history, mental patterns, religious and ethical beliefs, images of body, mind, and spirit and their integration, race, ethnicity or multiple ethnicities, kinship groups and family structures, and structures of society and community.

There are differences in the cultural history and beliefs about medicine and nursing, thus, different ways in which ideologies between physicians and nurses are formed and communicated. Beliefs, values, and attitudes are communicated differently to patients and patients' family members or significant others just as they are communicated differently to professionals. The transcultural communicative caring process is a multiplex of ideologies (Appiah, 1994; Coffman, 2006, 2014; Helman, 1997; Ray, 1989b, 2005; Ray & Turkel, 2014, 2015; Turkel 2007). Through communicative caring, the transcultural caring nurse needs to be open to learn about the team members' (i.e., physicians and other health-care professionals) and patients' cultural history, ideological and religious systems, and symbols or meanings that may affect their values, beliefs, attitudes, and behaviors about health and patterns of care and caring.

DIFFERENT SYMBOLS AND MEANING OF REALITY AND HEALTH

Symbols are a means of communication at every level of reality. Reality is something that has a life of its own—a meaning system that can expand limitlessly based upon what is valued. As such, "[s]ymbols are images, words, or behaviors that have multiple levels of meaning . . . stand for concepts that are too complex to be stated directly in words" (Womack, 2005, pp. 1–2). Signs on the other hand stand for one possible meaning, a fixed meaning. In health care, signs usually are a physical of psychological representation of a patient's disease or illness. Symbols produce action (Turner & Bruner, 1986; Wolf, 2014). Usually the meaning of a particular symbol is culturally assigned. "Man [woman] lives in the meaning he [she] is able to discern" (Polanyi & Prosch, 1975, p. 66). Symbols organize our perception of reality by imposing order onto disorder in our experience. Symbols represent cultural values and beliefs. Symbols for patients may be in represented in the form of religious symbols, such as a *Bible* on a bedside table or a medal around the neck; they may be in the form of a picture representing Chinese or Japanese linguistic symbols of joy and happiness; they may be in the type of clothing worn representing wealth or poverty; or jewelry representing a state in life, such as a wedding ring. Symbols in professional nursing culture are complex and convey multiple meanings—Roach (2002) called them comportment, one of her 6Cs of caring. The hiddenness of caring symbols come to life visually in actions—eyes, voice, and gestures (i.e., looks, how one speaks, and touches [physically and spiritually touches the patient, for example]). Symbols are also visible culture itself and also signify meaning; they may be in the form of a uniform, or colorful scrubs; a white uniform or laboratory coat; a pin representing where a nurse has achieved the recognition of a college degree; a name tag designating a nurse as a registered nurse, a bachelor of science in nursing (BSN), a charge nurse or nurse manager; a stethoscope around the neck symbolizing power and the ability to assess a patient. Symbols have deep meaning and represent symbolic interaction that determines what is valued and what is valuable in culture.

LANGUAGE AND COMMUNICATION

When assessing a patient from another culture, transcultural nurses recognize that communication is reciprocal (Blunter, DeHoop, & Hendriks, 2006).

Language is complex with diverse linguistic forms, such as the languages of English, Spanish, French, Chinese, Russian, German, and multiple other languages and diverse dialects. Language also is syntax, grammar, semantics, and interpretations. Communication is contextual and, as such, is a cocreative process of meaning and represents diverse cultures, and symbolisms. Ways of communicating are symbolic of a culture or multicultures. Today, there also is the language of technology—the computer, social media, and robotics—which has its own forms and symbols (Ess, 2014; Locsin, Purnell, Tanioka, & Osaka, 2011). In the contemporary era, digital communication has altered the way in which we value, learn, interact, behave, and ultimately know the world of the other. It is important to note that digital communication has been advanced by individuals who are knowledgeable about linguistics or communicating formally but perhaps not optimally. Often, miscommunication is apparent by differences in the meaning structure of language(s), symbolic interaction, and digital communication and how the meaning is conveyed from one to another. Communication is symbolic interaction and linguistic wherein meaning is interpreted through what language represents, including sign language for the hearing impaired, or Braille for the seeing impaired, diverse dialects, secret languages used by families or lovers, even "street language." When languages between the professional nurse and the patient are different, there often exist communication barriers that lead to misunderstanding on both sides of the relationship. Awareness and understanding and choice become more difficult. Often an interpreter, either in person or through the telephone system or an electronic digital system must be sought to mediate the data-gathering process and the development of the transcultural nursing care plan. It is important to remember that when using an interpreter in person or electronically, much may be lost in translation but also, much can be gained.

The universal in the communication process, however, is caring (i.e., compassion, conscience, commitment, confidence, competence, and comportment [Roach, 2002]) and communication (i.e., linguistic sensitivity to languages and meaning systems). People do understand and respond to the intricacies of the caring interrelationship for the meaning of authentic presence. Symbolic interaction is a message, meaning that is sent and received through interpretation. Symbolic interaction carries

with it all the phenomena of meanings associated with ethnocentrism, prejudice, marginality, stereotyping, and unequal relationships from socioeconomic or socioeducational positions of power (Brown, 2002; Coleman, 2006; Dennis, 2005). Body language and narrative communication convey ways of caring as concern for or disconnection from the other. Certain body language, such as eye contact and touch must be culturally thoughtful and appropriate.

DIFFERENT CULTURAL RITUALS

Transcultural nurses encounter many cultural rituals of diverse patients in practice. Many rituals also are embedded within the nursing profession itself (Wolf, 2014). Rituals reveal values at their deepest level. People express in ritual what "moves" them the most, and since the form of expression is standardized and compulsory in most situations, it is the values of the group that are revealed. Rituals give us clues to and understanding of the essential makeup of human societies (i.e., families, communities, nations, organizations, professions, professional organizations, political parties, religions, age, gender, and so forth). Rituals are a form of respect for a king, elder, or person of stature, such as the *Wai*, the Thai greeting of holding the hands together and bowing the head; or the hand salute of enlisted personnel to senior officers in the military. Rituals are ever present in religions in the form of services, such as the Catholic Mass, or praying the rosary with beads; the *Book of Common Prayer of Anglicans* or Episcopalians, the *Book of Worship* prayed by Lutherans, or for Muslim prayer, the *Salah* (praying 5 times a day on a decorative mat [*Sajjada* or *Musallah*] in the direction of Mecca in Saudi Arabia). Ritual activity eventually achieves structure or organization with rites, and norms that oversee and manage relationships. Structure is found at all stages and levels of culture and society. Rituals become social structures to assist in connecting people to their past and illuminate how a group maintains its cultural form over time. Rituals always include some type of status elevation, change, or transformation, such as a marriage ceremony in a church or courthouse, a commencement ceremony in high school or college, or a pinning ceremony in nursing with the recitation of Nightingale's or Jeanne Mance's pledge. Contemporary ideas of ritual are beginning to move us to reflect upon Buber's (1958, 1965) notion of a "life of dialogue" in the evolution of the *meaning* of community and culture.

ETHNOCENTRISM

Ethnocentrism is a belief in the superiority of one's own ethnic group or looking down upon people who are different. People tend toward self-interest while in the context of otherness, thus, ethnocentrism overall focuses on ethnic self-interest. Ethnocentrism can be acted out as dominance or intolerance from individual to individual, group to group, region to region, and nation to nation.

In recent history, in many multicultural Western nations, ethnic boundaries that had mattered most in the past have undergone a fundamental transformation, such that the average person no longer thinks of himself or herself solely in ethnic terms. A person or a new immigrant to a nation may continue to secure his or her identity by continuing to embrace traditions and customs of his or her original culture. But, to identify ethnically, to make it a prominent feature of one's identity in the West, for the most part, requires a conscious choice (Tuan 1998). In recent years, ethnocentrism has begun to show itself through behaviors reminiscent of hegemony and past hatreds, such as hatred for particular religious groups, or radical behaviors.

Cultural superiority or hegemony is not only at the individual or group level but also at the national level. It affects the way in which one conducts one's affairs in the company of others and on the world stage. For example, according to Reinhard, President of the Business for Diplomatic Action (*C-SPAN*, August 23, 2006), the world is becoming increasingly anti-American. Images of the past as a vision of heroism in World War II or a "can-do and optimistic nation" have been replaced by many other images, such as "stupid is so American" or entertainment products from the United States that are transported around the world that portray images that are criminally violent and sexually explicit. Also, because of different images of violence, war, and intolerance for the values, languages, and cultures of others, the United States has lost the respect that it used to enjoy. However, hope does spring eternal and within a democracy, change is ever present. Now people around the world are becoming increasingly optimistic about how the United States will resume its leadership position but with a cooperative spirit, and creativity and begin to influence again other nations toward democratic principles, attention to human rights, and the development of new forms of energy and growing the economy in the new "green" world that is emerging (Henderson, 2006).

STEREOTYPING

Stereotyping, closely related to prejudice, is alienating, typecasting, labeling, and classifying another person or group or culture in one way or another that may intentionally or nonintentionally offend the other (Congress & Gonzalez, 2005). In stereotyping, actions of one person, one community, one social class, one organization, or one government body may be considered representative of the whole culture. Concepts such as third-world countries, terrorists, ugly Americans, white trash, gringos, and patients referred to as noncompliant, or "frequent fliers" may indicate stereotyping or classifying that conjure up negative emotions and/or may misrepresent someone or something.

SOCIAL CLASS

Social class or socioeconomic status is a term in a culture that indicates personal history, family, upbringing, and social-economic circumstances. The class structure in the West is usually indicated by lower, middle, and upper class and the designations generally relate to economics and what is considered valuable in the culture. Although social class is usually designated by money and the acquisition of goods, other factors that are more invisible or symbolic are interwoven its meaning (Tuan, 1998). Attention has been given to the study of the culture of poverty, including how ethnic groups, through cultural heritage or discrimination are situated and/or remain in the culture.

In other parts of the world, such as in India, the Hindu caste system that dominated the culture and was organized to include or exclude groups around the nature of status, continues to hold considerable influence in the designation of social and economic status, marriage arrangements, and other cultural work activities. The lower class and lower castes give rise to vulnerable populations wherein health disparities are evident—lower caste correlates with poor nutrition, lack of clean water, inadequate education, and lack of access to individualized health care.

History, ethnicity, and the cultural or geographical contexts play a significant role in the evolution of class care in health-care organizations. Class care is evident by certain behaviors of professionals toward those without health insurance, immigrants, or the poor and toward those in emergency departments, where people who visit often are called "frequent fliers," for example.

MARGINAL STATUS

Marginality refers to a perceived lack of social connectedness and integration with the dominant culture. It highlights individuals who are stigmatized and discriminated against for various reasons in a culture (Andrews & Boyle, 2003, 2015; Dennis, 2005). Although against the law, a culture group may be marginalized because of race even though they have been born and raised in a particular nation-state (e.g., African Americans, Asian Americans, or Hispanic Americans). Also in some geographic regions of nation-states around the world, people are marginalized because of their religions. Certain groups choose to be marginalized because of diverse ideologies inconsistent with a dominant culture's rules of law and they then can be considered breaking the law (e.g., polygamists).

GENDER

Gender relates to sexual categories of masculinity and femininity, and includes the sexual diversity of male, female, heterosexual, homosexual, lesbian, gay, bisexual, and transgender categories (LeBesco, 2004; Winick, 1970). In the potential for culture-value conflict, the withholding of recognition of anyone in a group relates to the denial of the understanding of identity and equal recognition, which leads to oppression or denunciation (Habermas, 1994).

Gender also is a classification system from a linguistic standpoint important in transcultural communication. It is most often evident in Indo-European (i.e., Germanic, Italic, Celtic, Baltic, Slavic, Albanian, Greek, or Indo-Iranian subfamilies), and Semitic Hebrew, Arabic, Maltese, and Ethiopian) languages and shows the differences between male and female or neuter, animate, or inanimate gender characteristics of the above named languages (Winick, 1970).

INTERGENERATION AND INTERACTION

Intergenerational or multigenerational conflict occurs when there is a difference of values and the meaning of social construction of ethnicity or cultural conditioning on the part of children or kin (blood relations) of traditional families from a specific culture group (Winick, 1970). In the West and now in many developing nations, the social construction of ethnicity

entails having choices to participate in some cultural traditions and not in others (Tuan, 1998; Waters, 1990). Parents from diverse ethnic groups may believe that children who participate fully in a dominant culture could weaken the cultural transmission of values, beliefs, and attitudes about the traditional culture of birth. Younger generations seek choice in the adoption of views, values, and behaviors, often to avoid racial or cultural discrimination or hostility or to fit in with the dominant or digital cultures.

In patient care situations, transcultural nurses need to be very sensitive to understanding the differences in generations of patients and their coworkers. In nursing in North America, there tends to be multigenerational conflict among nurses themselves now that the ages for the practice of nursing are wide-ranging (see Box 6–1).

The multigenerational and multicultural conflict may occur when nurses from different eras try to relate together either in clinical practice or educational arenas. Again, misunderstanding related to values, beliefs, attitudes, behavior, and communication patterns can occur. The new generation of millennial nurses in general is considered computer literate yet realistic and collaborative while the veterans are loyal and follow a chain of command. The baby boomers are optimistic and follow a chain of command while the Generation Xers are skeptical and self-commanding. The digital Facebook/social media generation is a community that desires to communicate and make decisions almost immediately often demanding great efficiency and few mistakes but at the same time can potentially violate principles of individual and collective ethics. Behar (2013) referred to this group as the F generation (Facebook/social media) and noted that as a culture we are moving from Homo Sapien to Homo Socialicus. Floridi (2014) calls this process

---

BOX 6–1 ❖ Generational Names

- Veterans (1925–1945)
- Baby Boomers (Me Generation) (1946–1964)
- Generation X (Latchkey, MTV, Nexters) (1965–1980)
- Generation Y (Millennial Generation Y, Digital, Internet Generation, Infosphere Generation F [Facebook/Social Media])

(Behar, 2013; Duchscher & Cowin, 2004; Floridi, 2014)

the fourth revolution—how the infosphere is "reshaping human reality and changing our sense of self, relationships, society, politics, wars, and managing the environment" (pp. vi–x). Rosen (2012) calls this culture group the I generation. At the same time, this revolution is going on, for people in general and for health care professionals in particular, there is a growing trend in the technology culture toward addiction or "internet disorder and internet gaming disorder." listed now as a psychiatric diagnosis or mental health issues by the American Psychiatric Association (DSM-5, 2013). Openness to learning from one another in all environments becomes a priority.

PREJUDICE

As nurses, transcultural spiritual-ethical caring illuminates the need to avoid prejudice (prejudging people from a one-sided view), discrimination, or intolerance, and to listen and communicate in fairness, and understanding of the differences that may be exhibited by the patient, family members, or significant others. Gadamer (Outhwaite, 1985) reminds us, however, that to make judgments or decisions it involves prejudgment, that is, we come to each situation from our own living history—what we know and have stored in consciousness. When we interact with others and through education, we are continually learning and adding to our body of knowledge, hopefully mindful of and wise to the value of differences. Sometimes this knowledge is unreflective, however, and leads to decisions that are thoughtless, disrespectful, and hurtful to others. Caring thus is clouded by self-interests or self-centeredness.

FEAR

Cultural variation and diverse practices often generate fear in professionals who fail to seek understanding and recognize the other. Fear often generates a "fight-or-flight response" due to a heightened feeling of threat. People may seek comfort by staying among themselves or fleeing into their own areas of safety or requesting protection from law enforcement. People may react by perpetrating violence against another. Ghettos are formed or people are driven to or retreat into areas where similar cultural values will be respected and upheld. This can even apply to culture groups perpetrating the drug trade (Morris, 2012). Today many areas populated by one cultural group or another are now populated by similar socioeconomic

classes. Here again there is complexity. The areas that once were considered ghettos can now be part of re-gentrification where new groups, often of a higher socioeconomic class are moving into and changing areas. Concern is now for the vulnerable, poor, and disenfranchised. Where do people go when they are not recognized for what they can give to a community, or if they are immigrants fleeing violence and persecution? All people desire some type of rootedness, security, recognition, and transformation. Habermas (1994) stated that we are formed by recognition. When this does not occur, mistrust and fear ensue and continue to affect the way of being of the other. The demand for respect by one group goes hand in hand with the failure of cultural recognition on the part of the other. This failure generally is connected with gross social discrimination by subsequent cultural superiority of persons toward people of another race, ethnic group, or culture (Habermas, 1994). To participate fully in seeking the good of or care for another requires a framework of mutual respect and compassion founded on the intrinsic worth of all people in all cultures (Rockefeller, 1994; Wolin, 2005).

TIME

As a transcultural nurse, time is a factor in the practice of transcultural spiritual-ethical caring. Everything we do is associated with time, with most references to a 24-hour clock, 7 days a week (24/7), however time itself is an illusive concept in modern science and in the modern world (Hawking, 1998). In the healthcare arena and perhaps in all business, time is considered money. As nurse-patient ratios increase and transcultural needs increase, time becomes a critical factor in decisions about transcultural caring and the quality of culturally relevant care. Many nurses claim that they do not have time to care or provide transcultural caring to patients and their families or significant others.

DIVERSE MODELS OF HEALTH CARE

People of different cultures embrace different health-care systems or folk practices to deal with their health and illness care needs. The "health-belief model" to a large extent determines or influences the nature of disease, health, healing, and the human condition. These health-belief models can be the Western biomedical model, Eastern, or traditional views of health and healing that highlight systems related to holistic, complementary, alternative, or integrated medical/health-care practices.

The personal, social, and religious meaning and cultural practices of health and illness play a major role in the creation and interpretation of diseases or illness, vulnerability of pain, and suffering, pain reactions, treatment practices and codes of behavior, stigma of disease, food practices, coping with chronic illness, the environment, hot-and-cold systems of folk practices, and the understanding of health, healing, dying, and death rites (Helman, 1997; Kleinman, 1980, 1998; Coffman, 2006, 2014; Ray, 1998a, 2001c 2010a, 2010b, 2010c). The dominant health-care model in the West is a Western model of health care with a focus on empirical science, technology, and digital and social media communication (i.e., computer technology, smart phones, Instagram, Pinterest, Twitter, etc.).

Although cultures in the developing world do embrace their own traditional practices, for example, holistic Eastern practices of mind, body, and spirit integration and ethnomedicine, Western scientific medicine with technological and pharmacological therapeutics is making a big effect. On the horizon are emerging technologies, such as nanotechnologies, robotics, and bioenergetics that are being evaluated in relation to health and healing practices (Dossey, Keegan, & Guzzetta, 2005; Locsin, Purnell, Tanioka, & Osaka, 2011).

Gadow adopted the belief that "the nurse [more than any other health-care professional] attends the patient as a whole, not just as a single problem or system" (1980, p. 81). The nurse attends first to the ordinary intimacies of everyday life, thus, experiencing the person as a unique individual in his or her cultural complexities, weaknesses, strengths at the same time using his or her professional and scientific knowledge. Advocacy in Gadow's view is based upon the assumption of self-determinism—about what individuals want to do or how they choose. Self-determination or choice is the most fundamental and valuable human right (Gadow, 1980) and in the process of caring, to advance choices in health and illness care, transcultural nurses are challenged to be knowledgeable about the complexity of different cultures, and seek understanding of the multiple meanings of health and illness communicated by people of diverse cultures. Only then can transculturally relevant care be provided and transcultural competency be achieved.

LEGISLATION

The awareness and understanding of culture has been legislated throughout history. In nation-states,

comprehensive political processes over time have illuminated principles that reflect a culture's basic values and beliefs. Legislation deals with the process of understanding the spirit of or theories of the law within nations or organizations and enacting and judging principles as rules or the force of law. In a globalizing world, the theories need to be deemed valid, built upon the politics of recognition and genuine respect. In the West, often laws or policies grounded in the quest for diversity in culture or multiculturalism produce a homogenizing effect or making everyone the same (Taylor, 1994), for example, "political correctness" or hyper-tolerance, desiring not to offend anyone. By virtue of media communication, especially television and social media, political correctness or hyper-tolerance is fast becoming the norm. As in all investigation, backlash is advancing in the form of increased racism, multicultural fatigue, increased disrespect, and increased hatred and violence, and other negative factors.

In coming to terms with the integration of the cultures and laws of many nation-states or member nations, the European Union (EU) advanced a commitment to recognizing human rights, sustainability of development, promotion of social justice, protection of equality, solidarity between generations, and protecting children (Rifkin, 2004). The constitution of the EU has a single foreign minister responsible to conduct foreign and defense policies. Policies designed to blend immigration and refugee and asylum issues are decided by majority vote (Rifkin, 2004).

In the world, legislation enacted at the political level may be paradoxical. Principles of justice or fairness are the norm in the West or postcolonial nations. In some nations, such as India, newer legislation regarding the caste system has been enacted. Yet, in many instances, long-standing cultural traditions of the sociocultural/economic system overrule the law (Czerenda, 2006). In some smaller nations, rules are created at times by military force or, in part, by consensus thinking of small ethnic, religious, or tribal groups who may or may not have the interests of the diversity of a whole society in mind.

In larger societies in North America in the United States and Canada for example, democracy and justice have been strong principles. In the United States, the proclamation from the *Declaration of Independence* of ". . . We hold these truths to be self-evident, that all men are created equal, that they are endowed by their Creator with certain unalienable Rights, that among these are Life, Liberty and the pursuit of

Happiness. . . ." (in Congress, July 4, 1776), and the *United States Constitution* and its *Amendments* (Link & Coben, 1972) secure the values and beliefs of democracy as a force of law. In Canada, for example, *The Canada Act* with the subsequent *Canadian Charter of Rights* (1981) secured the constitution of Canada from the United Kingdom as the force of law for and in Canada (Milne, 1982). These constitutions are founded on the supremacy of God and principles that uphold the rule of law in relation to democratic principles of individualism, equality, and freedom.

The United Nations adopted its Charter on June 26, 1945 and entered into law, October 24, 1945 to provide opportunities to achieve international cooperation in solving international problems of an economic, social, cultural, or humanitarian nature and refraining from the threat or use of force (retrieved August 19, 2006). Continued attempts to operationalize democratic principles and the rule of law have involved negotiations, different movements and even a civil war in the United States and ongoing discussions and legislation to recognize the rights of citizens. In different nation-states and collectively within the United Nations, legislation deals with the process of understanding the spirit of the law and enacting it into rules or force of law. Capitalism and economic competition have been the hallmarks of many Western nations and now many non-Western nations. In the contemporary world of culture and the globalizing world, views of economic justice and democracy (Hahnel, 2005; Harman, 1998) are challenging people to move away from values of individualism and competition to values of participation and cooperation. But can diversity of culture within the notion of serving the good of a common humanity or the acceptance of multiculturalism within a globalizing world be legislated and accepted in different nation states? The United Nations Educational, Scientific and Cultural Organization (UNESCO) looks to how legislation helps to assist in interpreting the nature of new thought to cultural understanding and choice for all people. Recently, the World Health Organization has declared that the concept of health should be in every policy for the world community, which would involve consensus and enacting new rules of *law* within nation-states (WHO.org). Multiculturalism in many nations has already been discussed, experimented with, or enacted into law. Health in every policy is yet to be fully discussed or enacted; however,

the directive is being considered in Canada. The Canadian Nurses Association has taken a positive stand on this WHO directive.

In a globalizing world, there is a need for a self-reflective political culture so that recognition, honor, and respect are afforded all persons. Building of the global civic culture requires the following practices to assist in the recognition of the meaning of relationship and the equal worth of all people: communicative action that is caring, consensual, and culturally and religiously inclusive; health and security—the provision of essential benefits for life, liberty, and the pursuit of happiness; and information and actions that are subjected to sensitivity and continuing critical examination through dialogue and unmanipulated debate (Chinn, 2013; Economy & Levi, 2014; Fishkin, 1992; Habermas, 1995; Hahnel, 2005; Rifkin, 2004).

Legislation in Nursing and Medicine

In nursing, regulatory bodies, such as the state boards of nursing medicine or provincial colleges of nursing and medicine are designed for public safety to protect patients and caregivers by designing standards of practice and issuing licenses or certificates of competence of professionals to legally practice (Dittman, 2007; Turkel, 2006a, 2006b). Other organizations, such as the International Council of Nurses, the American Nurses Association, or the Canadian Nurses Association also set standards of practice that incorporate standards and codes of ethics to assist with the promotion of culturally appropriate care. Although not legislative per se, commissions, such as The Joint Commission in the United States, provide standards to promote safety and culturally and linguistically appropriate health care (2006). The Joint Commission has several standards, the 2006 Standards for Hospitals, Ambulatory, Behavioral Health, Long-Term Care and Home Care that also are cross-linked to the standards of the Office of Minority Health National Culturally and Linguistically Appropriate Services (CLAS). These standards support the provision of care and services that are conducive to the cultural, language, literacy and learning needs of individuals and advance understanding and competency in professional health-care interactions in health-care organizations.

In addition, congressionally mandated annual reports on health-care disparities in the United States, are submitted to the Agency for Healthcare Research and Quality to understand the affect of

stereotyping on medical decision making and improve models for health assessment and service
(http://www.qualitytools.ahrq.gov/disparitiesreport/
browse.aspx). Moreover, in the United States, the Patient Protection and Affordable Care Act (2010) may
facilitate more effectively how health care disparities
may be addressed and reduced (http://housedocs.
house.gov/energycommerce/ppacacon.pdf).

Dynamics of Transcultural Caring Tool for Choice

In this tool (see Fig. 6-6), Phases I–IV, cocreative
choices are made by building and understanding the
intricate meaning of the transcultural communicative
ethical relationship (see Ray's CARING Tool, the Culture-Value Conflict Tool) between the nurse and the
patient, the family, or significant others. In Phase I,
transcultural communicative spiritual-ethical caring
and advocacy recognizes first the unequal power of
the professional nurse-patient relationship as a
process of mutual interaction. In home care, the patient, although in a more powerful position because he
or she is within the home, will still defer to the nurse
to appreciate what is going on in his or her life. The
nurse must recognize the influence of his or her power,
or potential for power over the patient in any situation. Power is a relational process of dynamic energy
flow between one and the other. Power can be destructive or it can be a process of transcultural caring to
empower the self and others to know, listen, learn,
understand, heal, and transform. Recognition of the
empowering process of the nurse-patient relationship
as cocreative and a life force can assist the patient

to make choices that are valuable for his or her life
and move in the direction to what is necessary for
healing.

The relationship between the nurse as a transcultural professional and the other also encompasses an
ethic of accountability and responsibility (see Phase II
of the tool). Ethics of accountability and responsibility are found in consciousness and conscience, what
we know about and reflect upon when seeking the
good of the self and other, what we can reason and
discern based upon knowledge and experience, what
we *actually* experience, and the ongoing recognition
of the meanings of ethical communicative action that
could not have been known in advance but are being
revealed (cocreative emergence) in the living present
(what we continually anticipate) (Mead in Griffin,
2002). The nurse may elicit help through prayer, or
relinquish some aspects of care to other professionals
to deal responsibly with some challenging patient
care situations that are not within his sphere of
knowledge and experience, or what he or she chooses
to be a part of. For example, some nurses may choose
not to go into neighborhoods that pose a danger to a
nurse, not to give a particular medication that a doctor has ordered that he or she thinks is incorrect, or
participate in abortions. Although the large-scale systems of a hospital, clinic, or community organization
may figure into the paradoxes of human interaction,
it is the intricacy of the emerging relationship where
the tension of conflict and caring are played out and
where power, control, and the empowering of the
other through caring can be truly experienced and
understood.

Dynamics of Transcultural Caring Tool for Choice

Phase II
Ethic of Caring
• Responsibility (Mutual)
   and
• Accountability (Personal)
  for Potential Decision
  Conflict Resolution

Phase III
Ethic of Communication
• Respect
• Trust
• Compassionate/Existential
  Advocate for Negotiation

Phase I
Unequal Power
• Authority
• Knowledge
• Access to Privileged Information
• Influence
• Language/Cultural Customs

Phase IV
Ethic of Reconciliation
• Agreement
• Understanding
• Compromise/Choice

Figure 6-6: Dynamics of transcultural caring tool for choice.

Phase III illuminates the phenomena of emergence, the living present encompassing respect, trust, interaction, and compassion for negotiation exchange. Griffin (2002) claimed that "[i]t is the living present that we emerge as persons;" where "in the conflictual present . . . we are negotiating our aims and goals as construction of our future" (p. 193). "To be at the living edge is to search out the simplicity on the other side of complexity" (DePree, 1989, p. 22).

Phase IV identifies the living present as construction, of the future, the anticipated or hoped for future, the simplicity on the other side of complexity, through the ethic of reconciliation, the agreement, understanding, or compromise that is achieved by virtue of grasping in an immediate way the significance of the meaning of the art of choosing in what has happened or what is happening in the nurse-patient situation.

Transcultural Caring Negotiation Tool

The transcultural caring negotiation tool (see Fig. 6-7) is a synopsis of the all the tools in the art of negotiation in relation to the meaning of reality for the patient and family. The art of transcultural communicative caring is a dynamic process of sharing, acting and responding. Ethical caring plays a significant role of respect for persons, justice, and reconciliation. Transcultural nurses act in the role of culturebroker or engage with a culture broker (e.g., a linguistic or cultural family member or other professional). A culture broker is a middleperson who, according to anthropologists is one of the most powerful roles when negotiating between two or more people from diverse cultures.

The culture broker in nursing serves as a mediator or broker between the patient and other healthcare professionals to support the patients' cultural beliefs and values (Tripp-Reimer, 1985). In this process, the nurse must recognize his or her power in the relationship and have as a central purpose, empowering the patient to make choices that are consistent with his or her cultural values. Often, there is a tension or conflict, but as a transcultural caring nurse, resolution of tension is a priority (Gendron, 1988). **Negotiation ultimately concludes with the ethic of reconciliation (i.e., understanding, agreement, and compromise).** The real mission of transcultural caring negotiation is the symbolism of awakening a shared consciousness of understanding through its own expressive power (Gadamer, 1986). In this compassionate and cocreative act, the patient and the nurse experience a sense of the beautiful, the harmony of body, mind, and spirit (Watson, 1988, 2005, 2008).

Summary

Through exploration of caring as transcultural, spiritual, and ethical communicative action, competency, and transcultural tools to guide practice, research, and education, the following points have been made.

- Transcultural caring is knowledge-in-process and incorporates the Theory of Transcultural Caring Dynamics in Nursing and Health Care—caring as the essence of nursing, transcultural caring

Learn More

Ensuring Transcultural Competence

- Transcultural Caring as a Way of Being
- Knowledge/Professional Development
- Knowledge-in-Process/Reflective Practice
- Understanding and Discernment about Categories of Information
- Cultures/Technological Cultures
- Society/Communities
- Political Structures/Social Networks
- Economic Structures/Allocation of Resources
- Policies/Culture Brokering
- Practical Wisdom (Spiritual-Ethical Caring Authenticity)
- Clarification of Patient Values (Existential Advocacy)
- Caring Practice Evaluations (Patient and Peer)

Figure 6-7: Transcultural caring negotiation tool.

ethics, transcultural context, and universal sources (spirituality).

- Transcultural caring is cocreative emergence.
- Transcultural caring embodies awareness, understanding, and choice.
- The process of choice is not only the integration of the personal knowledge of the patient's story, scientific knowledge, and the art of transcultural caring in nursing (Chase, 2004), but also, the personal story of the nurse as a caring person and how she or he understands and interprets meaning of cultural health, illness, dying or death, and healing with the patient (Smith & Liehr, 2014).
- The intricate story of the nurse is often hidden, taken for granted, or not understood but it is always being put to work as practical wisdom.
- "What is required in the concrete situation [transcultural caring situation] is the kind of practical insight and knowledge [practical

wisdom] whose special merit is its ability to grasp what is demanded by the circumstances at hand" (Caputo, 1987, pp. 109–110).

- Practical wisdom is a mode of revealing meaning; it is *awareness* of caring for self and others, understanding of knowledge-in-process, and facilitation of *choice* in transcultural nursing situations and health care.
- Practical wisdom facilitates *understanding* of how a patient arrives at a *choice* and how the nurse and patient self-transcend or transform. The ethics of accountability and reconciliation illuminate the transformative process.
- Choice as understanding, agreement, and compromise completes the circle of transcultural caring.
- The essence or mode of revealing meaning relates to how individuals, through choice, are transformed through cocreative emergence in new and energetic ways.

Transcultural Nursing in Practice
Transcultural Caring Experiences

Mrs. Sherry Acton and Jennifer Linden RN

Jennifer, a new graduate nurse, is admitting a patient, Mrs. Acton, to the oncology unit of the Kensington General Hospital with a severe blood dyscrasia from chemotherapy. Her hemoglobin is 7. Mrs. Acton recently had been diagnosed with stage IV ovarian cancer. She did not have surgery and only once was admitted to the hospital for evaluation. She started chemotherapy weekly 3 weeks ago in her oncologist's cancer center. Upon admission to the emergency department (ED), she was fatigued and in severe abdominal pain. The ED physician ordered pain medication and a crossmatch and type for 2 units of blood to be given STAT upon admission to the oncology unit. After conducting a thorough transcultural nursing assessment after admission to the unit, Jennifer learned that Mrs. Acton is a Jehovah's Witness. Jennifer and Mrs. Acton are in great distress about the gravity of her health-care situation and her quality of life. Mrs. Acton tells Jennifer that her religion does not permit the giving of blood products and she cannot take blood of any kind. Jennifer was aware of the Jehovah's Witness religion and its beliefs but still does not understand why, under these dire circumstances, Mrs. Acton will not accept the blood transfusion. Jennifer is very nervous about talking further with Mrs. Acton, discussing the situation with her nurse manager, calling the ED physician and Mrs. Acton's oncologist about the situation. When the chart arrives on the floor, there is no indication that blood should not be given. Jennifer would like to give the blood as ordered but she knows that she does need to act on the patient's behalf.

QUESTIONS FOR TRANSCULTURAL CARING REFLECTION

- Based upon the Theory and Model of Transcultural Caring Dynamics of Nursing and Health Care, Ray's Transcultural Communicative Spiritual-Ethical CARING Tool, the Culture-Value Conflict Assessment Tool, and the Dynamics of Transcultural Caring for Choice Tool, identify what characteristics of the theoretical model and tools need to be taken into consideration to determine how Jennifer should embrace the transcultural nursing situation.

- Name the features of the theoretical model and tools that are most significant.
- Using the Internet and other religious books or documents, identify the central tenets of the Jehovah's Witness religion. What religious and social cultural rituals can be identified in the Jehovah's Witness religion?
- Identify what the potential conflict or tension is for Jennifer, for the ED physician and the oncologist. Identify your priorities. Where would you glean your cultural and religious knowledge to facilitate choice making for the patient?
- Use Ray's Transcultural Communicative Spiritual-Ethical CARING Tool and the Dynamics of Transcultural Caring Tool for Choice to show how Jennifer may communicate with Mrs. Acton, the nurse manager, the physician in the ED, and the oncologist?
- What steps would you take on a professional level to advocate and negotiate for this patient?
- How would you cocreate a process for health, healing, dying, and transformation?

Mr. Joseph Martinez and Daniel Barth, RN

Mr. Joseph Martinez, a 65-year-old man, was admitted at 6:30 p.m. from home to the medical-surgical unit through the admissions' department with gastrointestinal pain, at this time, of an unknown origin. Daniel was assigned to the patient for the 7 p.m. to 7 a.m. shift. Daniel came on the unit about 6:45 p.m. He received report from Joan who stated that she did not have time to admit Mr. Martinez yet. Daniel proceeded to the room. When Daniel saw the patient, he was still in his street clothes of jeans and a worn cotton shirt. Right away, Daniel raised his voice at the patient, thinking because of his Hispanic/Latino surname that he did not speak English. He started to tell the patient in a loud voice to get into the gown at the foot of the bed, pointing to it and said he would be back in a few minutes. Mr. Martinez put on the gown. He was in a lot of pain and just wanted to lie down and rest. He recalled that he had not had any pain medication since he left the doctor's office; his appointment was at 1 p.m. He was thirsty but there was no water glass beside the bed. He also had been nauseated and vomited a few times in the afternoon. Daniel came in the room with another nurse, Marta Rodriquez. Daniel got upset because Mr. Martinez had the gown on backward. Mr. Martinez did not have a chance to say anything. Marta spoke to the patient in Spanish but he could barely understand her.

QUESTIONS FOR TRANSCULTURAL CARING REFLECTION

- What occurred in this scenario?
- What aspects of the Culture-Value Conflict Assessment Tool were exhibited? Give a brief explanation of the dimensions and their meaning in this situation.
- What symbolic behavior (perceived meaning of conduct or comportment) was exhibited on the part of Mr. Martinez?
- What symbolic behavior (perceived meaning of conduct or comportment) was exhibited by Daniel and Marta?
- Identify issues within the organizational culture of the unit.
- Identify why intergenerational conflict may be arising.
- What are the patterns of communication? Although not identified in this scenario, reflect upon the many diverse forms of communication, such as the use or overuse of social media, that are facing health care professionals, either as individuals or in their practices, especially with young people or in mental health practice.
- What issues of language were presumed in this transcultural nursing situation?
- How can one practice spiritual-ethical caring when time and nurse-patient ratios are a problem in contemporary nursing?
- How does the model in this book and the different assessment tools presented in this chapter assist with issues identified in this scenario?

Mr. Tommy Washington and Latitia Brooks, RN

Latitia, a hospice nurse, was assigned to care for Mr. Tommy Washington, 59 years old, in his home in Freedom Village, Florida. Mr. Washington has a diagnosis of end-stage cancer of the esophagus with metastasis to the occipital area of the brain. He had had surgery and radiation, and was taking chemotherapy for the past 8 months. He, with the help of the oncologist, discharge planning nurses of the local hospital, and his family (wife and two sons) made the decision to transfer Mr. Washington to hospice care. Latitia was going to do a full physical assessment, including a cultural assessment to become more knowledgeable about the suffering that Mr. Washington was undergoing and the concerns of his family. Latitia was preparing her bag to include morphine sulfate medication for pain, intravenous therapy that had been ordered by the doctor, dressings, and a chalkboard so that Mr. Washington could write down his concerns. She thought that he may not be able to speak considering his diagnosis. Latitia also was prepared to be in the home to teach and comfort the patient and family. With her experience, she thought that Mr. Washington and his family may be frightened about the dying process. She also wondered about what family rituals, religious beliefs, and practices the family may have. When packing her bag, Latitia thought about herself. She became somewhat frightened to go to the home of Mr. Washington. She had never been assigned to a patient in a part of the city that was considered dangerous because of drug trafficking. She was familiar with the narcotic count that hospice nurses had to do in the home in what and how much was administered to the patient. She knew that the area was known for an attack on a nurse who carried narcotics. Latitia wondered if one of Mr. Washington's sons who was "physically challenged" after an automobile accident (she had read that in the hospital discharge notes) may be on pain medication. Would he take some of Mr. Washington's medication for pain? Latitia notified her supervisor that she was leaving and asked her to call her on her cell phone in an hour. She picked up her bag and headed for her car.

QUESTIONS FOR TRANSCULTURAL CARING REFLECTION

- What is occurring in this scenario? What physical and cultural processes are exhibited?
- What aspects of the Culture-Value Conflict Assessment Tool were exhibited? Give a brief explanation of the dimensions you identify and their meaning in this situation.
- What symbolic behavior (perceived meaning and comportment) was exhibited on the part of Latitia?
- Identify issues within a cultural community that present challenges to a community home care health/hospice nurse. Identify potential sociocultural, sociopolitical, and socioeconomic issues.
- Identify personal and professional fears that have been exhibited.
- Identify ways in which Latitia could deal with her fears in this home care nursing situation.
- What patterns of communication could be developed?

FURTHER REFLECTION

Do you feel that issues of ethnocentrism or prejudice are part of this transcultural caring experience?
- Are there legal issues that have to be confronted in this transcultural caring situation?

References

American Psychiatric Association (2013). *Diagnostic and statistical manual of mental disorders* (5th ed.). Arlington, VA: American Psychiatric Publishing.

Andrews, M., & Boyle, J. (Eds.). (2003). *Transcultural concepts in nursing care* (4th ed.). Philadelphia: Lippincott Williams & Wilkins.

Andrews, M., & Boyle, J. (Eds.). (2015). *Transcultural concepts in nursing care* (7th ed.). Philadelphia: Wolters Kluwer Health.

Appiah, K. (1994). Identity, authenticity, survival. In A. Gutmann (Ed.), *Multiculturalism* (pp. 149–163). Princeton, NJ: Princeton University Press.

Appleton, C. (2005). *The experience of reconciling conflict.* PhD Dissertation, Nova Southeastern University, Ft. Lauderdale, FL.

Arrien, A. (1993). *The four-fold way: Walking the paths of the warrior, teacher, healer and visionary.* San Francisco: HarperSanFrancisco.

Asante, M., & Gudykunst, W. (Eds.). (1989). *Handbook of international and intercultural communication.* Newbury Park: Sage Publications.

Baldwin, J., Faulkner, S., Hecht, M., & Lindsley, S. (2006). *Redefining culture: Perspectives across the disciplines.* Mahwah, NJ: Lawrence Erlbaum Associates Publishers.

Bee, R. (1974). *Patterns and processes: An introduction to anthropological strategies for the study of sociocultural change.* New York: The Free Press.

Behar, M. (2013). *Generation F.* Bulgaria: Alto Communications Publishing Ltd.

Bernstein, R. (1986). *Philosophical profiles: Essays in a pragmatic mode.* Philadelphia: University of Pennsylvania Press.

Blunter, R., DeHoop, H., & Hendriks, P. (2006). *Optimal communication.* Stanford, CA: CSLI Publications.

Boulding, E. (1988). *Building a global civic culture.* New York: Teachers College Press.

Boykin, A., & Schoenhofer, S. (2001). *Nursing as caring: A model for transforming nursing practice.* Boston: Jones and Bartlett.

Brown, C. (2002). A theory of the process of creating power in relationships. *Nursing Administration Quarterly, 26*(2), 15–33.

Brown, P. (1998). *Understanding and applying medical anthropology.* Mountain View: Mayfield Publishing Company.

Bronowski, J. (1978). *The visionary eye: Essay in the arts, literature, and science.* Cambridge: The MIT Press.

Buber, M. (1958). *I and thou.* New York: MacMillan Publishing Company.

Buber, M. (1965). *Between man and man.* New York: The Macmillan Company.

Capra, F., Steindl-Rast, D., with Matus, T. (1991). *Belonging to the universe.* San Francisco: HarperSanFrancisco.

Caputo, J. (1987). *Radical hermeneutics.* Bloomington: Indiana University Press.

Carper, B. (1978). Fundamental patterns of knowing. *Advances in Nursing Science, 1*(1), 13–24.

CGFNS International, Inc. [Bilingual Credential Evaluation rganization].www.news@cgfns.org

Charter of the United Nations. Retrieved August 19, 2006, from http://www1.umn.edu/humanrts/instree/aunchart.htm

Chase, S. (2004). *Clinical judgment and communication in nurse practitioner practice.* Philadelphia: F. A. Davis Company.

Chinn, P. (2013). *Peace and power: New directions for building community* (8th ed.). Burlington, MA: Jones & Bartlett Learning.

Coffman, S. (2006). Marilyn Anne Ray, theory of bureaucratic caring. In A. Marriner Tomey & M. Alligood (Eds.), *Nursing theorists and their work* (6th ed., pp. 116–139). St. Louis: Mosby-Elsevier.

Coffman, S. (2014). Marilyn Anne Ray, the theory of bureaucratic caring. In M. Alligood (Ed.), *Nursing theorists and their work* (8th ed., pp. 98–119). St. Louis: Elsevier.

Coleman, P. (2006). *Attracted to conflict: A dynamical systems approach to the study of protracted social conflict.* Paper presented at Florida Atlantic University, Center for Complex Systems and Brian Sciences, March 30, 2006.

Congress, E., & Gonzalez, M. (2005). *Multicultural perspectives in working with families* (2nd ed.). New York: Springer Publishing Company.

Czerenda, A. (2006). *The show must go on: A caring inquiry into the meaning of widowhood and health for older Indian widows.* Doctor of Nursing Science (DNS) Dissertation, Florida Atlantic University, Boca Raton, FL.

Davidson, A., & Ray, M. (1991). Studying the human-environment phenomenon using the science of complexity. *Advances in Nursing Science, 13*(2), 73–87.

Davidson, A., Ray, M., & Turkel, M. (2011). *Nursing, caring, and complexity science: For human-environment well being.* New York: Springer Publishing Company.

Dennis, R. (Ed.). (2005). *Marginality, power and social structure (Vol. 12): Issues in race, class, and gender analysis (research in race and ethnic relations).* London: JAI Press.

DePree, M. (1989). *Leadership is an art.* New York: Dell Publishing.

de Vries, H., & Sullivan, L. (2006). *Political theologies: Public religions in a post-secular world.* New York: Fordham University Press.

Dittman, P. (2007). *Men in recovery returning to community.* DNS Dissertation, Florida Atlantic University, Boca Raton, FL.

Dossey, B. Keegan, L., & Guzzetta, C. (Eds.). (2005). *Holistic nursing* (4th ed.) Boston: Jones and Bartlett.

Duchscher, J., & Cowin, L. (2004). Multigenerational nurses in the workplace. *Journal of Nursing Administration, 34*(11), 493–501.

Economy, E., & Levi, M. (2014). *By all means necessary: How China's resource quest is changing the world.* Oxford: Oxford University Press.

Eriksson, K. (1997). Caring, spirituality and suffering. *Caring from the heart: The convergence of caring and spirituality.* (pp. 68–84). New York: Paulist Press.

Eril, A., Nunning, A., & Young, S. (2010). *A companion to cultural memory studies.* Berlin: Walter de Gruyter.

Ess, C. (2014). *Digital media ethics.* Cambridge, UK: Polity Press.

Fishkin, J. (1992). *The dialogue of justice: Toward a self-reflective society.* New Haven: Yale University Press.

Frankl, V. (1984). *Man's search for meaning.* New York: Washington Square Press.

Gadamer, H. (1986). *The relevance of the beautiful and other essays.* (N. Walker, Trans.). Cambridge: Cambridge University Press.

Gadamer, H. (1990). *Truth and method* (2nd rev. ed., J. Weinsheimer & D. Marshall, Trans.). New York: Crossroad.

Gadow, S. (1980). Existential advocacy: Philosophical foundation of nursing. In S. Spicer & S. Gadow (Eds.), *Nursing: Images and ideals, opening dialogue with the humanities* (pp. 79–101). New York: Springer.

Gendron, D. (1988). *The expressive form of caring.* (*Perspectives in Caring Monograph 2*). Toronto: University of Toronto.

Griffin, D. (2002). *The emergence of leadership: Linking self-organization and ethics.* London: Routledge.

Grumime, V., Barry, C., Gordon, S., & Ray, M. (under review for publication). On virtual presence. *Advanced Nursing Science.*

Gudykunst, W. (2005). *Theorizing about intercultural communication.* Thousand Oaks: Sage Publications, Inc.

Gutmann, A. (1994). *Multiculturalism.* Princeton, NJ: Princeton University Press.

Habermas, J. (1986). *The theory of communicative action: Reason and the rationalization of society* (Vol. 1). Boston: Beacon.

Habermas, J. (1987). *The theory of communicative action: Lifeworld and systems: A critique of functionalist reason* (Vol. 2). Boston: Beacon.

Habermas, J. (1994). Struggles for recognition in the democratic constitutional state. In A. Gutmann (Ed.), *Multiculturalism* (pp. 107–148). Princeton, NJ: Princeton University Press.

Habermas, J. (1995). *Theory of moral consciousness and communicative action.* Cambridge, MA: The MIT Press.

Habermas, J. (2006). On the relations between the secular liberal state and religion. In H. de Vries & L. Sullivan (Eds.), *Political theologies: Public religions in a post-secular world* (pp. 251–260). New York: Fordham University Press.

Hahnel, R. (2005). *Economic justice and democracy.* New York: Routledge.

Harman, W. (1998). *Global mind change* (2nd ed.). San Francisco: Berrett-Koehler Publishers, Inc.

Hawking, S. (1998). *A brief history of time.* New York: Bantam Books.

Heidegger, M. (1962). *Being and time* (J. Macquarrie & E. Robinson, Trans.). San Francisco: Harper SanFrancisco.

Heidegger, M. (1972). *On time and being.* (J. Stambaugh, Trans.). New York: Harper & Row, Publishers.

Heidegger, M. (1977). *The question concerning technology and other essays.* (W. Lovitt, Trans.). New York: Harper & Row, Publishers.

Helman, C. (1997). *Culture, health and illness* (3rd ed.). Oxford, UK: Blackwell Science.

Henderson, J., with S. Sethi (2006). *Ethical markets: Growing the green economy.* White River Junction, VT: Chelsea Green Publishing Company.

Huyssen, A. (2003). *Present pasts: Urban palimpsests and the politics of memory (cultural memory in the present).* Stanford, CA: Stanford University Press.

Jeffreys, M. (2006). *Teaching cultural competence in nursing and health care: Inquiry, action and innovation.* New York: Springer Publishing Company.

Kalifon, S., & Mollov, M. (2006). Changing perceptions of the "other": A field experiment. *Practicing Anthropology, 28*(3), 4–7.

Kehoe, A. (1998). *Human: An introduction to four-field anthropology.* New York: Routledge.

Kim, Y. (1989). Intercultural adaptation. In M. Asante & W. Gudykunst (Eds.), *Handbook of international and intercultural communication* (pp. 275–294). Newbury Park: Sage Publications.

Kleinman, A. (1980). *Patients and healers in the context of culture.* Berkeley: University of California Press.

Kleinman, A. (1998). Do psychiatric disorders differ in different cultures? In P. Brown (Ed.), *Understanding and applying medical anthropology.* London: Mayfield Publishing Company.

Kurzweil, R. (2005). *The singularity is near.* New York: Viking Penguin.

LeBesco, K. (2004). *Revolting bodies.* Amherst, MA: University of Massachusetts Press.

Lederach, J. (1999). *The journey toward reconciliation.* Scottdale, PA: Herald Press.

Leininger, M. (1970). *Anthropology and nursing: Two worlds to blend.* New York: John Wiley Company.

Leininger, M. (1978). *Transcultural nursing: Concepts, theories, and practices.* New York: John Wiley and Sons.

Leininger, M. (Ed.). (1991). *Culture care diversity & universality: A theory of nursing.* New York: National League for Nursing Press.

Leininger, M. (1995). *Transcultural nursing: Concepts, theories, research and practice.* Columbus, OH: McGraw-Hill.

Leininger, M. (1997). Transcultural nursing research to transform nursing education and practice: 40 years. *Image: The Journal of Nursing Scholarship, 29*(4), 341–354.

Leininger, M., & McFarland, M. (Eds.). (2006). *Culture care diversity and universality: A worldwide theory of nursing* (2nd ed.). Sudbury, MA: Jones and Bartlett.

Link, A., & Coben, S. (1971). *The democratic heritage: A history of the United States* (Vol. 2). Waltham, MA: Ginn and Company.

Lipson, J., & DeSantis, L. (2007). Current approaches to integrating elements of cultural competence in nursing education. *Journal of Transcultural Nursing, 18(*1), 10S–20S.

Lonergan, B. (1958). *Insight: A study of human understanding.* San Francisco: Harper & Row, Publishers.

Lonergan, B. (1972). Method in theology. New York: Herder and Herder.

Lowe, J., & Crow, K. (2009). Utilization of a Native American nursing conceptual framework to transform nursing education. *International Journal for Human Caring, 13*(3), 56–64.

Lowe, J., & Nichols, L. (2014). Utilisation of a Native American nursing conceptual framework: Implications for practice and research. *Australian Journal of Advanced Nursing, 31*(2), 13–22.

Mason, D. (1998). *Whairora Maori health development.* Auckland, NZ: Oxford University Press.

McFarland, M. (2006). Madeleine Leininger: Culture care theory of diversity and universality. In A. Marriner

Tomey & M. Alligood (Eds.), *Nursing theorists and their work* (pp. 643–662). St. Louis: Mosby-Elsevier.

McFarland, M., & Wehbe-Alamah, H. (2015). *Leininger's culture care diversity and universality: A worldwide theory of nursing* (3rd ed.). Burlington, MA: Jones & Bartlett Learning.

Milne, D. (1982). *The new Canadian constitution.* Toronto: James Lorimer & Company, Publishers.

Morris, E. (2012). Respect, protection, faith and love: Major care constructs identified within the subculture of selected urban African American adolescent gang members. *Journal of Transcultural Nursing, 23*(3), 262–269.

Newropeans Magazine, *Global Europe 2020,* Retrieved August 2006, from http://www.newropeans –magazine.org/

Nightingale, F. (1969). *Notes on nursing: What it is and what it is not.* New York: Dover. (Original work published 1860)

Nightingale, F. (1992). *Notes on nursing: What it is, and what it is not.* Philadelphia: J.P. Lippincott.

Office of the Legislative Council (2010). Compilation of Patient Protection and Affordable Care Act, Retrieved from http://housedocs.house.gov/energycommerce/ppacon.pdf

O'Murchu, D. (1997). *Quantum theology.* New York: The Crossword Publishing Company.

Outhwaite, W. (1985). Hans Georg Gadamer. In Q. Skinner (Ed.), *The return of grand theory in the human sciences.* New York: Cambridge University Press.

Palmer, P (1993). *To know as we are known: Education as a spiritual journey.* San Francisco: HarperSan Francisco.

Peacock, J. (1986). *The anthropological lens.* Cambridge: Cambridge University Press.

Peat, F. (2002). *From certainty to uncertainty: The story of science and ideas in the twentieth century.* Washington, DC: Joseph Henry Press.

Polanyi, M., & Prosch, H. (1975). *Meaning.* Chicago: The University of Chicago Press.

Pollock, M. (2006). Everyday antiracism in education. *Anthropology News, 47*(2), 9–10.

Purnell, L., & Paulanka, B. (2008). *Transcultural health care* (3rd ed.). Philadelphia: F. A. Davis Company.

Ray, M. (1981). A study of caring within an institutional culture. *Dissertation Abstracts International, 42*(06). (University Microfilms No. 8127787).

Ray, M. (1989a). Transcultural caring: Political and economic visions. *Journal of Transcultural Nursing, 1*(1), 17–21.

Ray, M. (1989b). The theory of bureaucratic caring for nursing practice in the organizational culture. *Nursing Administration Quarterly, 13*(2), 31–42.

Ray, M. (1991). Caring inquiry: The esthetic process in the way of compassion. In D. Gaut & M. Leininger (Eds.), *Caring: The compassionate healer* (Pub. No. 15-2401, pp. 181–189). New York: National League for Nursing Press.

Ray, M. (1992). Critical theory as a framework to enhance nursing science, *Nursing Science Quarterly, 5*(3), 98–101.

Ray, M. (1994a). Transcultural nursing ethics: A framework and model for transcultural ethical analysis. *Journal of Holistic Nursing, 12*(3), 251–264.

Ray, M. (1994b). Complex caring dynamics: A unifying model of nursing inquiry. *Theoretic and Applied Chaos in Nursing (Complexity and Chaos in Nursing), 1*(1), 23–32.

Ray, M. (1997a). Illuminating the meaning of caring: Unfolding the sacred art of divine love. In M. Roach (Ed.), *Caring from the heart: The convergence of caring and spirituality* (pp. 163–178). New York: Paulist Press.

Ray, M. (1997b). The ethical theory of existential authenticity: The lived experience of the art of caring in nursing administration. *Canadian Journal of Nursing Research, 20*(1), 111–126.

Ray, M. (1998a). A phenomenologic study of the interface between caring and technology: A new reflective ethics in intermediate care. *Holistic Nursing Practice, 12*(4), 71–79.

Ray, M. (1998b). Complexity and nursing science. *Nursing Science Quarterly, 11*, 91–93.

Ray, M. (1999a). Critical theory as a framework to enhance nursing science. In E. Polifroni & M. Welch (Eds.), *Perspectives on philosophy of science in nursing* (pp. 382–386). Philadelphia: Lippincott.

Ray, M. (1999b). Transcultural caring in primary health care. *National Academies of Practice Forum, 1*(3), 177–182.

Ray, M. (2001a). The theory of bureaucratic caring. In M. Parker (Ed.), *Nursing theories, nursing practice* (pp. 421–431). Philadelphia: F. A. Davis Company.

Ray, M. (2001b). Complex culture and technology: Toward a global caring communitarian ethics of nursing. In

R. Locsin (Ed.), *Advancing technology, caring, and nursing* (pp. 41–52). Westport, CT: Auburn House.

Ray, M. (2001c). Transcultural assessment. In S. Koch & S. Garratt (Eds.), *Assessing older people: A practical guide for health professionals* (pp. 35–40). Sydney: MacLennan & Petty.

Ray, M. (2005). The theory of bureaucratic caring. *Nursing theories and nursing practice* (2nd ed., pp. 421–431). Philadelphia: F. A. Davis Company.

Ray, M. (2007a). Technological caring as a dynamic of complexity in nursing. In A. Barnard & R. Locsin (Eds.), *Technology and nursing: Practice, concepts , and issues.* United Kingdom: Palgrave MacMillan.

Ray, M. (2007b). Caring scholar response to "Achieving compassionate excellence: A cooperative accelerated BSN program." *International Journal for Human Caring, 12*(2), 39–41.

Ray, M. (2010a). *Transcultural caring dynamics in nursing and health care.* Philadelphia: F. A. Davis Company.

Ray, M. (2010b). *Caring within an institutional culture: The discovery of the Theory of Bureaucratic Caring.* Germany: Lambert Academic Publishers.

Ray, M. (2010c). Creating caring organizations and cultures through communitarian ethics. *Journal of the World Universities Forum, 3*(5), 41–52.

Ray, M., & Turkel, M. (2001). Culturally based caring. In L. Dunphy & J. Winland-Brown (Eds.), *Primary care* (pp. 43–55). Philadelphia: F. A. Davis Company.

Ray, M., & Turkel, M. (2014). Caring as emancipatory nursing praxis: The theory of Relational Caring Complexity. *Advances in Nursing Science, 37*(2), 132–146.

Ray, M., & Turkel, M. (2015). Marilyn Anne Ray, the theory of bureaucratic caring. In M. Smith (Ed.), *Nursing theories and nursing practice* (4th ed.). Philadelphia: F. A. Davis Company.

Ray, M., Turkel, M., & Marino, F. (2001). The transformative process for nursing in workforce redevelopment. *Nursing Administration Quarterly, 26*(2), 1–14.

Ratzinger, J. (2007). *On conscience.* San Francisco: Ignatius Press.

Reeder, F. (1984). Philosophical issues in the Rogerian science of unitary human beings. *Advances in Nursing Science, 8*(1), 14–23.

Reeder, F. (1992). Conceptual foundations of science and key phenomenological concepts. In J. Poindexter (Ed.), *Nursing theory, research, and practice: Summer research monograph* (pp. 177–187). Detroit, MI: Wayne State University Press.

Reeder, F. (2007). What will count as evidence in the year 2050? *Nursing Science Quarterly, 20,* 208–211.

Reinhard, K., President of the Business for Diplomatic Action (HQ 437 Madison Ave., 11th Floor, New York, New York 10022), *C-SPAN,* August 23, 2006.

Rifkin, J. (2004). *The European dream.* New York: Jeremy P. Tarcher/Penguin.

Roach, M. (2002). *The human act of caring* (rev. ed.). Ottawa: Canadian Hospital Association.

Rockefeller, S. (1994). Comment to the articles on multiculturalism. In A. Gutman (Ed.), *Multiculturalism.* Princeton, NJ: Princeton University Press.

Rosen, L. (2012). *iDisorder: understanding our obsession with technology and overcoming its hold on us.* New York: Palgrave Macmillan.

Smith, B. (1998). *On the origin of objects.* Cambridge, MA: MIT Press.

Spector, R. (2008). *Cultural diversity in health and illness* (7th ed.). Upper Saddle River, NJ: Pearson Prentice Hall.

Stoll, D. (2006). The value of liberalism and truth standards. *Anthropology News, 47*(6), 7.

Sumner, J. (2006). Concept analysis: The moral construct of caring in nursing as communicative action. *International Journal for Human Caring, 10*(10), 8–16.

Sumner, J. (2008). *The moral construct of caring in nursing as communicative action: A theory for nursing practice.* Saarbrüken, Germany: VDM Verlag Dr. Müller.

Taylor, C. (1989). *Sources of the self: The making of modern identity.* Cambridge, MA: Harvard University Press.

Taylor, C. (1991). *The ethics of authenticity.* Cambridge, MA: Harvard University Press.

Taylor, C. (1994). The politics of recognition. In A. Gutmann (Ed.), *Multiculturalism* (pp. 25–73). New Jersey: Princeton University Press.

The New American Bible. (1970). New York: Catholic Book Publishing Co.

Thompson, E. (2006). The problem of "race as a social construct". *Anthropology News, 47*(2), 6–7.

Tjittas, M. (1998). Psychoanalysis, public reason, and reconstruction in the "New" South Africa. *American Imago, 55*(1), 51–75.

Tripp-Reimer, T. (1985). Expanding four essential concepts in nursing theory: The contribution of anthropology (pp. 91–103). In J. McCloskey & H. Grace (Eds.), *Current issues in nursing.* Boston: Blackwell.

Tuan, M. (1998). *Forever foreigners or honorary whites?* New Brunswick: Rutgers University Press.

Turkel, M. (2006a). What is evidence-based practice? In S. Beyea & M. Slattery (Eds.), *Evidence-based practice in nursing: A guide to successful implementation.* Marblehead, MA: HcPro Publishing.

Turkel, M. (2006b). Integration of evidence-based practice in nursing. In S. Beyea & M. Slattery (Eds.), *Evidence-based practice in nursing: A guide to successful implementation.* Marblehead, MA: HcPro Publishing.

Turkel, M. (2007). Dr. Marilyn Ray's theory of bureaucratic caring. *International Journal for Human Caring, 11*(4), 57–70.

Turkel, M., & Ray, M. (2009). Caring for the not so picture perfect patient: Ethical caring in the moral community of nursing. In R. Locsin & M. Purnell (Eds.), *A contemporary nursing process: The (un)bearable weight of knowing persons* (pp. 225–249). New York: Springer Publishing Company.

Turner, V., & Bruner, E. (1986). *The anthropology of experience.* Urbana: University of Illinois Press.

Volkan, V. (1998). *Bloodlines: From ethnic pride to ethnic terrorism.* Boulder, CO: Westview Press.

Waters, M. (1990). *Ethnic options: Choosing identities in America.* Berkeley: University of California Press.

Watson, J. (1979). *Nursing: The philosophy and science of caring.* Boston: Little Brown.

Watson, J. (1988). *Human science, human care.* New York: National League for Nursing. (Original work published 1985)

Watson, J. (1992). Notes on nursing: Guideslines for caring then and now. In F. Nightingale, *Notes on nursing: What it is, and what it is not* (pp. 80–85). Philadelphia: J. P. Lippincott.

Watson, J. (2005). *Caring science as sacred science.* Philadelphia: F. A. Davis Company.

Watson, J. (2008). *Nursing: The philosophy and science of caring* (rev. ed.). Boulder, CO: University Press of Colorado.

Wilson, R. (2006). The moral imperialism critique is not valid. *Anthropology News, 47*(6), 7.

Winick, C. (1970). *Dictionary of anthropology.* Totowa, New Jersey: Littlefield, Adams & Co.

Wolf, Z. (2014). *Exploring rituals in nursing: Joining art and science.* New York: Springer Publishing Company.

Wolin, R. (2005). Jurgen Habermas and post-secular societies. *The Chronicle of Higher Education, September, 23, 2005*, Section B, B16–B17.

Womack, M. (2005). *Symbols and meaning*. Walnut Creek: AltaMira Press.

Wu, C.J., & Ray, M. (in press). Technological caring for healthcare complexities of patients with cardiac disease comorbid with diabetes. *International Journal for Human Caring*.

Yapple, P., & Korzenny, F. (1989). Electronic mass media effects across cultures. In M. Asante & W. Gudykunst (Eds.), *Handbook of International and Intercultural Communication* (pp. 295–317). Newbury Park: Sage Publications.

Young, K., & Nabuco de Abreu, C. (Eds.) (2010). Internet addiction: *A handbook and guide to evaluation and treatment*. New York: Wiley.

Bibliography

United Nations Millennium Goals 2015 and post 2015. Retrieved August 19, 2015 from unitednations.org/undp

World Health Organization. Retrieved August 19, 2015 from who.org

Transcultural Caring Experiences

Overall Objectives

1. To highlight the Transcultural Caring Dynamics in Nursing and Health-Care Theoretical Model and the assessment and planning tools by identifying the transcultural caring-based learning (TCCBL) approach for achieving transcultural caring competency (responsibility and accountability) in transcultural experiences in culturally dynamic communities outlined in this Section 2, Chapters 7 to 33.

2. To highlight the TCCBL process for **awareness** of the meaning of dialogue in transcultural communicative spiritual-ethical caring action.

3. To present the concept of transcultural caring evidence-based practice—cocreative dialogue, assessment, planning, **understanding,** and facilitation of **choice** in practice.

4. To present the concepts of transcultural caring competence (and incompetency) for accountability and responsibility by outlining the meaning of the critical caring inquiry (reflection and transcultural communicative spiritual-ethical caring dialogue process to address transcultural caring experiences).

5. To identify the pattern-identification process (i.e., pattern seeing, pattern mapping, pattern recognizing, and pattern transforming).

6. To show through critical caring inquiry how pattern identification is to be applied to the transcultural caring experiences in practice and outlined in this section.

CHAPTER 7

Transcultural Caring Competency in Transculturally Dynamic Communities

Achieving transcultural caring responsibility and accountability in nursing practice (transcultural caring competency) is a cocreative process of awareness of communicative spiritual-ethical caring action. The process involves respecting others through compassion and justice; seeking knowledge and understanding of the holistic nature of people from diverse cultures and ethnicities with diverse health and caring needs; securing evidence from various literary and electronic/Internet/social media sources; recognizing complex health-care organizations community and home health contexts as small cultures; engaging with simulated nursing situations as a means of improving cultural awareness and decision-making; sustaining collaboration, including interprofessional collaboration, across languages, media, cultures/ethnicities, and borders, even in outer space; building partnerships within local, global, civic, and bureaucratic communities; and facilitating the choices for health, caring, healing, well-being, and a peaceful death. (Marilyn A. Ray)

Chapter Objectives

1. To outline the meaning of transcultural caring competency
2. To present the transcultural caring-based learning (TCCBL) approach.
    2.1 To outline the pattern-identification process.
    2.2 To discuss patterns of relationships, including interprofessional relationships and simulated nursing situations.
    2.3 To express the meaning of self-care in the TCCBL approach.
3. To highlight the critical caring inquiry process as communicative ethical-spiritual caring action.
4. To present the notion of transcultural caring evidence.
5. To outline transcultural caring competency as accountability and responsibility in nursing practice.
6. To identify diverse transcultural caring experiences.

KEY WORDS

Transcultural caring
• transcultural caring competency • responsibility and accountability
• transcultural caring evidence • transcultural caring-based learning (TCCBL) process
• complexity sciences
• critical caring inquiry
• transcultural communicative spiritual-ethical caring • pattern identification (pattern seeing, pattern mapping, pattern recognizing, pattern transforming and creative applications of simulation, internet, and social media)
• transcultural caring experiences • culturally dynamic communities

*C*ulturally dynamic communities illuminate the changing sociocultural environment in North America and around the world. Many culturally dynamic communities exhibit the changing nature and complexity of societies, social networks, demographics, and intercultural interaction. Contemporary local and global cultures are transforming as people interact. Nurses and other professionals must be continually aware of their responsibilities to provide competent transcultural care, understand diverse ways of caring, and appreciate the changing contexts, including family, community, national, geopolitical, and organizational systems where nursing and health care are practiced. The transcultural caring experiences outlined in Section 2 and Chapters 7 to 33 manifest the complexity and examples of culturally dynamic communities and health and nursing and other professional care needs, such as the ideological evolution of change in the Mexican American relationship, historical changes of blacks in American culture, and farmworker issues of a Guatemalan-Mayan (Central American) subculture in the United States, and the Ebola crisis in Africa.

The transcultural experiences present nurses and other professionals with stories (case studies, nursing and health-care situations) that evoke many questions and cross-cultural comparison and peak awareness and heighten understanding of social networks, migration, intermigration, panethnicities, and the choices for health, healing, or dying that nurses facilitate.

Section 2 uses practical transcultural caring experiences because these help us to discover the reality that gives expression to our commitment (Knowlden, 1990; Smith & Liehr, 2005, 2014). Nurses' commitment is the desire for knowledgeable caring and competency in transcultural nursing practice. From a caring perspective, Roach (2002) identified *competence* as one of her 6Cs of Caring and defined it ". . . as the state of having the knowledge, judgment, skills, energy, experience and motivation required to respond adequately to the demands of one's professional responsibilities" (p. 54). Professional responsibilities for competency specific to nursing relate (1) to the moral ideal of the preservation and enhancement of human dignity; (2) to the professional and legal scope of practice defined by various nurse practice acts in nursing's diverse roles in health assessment, nursing and health-care management and therapeutic interventions, health promotion and disease prevention, and patient safety; and (3) to appreciating cultural diversity (Breda, 2009; Burkhardt & Nathaniel, 2008; Leininger & McFarland, 2006; McFarland & Wehbe-Alamah, 2015; Watson, 2005). Transcultural caring competence reflects the ideals of personal accountability and ethical responsibility for understanding oneself as a cultural/multicultural being, supporting nurse-patient and family relationships, being present to, compassionate, caring, and just in upholding the dignity of the other, seeking the meaning of diverse values, beliefs, attitudes, and opinions, acquiring and applying professional nursing, medical, and organizational knowledge, and considering the living history and challenges of cultural changes in a global society (Ray, 2010a).

In Section 2, each chapter contains a transcultural caring experience (story, case study, nursing and health care situation), an introduction, and story that reflects culture as dynamic complexity, multiculturalism, interculturality, and panethnicity. In the transcultural caring experiences, the members of the transcultural caring-based learning (TCCBL) dialogue group (i.e., student, faculty member, or other professional) will apply the *Transcultural Caring Dynamics in Nursing and Health-Care Theory and Model*, and the assessment tools discussed in Chapter 6 that **best** assist with learning and assessment of the experiences:

- Transcultural Caring Dynamics Assessment Tool
- Culture-Value Conflict Assessment Tool
- Ray's Transcultural Communicative Spiritual-Ethical CARING Tool for Cultural Competency
- Dynamics of Transcultural Caring Tool for Choice
- Transcultural Caring Negotiation Tool

The model and tools used in conjunction with critical caring inquiry—reflective thinking and communicative spiritual-ethical caring action—which is a pattern-identification approach for engaging in the TCCBL process, will assist in developing transcultural competency (accountability and responsibility) within the transcultural caring experiences. The following discussion will address the general learning approach using the TCCBL process, the critical caring inquiry, the pattern-identification process, and the directions for engaging in the group dialogue.

Transcultural caring competence reflects the ideals of personal accountability and ethical responsibility for:

- Understanding oneself as a cultural/multicultural being
- Being compassionate, caring, and just in upholding the dignity of the other
- Supporting the nurse-patient and family relationships
- Seeking the meaning of diverse values, beliefs, attitudes, and opinions
- Acquiring and applying professional nursing, medical, technological, and organizational knowledge
- Considering the living history and challenges of cultural changes in a global society

Transcultural Caring-Based Learning Approach

The learning approach to this section is TCCBL that is modeled, in part, on the problem-based learning (PBL) and continuing competence model (Cunningston, 2001; Norman, Klass, & Wenghofer, 2008; Solomon, 1999) now used in manymedical schools and some nursing schools in North America. Students, in small groups of 2 to 12, which can include online groups, and with the facilitation of a tutor (either a teacher or designated student or other professional), cocreate their *own* understanding as they dialogue with other members of the group, use critical caring inquiry, and seek and apply evidence from study of the literature and Internet information/data or other media (transcultural evidence). With the TCCBL approach, transcultural evidence is gleaned through critical caring and problem-solving inquiry (i.e., reflection and transcultural communicative spiritual-ethical caring), and a process called pattern identification. Life patterns include all human-environment or human field processes. The forms or structures of life processes are expanded ways of knowing in nursing—personal and relational, biophysical, neurological-psychological-immunological, ethical, spiritual, aesthetic (art), and empirical (observational phenomena). Moreover, the forms are historical and sociocultural—technological, legal, economic, political, organizational, educational, and social (Ray, 2011). In the area of educational challenges, pattern identification processes can be initiated within interprofessional groups, such as with medical students, physicians,social workers, medical anthropologists, and so forth. In the contemporary age of networking, social media and leadership skills for creative problem solving and caring communication are critically important. Thus, pattern identification can be used not only in the context of simulation scenarios grounded in caring science, integrating technology into curricula (Eggenberger, Keller, & Locsin, 2010), but also it can be used via other forms of technological applications, such as for patients in the area of discharge planning with virtual presence--ongoing phone calls, video-conferencing, Skype, and other social media, such as Facebook, Facetime, Instagram, Twitter, and so forth. As well, TED (Technology, Entertainment Design--ideas worth communicating) TED-like talks, space education, and anything creative where understanding patterning can be developed (Barry, Gordon, & King, 2015; Eggenberger et al., 2010; 2013; Gallo, 2014; Grumime, Barry, Gordon, & Ray [in press]; Hatfield, 2013; Kaku, 2014; Stone, 2014; Wu & Ray (2016). Pattern identification involves:

- Pattern seeing
- Pattern mapping
- Pattern recognizing
- Pattern transforming

THE PROCESS OF UNDERSTANDING CRITICAL CARING INQUIRY FOR TRANCULTURAL CARING-BASED LEARNING

In a complex multicultural or panethnic world, one person cannot solve problems alone, but groups or organizations of people dedicated to human caring, the public good, and protection of animals and the environment can if they know how to work together. The first step is to begin thinking and reflecting about interdependence and caring communication—how people of diverse cultures or groups affect each other and how they make choices. What happens when one member of a family, group, or community does *not* interact or is silenced in some way? Does it matter which group member is silenced or which component or part of a cultural organization does not have a voice? Contemplating questions of interconnectedness and its affects provides a view of the complexity of relationships and relatedness (Bar-Yam, 2004) and helps us to understand the meaning of transcultural spiritual-ethical caring communication.

NETWORKS OF RELATIONSHIPS

Advanced technology, the global economy, and world politics, including war, religious sectarianism, and terrorism, have influenced specific cultures, and changed the nature of societies, intercultural relationships, and environments. Binational and multinational participation is interlinked with human interaction, politics, economic trade, and technology. Today, local communities and the world are dominated by networks ofrelationships energized by not only competition for material and nonmaterial resources but also by cooperation that shows the benefits of intercultural, interracial, and national and international participation. Business, education, travel, military service, and the virtual world of the Internet social media have helped people to develop new partnerships and bonds, often leading to multinational treaties, religious understanding, new business relationships, friendships, marriages, and the intermingling of families of diverse cultures. Despite the seemingly unending cycles of violence and competition for power and authority, we are increasingly becoming a more unified human culture.

In the process of experiencing the benefits of participation, however, many culturally dynamic communities also exhibit conflict. Diversity of values, beliefs, and attitudes often increase pressures to remain the same. Clashes about what is valued and valuable can create the conditions for new conflicts or prolonged conflict and even war. Past histories and present assessment of problems about the future can affect intercultural interaction. Religious disputes, the transmission of diseases, old prejudices, land and border disputes, migration patterns, and immigration issues tend to keep people from forming the bonds that are necessary to build healthy relationships and ultimately, the global civic culture (Berman, 2004; Boulding, 1988; Economy & Levi, 2014; Eisler, 2007; Henderson, with Sethi, 2006; Kurzweil, 2005; Wolfe, 2012). Developing awareness and seeking understanding to make the right choices are the foundations for effective change and transformation. Included in the process is how nursing and health care is understood transculturally. The provision of transcultural nursing care, understanding transcultural caring, and the distribution and provision of quality health care move forward by means of understanding ourselves as cultural and multicultural beings, by interacting with people of different cultures, and by engaging in communicative spiritual-ethical caring action (Boykin, Schoenhofer, & Valentine, 2014; Davidson, Ray, & Turkel, 2011; Smith, Turkel, & Wolf, 2013).

INTRICACIES OF THE TRANSCULTURAL CARING-BASED LEARNING PROCESS

Within the learning process, different people coming from different cultural backgrounds will have different basic values, beliefs, attitudes, assumptions, and opinions about the meaning of their world (Wilhelm & Zlotnick, 2014). As open as people can be to diverse ideologies, and situations, we often defend our own opinions either consciously or subconsciously. Nurses have diverse views about the nature of their lives, ethnicities, nursing care and caring, the nursing culture, and its expression in everyday practice. Conflicts or struggles of views often take place. Our individual cultural meanings of our own and diverse cultures can hinder rather that facilitate dialogue.

THE PROCESS OF SELF-CARE IN TRANSCULTURAL CARING-BASED LEARNING

Before forming a TCCBL group, the learners need to take time for self-care, self-reflection, and self-renewal to awaken their creative selves to cocreate communities of caring (Barry, Gordon, & King, 2015; Turkel & Ray, 2004; Turkel, Ray, & Kornblatt, 2012). When the learners take time for self-care and renewal, and understand the oneness of humanity and the uniqueness of individuals, the learning group will form a true community.

Ways to accomplish self-care include the following (adapted in part from Brown, 2006; Turkel & Ray, 2004):

- Recognizing that our lives are grounded in creativity and a spiritual-ethical consciousness
- Taking time for personal relaxation, exercise, and meditation
- Contemplating our own worldview
- Reflecting on our own theories of life
- Contemplating our ways of life as artistic, imaginative, and inventive
- Reflecting on reflection itself—that in nursing, reflective practice is a reflection-in-action and the core of professional artistry (Jarvis, 1991; Turkel & Ray, 2004)
- Meditating on who we are as creative beings, cultural/multicultural beings, caring persons, and transcultural nurses, and transcultural caring experiences (Ray, 2010a, 2010b, 2010c)
- Reflecting on others as caring people
- Engaging our imagination and contemplating how one would feel as a person who is different, from another community or country, engaged in different roles, struggling for a "place in the world," and speaking a different language
- Becoming aware that creative selves need acknowledgment, respect, and nurturing
- Reflecting on how individual values, beliefs, attitudes, social media, and opinions influence behavior, group behavior, society, and culture
- Recognizing that each group forms a unique culture and community of caring
- Recognizing that every choice supports, enhances, or diminishes our creative selves

CRITICAL CARING INQUIRY: REFLECTIVE PRACTICE IN TRANSCULTURAL COMMUNICATIVE SPIRITUAL-ETHICAL CARING ACTION

Genuine dialogue grounded in a universal caring perspective of compassion and justice (critical caring inquiry) is not just analysis or even exchanging opinions. It entails *reflective practice* (reflection-in-action)—suspending our beliefs and looking at our own and other's beliefs, attitudes, values, and opinions and seeing and touching with a compassionate heart through reflective caring action, what something may mean. If we can see in the best possible way, what all of our values, beliefs, attitudes, and opinions mean, then we can begin to understand our moral conscience or responsibility and begin to share in the understanding of the common conscience of humankind, and thus authentically care for others transculturally. This common responsibility involves serving the "good" of each other, a transforming communicative spiritual-ethical caring action that manifests compassion and justice for the protection and enhancement of human dignity (Ray, 1989, 1998, 2010a, 2010b, 2010c; Ray & Turkel, 2014; Watson, 1988, 2005). Our common understanding of what it means to be human, caring, ethical, and spiritual can "shed more light" upon the communicative narrative, and the narrative that is communicated in the transcultural caring experiences in Chapters 8 to 33 in this section.

THE COCREATIVE PROCESS OF SEEKING MEANING

For a deeper understanding of seeking meaning, we can focus on the meaning of "light." Bohm (1990) stated that ordinary light is incoherent; it goes in many directions. Laser light, on the other hand, is directive; it is coherent. The light waves build up an intense beam with tremendous power, a coherent communicative energy to affect some type of change. Human beings in authentic dialogue are like laser light. They can think together cocreatively and radiate tremendous power; there is a coherent movement in communication. This type of communication illuminates understanding and takes the group members beyond opinions. It is participatory consciousness that is aware and sensitive to what is happening, and then through seeking understanding builds a form of transformative consciousness and conscience where the flow of meaning that is shared and cocreated holds people together to make potential ethical choices that are compassionate and just. The flow of meaning is transculturally dynamic, always emerging through transcultural communicative spiritual-ethical caring interactions.

Transcultural communicative spiritual-ethical caring action increases awareness of the needs of another. We move more cocreatively in authentic dialogue. We can share an appreciation of the meanings being expressed. In this way, not only communication can take place by group participation and authentic dialogue, but also evaluation. The group can encourage supportive initiatives that enhance learning or help people who may be retarding learning in the group (Cunnington, 2001; Turkel & Ray, 2004). In this TCCBL process, the Transcultural Caring Dynamics in Nursing and Health-Care Theory and Model and the transcultural caring tools are used as guides for analyzing the following transcultural caring experiences. Students are encouraged to use the model and tools and all literature and Internet data as transcultural caring evidence to enhance self-reflection and dialogue. Through dialogue, students will determine or evaluate when their learning is adequate for understanding or transcultural caring competency is beginning in relation to each transcultural experience presented. The task of the teacher (tutor) is not to impart knowledge but to encourage reflection on each experience and evidence-seeking from multiple sources, to facilitate dialogue, and to coach participants.

As stated, everyone in the group is to take responsibility for the evaluation of the learning process. The cocreative process requires a system of checks-and-balances whereby each group member

---

Reflective Practice in Transcultural Spiritual-Ethical Caring Communicative Action

- Suspend one's own beliefs.
- Look at the other's beliefs, attitudes, values, and opinions.
- Contemplate what it means to share a common humanity.
- See and touch with the heart of compassion what the other is communicating either orally and/or symbolically.
- Contemplate what the communication may mean.
- Filter one's own beliefs, attitudes, and opinions in relation to the communication.
- Reach out in a morally responsible way to seek meaning with the other through spiritual-ethical communicative caring action (use Ray's Transcultural Communicative Spiritual-Ethical CARING Tool as a guide).

---

reads the transcultural caring experience, engages in critical caring reflection and initial self-directed evidence gathering, synthesizes data, and then communicates his or her interpretation of the meaning of the transcultural nursing situation to and with the group. In individual and group evaluation, the TCCBL process helps students and teachers (tutors) to gather the most important evidence from the patient's experience and use the data to facilitate understanding and responsibility for beginning transcultural caring competency.

Transcultural Caring Evidence and Competency in Nursing

Transcultural caring evidence and competency in nursing involves innovation (Jeffreys, 2006; Smith, Turkel, & Wolf, 2013; Turkel, Ray, & Kornblatt, 2012), and the *intent* to make a difference in the lives of others through *knowledgeable* caring or communicative spiritual-ethical caring. This intent is not power over the cultural other but a caring presence that fosters listening to the experience, compassion, and choice toward an improved life of possibilities while dealing with the differences and contradictions of everyday life. Every interaction in nursing involves a moral choice to do good—to commit to the other, to be accountable to self and other as multicultural beings, and to be responsible for improving the life of self and the other. Even in the technological world of gathering and sharing information, a transcultural caring nurse is prompted by thoughtful insight rather than by only technical skill (Wu & Ray, 2016, in press). Transcultural caring evidence demands competency, that is, the ethical demand exhibited by love, hope, trust, and responsibility that will promote a present and future of understanding, healing, and transformation.

TRANSCULTURAL CARING EVIDENCE

Transcultural caring experience in nursing embraces caring as a universal phenomenon in all relationships (Turkel, 2007). It includes evidence-based practice content, and sociocultural traditions and rituals about the meaning of health, healing, and illness communicated by patients and professionals as they relate together (Leininger & McFarland, 2006; McFarland & Wehbe-Alamah, 2015). In a sense, gathering transcultural evidence is ethnographic, that is, engaging with others and their practices to understand their social world (Kleinman & Benson, 2006; Ray, Morris, & McFarland, 2014). The holistic transcultural view of evidence gathering includes communicative spiritual-ethical caring interaction, description and observation of patient and family experience, and what can be gleaned from the literature, the Internet, and other information sources. The most important evidence is (1) what is given by people about their own values, beliefs, and attitudes about life, caring, health, and healing, dying, death and (2) what is learned through research. Seeking knowledge through quantitative research studies presents valid objective evidence of nursing and sociocultural situations; seeking knowledge through qualitative human science research presents subjective evidence, forms of narrative evidence that contribute to understanding the real-world experience by interpreting meaning from the actual narratives or stories of people of diverse cultures. All forms of evidence help transcultural nurses to be more aware so as to facilitate understanding and choice making in the professional-patient interaction. Because transcultural caring and, especially transcultural communicative caring interaction, is relational and holistic, it is a spiritual-ethical *lived* experience. In the real world and through the TCCBL process, the transcultural caring experience unfolds as a life story or living history, and meanings are cocreated. Stories help us to discover the reality that gives expression to our

commitments, illness, and suffering (Kleinman, 1988; Knowlden, 1990; van Manen, 2014). As Gadow remarked, "we compose storied lives, experience is structured as plot [sequence of events], a life becomes *my* life by my weaving the events into a coherent whole" (1996, p. 8). Thus, "Story theory . . . describes story as a narrative happening of connecting with self-in-relation . . ." (Smith & Liehr, 2005, p. 273). Body, mind, and spirit in a transpersonal relationship are woven together—a speaking together, a harmony that makes us one (Watson, 1988, 2005).

Conversely, storied lives can become hidden. In attempting to attain transcultural caring competence, there can be a danger in the evidence-based practice movement. Theories, codes, standards of practice, and so forth can become impersonal or even coercive by assuming the authority of general statements or research data over the personal description of the patient. Theories, codes, and so forth, can be so stereotypical that they silence the true-life experiences of persons. At the same time, however, the recognition of patient-centered care should not be developed at the expense of professional knowledge and caring-centered care. Gadow (1996) claimed that nurses must not lose sight of the fact that both perspectives of the relationship are necessary, the moral voice of the patient and the moral voice of the professional nurse as they cointerpret and cocreate choices for the good, human dignity of each, and the entire moral community (Ray, 1998, 2007).

The Silent and the Visible Voice

As part of the moral voice in transcultural nursing, language understanding, verbal and nonverbal symbolic interaction is necessary for understanding. If a patient or family member, including persons who are deaf or blind, cannot communicate adequately in a language that can be understood by the health-care professional, then it is necessary to secure the services of an interpreter. A family member may be used as an interpreter if necessary. As nurses are legally responsible to generate the most accurate holistic data possible, there is a need to determine how to secure information. Verbal and nonverbal communication, comportment, one of Roach's 6Cs of Caring (2002) convey meaning. Relating symbolically means that transcultural nurses are morally responsible for understanding both the "silent and the visible voice" of the other. The nurse should make a logical connection between signs and symbols even though a particular language is or is not being used. This is particularly true when patients are unconscious or semiconscious (Ray, 1998, 2007; Wolf, 2014). Transcultural nurses must be vigilant in trying to understand the multivocality or many meanings of something communicated by patients that may not be easily defined or shared (Womack, 2005).

TRANSCULTURAL CARING COMPETENCY: ACCOUNTABILITY AND RESPONSIBILITY

DelVecchio Good (1995) remarked that competence is a core symbol of professionalism. The idea of competence carries with it diverse meanings for different professional groups. Competence varies according to standards of practice, different philosophies, and changes over time. From an anthropological perspective, cultural competence is considered "an essentially contested domain" (Good, in Fitzgerald, Williamson, Russell, & Manor, 2005, p. 334). For example, the anthropologist Green (2006) stated that because of the general focus on cultural needs of vulnerable people, cultural competence is now promoted to meet state and federal requirements for continued funding, or to meet specific governmental or organizational standards of practice (p. 3). Professionals often presume cross-cultural insight, invoking the ideas and language of anthropology, such as culture or ethnography (a cross-cultural research method) without knowledge of or having lived the experience in culturally diverse settings. The same can be true of nurses who invoke knowledge of transcultural nursing without an understanding of what it means to reflect upon and live the meaning of transcultural caring in practice. In nursing, cultural competence has become one ". . . mantra of contemporary nursing practice" (Dreher, Shapiro, & Asselin, 2006, p. 5). Transcultural nursing scholars *have* responded, however, to the issue of cultural competence. Leininger (1991; Leininger & McFarland, 2002, 2006; McFarland & Wehbe-Alamah, 2015; Jeffreys, 2006; and Purnell and Paulanka, 2008) referred to cultural competence as awareness, sensitivity, and transcultural knowledge and skill to provide culturally congruent care for clients by addressing their culture care needs. In the *American Academy of Nursing Expert Panel Report* (Giger et al, 2007) scholars addressed cultural competence by presenting issues and making recommendations to deal with health disparities in ethnic minority populations. Transcultural nursing educators, Lipson and DeSantis

(2007), and many other scholars published in the *Journal of Transcultural Nursing,* discussed the current concerns related to the inclusion of the culture concept and cultural competence in nursing education. They addressed the integration of multiple elements and meanings of cultural competence by presenting a variety of teaching-learning methods to incorporate in nursing curricula.

Definition of Transcultural Caring Competence

In a clearer definition of *cultural competency* for health professionals, Fitzgerald et al (2005) identified three forms: culture-general, intercultural, and culture-specific. The *culture-general* recognizes that universally all persons and relationships are multicultural. The *intercultural* recognizes that professionals have the ability to work with persons who are culturally and linguistically diverse. The *culture-specific* relates to understanding the meaning of diverse relationships as people relate in context or function in experience.

To reiterate, from a *caring* perspective, Roach (2002) identified competence as one of her 6Cs of Caring and defined it ". . . as the state of having the knowledge, judgment, skills, energy, experience and motivation required to respond adequately to the demands of one's professional responsibilities" (p. 54). As a unique process *in* nursing, caring integrates not only competence but also, commitment, compassion, conscience, confidence, and comportment (Roach, 2002). The *transcultural caring dynamic* of competency articulated in this book is universal and specific: caring is spiritual (loving) and ethical, cocreative, and emergent as it is lived in the experience of transcultural communicative caring action. In essence, transcultural caring competence relates to personal accountability for self and professional responsibility for others within the ethics of caring and love as well as justice to facilitate right action and choice making in culturally dynamic relationships and communities (Ray, 2010a).

Cultural Incompetence

Anthropologists Fitzgerald et al (2005) remarked on the idea of cultural incompetence by stating that "[t]o behave in ways considered culturally incompetent could mean that a person loses the opportunity, sometimes even a right, to make decisions for oneself or others and to have one's decisions honored and supported" (p. 332). Leininger (1991; Leininger & McFarland 2006 referred to cultural competence as the provision of culturally congruent care that engages the "cultural" other respectfully and with transcultural knowledge and skill to facilitate decisions and actions to preserve and maintain, to accommodate and negotiate, or to repattern or restructure care (Douglas et al, 2011; Miller et al. 2008). Anything else or less than the behavior referred to in this perspective is cultural imposition (Leininger & McFarland, 2006; McFarland & Wehbe-Alamah, 2015) or cultural incompetence.

Transcultural incompetence implies that, the caregiver forming a relationship who does not honor, respect, and seek understanding of the value of culture or transcultural communicative spiritual-ethical caring, is an incompetent one. When a patient, family member, or any other person including professionals in the relationship are dishonored by name calling, ignorance, prejudice, or lack of protection, the relationship is damaged. In transcultural spiritual-ethical communicative caring, to move toward the dynamics of transcultural caring choice, there is an ethic of caring that includes mutual responsibility and personal accountability (see the Dynamics of Transcultural Caring Tool for Choice Tool on pg. 188). Spiritual-ethical accountability and responsibility cocreate the conditions for ethical transcultural interaction and justice or right action in the processes of health, illness, healing, dying, and death (Ray & Turkel, 2014).

Directions for Using the Transcultural Caring-Based Learning Process

The TCCBL process is designed to assist with the development of critical transcultural caring inquiry in the transcultural caring experiences that are presented in Chapters 8 to 33. Included in this TCCBL process is the movement from a focus only on teaching and learning in nursing toward interprofessional teaching and learning perspectives. The idea of culture as dynamic complexity and the profession of nursing as grounded in complexity science illuminates the need for a broader approach to education in transcultural caring for all disciplines who are engaged in the health and social sciences (Byrne & Callaghan, 2014; Davidson, Ray, & Turkel, 2011; Espinoza, Ukleja, & Rusch, 2010; Ray & Turkel, 2014; Ray & Turkel, 2015). The TCCBL process engages small groups of students (2 to 12; it can be more if necessary) from nursing and other disciplines with a teacher who together cocreate understanding of the meaning of a transcultural caring experience or

situations through authentic dialogue by way of critical caring inquiry. As mentioned earlier, learners gather transcultural evidence to understand their own group process and that of the transcultural caring experience being presented through **pattern identification**—pattern seeing, pattern mapping, pattern recognizing, and pattern transforming. This group process of critical caring inquiry (i.e., reflection and transcultural communicative spiritual-ethical caring dialogue) is cocreative. For example, students or others can set up a simulated dramatic scene whereby they can select who plays the diverse roles in the transcultural caring experiences. As a learning tool to assist with transcultural communicative spiritual-ethical caring analysis, to evaluate, or critique the communicative caring process, the sessions can be videotaped. A Webcam may be used if the process is used within an online course. Evaluation then becomes an art form to observe patterns of human interactions, the self-in-relationship using the TCCBL approach. The following pattern-identification process is used as the central characteristic of TCCBL.

PATTERN-IDENTIFICATION PROCESS

Each transcultural caring experience that follows will be oriented to a critical caring inquiry, a communicative spiritual-ethical caring process of thinking, and pattern identification for transcultural caring competency. Critical caring inquiry and thinking are complex reflective and communicative problem-solving activities that can be described in many different ways (Alfaro-LeFevre, 2006, 2009). The critical caring inquiry used in the TCCBL process is a dialogical transcultural caring approach to seeking evidence—transcultural communicative caring action that is first reflective in a spiritual and ethical (compassionate and just) sense followed by the use of the pattern-identification process. The dialogue initiated by learners encourages not only reflection but also the use of the theory and model of this book to guide the content and the use of the various tools as described in Chapter 6. Following is the pattern identification: pattern seeing, pattern mapping, pattern recognizing, and pattern transforming to aid in the TCCBL process.

Pattern Identification

Pattern identification is a process of pattern seeing, pattern mapping, pattern recognizing, and pattern transforming in the dialogic encounter of learners to illuminate transcultural competency in the context of the transcultural caring experiences. Pattern identification captures and weaves many aspects of life stories of persons or groups of diverse cultures into convincing descriptions or holistic portraits around these stories to facilitate awareness, understanding, and choice.

To identify patterns in the transcultural caring experiences in the following chapters, the reader must become involved with the story and his or her lifeworld. The reader also must become involved in his or her mind with other members of the group when the group learning process begins. Each experience illuminates a particular ethnicity or panethnic/sociocultural or professional group in a cultural context for reflection, assessment, and interpretation and potential problem-solving. Students should review the TCCBL process, the Transcultural Caring Dynamics in Nursing and Health-Care Theory and Model used to guide the content of the book, and the transcultural caring tools for assessment (see Chapter 6) before approaching the learning situation. The following make up the pattern-identification process.

Pattern Seeing

Pattern seeing is a process of visualizing caring and the transcultural caring relationship. Pattern seeing is the movement in the transcultural caring relationship that captures (1) the lived experience, (2) other forms of evidence, and (3) the meaning of the life story that helps in weaving together the story of individuals and family members or significant others from diverse cultures. The following list will help us to understand pattern seeing.

- Focus on the meaning of transcultural compassion and justice. What "touches" the heart and what is justice in the human relationship (Ray & Turkel, 2014)?
- Develop an awareness of the meaning of transcultural caring from reviewing the content of the chapters and your own perspective.
- Dialogue (relate and reflect through transcultural communicative spiritual-ethical caring) about the transcultural experience presented in nursing and sociocultural situations, including relationships with other disciplines.
- Outline the dominant aspects of the transcultural caring experience of the person in the sociocultural context. What is the meaning of the person in relationship to family, community, other professions, organization, culture, or world?

- Relate the experience to the Transcultural Caring Dynamics in Nursing and Health-Care Theory and Model developed in this book.
- Relate the experience to other tools in the book:
  - Culture-Value Conflict Assessment Tool
  - Transcultural Caring Dynamics Assessment Tool
  - Ray's Transcultural Communicative Spiritual-Ethical CARING Tool for Cultural Competency
  - Dynamics of Transcultural Caring Tool for Choice
  - Transcultural Caring Negotiation Tool

Pattern Mapping

Pattern mapping is a way of looking at and interpreting the content and meaning of the descriptions or portraits of pattern seeing to agree on a way to understand the persons or groups in the context of their life experiences. The following will help us to understand a process of pattern mapping.

- Collect or generate *patterns* of evidence (i.e., experience of person in his or her cultural context or lived world), and evidence collected from literature and the Internet and others in the learning group.
- Appreciate whether or not there may be a difference in linguistic (language) or symbolic interaction, signs, or symbols in the experiences.
- Determine *all* the forms of evidence in the transcultural caring experience (i.e., nursing and medical evidence, transcultural nursing/caring evidence, and social and historical evidence from participants, literature and Internet sources).
- Cluster the patterns (descriptions) of sociocultural and transcultural nursing and other disciplinary evidence.
- Plot the sequence of events of the patterns that are *relevant* to the experience and as you related them to the theory and model or tools developed in this book or the literature and other information sources.

Pattern Recognizing

Pattern recognizing is a process of reflection, interaction, and dialogue to facilitate increased awareness, identification, acknowledgment, validation, and un-derstanding of patterns in the pattern-seeing and pattern-mapping interpretive processes (Byrne & Callaghan, 2014; Turkel, Ray, & Kornblatt,

2012). The following will help us to understand pattern recognizing.

- Reflect on the patterns of clustered data as they relate to the dimensions in the theory and model and any of the other assessment tools in the book and seek knowledge from each other.
- Determine what else may be needed to discover more about the experience, as you synthesize the data (more specific culture-history, medical, or socioeconomic aspects).
- Research the sources of data—other literature and Web sites on caring, society, culture, health, illness, healing, and other scientific knowledge.

Pattern Transforming

Pattern transforming of meanings by rereflection and interpretation is a way of synthesizing all the transcultural caring patterns to reveal opportunities for choice for patients, families, significant others, and professionals. The following is a means to facilitate choice making for transformative processes: caring, healing, health, dying, or a peaceful death.

- Identify and seek understanding of the strengths and weaknesses of the dominant health-care system in your community in meeting different cultural needs of patient and families.
- Identify *all* possible choices for health, healing, and transformation that can be cocreated or projected based on the evaluation of the potential shared meaning-making of the health-care professional(s) and the person, family, community, organizations, and the health-care systems in the experience.

Directions for Forming a Transcultural Caring-Based Learning Group

Forming a TCCBL group is an artful practice of teaching and learning. Teaching and learning is pedagogy of thoughtfulness and communicative spiritual-ethical caring action in the discipline and profession of nursing and other health-care professionals (Eggenberger et al 2013; France & Ray, 2014). "The term, *discipline* is related to the notion of disciple (someone who follows a great teacher [or tutor] or a great example), and also to the notion of *docere* (meaning to teach), and to the term *doctor* (a learned person)" (van Manen, 1991, pp. 198–199). The term *profession* is commitment to the science and art (experience) of professional practice (Parker, 2006; Smith & Parker (Eds.), 2015; van Manen, 2014). In this following discourse, the

TCCBL is a method of integrating students, a tutor, a body of knowledge (i.e., transcultural caring experience) with a relational caring experience that fosters participation for the purposes of cocreative teaching and learning.

1. Formulate a learning group of students with a teacher (tutor) or selected student.
2. Reflect on oneself as a multicultural being and the meaning of self and one's identity.
3. Reflect on the meaning of compassion for oneself and within and for each other in the learning group.
4. Reflect on the participants in the transcultural caring experience after reading.
5. Reflect on the meaning of transcultural caring (compassion and justice) in all transcultural communicative actions with participants in the story *and* the members of the learning group.
6. Review the Transcultural Caring Dynamics in Nursing and Health-Care Theory and Model and corresponding data presented in chapters in this book.
7. Discover ways of applying the model and any of the five transcultural caring assessment negotiation tools to the transcultural caring experiences.
8. Describe the culture(s) in the transcultural caring experience.
9. Interpret individually the meaning of the transcultural caring experience by using the pattern-identification process—pattern seeing, pattern mapping, pattern recognizing, and pattern transforming.
10. Dialogue as a group about the meaning of the transcultural caring experience and the patterns that you individually identified. Focus on interpersonal and cross-cultural comparison by using the following (video the process for future analysis):
    - Application of critical caring inquiry.
    - Consideration of the pattern-identification process as a collective group.
    - Compare and contrast the pattern-identification process.
11. Begin to describe as a whole, the complex culture of the transcultural caring experiences.
    - Describe the dynamics/styles of leadership in the learning group.
    - Identify the potential conflicts of values, beliefs, attitudes, and opinions of each person in the group that unfolded.

- Identify ways to arrive at compromise, agreement, or reconciliation of diverse values and beliefs within the group.
12. Reformulate the transcultural caring experience/story/case study with knowledge and skill learned through the TCCBL process.
13. Identify potential needs for nursing, health care, and social system intervention.
14. Identify what would be the responsibility of a transcultural nurse or other health-care professional.
15. Evaluate the TCCBL process for each student participant.
16. Identify what transcultural caring competencies were gleaned from group participation and using the TCCBL process, and online learning if appropriate.

Transcultural Caring Experiences and the Transcultural Caring-Based Learning Process

The ultimate purpose of the transcultural caring experiences for students and others is not to find all the answers in the contents of this book, but to collect all evidence, discover, and gain insight through reflection on the stories and the commentaries, and apply the TCCBL process. By participating with the transcultural caring experiences as students, faculty, or clinical practitioners, the information sharing is individually creative and collectively cocreative. When reflected upon and dialogued about, students and others can deal with potential differences of values and opinion, and move toward a participatory consciousness that captures new ideas and generates modes of helping through compassion and justice for the people representing diverse culture(s) in each story *and* for members of their own learning group. Students may come to an agreement or compromise about the meaning(s) of the experiences and what choices should or could be made.

Engaging consciously through transcultural communicative spiritual-ethical caring with authentic dialogue in each experience, student nurses and others become aware of and are sensitive to what has happened in the story, what is happening within a particular culture or diverse culture/panethnic group, and what is happening within one's own learning group as they interact and form a particular type of learning culture. Within each small group, each person will begin to recognize his or her own individual multicultural being, his or her own culture/ethnicity, and his or her own creative style as people participate together. Learners will ultimately find how one, as a caring nurse, nursing student, or other professional, begins to understand oneself, and discovers and interprets the meaning of the experiences of the diverse people in the context of the cultures or social, nursing, or health-care situations presented. Simultaneously, the TCCBL process not only will foster interaction, authentic dialogue, and collaboration with group members, but also will encourage seeking evidence, enhancing insight, and gaining competency through the contents of the book information itself, the literature, and Internet sources. In this way, group members can become more aware and seek understanding and facilitate choices for potential health, healing, and well-being of the vulnerable people (e.g., patients, families, communities, and nations) presented in the transcultural caring experiences. By this learning process, students or other learners realize that no one exact cultural outcome for specific ethnicities or culture groups emerges. Interpretation yields different insights. Learners will recognize that the meaning of "health" of people is always dynamic and emergent; it is interconnected fully with their environment (i.e., the context), the self in relation to others, and to life-world experiences. Learning is open and emergent as is the meaning of culture. Learning about the transcultural caring experiences in this book as a foundation for dialogue that facilitates critical caring thinking, communication, and ways of understanding will help students and other professionals deal with complex choices that they, as transcultural nurses, will face with *actual* patients, families, and significant others in nursing and health care, or sociocultural situations or systems. Faculty, students, and other health-care and social science professionals may also contemplate what it is like to engage with simulated patients, potential robots, patients and clients over the internet/webcam/social media sites, including Facebook, Facetime, Skype, Twitter, and so forth (Byrne & Callaghan, 2014; Davidson, Ray, & Turkel, 2011; Eggenberger et al, 2010, 2013; Espinoza, Ukela, & Rusch, 2010; Losin, Purnell, Tanioka, & Osaka, 2011; Skype Communications S.a.r.l.; Stone, 2014; Wu & Ray, 2016, in press).

References

Alfaro-LeFevre, R. (2006). *Applying the nursing process: A tool for critical thinking* (6th ed.). Philadelphia, PA: Lippincott Williams & Wilkins.

Alfaro-LeFevre, R. (2009). *Applying nursing process: A tool for critical thinking* (7th ed.). Lippincott Williams & Wilkins.

Bar-Yam, Y. (2004). *Making things work: Solving complex problems in a complex world.* Boston: Knowledge Press.

Barry, C., Gordon, S., & King, B. (2015). *Nursing case studies in caring.* New York: Springer Publishing Company

Berman, P. (2004). *Terror and liberalism.* New York: W. W. Norton & Company.

Bohm, D. (1990). *On dialogue.* Ojai, CA: David Bohm Seminars.

Boulding, E. (1988). *Building a global civic culture.* New York: Teachers College Press.

Boykin, A., Schoenhofer, S., & Valentine, K. (2014). *Health care system transformation for nursing and health care leaders.* New York: Springer Publishing Company.

Breda, K. (2009). *Nursing and globalization in the Americas: A critical perspective.* Amityville, NY: Baywood Publishing Company.

Brown, C. (2006). *Caring for self for nursing leaders: Climbing to the mountain peak.* Doctoral Dissertation (Proquest AAT, 3209569), Florida Atlantic University, Boca Raton, FL.

Burkhardt, M., & Nathaniel, A. (2008). *Ethics issues in contemporary nursing practice* (3rd ed.). Clifton Park, NY: Thomson Delmar Learning.

Byrne, D., & Callaghan, G. (2014). *Complexity theory and the social sciences.* London: Routledge.

Cunnington, J. (2001). Evolution of student evaluation in the McMaster MD programme. *Pedagogue: Perspectives on Health Sciences Education, 10,* 1–9.

Delvecchio Good, M. (1995). *American medicine: The quest for competence.* Berkeley, CA: University of California Press.

Dreher, M. Shapiro, D., & Asselin, M. (2006). *Healthy places, healthy people: A handbook for culturally competent community nursing practice.* Indianapolis: Sigma Theta Tau International.

Douglas, M., Uhl-Pierce, J., Rosenkoetter, M., et al. (2011). *Standards of practice for culturally competent care: 2011 update.* Journal of Transcultural Nursing, 22(4), 317–333.

Economy, E., & Levi, M. (2014). *By all means necessary: How China's resource quest is changing the world.* Oxford: Oxford University Press.

Eggenberger, T., Garrison, J., Giovengo, K., & Hilton, N. (2013). *Discharge phone calls: Using person-centered communication to improve outcomes.* Journal of Nursing Management, 21, 733–739.

Eggenberger, T., Keller, K., & Locsin, R. (2010). *Valuing caring behaviors within simulated emergent nursing situation.* International Journal for Human Caring, 14(2), 22–28.

Eisler, R. (2007). *The real wealth of nations: Creating a caring economics.* San Francisco: Berrett-Koehler Publishers, Inc.

Espinoza, C., Ukleja, M., & Rusch, C. (2010). *Managing the Millennials: discover the core competencies for managing today's workforce.* New York: Wiley.

Fitzgerald, M., Williamson, P., Russell, C., & Manor, D. (2005). Doubling the cloak of (in)competence in client/therapist interactions. *Medical Anthropology Quarterly, 19(3),* 331–347.

Floridi, L (2014). *The 4th revolution: How the infosphere is reshaping human reality.* Oxford: Oxford University Press.

France, N., & Ray, M. (2014). Studying caring science in nursing: The foundation of the discipline and profession of nursing at Florida Atlantic University. In K. Vaiyda (Ed.). Nursing for the curious: Why study nursing? Camberra, Australia: Curious Academic Publishing (Kindle version).

Gadow, S. (1996). Ethical narratives in practice. *Nursing Science Quarterly 9(1),* 8–11.

Gallo, C. (2014). Talk like TED: The world's public-speaking secrets of the world's top minds. New York: St. Martin's Press.

Giger, J., Davidhizar, R., Purnell, L., Harden, J., Phillips, J., & Strickland, O. (2007). American Academy `of Nursing expert panel report: Developing cultural competence to eliminate health disparities in ethnic minorities and other vulnerable populations. *Journal of Transcultural Nursing, 18(2),* 95–102.

Green, J. (2006). On cultural competence. *Anthropology News, 47(5),* 3.

Grumime, V., Barry, C., Gordon, S., & Ray, M. (2016, in press). On virtual presence. *Advances in Nursing Science.*

Hatfield, C. (2013). An astronaut's guide to life on earth: What going to space taught me about ingenuity, determination, and being prepared for anything. New York: Little, Brown & Company.

Henderson, H., with Sethi, S. (2006). *Ethical markets: Growing the green economy.* White River Junction, VT: Chelsea Green Publishing Company.

Jarvis, P. (1991). Reflective practice and nursing. *Nurse Education Today, 12,* 174–181.

Jeffreys, M. (2006). *Teaching cultural competence in nursing and health care: Inquiry, action and innovation.* New York: Springer Publishing Company.

Journal of Transcultural Nursing. (2007). *18*(1), 5S–90S. (Suppl. to Vol. 18, No. 1)

Kaku, M. (2014). The future of the mind: The scientific quest to understand, enhance, and empower the mind. New York: Doubleday.

Kleinman, A. (1988). *The illness narratives: Suffering, healing & the human condition.* New York: Basic Books, Inc.

Kleinman, A., & Benson, P. (2006). Anthropology in the clinic: The problem of cultural competency and how to fix it. *PLOS.* Retrieved July 6, 2009, from http://www.plosmedicine.org/article/info:doi/10.1371/journal/pmed.0030294

Knowlden, V. (1990). The virtue of caring in nursing. In M. Leininger (Ed.), *Ethical and moral dimension of care* (pp. 89–94). Detroit: Wayne State University Press.

Kurzweil, R. (2005). *The singularity is near.* New York: Viking.

Leininger, M. (Ed.). (1991). *Cultural care universality and diversity: A theory of nursing.* New York: National League for Nursing Press.

Leininger, M., & McFarland, M. (Eds.). (2002). *Transcultural nursing: Concepts, theories, research and practice* (3rd ed.). New York: McGraw-Hill Medical.

Leininger, M., & McFarland, M. (2006). *Culture care diversity and universality: A worldwide theory of nursing.* Sudbury, MA: Jones & Bartlett Publisher.

Lipson, J., & DeSantis, L. (2007). Current approaches to integrating elements of cultural competence in nursing education. *Journal of Transcultural Nursing, 18*(1), 10S–20S.

Locsin, R., Purnell, M., Tanioka, T., & Osaka, K. (2011). Human rights and humanoid relationships in nursing and complexity science. In A. Davidson, M. Ray, & M. Turkel (Eds.), Nursing, caring, and complexity science: For human-environment well-being. New York: Springer Publishing Company.

McFarland, M., & Wehbe-Alamah, H.(2015). Leininger's culture care diversity and universality: A worldwide

nursing theory (3rd ed.). Burlington, MA: Jones & Bartlett Learning.

Miller, J., Leininger, M., Leuning, C., Andrews, A., Ludwig-Beyer, P., & Papadopoulos, I. (2008). Transcultural Nursing Society Position Statement on Human Rights. *Journal of Transcultural Nursing, 19*(1), 5–7.

Norman, G., Klass, D., & Wenghofer, E. (2008). Predicting doctor performance outcomes of curriculum intervention: Problem-based learning and continuing competence. *Medical Education, 10,* 1365–2923.

Parker, M. (2006). *Nursing theories, nursing practice* (2nd ed.). Philadelphia: F. A. Davis Company.

Purnell, L., & Paulanka, B. (Eds.). (2008). *Transcultural health care* (2nd ed.). Philadelphia: F. A. Davis Company.

Ray, M. (1989). Transcultural caring: Political and economic visions. *Journal of Transcultural Nursing, 1*(1), 17–21.

Ray, M. (1998). A phenomenologic study of the interface of caring and technology in intermediate care: Toward a reflexive ethics for clinical practice. *Holistic Nursing Practice, 12*(4), 69–77.

Ray, M. (2007). Transcultural caring as a dynamic of complexity in nursing practice. In A. Barnard & R. Locsin (Eds.), *Technology and nursing: Practice, concepts and issues* (pp. 174–190). United Kingdom: Palgrave MacMillan.

Ray, M. (2010a). *Transcultural caring dynamics in nursing and health care.* Philadelphia: F. A. Davis Company.

Ray, M. (2010b). *A study of caring within the institutional culture: The discovery of the Theory of Bureaucratic Caring.* Germany: Lambert Academic Publishers.

Ray, M. (2010c). Creating caring organizations and cultures through communitarian ethics. Journal of the World Universities Forum, 3(5), 41–52.

Ray, M. (2011). Complex caring dynamics: A unifying model of nursing inquiry. In A. Davidson, M. Ray, & M. Turkel (Eds.). *Nursing, caring, and complexity science: For human-environment well-being* (pp. 31–52). New York: Springer Publishing Company.

Ray, M. & Turkel, M. (2014). Caring as emancipatory nursing praxis: Theory of relational caring complexity. *Advances in Nursing Science,* 37(2), 132-146.

Ray, M. & Turkel, M. (2015). Marilyn Anne Ray's theory of bureaucratic caring. In M. Smith M. Parker (Eds.),

Nursing theories and nursing practice (4th ed.). Philadelphia: F. A. Davis Company.

Roach, M. (2002). *Caring, the human mode of being.* (2nd rev. ed.). Ottawa, ON: CHA Press.

Smith, M., & Liehr, P. (Eds). (2003). *Middle range theory for nursing.* New York: Springer Publishing Company.

Smith, M., & Liehr, P. (2005). Story theory: Advancing nursing practice scholarship. *Holistic Nursing Practice, 6,* 272–276.

Smith, M., & Liehr, P. (2014). Middle range theory for nursing (3rd ed.). New York: Springer Publishing Company.

Solomon, P. (1999). Adapting to problem-based learning. *Pedagogue: Perspectives on the Health Sciences Education 9,* 6–9.

Stone, B. (2014). Things a little bird told me: Confessions of the creative mind. New York: Grand Central Publishing, Hachette Book Group.

The New American Bible. (1987). Nashville: Thomas Nelson Publishers.

The Kingdom of Saudi Arabia. (1993). (9th ed.). London: Stacey International.

The Quran (Mahmud Y. Zayed, Checked and Revised). (1980). Beirut: Dar Al-Choura.

The Southwest Indian Foundation Catalogue. (Late Autumn, 2006). Gallup, New Mexico.

Turkel, M. (2007). *Evidence based practice.* Marblehead, MA: HC Pro, Inc.

Turkel, M., & Ray, M. (2004). Creating a caring practice environment through self-renewal. *Nursing Administration Quarterly, 28*(4), 249–254.

Turkel, M., Ray, M., & Kornblatt, L. (2012). Instead of reconceptualizing the nursing process: Let's rename it. Nursing Science Quarterly, 25(2), 194–198.

Van Manen, M. (1991). *The tact of teaching: The meaning of pedagogical thoughtfulness.* Albany: State University of New York Press.

Van Manen, M. (2014). Phenomenology of practice. Walnut Creek, CA: Left Coast Press.

Watson, J. (1988). *Nursing science and human care.* New York: National League for Nursing Press.

Watson, J. (2005). *Caring science as sacred science.* Philadelphia: F. A. Davis Company.

Wilhelm, D., & Zlotnick, C. (2014). Nursing students in a global learning environment: Creative teaching methods on culture, emotion, and communication. Journal of Transcultural Nursing, 25(3), 296–302.

Wolf, A. (2014). Exploring rituals in nursing: Joining art and science. New York: Springer Publishing Company.

Wolfe, A. (2012). Political evil: What it is and how to combat it. New York: Vintage Books.

Womack, M. (2005). *Symbols and meaning.* Walnut Creek: AltaMira Press.

Wong, T., & Pang, S. (2000). Holism and caring: Nursing in the Chinese health care culture. *Holistic Nursing Practice 15*(1), 12–21.

Wood, A. (2004). *On the border: Society and culture between the United States and Mexico.* Boulder, CO: SR Books.

Wu, J. & Ray, M. (2016). Technological caring for healthcare complexities of patients with cardiac disease comorbid with diabetes. *International Journal for Human Caring,* 20(2).

Select Bibliography

Audinet, J. (2004). *The human face of globalization: From multicultural to mestizaje* (F. Dal Chele, Trans.). Lanham, MD: Rowman & Littlefield Publishers, Inc.

Bronson, R. (2006). *Thicker than oil: America's uneasy partnership with Saudi Arabia.* Oxford: Oxford University Press.

Hidden history of the Kovno ghetto. United States Holocaust Museum (1997). Boston: Little, Brown & Company.

Jahoudi, M. (1993). *Christian & Islamic spirituality.* New York: Paulist Press.

Jenkins, R. (1998). *Questions of competence: Culture, classification and intellectual disability.* New York: Cambridge University Press.

Smith, H. (1991). *The world's religions.* San Francisco: HarperSanFrancisco.

Sparks, I. (1991). *Exploring the world's religions.* San Francisco: HarperSanFrancisco.

Toward evidence-based nursing. (2003). Washington, DC: The Advisory Board.

CHAPTER 8

The Border and Pueblo: An American Mexican Cultural Experience

*M*exico is one of the three countries of North America. Each nation's record is a living history of multiple cultures; native or indigenous peoples; diverse languages, locations, and geography, exploration; conflict, war, and conquests; migration; and the building of nation-states. Each nation is important to each other in growth, friendships, improving relationships of diverse cultures, engaging in peaceful dialogue, exercising wisdom in politics to understand diverse ways of life, improving economic well-being by addressing issues of globalization, human and material resources, trade, technology, military defense and support, the drug trade, violence, legal and illegal immigration, and respecting laws governing the ways of life. The following story is a transcultural caring experience that the author had when studying for a master of arts degree in cultural anthropology. The following has story excerpts, reflections, and commentary from the author, and questions for your reflection and evaluation.

AUTHOR'S REFLECTION

I was very excited about studying in Mexico, about culture and health first introduced to me in my master of science degree in nursing by Dr. Madeleine Leininger, the first nurse-anthropologist and "mother" of the discipline of transcultural nursing. Dr. Leininger had written a book in 1970 on *Nursing and Anthropology: Two Worlds to Blend*. I had taken a course in Spanish in university. I had studied a little about Mexico and was interested in the anthropologist Redfield's (1989) work and modeling on community development in Mexico. To this day, I continue to use Drs. Leininger and Redfield's ideas in my own research on organizations as small cultures and complex transcultural caring dynamics.

Marilyn's Story: The Nurse-Anthropology Student

I was so excited. I learned that 10 colleagues and I had been selected to do fieldwork in cultural anthropology studying culture, health, health care, and the family structure in Mexico. The class was divided into cultural anthropologists, archaeologists, physical anthropologists, and linguists coming from nursing, social work, and pure anthropology backgrounds. We were divided into small groups. My group consisted of two nurses, a social worker, and a nutritionist. We were going to Mechoacanejo, a small pueblo near Teocaltiche, in the state of Jalisco, the same state as Guadalajara. I didn't speak Spanish well but one woman in our small group was fluent. As anthropology students, we were going to do ethnography, participant observation in another country. We were given instructions that we would have to "live the culture," taking with us only the bare essentials of some clothing for everyday use, a sleeping bag, two towels, and some toiletries. Four of us drove in the professor's dilapidated white van; he traveled by plane. We drove from San Francisco, California winding our way sometimes along the freeway and sometimes along the beautiful Pacific Coast Highway to San Diego where we were to cross the border. It was my second time crossing the U.S.-Mexican border. The notion of a border has much symbolism to me. I was born in Canada near the border with the United States. We crossed the border to the United States many times for shopping or vacations. There was always something quite exciting but, at the same time, frightening about it—flags on the bridge; police; immigration buildings with their officials; identification cards; customs stalls on both sides of the border; customs agents who asked who we were, where we were from, where we were going, and what were we bringing across.

We made it through the maze of officials. We hoped that the old van would hold up because we were going through unfamiliar territory. One night we had to sleep on benches in one of the old towns. I can't really remember why that happened. We were all together, though, so we figured we could all protect each other. I do remember that there were a lot of cockroaches and flies in the bathroom. We finally made it to a little village or pueblo of Mechoacanejo after spending some time in Guadalajara, the capital city of Jalisco, the *Perla del Occidente* (Pearl of the West) and now referred to as the "Silicon Valley" of Mexico. Our new home was a "museum" made of mud and multicolored glass from broken pop bottles. The museum was

AUTHOR'S REFLECTION

Borders reveal much about a nation-state. What is the lifeworld like for the people living beyond the borders? Borders illuminate the meaning of the importance of some things, especially the laws and rules, or even the nature of officials. Are the border agents strong and intimidating? Are the buildings beautiful or rundown? Is the landscaping perfect or lacking? The U.S.-Mexican border seemed ominous. This one had a small fence at that time and more border guards than I had ever seen. The contrast between the suburbs of San Diego and San Ysidro where the border was and the city of Tijuana, Mexico was very sharp. The structures tell the story of the struggles of the people who try to come to the United States and the guards and agents who try to keep them out. Many Latinos work as inspectors on both sides of the border.

There is a whole culture at the borderlands, a history, heavy with meaning, some good, some bad. To people fleeing violence, borders represent freedom or oppression, or even slavery or imprisonment. This Mexican-U.S. border is the most heavily crossed land port in the world. Over the years, alcohol, prostitution, drugs, and gambling proliferated and Tijuana seemed to become "a regulated vice haven for foreigners" (Cabeza de Baca & Cabeza de Baca in Wood, 2004). The stereotypes created by this image do not go away easily.

built by the townspeople to house the pre-Columbian artifacts of the region that the local priest, Father Lopez (pseudonym), collected in his travels to the remote villages. What a sight. Inside, besides the ancient artwork, there were dirt floors and a huge stone fireplace, some chairs, and little cots for the four of us. There was an impaled butterfly collection on one wall. We met the family who would take care of us, a widow, Luz, the sister of Father Lopez, her six children, and their grandmother, *Abuela*.

We learned a lot about village life. Most of the people in the village were Mestizos, a blend of Spaniard and Amerindian, and were Catholic. We were anthropology students, but two of us were nurses *las enfermeras*, so were asked to go to other pueblos to just "be there" and provide as much support as possible for the people who did not receive much care because of the remoteness of their location. We went with Father Lopez on horseback. I remember how hot the sun was, how he wore his sombrero (priests weren't allowed by the government in those days to wear their priestly garb), sang to the people who plowed the fields, and gave coins to the little children who lined the path. No one spoke English in the village so our Spanish improved over time. We did speak with the heart though, exchanging smiles and nods and sometimes hugs. I was always happy to speak in English with my colleagues at night. At times, I suffered from bad headaches trying to translate Spanish words into English and then give a response back in Spanish. It seemed to take forever to communicate. I wasn't at a point where I could actually think in the language but felt like I was getting there. Each evening the chief of police, called *El Jefe*, watched over the museum where we slept. Many nights we were serenaded by the local villagers with mariachi music. (Guadalajara was the birthplace of mariachi music.)

The population comprised mostly elderly people or children. Old men, skin sun-drenched from work in the fields, sat outside small houses close to the narrow roads and talked. Children played and helped their mothers and the elderly. Women were dressed in colorful skirts and blouses. Women washed, and cleaned, and prepared meals with mostly eggs and vegetables, and made alfalfa juice drinks, which took some getting used to but were a good source of vitamins and minerals. There wasn't much meat; chicken was prepared for special occasions. Government-sponsored dried fish, stored at the health clinic, was given to the people every Monday. There was a volunteer at the clinic and the doctor came once a week. All physicians after graduation had to spend 1 year caring for people in small pueblos, if they could reach them by car.

Most of the young men in the village were not there. We were told that they went to the United States to find work and make money. They bused from their homes and made it across the border either at Tijuana or areas in Arizona or Texas to work in the fields for at least 6 months out of the year to earn money to help their families. We learned that it was a multigenerational thing in this village. Young men went away when they came of age. Sometimes they didn't come home; they became undocumented workers or even illegal immigrants of the United States. Some went to Canada. Some came home to gather their families to try to cross at the borders of the states with Mexico or to get across the Rio Grande.

Transcultural Caring-Based Learning Approach

Please review the information about the Transcultural Caring Dynamics for Nursing and Health-Care Model, the assessment tool, the transcultural caring-based learning (TCCBL) approach, the transcultural caring inquiry information explained in previous chapters of this book, and any other relevant literary and Internet information before dialoguing about this transcultural caring experience. In your small group, apply the TCCBL approach; critical caring inquiry; and the purpose, goals, and objectives in relation to your transcultural caring situation for pattern identification (i.e., pattern seeing, pattern mapping, pattern recognizing, and pattern transforming). Use dimensions of the Transcultural Caring Dynamics in Nursing and Health-Care Theory and Model and use the most appropriate assessment tools for transcultural evidence gathering. The "Reflections with Questions" section that follows is a

AUTHOR'S REFLECTION

The people of the pueblo were poor but rich in spirit. Overall, I noticed that people were happy, smiling and talking with each other. Some were very thin and unhealthy looking; others were very healthy and well nourished. Our nutritionist found that although there was not much protein from meat, protein was secured through vegetables. Fruits and vegetables to be sold hung from stalls in the narrow streets. Often there were flies on the fruit. Women had many children back then. Many young women were pregnant and their husbands were away working in the United States or Canada. They relied on the money that the men would make and bring home after working far away. I noticed that young people liked to play and sing songs. They even imitated my colleagues and me, which was so much fun. Old people liked to visit with each other on their doorsteps or in the post office. I found out a lot about the culture and people by sitting in the post office, and engaging in participant observation. The same things that plague each of us about human relationships, past hurts, resentments, lack of resources, differences of opinion, and lack of understanding, and love relationships also plagued the people of the pueblo.

guide that will assist you individually and collectively in your learning group with dialogue and interpretation of what is happening in the story; what is happening now in the international relationship between the United States, Mexico, Central America, and Canada; and what your responsibilities as a transcultural nurse should be.

Reflections with Questions

Mexican culture is critically important within the United States and to the relationships between Mexico and the United States. As a group of nursing students, reflect upon the story of crossing the border and living among the village people, their living history, and their transcultural and transnational relationship then and now with the United States. Reflect also on what is occurring between Central America (Guatemala, Honduras, and El Salvador) and Mexico, and the United States and Canada. What is the difference between a refugee and an undocumented immigrant? What status is afforded people who have diverse classifications of status (As an example, see, http://www.forbes.com/sites/andyjsemotiuk/2014/07/31/the-refugee-crisis-unfortunately-our-best-will-never-be-enough/.)

Transcultural Nursing Reflections

- As a transcultural nurse, what are your thoughts as you read and reflect upon this story? What does the story bring to mind about culture, relationships, cultural differences, intercultural relationships, villages, religion, nutrition, sense of community, undocumented workers, and so forth?
- How do you define health? How do you define cultural health and/or illness?
- Imagine yourself in diverse ways, for example, a nurse without Mexican or Spanish heritage living in the Northeast of the United States, a Mexican American nurse living in California, a Mexican nurse living in Tijuana, or an American or Canadian nurse living in Mexico and living with the people of a particular Mexican cultural community. Think about the challenges of speaking and understanding a different language, of learning and speaking either Spanish or English, and of communicating professionally in another language. Consider how we learn languages and how we build or have confidence to address nursing, health care, and social problems when able to speak another language.
- Reflect upon migration in general. What is the relationship between migration and violence, migration and poverty? Reflect on the socioeconomic and geopolitical issues. Is

migration a health issue? Are there diseases that may exist in one country and considered minimal in another? What are the United Nations' Millennium Goals post 2015, and how would Mexico and other Central American nations be a part of those developments?

- This transcultural caring experience occurred many years ago. What has changed with respect to the issues that face the United States and Mexico? The experience demonstrates the nature of the border, border communities, and communities within Mexico and California. Discuss also the issues of the border states of Arizona and Texas. Contemplate the southern border of Mexico and the boundary between North and Central America. How permeable is Mexico's southern border of migration patterns to the United States? Why are so many unaccompanied children coming to the border between Mexico and the United States? Where are the children and others from? What are "coyotes"? How did they get that name and become so influential in immigration issues? What is the "train of death" (nicknamed The Beast) traveling north toward the U.S border from the Guatemalan-Mexico border? Why has human/sex trafficking/smuggling increased worldwide? What are "Snakeheads"?

- Contemplate the northern border between Canada and the United States. What is the North American Free Trade Agreement (NAFTA)? How important are the northern and southern borders in the NAFTA? What is the significance of health and well-being for people of North America in the NAFTA? Compare and contrast varying viewpoints in terms of free trade, economics, globalization, poverty, immigration, and health care.

- What is the meaning of immigration, legal or illegal? What is an undocumented worker? What perceived or actual jobs need to be filled that "invite" people from Mexico to the United States or Canada? What is facing the Mexican people in poverty and health, and the need for education and work and economic development? What are the immigration laws in Canada and the United States? How are they changing? How does money and education versus poverty and lack of education impact the immigration laws? What do we mean by human rights and justice in developing countries versus developed countries?

- Multigenerational migration is a living history from this story. What is the cultural patterning in multigenerational migration? What does it mean for transcultural transmission of values from one generation to the other? Reflect upon why some pueblos in Mexico would promote migration to the United States while others do not. Are there gender differences in migration patterns?

- What is our moral obligation as transcultural nurses to speak on behalf of or for disenfranchised or vulnerable people, not only migrants from Mexico or Central America but also migrants from any part of the world? Does a transcultural nurse have a responsibility to examine the resources and facilitate improvement of health to migrant people, legal or illegal? Examine the Human Rights document of the Transcultural Nursing Society (Douglas et al, 2011; Miller et al, 2008) from the *Journal of Transcultural Nursing Society* and its Web site and determine if or how the precepts are put into practice within the views identified in this transcultural caring scenario.

- Identify the differences, if any, between fundamental human rights in Mexico and in the United States. What are the transnational migration patterns that affect different communities in the Southwest, especially California, Arizona, and Texas?

- Are you aware of the history of Mexico in relation to the United States? Compare and contrast, for example, the cultures of the Rio Grande Valley of Texas and Southern California. How have things changed over time?

- How strong is the culture of poverty in Mexico and in the United States? Can you discover what government leaders are doing in creating jobs and reducing poverty, providing for health care and education; and improving land development, sanitation, water safety, and nutrition in Mexico and the United States?

- What socioeconomic, spiritual, and population issues face the borderlands? Do you think that building a fence in the southern United States helps or hinders the effort to deal reasonably and effectively with the problems that face the two nations? What does homeland security mean? What is its formal name in the United States? What is the formal name for immigration and naturalization in the United States? What is the history of the borderlands and cities on both sides of the border? What is the meaning of vice (i.e., drugs and prostitution) rings within or at the borders?
- What have you read about the drug and sex trafficking that occurs at the border? What do you think has escalated the border problems in the past decade?
- In the United States and especially in the border cities and states, different organizations, such as the United Farmworkers of America have helped Americans or Mexicans achieve some equity in the workplace. What are your thoughts about these organizations?
- What is the population of Latinos in the United States? Can babies of illegal immigrants be given United States citizenship if they are born in the United States? What are the migration patterns of Mexicans and Central Americans within the United States? How can people of Mexican heritage who are in the United States legally help the immigration issues that face both nations?
- Are you aware of the migration patterns of Mexicans and Central Americans to Canada? Is there a difference between Canada and the United States in how they deal with immigration and health care for Mexicans and Central Americans? How are immigration, health care, and welfare needs handled?
- What is the state of women migrating to the United States and Canada from Mexico? Are there statistics that determine the number of women migrating without their children and children migrating without their mothers or fathers?
- Examine through the World Health Organization's (WHO) Web site and other literature, what are the major health needs of the Mexican people. What are the WHO concerns regarding the H1N1 virus or other viruses, such as Ebola, or bacteria? Compare this virus or any other virus from a public health standpoint with the Ebola virus of west and central Africa. What is the position of the World Health Organization, the U.S. Centers for Disease Control and Prevention (CDC), and the United Nations (UN) regarding diseases across borders/nations? What is meant by the UN Millennium Development Goals 2015 and beyond? Do Mexican people as undocumented people have a right to health care in the United States? Do they have the right to health care in Canada?
- What policies affect nurses and physicians in caring for undocumented workers at a U.S. health clinic or hospital? Should nurses who are transcultural in spirit be obliged or be willing to speak Spanish when caring for people of Hispanic heritage in the United States?
- Consider the idea of microcredit, such as that started in Bangladesh for women developed by the 2006 Nobel Peace Prize winner Mohammed Yunus of the Grameen Bank. It made available small amounts of money on credit so that women would be able to use their talents and gifts to develop small businesses to assist their families and the nation. Do you have any new economic ideas that would encourage respect for persons and economic development, especially in relation to women, to enhance the abilities of the people of Mexico (and other developing nations) so that Mexico and other countries may become more economically viable as nations?

Select Bibliography

Douglas, M., Uhl-Pierce, J., Rosenkoetter, M., et al. (2011). Standards of practice for culturally competent care: 2011 Update. *Journal of Transcultural Nursing,* 22(4), 317–333.

Gonzalez, F., Huynh-Nhu, L., & Perry, D. (2014). Using an optimality index to understand perinatal health disparities: A pilot study with Latina immigrants. *Journal of Transcultural Nursing,* 25(3), 265–272.

Koch, P. (2006). *The Aztecs, the Conquistadors, and the making of Mexican culture.* Jefferson, NC: McFarland & Company, Inc., Publishers.

Kovic, C. (2008). Jumping from a moving train: Risk, migration and rights at NAFTA's southern border. *Practicing Anthropology, 30*(2), 32–36.

Leininger, M. (1970). *Nursing and anthropology: Two worlds to blend.* New York: John Wiley & Sons, Inc.

Miller, J., Leininger, M., Leuning, C., Pacquiao, D., Andrews, M., Ludwig-Beymer, P., & Papadopoulos, I. (2008). Transcultural Nursing Society position statement on human rights. *Journal of Transcultural Nursing, 19*(1), 5–7.

Redfield, R. (1989). *The little community and peasant society and culture.* Chicago: University of Chicago Press. (Midway reprint ed.) (First published 1956)

Semotiuk, A. (2014). A promise kept: A tribute to a mother's love. North Charleston, SC: Create Space Independent Publishing Platform.

Speed, S. (2008). Human rights and the border wall. *Anthropology News, 29*(9), 25.

Sternberg, R.M., & Barry, C. (2011). Transnational mothers crossing the border and bringing their health care needs. *Journal of Nursing Scholarship, 43*(1):64–71.

Stephen, L. (2007). *Transborder lives.* Durham: Duke University Press.

Vila, P. (2003). *Ethnography at the border.* Minneapolis, MN: University of Minnesota Press.

Wood, A. (Ed.). (2004). *On the border: Society and culture between the United States and Mexico.* Boulder, CO: SR Books.

CHAPTER 9

A Vibrant African American Community: The 49ers and the Quest for Justice

*A*frican American culture is composed of a culturally dynamic number of communities that illuminate a living history of life as slaves to becoming free. The living history captures the past and the future in the present. The present highlights the changing sociocultural environment in North America, the Caribbean, South America, and other nations. The African American culture exhibits deep historical and social bonds, and global social networks since the time of the slave trade and the great Diaspora from Africa, which often resulted in forced migration, overpowering intercultural interaction, challenging geopolitical realities, and significant human rights issues. The African American culture in the United States is an integration of Africans from around the world. The African American 49ers in the following story illuminate the integration of the lives of African Americans and African Caribbeans. The African American 49ers have experienced discrimination; the changing nature of racism; the quest for justice; the changing family structure; and the challenging educational, legal, economic, and health systems. The following transcultural experience presents nurses and others with a story of courage and strength that brings to life the value of deep social bonds and unity and what that means for the contemporary world of vulnerable populations, health, and healing.

The African American 49ers' Story and Their Experiences in the Quest for Justice

The "49ers," is a group of seven African Americans, four men (formerly five with the passing of the Beloved Harold Braynon, JD in 2011) and three women in Miami, Florida. They have been meeting together and socializing for more than five decades. The group agreed to meet

223

with me in their meeting place, a restaurant near Little Haiti in Miami, Florida. The 49ers have been a community since attending and graduating in 1949 from Booker T. Washington High School, named after the prominent African American champion for African American education in the mid- to late 1800s. An African American nurse colleague of mine introduced me to them. Her mother is one of the 49ers. These fascinating people have lived and learned through their families' stories about slavery, their own lives of segregation and racism, the African American freedom struggle during the 1950s, the 1954 landmark legal decision of *Brown v. Board of Education*, the civil rights movement of the 1960s, the passing of the Civil Rights Act of 1964 (Pub.L. 88-352, 78 Stat/241, which outlawed discrimination on the basis of race, color, religion, sex, or national origin), the passing of the Voting Rights Act of 1965 (42 U.S.C.1973-1973bb-1, which prohibits racial discrimination, with changes most recently June 25, 2014 [http://www.thetakeaway.org/story/301459-voting-rights-act/]), and an African American running for and becoming the 44th President of the United States in 2009 and reelected in 2013.

Although their community and neighborhoods have changed, the 49ers gather from different parts of the city of Miami and region once a month for lunch to discuss the business of the organization of the 49ers, talk about the concerns of the day and the future, and reminisce about the past. They enjoy staying healthy and do many things to keep themselves in good health: fellowship, prayer, family gatherings, good food, visiting their doctors when necessary, taking medications as appropriate, continuing education, socializing with others, and traveling. Judge Harold Braynon, a former state of Florida assistant attorney general and judge and one of the 49ers, died in 2011. He left a lasting legacy for his family, community, the 49ers, and the state of Florida through his commitment to improving the lives of African Americans and others by protecting civil rights.

Bonding started early; they were always together from childhood and wanted to stay connected. As the members of the 49ers stated, they have and always have had a deep faith in God, in family, and in each other. One can see that they genuinely love each other as they interact together. They are an authentic community who enjoy talking, laughing, smiling, telling stories, and sharing jokes. The sensitive stories of family experiences of the great Diaspora from western Africa to the southern United States, to and from the Bahamas and other Caribbean nations, and finally to the city of Miami were gripping. Stories about education abounded because they were retired educators, counselors, a principal, coaches, a military officer, a state commissioner, and a lawyer; they also share memories from the life of late judge and former state of Florida Assistant Attorney General Braynon. They were highly influenced by their teachers at Booker T. Washington High School—teachers who always encouraged them no matter how hard the struggle to continue to have faith, to stay disciplined, and to pursue an education. The 49ers stated that before 1928, if black children wanted to go to high school, they would have had to leave home in Miami and go to Jacksonville, Florida. The north of Florida was considered in many ways to be the black South. Children could attend high school. However, in the black South at harvest time, schools were closed so children could work in the fields. At Booker T. Washington High School in Miami, the 49ers were proud that they did have their own high school despite the fact that they didn't have enough supplies and books. They were given "hand-me-downs" from the white schools. The group pointed out that they did not know that they were "disadvantaged or living in a ghetto" until they went to college and found out.

There was discrimination in what neighborhoods that they could go into, the kind of water fountain they could drink from (it was called colored water), the kinds of bathrooms they could use, or the kinds of businesses they could enter. Their educational home, Booker T. Washington High School, was a sanctuary for hope. It was similar to what Martin Luther King, Jr. said in 1963, that the South could hew "a stone of hope from segregation's mountain of despair." President Kennedy in a speech in 1963 stated that a "Negro" baby born in America had about

AUTHOR'S REFLECTION

Community is what is woven throughout the 49ers' stories and in their conversation. Community has many symbols and definitions. It is culture. It involves choice; it involves human relationships; it can be a location, a boundary, a place, or place making; it can be home to one or many; it can be where groups of people come together to negotiate competing visions for a particular goal or solve problems; and community can be an idea, a dream; and hope for the future (Cohen, 1989; Wirtz, 2008). For the 49ers, community meant human relationships. The motto of the 49ers is "Human relations is still the key to survival."

one-half as much chance of completing high school as a white baby born on the same day. This community of students showed that they could not only complete high school but also attend college because of sheer determination and commitment, even before the legislative reforms of the Civil Rights Act of 1964. They hope that this will be the same destiny for Booker T. Washington High School students today, for the Latinos who are the new immigrants from Central and South America.

Today, there is equal education, but when the 49ers were students, the motto was "separate but equal." In reality, it was "separate and unequal." As students and young people before the historical changes for equality and equal protection under the law, there was a sense of pride and respect for African American people in authority, ministers of the church, their parents, the principal, and their teachers, and tolerance to some degree for others. The 49ers are perplexed that despite success through the civil rights struggle and legislation, the ethics and morals of the black community have changed. They think that there is a breakdown in the family ("babies having babies"), in discipline, and in the value of education. Because the struggle is over, there is no longer motivation, one 49er said. The 49ers remarked that new generations of blacks do not believe what blacks went through because they have not experienced fierce discrimination, suffering, and challenges for equality. (However, we do see today that racial discrimination is very much "alive and well" and shows up in so many different components of society, such as the voting rights arena and within law enforcement.) The 49ers said that blacks do not have much of a community anymore, a community like they have experienced and supported for so many years. Overall, there is a lack of respect for teachers, one of the group remarked. The black teacher is no longer at the top of the pyramid for emulation as in days of old. There is a focus on money—money is what is fueling the dissension, and the drug trade.

As the 49ers reiterated, "discipline and respect start at home." If the child was disciplined at home, there would not be the problems of today. "Yes, Mother" is not as important as it once was. As a group, the 49ers are meeting each month, rededicating themselves to God and each other, and setting up scholarships for children and worthy organizations, such as the United Negro College Fund, and the Booker T. Washington High School Fund, and providing funds for organizations to conquer sickle cell anemia. In July 2009, the 49ers celebrated their 60th anniversary of community by attending many church services; enjoying a banquet; revisiting Virginia Beach, the only Atlantic Ocean beach in south Florida where, prior to civil rights' legislation, black people could swim; receiving awards and proclamations from councilpeople from the city of Miami and the governor of the state of Florida; and the promise to be honored at the White House under the direction of the staff of President Barack Obama, the first black President of the United States. (I was privileged to have been invited to the 49ers banquet and to be introduced to the group of class members who attended as a professor who was sharing their story of courage and hope with the world.) Their legacy lives on through their motto, "Human relations is still the key to survival!"

AUTHOR'S REFLECTION

The 49ers are members of a southeast Florida African American group who went to school together and remained a viable community ever since their graduation in 1949. As a group, they established a living history, a community of caring where they shared beliefs, values, opinions, and the lifeworld. They are representatives of the African American Diaspora, who were brought from Africa to the New World as slaves, and then migrated to different parts of the United States, the Caribbean, and other regions. The 49ers lived through many historical eras that marked their quest for justice: tolerating yet challenging the way in which all African Americans had to deal with discrimination and prejudice, changes in national policies, changes in family structure, and changes in paths to education and prosperity. Throughout all their struggles, the 49ers maintained their compassion for each other, their community, and the nation in which they live.

Transcultural Caring-Based Learning Approach

Please review the information about the Transcultural Caring Dynamics for Nursing and Health-Care Model, the assessment tools, the transcultural caring-based learning (TCCBL) approach, and the transcultural caring inquiry information explained in previous chapters of this book, including the purpose, goals, and objectives outlined in Section 2, Chapter 7, any other relevant literary and Internet information before dialoguing about this transcultural caring experience. In your small group, apply all the processes of the TCCBL approach and the transcultural caring inquiry in relation to this transcultural caring situation for pattern identification (i.e., pattern seeing, pattern mapping, pattern recognizing, and pattern transforming). Use dimensions of the Transcultural Caring Dynamics in Nursing and Health-Care Model and use the most appropriate assessment tools for transcultural evidence gathering.

Reflections with Questions

The reflections with questions that follow are guides that will assist you individually and collectively in your learning group with dialogue and interpretation of what is happening in the story; what is happening now in the African American community in Florida and around the United States, the Caribbean, and Canada; and what your responsibilities as a transcultural nurse should be.

Transcultural Nursing Reflections

- As a transcultural nurse, through compassion and the understanding of justice (i.e., fairness, human rights, representation, and political dialogue) contemplate how you can pursue knowledge of the history of segregation, racism, prolonged prejudice, and ways to initiate change and reconciliation by reflecting on the 49ers. How can transcultural nurses affect change that will improve the lifeworld of African Americans? How does a transcultural nurse become culturally competent (responsible) in the African American community? Imagine yourself as an African American going through slavery, separation from family and community, segregation, racism, prejudice, and struggles for civil rights. Also, imagine yourself as a white American at the time of the Civil War, during the time of reconstruction. Imagine yourself as a lawyer who is engaged in the fight to impede or improve legislation for equal protection under the law and equal rights. How do those personas speak to you?
- What do the concepts of being just and justice mean to you in African American history? What is the meaning of civil rights and how does that term differ from human rights? Do civil rights affect health care or nursing care?

- How can a transcultural nurse affect the political arena to contribute to the establishment of more fair and equitable health and social care? Share your views of discrimination and in relation to voting rights.
- What changes have appeared in the general family structure and the African American family, in the educational system, its structure and the nation from the time of "Jim Crow" through *Brown v. Board of Education* and the Civil Rights Act? How has education changed? What does it mean to be separate but equal or separate andunequal? Why do you think that this has happened not only in the United States but also in many parts of the world?
- How does discrimination marginalize a culture? Are we separated primarily by prejudice and/or by socioeconomics?
- What does being a vulnerable population mean to you?
- What do you think about the term "people of color"? Is this discriminatory or a fair term?
- What is the meaning of community, first, in the examples that are shared in this story and second, to you?
- What does "black folk" culture mean to you?
- How does the church help to build community?
- How do you envision bonding among the community?
- How is the sense of family and community changing in African American society, in American society, and in world society?
- What is changing in the meaning of interculturality/transculturality in the national and world communities?
- Articulate the changing nature of transcultural relationships in the United States and around the world especially under the leadership of President Barack Obama, the first African American president. Do you think that American society will be different following subsequent elections in the United States?
- Contemplate the meaning of culture as a transgenerational phenomenon. What central cultural values prevail, for example, in your own family culture, in your professional culture, in a hospital where you have practiced? What values are changing in American culture, African American culture? Why are they changing?
- What do elders who have gone through struggles have to teach the younger generation? What type of effect do elders have on family development? Can elders have an effect on "gang" development? How do grandparents, especially grandmothers, contribute to African American culture? How important is understanding differences in communication and/or means of expression or language?
- In this story, human relationships, faith in God, and meeting with each other as a community kept the 49ers healthy. What is the meaning of the black church in African American culture? What genetic history, physical and emotional changes, is occurring in the African American community that contributes to a healthy or an unhealthy lifestyle today?
- Are there differences between males and females in health issues? What are the major health concerns from gender perspectives, such as pregnancy, sexually transmitted diseases, hypertension, and diabetes? How is the American health-care system helping to address the health-care needs in black communities?
- Are there syndromes or problems that are prevalent, such as nutritional problems, cardiovascular problems, diabetes, sickle cell anemia, and sexually transmitted diseases? How are African Americans affected by HIV/AIDS? Is the population affected more or less by HIV/AIDS than any other population (see the Centers for Disease Control and Prevention Web site for the current information regarding HIV/AIDS. http://www.cdc.gov/hiv/default.html/
- Are there differences between northern and southern African American people in the United States? Is there a difference of social identity? Are there preferred ethnic/racial labels for blacks living in Canada or from the nation of Haiti?

AUTHOR'S REFLECTION

Transgenerational values are critical in the development of a family, a community, a nation. A culture is sustained by the values, beliefs, and attitudes that are transmitted from one to the other in a group over time: a family, members of a profession, (Morris, 2012), an organization, and a nation-state. A dynamic culture is transformed by spiritual-ethical communicative caring action—choices for healing, health, and well-being—transformation for the best possible future.

- How do the Haitian American and other Caribbean Americans, including Cuban and Puerto Ricans, differ from American black and African communities in their understanding of culture, history, geography, and geopolitical decisions for equality and freedom? Are there differences in social identity? Are there preferred ethnic/racial labels of the groups living in the United States? What are the language differences?
- Can you envision a notion of distributive justice for health care? How can you as a transcultural nurse affect the quality of care in African American communities? How does economics fit into the picture? How do educational opportunities fit into the picture? What transcultural caring activities would you engage in to improve the health and well-being of African American people and their families?
- As transcultural nurses, do we have a moral responsibility to examine the resources and facilitate improvement of health to black people? Examine the Human Rights document of the Transcultural Nursing Society (2008) and its update in 2011 (Douglas et al, 2011) and determine if or how the precepts are put into practice within the views identified in this narrative.

Select Bibliography

Arrighi, B. (Ed.). (2007). *Understanding inequality: The intersection of race/ethnicity, class, and gender* (2nd ed.). Boulder, CO: Rowman & Littlefield Publishers, Inc.

Brown v. Board of Education, 347 U.S. 483 (1954).

Brown, D., & Webb, C. (2007). *Race in the American south: From slavery to civil rights*. Gainesville, FL: University Press of Florida.

Civil Rights Act of 1964, Pub. L. No. 88-353, 78 Stat. 241 (1964).

Civil Rights Act of 1964, 42, U.S.C. § 1971 *et seq.* (1988).

Cohen, A. (1989). *The symbolic construction of community*. New York: Routledge.

Douglas, M., Uhl-Pierce, J., Rosenkoetter, M., et al. (2011). Standards of practice for culturally competent care: 2011 update. *Journal of Transcultural Nursing*, 22(4), 317–333.

Dunn, M. (1997). *Black Miami in the twentieth century (Florida history and culture)*. Gainesville, FL: University Press of Florida.

Frymer, P. (2014). Uneasy alliances: Race and party competition in America. Princeton, NJ: Princeton University Press.

Miller, J., Leininger, M., Leuning, C., Pacquiao, D., Andrews, M., Ludwig-Beymer, P., & Papadopoulos, I. (2008). Transcultural Nursing Society position statement on human rights. *Journal of Transcultural Nursing*, 19(1), 5–7.

Morris, E. (2012). Respect, protection, faith and love: Major care constructs identified within the subculture of selected urban Agrican American adolescent gang members. *Journal of Transcultural Nursing*, April 3, 2012. doi: 10,1177/1043659612441014.

Ray, M., & Turkel, M. (2014). Caring as emancipatory nursing praxis: The theory of relational caring complexity. *Advances in Nursing Science, 37*(2), 132–146.

Robinson, E. (2011). *Disintegration: The splintering of Black America.* New York: Anchor Books.

Tarrant-Reid, L. (2012). *Discovering Black America: From the age of exploration to the twenty-first century.* New York: Abrams.

Voting Rights Act of 1965 (42 U.S.C. 1973m 1973bb-1), Enacted by the 89th Congress of the United States to enforce the 15th Amendment of the Constitution of the United States.

Wirtz, K. (2008). RACE: Are we so different: A community-wide collaboration. *Anthropology News, 49*(9), 15.

Woodward, C. (1955/2001). *The strange career of Jim Crow.* Oxford: Oxford University Press. (Commemorative Edition)

Web Listings

Centers for Disease Control and Prevention, Department of Health and Human Services, www.cdc.gov

U.S. Government, www.usa.gov

HIV surveillance special report: Behavioral and clinical characteristics of persons receiving medical care for HIV infection 2012. Retrieved from http://www.cdc.gov/hiv/pdf/library/reports/surveillance/cdc-hiv-hssr_mmp_2012.pdf

Voting Rights Act: Can Congress act to save it? The Take Away, June 26, 2014. Retrieved http://www.thetakeaway.org/story/301459-voting-rights-act/

CHAPTER 10

The Story of a Guatemalan Mayan Farmworker

Guatemalan Mayans are members of an ancient aboriginal culture with a diverse tribal cultural history, many dialects and languages, a complex civilization, and a rich intellectual foundation, which includes the calendar based upon the length of the day, great temples and edifices, exquisite ruins, a blend of traditional and Christian religions, sacred rituals, a healthcare system of the hot-and-cold theory of health and illness, and a courageous migration to the developed world. Guatemala borders southern Mexico, where many Guatemalans find themselves en route to the United States. Often they are affected by the immigration policies of Mexico and overwhelmed by the drug cartels and violence in the country as well as in all of Central America (including Honduras and El Salvador) (Kovic, 2008). Guatemalan-Mayans leave their native land to find work in the fields of North America, especially southeast Florida where they first contributed to farmworking by picking oranges and then began to accomplish other service-related occupations, such as lawn care, to make a living. The emigration of Guatemalan Mayans from Guatemala to find a better way of life began in the 1980s after a brutal civil war in Guatemala. Some of the people in the United States are undocumented while others are documented or legal immigrants. The following is the transcultural caring experience of Kinich, a young Mayan husband and father whose heritage is the ancient, aboriginal Quiche tribe (the Cakchiquel [Kaqchike]) and the Tzutuhil) from the highlands of western Guatemala. Many of Kinich's relatives are from the Yucatan Peninsula, where much migration took place before and after the Spanish conquest of the region in about 1532.

Kinich's Story

Kinich (a name from the Mayan god of the sun) left Guatemala for south Florida to earn a better living for his family by picking vegetables. When he said goodbye to his wife and his three children in Guatemala they were hoping that after he knew more about his new

230

community, he could bring them to live with him. (We do not know if Kinich is documented or undocumented in the United States.) Kinich missed his family so much, and at night after a 12-hour day, Kinich did not much care for the barracks-type living that he shared with other men next to the farm where they worked. (Not all people lived in barracks-type dwellings. Some Guatemalan families lived together in all age ranges in this area of southeast Florida, too. [See Mayan Ministry, Diocese of Palm Beach, Lake Worth, Florida, mayaministry@aol.com].). In the barracks, men huddled together to share stories of their lives "back home" in the many different small communities of Guatemala. They spoke with many Mayan dialects. Sometimes they could not understand each other, which did not help to build a unified community. But they still tried. They had a common bond of survival; the ability to endure pain and suffering; and from their past, a deep religious respect for ancestral bonds with the dead. They or their families all suffered from some kind of persecution by centuries-old oppression and guerilla tactics. And now, from what they had learned, many of the families in their home country were suffering from the negative influence of drug cartels and violence, including murder and rape. There were so many legends and mysteries of the ancient Mayan people that they had in their memories and they tried to talk as best they could with each other about them.

Sometimes they would talk about all the things they could buy after they were paid, especially the "high-tech" things. Sometimes the men, especially the Ladinos (people who reject the ancient Mayan traditions) would drink alcohol and occasionally fight. Kinich was afraid when drinking got out of hand. Their experiences in the fields, the long hours, and fear of the pesticides that were put on the plants and soil that they knew they were breathing when they picked the vegetables also became part of their storytelling. They even talked about how hard it was to have time to eat and use the bathroom. Their boss from the farm corporation was humane but strict.

In the barracks, there was even talk about prostitutes employed by the men. Kinich did not want to break his sacred vows of marriage. He had a strong faith that combined Catholicism with some of the ancient Mayan spiritual beliefs, especially of the hot-and-cold theory as the cause of or what influenced health and illness (disease). Kinich also was aware that some of the men in the barracks had already been infected with sexually transmitted diseases (STDs) and had to go to the Covenant of Caring Health-Care Clinic managed by nurse practitioners, nurses, doctors, dentists, and others. It was about a mile away from the farm. Kinich heard that there was even someone at the clinic who spoke his dialect of the Mayan language. He also heard that the clinic stayed open in the evening to help the farmworkers who needed care. Kinich had a chronic cough and bad teeth from smoking and no dental care throughout his life. He never really had much attention from a health-care professional or traditional healer in the past. Sometimes Kinich had toothaches and thought that maybe he could go to the clinic at some time. He heard that whoever worked at the clinic cared for everyone and never turned anyone away. He was scared though. Kinich decided to ask his supervisor if someone could drive him to the clinic. He wanted to get something for his cough, and get his teeth checked because he felt like they were causing him so much pain. When he spit, the mucus was greenish-brown. One day, one of the supervisors did take Kinich to the clinic. The staff was very friendly, a few spoke Spanish, and one of the nurses did speak the Mayan dialect that he knew. He was so happy. He could tell his story of his bad teeth, his cough and his loneliness for his family. He knew that he had to work in the fields to make money to live and send home. But he hated the barracks life and wanted to be safe with his wife and three children.

Transcultural Caring-Based Learning Approach

Please review the information about the Transcultural Caring Dynamics for Nursing and Health-Care Model, the assessment tools, the transcultural caring-based learning (TCCBL) approach, and the transcultural caring inquiry information explained in previous chapters of this book, and other relevant literary and Internet information before dialoguing about this transcultural caring experience. In your small group, apply the TCCBL approach, and all other processes in relation to your transcultural caring situation for pattern identification (i.e., pattern seeing, pattern mapping, pattern recognizing, and pattern transforming). Use dimensions of the Transcultural Caring Dynamics in Nursing and Health-Care Theory and Model and use the most appropriate assessment tools for transcultural evidence gathering.

Reflections with Questions

The reflections that follow are guides that will assist you individually and collectively in your learning group with dialogue and interpretation of what is happening in the story; what is happening now in the Mayan community and in the farmworker community in the United States, Guatemala, Honduras, El Salvador, Mexico, and Canada; what the ethnonursing method can do; and what your responsibilities as a transcultural nurse are or should be. Give attention to the ancient culture. Focus on migration patterns and on reasons why Central American migrants, especially Guatemalan Mayans, risk their lives to come to the United States. As a transcultural caring nurse, consider your responsibilities to understand human rights, the voices of the oppressed, immigration issues, immigration policy, and health-care problems of Guatemalan and other Mexican and Central American migrants in the United States.

Transcultural Nursing Reflections

For this transcultural caring experience, imagine yourself as student nurse researcher who has been selected to work with one's professor on a research study at the Covenant of Caring Health-Care Clinic. You have been asked to help conduct a mini-qualitative research study with your professor using Leininger's ethnonursing method (McFarland & Wehbe-Alamah, 2015; Ray, Morris, & McFarland, 2013).

The goal of the Covenant of Caring Health-Care Clinic is to provide health and nursing care, and dental services to the farmworkers in the immediate area. As a student in the clinic you have been asked to follow Kinich's case (with a staff nurse and your professor who is conducting qualitative research in environmental health in the clinic and from the farm itself).

Examine Kinich's story and determine what his health and nursing care needs might be. You have studied transcultural nursing and learned about the multicultural area of south Florida and other communities. Since the culture of the Guatemalan Mayan farmworker community in the area is unique, you are anxious to interact with Kinich and learn more about his culture. You and your staff nurse are being assigned an interpreter (fluent in the many Mayan dialects; there are more than 22) to assist you with communication. The interpreter will help you phrase questions and help you with "field notetaking" (a dimension of the ethnonursing methodology).

Along with discovering Kinich's physical and dental care needs and investigating his chronic cough and discolored sputum, you are asked to compile diverse information about the Guatemalan Mayan culture, the culture of farmworkers in south Florida and in the United States, the culture of poverty in America, and the migration patterns of the Mayan and other Central American people. You will be gaining experience in initial qualitative research. You will be using the late Dr. Madeleine Leininger's ethnonursing method (observation of the cultural environment [in this case, the farm where Kinich works and his living quarters], participation with the subject or respondent through interviewing and field notetaking, and reflection on and interpretation of the data collected [OPR]). This approach focuses on analysis of and reflection on the observations and interview data, followed by interpretation to generate themes and patterns of the culture to generate change or improvement in health and transcultural nursing care. You have some orientation to this approach to qualitative investigation in your research classes. You know that your professor has gone to the Institutional Review Board of the university to gain permission to conduct the ethnonursing study. You also know that your professor and you need informed consent to interview any subject. Your professor has designed about 10 research questions for you to use and a survey tool to collect population data about the Guatemalan Mayan people. You are excited about the reality of doing ethnonursing research and thinking about going with your professor to see the corporate owner to gain permission to observe the workers in the vegetable field and to discuss the farmworker community with Kinich. Given that the Institutional Review Board has given their consent to your professor and to you as a student research assistant, you also have approval to seek Kinich's story with an interpreter after informed consent signatures. Within the framework, you have permission to observe and collect data at the clinic. You have gone over the list of research questions to ask Kinich (with the interpreter) and, at the same time, have found a place in the clinic to do some participant observation.

- What do you think is contributing to Kinich's physical problems, his cough and the yellow-brown sputum caused by a chronic pulmonary condition? What do you think are his dental needs? What may be the unique health-care concerns of this Guatemalan Mayan man highlighted in this example, such as physical (especially respiratory and dermatological), dental, and nutritional needs?
- As a transcultural nurse, how much can or would you be prepared to support Kinich and speak to his needs and other farmworkers after the study is complete?
- What other issues, especially economic, could affect Kinich as an individual and his family who is not with him? What are the unique cultural, linguistic, and spiritual dimensions that are part of Kinich's life?
- What type of health-care system would you project is in force in the Covenant of Caring Health-Care Clinic?
- What is the function of a local clinic health-care system? Are there rules that link clinics to local public health departments? What is the state of the health insurance system in this area? What transportation services, if any, should be available at the clinic?
- What health and community resources would be available for Kinich and the other members of farmworker communities, especially those who may have contracted HIV/AIDS or STDs?
- What respiratory health problems might the farmworkers have contracted?
- Does a nurse have a responsibility to examine the resources and facilitate improvement of health care for people of migrant cultures? (See Goodman & Noriega's [2015] Guatemalan primary care guidelines and compare to United States' health care.)
- What is occupational health?
- What is the responsibility of nurses caring for the earth or understanding "ecological nursing"?
- Does a corporation have responsibility for occupational health—to protect people who are working for them and help people with their health problems if the job is contributing to the health-care problems? What type of health-care insurance might be available? What political and economic evaluative information of farmworker sociocultural communities would you seek? Is there farmworker health-care data available?
- How is the health-care system different in the farmworker community in the United States compared to another farmworker community, for example, in southern Ontario, Canada? Are there farmworker advocacy groups (i.e., grassroots organizations) to ensure more just actions for farmworkers?
- What is the North American Free Trade Agreement (NAFTA) about? What provisions of this agreement may affect this situation? What other laws in the United States or in North America affect migrant communities?

Select Bibliography

Andrews, M., & Boyle, J. (Eds.). (2007). *Transcultural concepts in nursing care* (5th ed.). Philadelphia, PA: Lippincott Williams & Wilkins.

Barry, C., & Kronk, P. (1993). *Nursing Guatemalan families using Leininger's culture care theory.* In M. Parker (Ed.), Patterns of nursing theories in practice (pp. 142–156). New York, NY: National League for Nursing Press.

Coe, M. (2005). *The Maya* (7th ed.). London: Thames & Hudson.

Goodman, R., & Noriega, S., (2015). *Culturally specific guidelines for primary care in rural Guatemala.* Columbus, OH: The Educational Publishers, Inc.

Herp, C. (1996). *Meaning of folk and professional health care experienced by Guatemalan Mayans in southeast Florida.* Master of science in nursing thesis, Florida Atlantic University, Boca Raton, FL.

Kovic, C. (2005). Mayan voices for human rights: Displaced Catholics in Chiapas, Mexico. Austin: University of Texas Press.

Kovic, C. (2008). Jumping from a moving train: Risk, migration and rights at NAFTA's southern border. *Practicing anthropology, 30*(2), 32–36.

Leininger, M., & McFarland, M. (Eds.). (2006). *Culture Care diversity and universality: A worldwide theory of nursing* (2nd ed.). Sudbury, MA: Jones & Bartlett Publishing Company. [Ethnonursing method included]

McFarland, M., & Wehbe-Alamah, H. (2015). *Leininger's culture care diversity and universality: A worldwide nursing theory.* Burlington, MA: Jones & Bartlett Learning.

Nazario, S. (2007). *Enrique's journey.* New York, NY: Random House, Inc.

North American Free Trade Agreement (NAFTA), January 1, 1994. Retrieved April 25, 2008, from http://www.fas.usda.gov/itp/Policy/NAFTA/nafta.asp

Ordonez, M. (2006). *The lived experience of health among older Guatemalan women.* Master of Science thesis. Florida Atlantic University, The Christine E. Lynn College of Nursing, Boca Raton, FL.

Purnell, L. (2001). Guatemalans' practices for health promotion and the meaning of respect afforded by health care providers. *Journal of Transcultural Nursing, 12*(1), 40–47.

Ray, M., Morris, E., & McFarland, M. (2013). Ethnonursing method of Dr. Madeleine Leininger. In C. Beck (Ed.). *Routledge international handbook of qualitative research.* London: Routledge.

Rogers, M. (1970). *An introduction to the theoretical basis of nursing.* Philadelphia: F. A. Davis Company.

Schuster, E., & Brown, C. (Eds.) (1994). *Exploring our environmental connections.* New York: National League for Nursing Press.

Sharer, R., & Traxlor, L. (2005). *The ancient Maya* (5th ed.). Stanford, CA: Stanford University Press.

Speed, S. (2006). At the crossroads of human rights and anthropology: Toward a critically engaged activist research. *American Anthropologist, 108*(1), 66–76.

CHAPTER 11

The Transcultural Social and Health Experience of an Asian Indian Widow

*T*he Asian Indian culture has been a source of great intrigue over the course of its history. India is the world's largest democracy and an international economic and technological culture. At the same time, many of its people continue to live in poverty and are illiterate. Major cultural phenomena have a great effect on the lifeworld of Indians within India and abroad: the Hindu religion, the oldest existing religion in the world of the non-Biblical tradition; the caste system, stable for more than 2 centuries, but now changing under Indian government rule; the configuration of linguistic regions in India; the traditional role of marriage that controls family, lineage, and kinship structure; the strength of the mother-son relationship; the changing role of women and widows in the new India; and the rise of the modern economic society since gaining independence from Britain. The following is a story of an Asian Indian widow who came to the United States for support and care from her son. Her story represents the changing role of widows in India and the traditional mother-son relationship in the Indian family structure.

Lakshmi's Story

Lakshmi, a 72-year-old Hindu woman from Hyderabad, India, became widowed 12 years ago when her husband died in her arms of a sudden heart attack. She was deeply grief-stricken. Two years into her widowhood, after being told she had three blocked coronary arteries that required surgical intervention, Lakshmi sold most of her belongings and moved to a home for the aged on the outskirts of the city. Very different from the grand home she shared with her husband's family, she lived in a one-room apartment with a hot plate to make tea and a small refrigerator where she stored those favorite foods not available in the

235

communal dining hall. She spent her days reading and entertaining friends from the home for the aged and a few visitors from her old neighborhood who were able to make the hour-long trip.

Once a well-known singer whose voice could be heard in many Hindi films, Lakshmi played her harmonium, an accordion-like instrument, and sang the old songs that made her famous. Her only child, a son living in Atlanta, Georgia, repeatedly urged her to come to the United States to have the cardiac surgery she needed and move in with him and his family. Although her mobility was severely restricted because of her heart condition, Lakshmi made the trip from India and was promptly admitted to the hospital for preoperative testing. Lakshmi expressed fear that she would not survive the surgery or, worse yet, that she would become a burden to her son and his family. She also understood from widow friends who have moved to the United States that Asian Indian widows, although treated well by most Americans, were often discriminated against by fellow Asian Indians when it came to participating in Hindu religious activities and other things. While Lakshmi felt the occasional sting of discrimination in India because of her widow status, for the most part, she was able to live her life as she liked and was surprised and disappointed to find that some Asian Indians had chosen to carry the "old ways" to their new home in the United States.

Transcultural Caring-Based Learning Approach

Please review the information about the Transcultural Caring Dynamics for Nursing and Health-Care Theory and Model, the assessment tools, the transcultural caring-based learning (TCCBL) approach, and the transcultural caring inquiry information explained in previous chapters of this book and any other relevant literary and Internet information before dialoguing about the transcultural caring experience. In your small group, apply the TCCBL approach, and other processes in relation to your transcultural caring situation for pattern identification (i.e., pattern seeing, pattern mapping, pattern recognizing, and pattern transforming). Use dimensions of the Transcultural Caring Dynamics in Nursing and Health-Care Model and use the most appropriate assessment tools for transcultural evidence gathering. The Reflections with Questions section that follows is a guide that will assist you individually and collectively in your learning group with dialogue and interpretation of what is happening to the Indian widow as she reflects on her past history and present situation.

Reflections with Questions

Reflect on the changing history of India and the changing history and migration patterns of Asian Indians in the United States and other parts of the Western world, and consider the need for advanced cardiac surgery and care. Focus some attention on the role of women and widows in India, and on the rich cultural heritage of India, including dress, languages, religion, foods, and health care. What are your responsibilities as a transcultural nurse in understanding the changing nature of Indian culture?

Transcultural Nursing Reflections

- In your small learning group, determine how you would interact with Lakshmi if you were her primary nurse (and discharge planner) in the cardiac clinic of the American hospital. What transcultural caring thoughts come to your mind about Lakshmi? What human and literary (also, Internet) resources would you use to assist you in your evaluation of the caring needs of Lakshmi?
- What actions (compassion and justice) were exhibited in this transcultural experience by Lakshmi's son and his family? Describe the kinship structure of India and, in particular, the role sons play with regard to Indian widows. When contemplating the process of Lakshmi's move from India to Atlanta, Georgia, what issues come to mind?

- What is the population of India? What is the level of poverty and illiteracy in India? Compare and contrast Hyderabad, India with other Indian cities, for instance, those in the north? What is the official language of India? What are the dominant languages spoken in Hyderabad; in the north of India? What are the main industries and compare them with Mumbai or New Delhi?

- Identify central precepts of the Hindu religion. As a Hindu woman, what are the dominant characteristics or tenets of Hinduism that would be important to Lakshmi in India and in the United States?

- What is the caste system (i.e., *varna*, *jat*, or social-ranking system for occupations) and what is its effect on Indian society? What is meant by scheduled caste and scheduled tribe? How has the caste system influenced the lives of Indian widows? How is the caste system changing in modern India?

- Discuss the changing roles of women in contemporary India, women's influence on society, and women's participation in the Indian music and film industries. How do these lifeworld experiences of Lakshmi differ from perceptions you may have had of Asian Indian women?

- Contemplate the changing nature of widowhood in India. What are some of the traditional images of widowhood in India and how have they changed over time? What are the images of widowhood that this story presents?

- What gerontological support systems are available in India for older Indian widows? How would the home for the aged where Lakshmi lived in Hyderabad differ from traditional living arrangements for Indian widows in India?

- When we examine Lakshmi's lifeworld, what are the losses she has endured and how might you expect she has coped with them? What are the laws and practices influencing remarriage in India?

- What are the migratory patterns of Asian Indians to North America (Canada and the United States)? What are potential discriminatory issues Lakshmi may face if she makes a permanent move to the United States? Where, in other parts of the world, are Asian Indians concentrated?

- Lakshmi has come for cardiac care and support at the urging of her son. Reflect upon yourself as a cardiac care nurse and rehabilitation nurse. As a cardiac care nurse, how would you engage in transcultural caring to assist Lakshmi? What is the meaning of "technological' caring? Project Lakshmi's health and nursing care needs with a diagnosis of "blocked coronary arteries" (coronary artery disease [CAD] or atherosclerosis). Discuss the effects of CAD. What are the signs and symptoms? What is angina pectoris? What is ischemia? What diagnostic tests would Lakshmi have to confirm a diagnosis? What is enhanced external counterpulsation (EECP); which may help in the care of Lakshmi? As a cardiac and vascular nurse, is this procedure recommended by cardiologists? Explain some central aspects of a balloon angioplasty with or without stents. What is transmyocardial laser revascularization or TMR? What is "angiogenesis," which can be used to trigger the heart to grow new blood vessels to increase blood flow to the heart muscle? What medications will Lakshmi have to take to assist her with CAD?

- What are the holistic nursing caring (i.e., body, mind, and spirit) needs of Lakshmi? Project the caring needs of Lakshmi in a cardiovascular intensive care unit. How should Lakshmi's spiritual needs be honored? What rehabilitative caring interventions can you identify that would benefit Lakshmi postprocedures or postsurgery?

- India has a rich cultural and religious history in South Asia. What are India's major religions other than Hinduism?

- What are the main languages spoken in India?

- What roles did the British, Dutch, Portuguese, and French play in Indian history? When did India gain its independence from Britain? And why?

- What influence did Mahatma Gandhi have on Indian history?
- Describe India's relationship with Pakistan.
- Who are the Sikhs and what is their role in Indian society? Where are the Sikhs most concentrated outside India?
- What is India's position in the globalizing world? What is India's relationship with western nations? What is meant by the term "outsourcing" and how does it relate to the Indian economy and globalization?
- How is the health-care system changing in India? Compare and contrast traditional Indian medical systems, such as ayurvedic medicine, with allopathic medical and health-care practices.
- What is the level of poverty in the country?
- How is the nursing profession perceived in India as compared with the United States or Canada? Are there many Indian Americans and Indian Canadians who have chosen nursing as their profession? Why are Indian nurses so important to the West? As the nursing shortage vacillates in the United States and Canada, how many nurses are recruited from India to each country? Are there ethical issues recruiting from India when the country itself is in a nursing shortage?

Select Bibliography

Barnard, A., & Locsin, R. (2007). *Technology and nursing: Practice, concepts and issues*. London: Palgrave Macmillan.

Cameron, M. (1998). *On the edge of auspiciousness: Gender and caste in Nepal*. Urbana & Chicago, IL: The University of Illinois Press.

Chen, M. (2000). *Perpetual mourning: Widowhood in rural India*. New Delhi: Oxford University Press.

Czerenda, A.J. (2006). *"The show must go on": A caring inquiry into the meaning of widowhood and health for older Indian widows*. Dissertation Abstracts International, 67B (06), AAT 3222085.

Czerenda, A. J. (2010). The meaning of widowhood and health to older middle-class widows living in a south Indian community. *Journal of Transcultural Nursing*, 21(4):351–360.

Huyler, S. (1999). *Meeting God: Elements of Hindu devotion*. New Haven, CT: Yale University Press.

Karve, I. (2002). The kinship map of India. In P. Uberoi (Ed.), *Family, kinship and marriage in India* (pp. 50–73). New Delhi: Oxford University Press. (Original work published 1993)

Klostermaier, K. (2003). *A Short History of Hinduism*. Oxford: Oneworld Publications.

Lamb, S. (2000). *White saris and sweet mangoes*. Berkeley, CA: University of California Press.

Locsin, R. (2005). *Technological competency as caring in nursing: A model for practice*. Indianapolis: Sigma Theta Tau, International.

Luce, E. (2012). *In spite of the gods: The rise of modern India*. New York: Doubleday, Anchor Books.

Rajadhyaksha, N. (2007). *The rise of India: Its transformation from poverty to prosperity*. Singapore: John Wiley & Sons (Asia), Pte, Ltd.

CHAPTER 12

The Cultural, Health-Care, and Intermigration Experience of a Filipino Nurse

*T*he Philippines is an important country in "New World" and Pacific Region explo-ration and development. It is a nation of many islands with a population of more than 88 million people. Their heritage is primarily Malay, Indonesian, and mainland Chinese and their religion is primarily Catholic because of the influence of Spain. The history of the Philippines is divided into four distinct phases: the pre-Spanish period before 1521; the Spanish period from 1521 to 1898; the American period from 1898 to 1946; and the postin-dependence period from 1946 to the present. Because the Philippines played a dominant role in United States history, especially during the World War II era, there is a close tie between the two countries. A quest for independence from the United States military enterprises at Clark Air Force Base and Subic Bay Naval Base brought many changes to the region; however, given the changes occurring in the geopolitics of the Pacific region, with regard to economics and security, an approach to co-creating new ways of interaction and under-standing is advancing. Also, the quest for independence on the part of Muslim groups in the southern islands is challenging the Republic of the Philippines. Again leaders are trying to find new ways of understanding how people who share diverse religious and cultural values can live and grow together peacefully.

Migration to the United States and other developed countries is continuous. Filipino nurses have been migrating to America for more than 5 decades and have contributed to nursing and have helped sustain the Philippine economy (PNAA, 2014). Filipino nurses have been significant to the profession of nursing in this country because of their advanced nursing education and their command of the English language. They have contributed greatly to providing nursing care in many hospitals and health-care agencies. However, *nurses from the United States and the Philippines currently are coming together to dialogue about how to ensure that the Philippine Health Services have an effective nursing workforce in the Philippines to put into practice the Human Resource for Health Master Plan (2005–2030—Reformulated) (The Philippine Nurses Association of America, 2014). In the following story, Agnes shares her life of courage, determination, hope, and integrity. While Agnes has achieved so much in her chosen country, she longs to return to the Philippines to serve the poor there with her love, commitment, and knowledge.*

Agnes' Story

Agnes was born in a small town in the Philippines, a country composed of many islands in Southeast Asia. Agnes was a member of a large Catholic family, the fourth child of nine children, seven brothers and one sister. Her father was a lawyer and a judge in the municipal courts of two towns. Her mother graduated in home economics and fulfilled her teaching role as a mother in the home. Agnes's parents emphasized family values of honesty, solidarity, humility, fairness, and righteousness. The children were all given responsibilities to accomplish.

Agnes's heritage is Chinese and Spanish; her father's kin came from China and her mother's from Spain. They spoke Tagalog and a dialect called Pangasinan at home and English at school. Their father insisted that they write letters in English. Agnes's father had the greatest influence on her life. As a humble, fair, and honest man, she learned so much from him. He served the poor and underserved by helping them with their legal problems or anything else that they needed to talk about. There were long lines at the house. He did not charge for his services and felt that serving the poor was serving God. The people thanked her father with gifts of fruit, vegetables, fish, and sometimes chickens. The best advice her father gave her was to value education. All the brothers and sisters were given the opportunity to go to school and their father always said that it was their ticket to start their own lives.

And Agnes did just that. After receiving her bachelor of science in nursing (BSN) in 1978, she volunteered for 6 months to work in one of the remotest/poorest areas of her hometown. She worked as a community health nurse, delivering babies and providing home visits to sick people. She also worked in a public health agency giving immunizations and educating people on health problems. From there, Agnes went to Manila and worked in a Catholic pediatric hospital where, after a few months, she became a charge nurse.

Overall, when Agnes was growing up, health care in the Philippines was difficult to access for both professional and poor people. It was expensive; there was no health insurance. Often the doctor came to the house and often did not charge for services. Agnes's mother cooked special food and delivered it to the doctor's house as a "thank-you" for the services to their family. When hospitalization was needed, rather than go to the one hospital in their town, they went to Manila because many of the doctors in the hospital were members of the family or were friends of the family. They either paid for the services in cash or received the services for free if they were family. Influence and corruption were big in the Philippines; however, things have been changing in the country in recent years because of increased economic development.

Agnes applied for a visa to the United States in 1980. She had only $100 in her pocket when she arrived in Florida to work in a nursing home. She did not have enough money to rent an apartment but soon, after living in a supervisor's home, and after securing a second job, she was able to get an apartment and buy a car (she had to learn to drive). One experience that prompted her to buy a car was when she was threatened at knifepoint by a former employee Agnes had terminated for sleeping on the job. Agnes had to adjust to cultural changes in the United States. She was married in 1984 to a Caucasian American and had three wonderful boys. When her boys were younger, they didn't understand their mixed cultural background of Filipino and Caucasian. When they went to school, Agnes told them that they are "Americano" people. The term gave them joy and a sense of identity. Agnes completed a master of science in nursing (MSN) program in nursing administration.

Agnes is always thinking about family back home. She set aside an emergency fund for her family in the Philippines. The money is available for family members either to borrow or use in any way. She has a system of "pay it forward" so that rather than paying it back, a family member who has borrowed the money can later "adopt" a brother, sister, niece, or cousin and assist him or her with tuition fees or medical expenses.

Agnes's dream is to return to the Philippines and serve the poor and underserved as her father did. Following in the footsteps of missionaries of the past who have served the poor, such as Saint Mother Teresa, Agnes would like to go a remote area and provide nursing, spiritual comfort, and social services to the needy. The needs are still as great as when she was young. The hospitals today, particularly in the city of Manila, are both private and public. Agnes said that if you do not have any money, you go to the public hospital; otherwise you have to pay for hospitalization at the private hospital. There is some health insurance coverage but, for the most part, people who have some money pay for their care. Physicians' fees are high in public hospitals as they are in the private hospitals. Nurses are educated with a BSN in the Philippines. But often, they want to leave for the United States, usually because they have family members in the country, or are recruited to come to the United States to fill the gap in the shortage of nurses. In the modern era, there are many cultural changes in the social and technological dimensions in the Philippines. There are a lot of courses in electronics and computer technology. Mostly everyone has a cell phone. The family life has changed, and women have gained more independence. There continues to be great emphasis on going abroad and earning money and sending financial assistance back home. But at the same time, there is a longing for home and family.

Transcultural Caring-Based Learning Approach

Please review the information about the Transcultural Caring Dynamics for Nursing and Health-Care Theory and Model, the assessment tools, the transcultural caring-based learning (TCCBL) approach, and the transcultural caring inquiry information explained in previous chapters of this book, and any other relevant literary and Internet information before dialoguing about this transcultural caring experience. In your small group, apply the TCCBL approach, and all processes in relation to your transcultural caring situation for pattern identification (i.e., pattern seeing, pattern mapping, pattern recognizing, and pattern transforming). Use dimensions of the Transcultural Caring Dynamics in Nursing and Health-Care Model and use the most appropriate assessment tools for transcultural evidence gathering.

Reflections with Questions

After reviewing the story of Agnes in your small group, reflect upon what would it be like to be Agnes, living in a small town in the Philippines, working with the poor, then leaving home and coming to the United States with little money, getting a nursing job, marrying an American, and raising biracial and bicultural children. Perhaps you have experienced leaving your country or place of birth, leaving family, and creating your own family far away; perhaps you have had similar experiences in language challenges; perhaps you have had your own transcultural challenges of nursing when working in a hospital in the United States or Canada.

Transcultural Nursing Reflections

* In your small group, what transcultural caring thoughts come to your mind about this story of Agnes? When contemplating the process of migration of Agnes to the United States,

what ideas come to your mind about her story, her immediate family, and her family in the Philippines? What is most significant of the migratory process from the Philippines? How would this compare with other Southeast Asian nations? What has been the significance for nursing and health care in the past 5 decades of emigration from the Philippines and immigration to the United States and Canada?

- Discuss the strength of nursing in the Philippines through information gleaned from the Philippine Nurses Association, university schools or faculties of nursing, and interaction with Filipino nurses.
- What are the bicultural images that this story presents?
- What caring actions (i.e., compassion and justice) were exhibited in this transcultural experience by Agnes for her family with her own children and her family in the Philippines?
- How do the spiritual values of the past influence the way in which Agnes lives her life and desires to cocreate her future by adding to her education and thoughts of returning to the Philippines to serve the poor people? What values continue to help her?
- Can you contemplate the meaning of "back home," "longing to return home," or the notion of "returning to roots" for an immigrant?
- How important is the meaning of community for an immigrant or a new citizen of the United States?
- What is the meaning of potentially having financial freedom from Agnes's viewpoint?
- What is unique about the Filipino American culture within cultures—Filipino American culture within the culture of the United States?
- What is the health-care system in the Philippines? Compare and contrast the system with the United States.
  What components advanced in the chapters in this book contribute to understanding Agnes and her Filipino American extended-family experience?
- Project what gerontological health needs may be forthcoming for Agnes's family in the Philippines.
- What are the kinship structures identified in Agnes's story—her own nuclear Filipino American family, her extended family in the Philippines, and projections for the future of serving the poor as a missionary from a religious community "back home"?
- What does poverty mean to you; to being poor in Canada or in the United States; to being poor in a developing country, such as the Republic of the Philippines?
- With the nursing shortage vacillating each year in the United States and Canada, approximately how many nurses per year may be recruited from the Philippines to each country in the West? What are the ethics of recruiting nurses from the developing world to serve the needs of people of means in the Western nations? What is the responsibility of the agencies that recruit nurses?
- How would you work with nurses from a different culture? How would you help nurses understand the multiculturalism of the United States? How would you deal with the potential culture-value conflict? How could you tap the resources of nurses from other cultures in flexibility or adaptation in U.S. or Canadian health-care systems?
- The Philippines has a rich history, influenced by China and Southeast Asia, Indonesia, Spain, and the United States. What is the connection of the Philippines with the histories of China and other Asian nations? What are the main cultural and religious groups in the Philippines? What are the past and current migration patterns of the people from the Philippines to the United States and Canada? What are the main languages spoken in the Philippines? How do languages and dialects influence cultural evolution? Why are education and the English language so important to the Filipinos?
- Why are the Philippines so important to the United States? Outline the relationship that the United States and the Philippines had before and have after World War II. Identify the role that American military nurses played and their contributions to the war effort

AUTHOR'S REFLECTION

In November 2012, I was invited to the Philippines by the Philippine Nurses Association. I was honored to keynote the International Qualitative Nursing Research Conference. In my experience, I was privileged to meet so many outstanding nursing professionals from the Philippine Nurses Association and deans and faculty of many Filipino universities who have changed the world of nursing and health care in the Philippines. I would like to acknowledge my colleagues, Sister Remy and Dr. Elizabeth Baua of St. Paul's University, Drs. Florenda Cabatit and Rozzano Locsin and others at Silliman University, and Dr. Erlinda Palangas, who have been instrumental in contributing to improving nursing and health care and creating caring communities in the Philippines and throughout the world through nursing education and research.

in the Philippines during World War II. How has the U.S. military presence changed in the Philippines? What has been the history of U.S. policy toward the Philippines? Are the Philippines an independent nation-state?

- Look into "Filipino comfort women" abducted during World War II by the Japanese and how they, as survivors, were able to tell their stories of rape and abuse after the war.

Select Bibliography

Doria, J. (2014). A culturally congruent education group: An evidence-based approach to improve prenatal care utilization. *Journal of Nursing Practice Applications and Reviews of Research (Philippine Nurses Association of America, Inc.), 4*(2), 94–101.

Emerson, E., Griffin, M., L'Eplatteneir, N., & Fitzpatrick, J. (2008). Job satisfaction and acculturation among Filipino registered nurses. *Journal of Nursing Scholarship, 40*(1), 46–51.

Locsin, R. (2005). *Technological competency as caring in nursing: A model for practice.* Indianapolis, IN: Sigma Theta Tau International.

Locsin, R., & Purnell, M. (2013). Professional nursing: Scientific practice or simple care? *Philippine Journal of Nursing, 83*(1), 34–36.

Mendoza, S. (2001). *Between the homeland and the diaspora: The politics of theorizing Filipino and Filipino American identities.* London: Routledge.

Web Listings

Philippine Journal of Nursing (Official Journal of the Philippine Nurses Association). Philippine Nurses Association. www.pna-ph.org

Philippine Nurses Association of America, http://www.mypnaa.org/index.php

Journal of Nursing Practice Application and Reviews of Research. Philippine Nurses Association of America, Inc. info@mypnaa.org

U.S. Department of State, http://www.state.gov

CHAPTER 13

Transcultural Diversity Within Unity in Jamaica: Out of Many, One People

*T*he Caribbean nation of Jamaica has a history of aboriginal and other culture group integration, including migration from different parts of Africa, Central America, South America, North America, the United Kingdom, and Europe. Jamaica formerly was under British rule but now has independence. It continues to be a member of the Federation of the British Commonwealth of Nations and CARICOM (Caribbean-Community). It is a nation in which its multiculturalism has emerged into a unity of people. It is a nation with a strong Ministry of Health that oversees the health-care system. All Caribbean nations, especially Jamaica, benefit too from the Pan American Health Organization's (PAHO) common goal of improving the public health and welfare of vulnerable people. In the past, there was immigration to the United Kingdom, but more recently, there has been increasing migration from Jamaica to the United States and Canada. The following story by Florence is a portrait of the nation of Jamaica with its rich history, music, food, dialects, orientation to Britain, pursuit of independence, multiculturalism, and emergence from many people into one people (Out of Many, One People—[the motto of Jamaica]).

Florence's Story

It was a hot November day, as usual in the tropics, and the 40 girls who were sitting in the classroom were surprised when the announcement came over the loud speaker:

"There will be a general assembly immediately; all classes should proceed to the meeting area outside of the rectory."

What could be so urgent that they were calling an assembly in the middle of the day? The girls were whispering to each other as they bustled out of their classrooms and started walking toward the assembly area. There at the top of the stairs was the headmistress, Sister Maureen Claire, looking very solemn. All the girls looked at each other; it had to be bad news. The headmistress could hardly choke back the tears as she spoke. "The president of the United States was shot and killed; school is dismissed today."

Some of the young ladies were delighted by the early dismissal. They proceeded to the office to call their parents to come and pick them up for the drive home. As a group of 3rd formers [3rd grade out of a total of five grades in Jamaican secondary education] started walking toward the bus stop they started to talk:

Flo: "I understand the president of the United States is a very powerful man but we are not Americans. Why should we care?"

Rosemarie: "I think Sister let us go home because he was a Catholic. You know how those nuns are."

Claudette: "Yes, and the class prejudice will always be here. They have no consideration for us. Now we have to go home in the middle of the day. My mother is working so I will not be able to get into the house. I have no maid to let me in."

Marcia: "I wish we had more 'roots people' teaching us. We have been independent for 1 year now and we are still crying over what is happening in America and England. I don't remember us getting off from school when the first Jamaican governor died."

Nancy: "Yes, but you must remember our motto, 'Out of Many One People.' We have a lot of American teachers here. With the exception of Sister Maureen Claire, all the nuns are Americans."

Flo: "You are right, I know what we should do. Why don't we start a new club where we could start finding out about our history. We could ask Mrs. Brown to help us. There is a rumor that she is a descendent of Nanny."

Claudette: "Who's Nanny?"

Marcia: "You fool-fool or something? Nanny was a very influential slave in Jamaica. It was rumored that she was the mother of a famous Ashanti chief from Kumasi, Ghana. On the way to the United States, she incited such a riot on the ship that they decided to take all the Ashantis on the ship to Jamaica. No one would buy those rebellious black people."

Nancy: "Well, you know my folks are from Shanghai, and my mother to this day cannot speak English. It was so funny, last week we went to the bank and my mother's patois was so bad the clerk thought she was speaking Chinese. Mom told me that her folks were brought here to work on the railroad because Nanny and the other slaves ran away into the hills as soon as the ship landed in Jamaica. But those Chinese people were smart. They were never going to work on any railroad; they were going to be merchants. As soon as they landed they opened a little shop and that's how we came to own that big supermarket."

Flo: "Well, coolie girl, what's your story?"

Marcia: "We are not coolies; we are descendents of Indians from East India. We brought the spices, such as curry, and mangoes to Jamaica. The poor unfortunate indigenous Arawak Indians died after the Spanish exposed them to so many diseases. My forefathers came as merchants along with the Syrians, Arabs, and Chinese. That's on my father's side. My grandmother is a white woman; her parents were English, Portuguese, and German."

The bus arrived at that moment and the girls all piled on the bus. The bus was crowded with women going to the market and the girls could not sit together. As they got off the bus at Half-Way Tree to change buses for the rest of the ride to their respective homes, they could smell the odor of the fresh baked patties coming from Tastee Patty Shop and in the distance there was the sound of reggae music. The voice of Bob Marley was trailing in from Derrick Harriot's the Musical Chariott's record store . . . "One love, one love. I say one love. As I sit in my yard in Trench town . . ." The music was contagious as was the beat of the drums, which provided the background for the song.

The girls were feeling so free, they were happy to be out of school. The end of the semester was just weeks away and they were looking forward to Christmas.

Flo: "Anybody game, let's go buy some patties and coco bread with our bus fares and walk the rest of the way home. I am in the mood for an ackee patty [Caribbean fruit from the Caribbean Ackee tree]."

Off they went to Tastee's. When they got out of the patty shop there was a store decorated for Christmas.

Nancy: "I hope I do well in my exams. Mummy promises me a trip to Miami if I get all As this semester."

Flo: "You are too privileged. Me, after church I'll go to Christmas market as usual with my two sisters and we'll hide from the Jonkonnus [African Jamaican figure called Anancy or Anansi who is dressed in a fantastic costume. The custom, especially popular at Christmas time, is based on story and rituals advanced from an oral tradition when "slaves" asked for gifts from "masters"]. The devil is so scary, I have always been afraid of the Jonkonnus ever since I was a little girl. Then when we get home we will drink sorrel wine and have rum cake. Christmas is my favorite time of the year."

Claudette: "Speaking of church, do you think they'll have a nine night for the president? When my grandmother got sick last year, they rushed her to University hospital. The doctor said she had kidney failure. My poor mother asked if she could have dialysis. The doctors laughed so hard. 'Ma'am, we only have two dialysis machines on the Island, your mother is 70 years old.' So we brought her home to die, the nine nights of singing, dancing, and eating was something else. I would have invited you all but my mother said this was big people affair."

Rosemarie: "Maybe your mother should have called the Ministry of Health. Do you believe that was right that because your grandmother was old she should not get care?"

Marcia: "Girl, get with it. You think that because we are independent now and the Prime Minister say 'Out of Many, One People' that 'a so it go!' My great-grandmother, the one who is descended from the famous pirate Anne Bonny and is related to Marcus Garvey, always used to say 'me come er fe drink milk no fe count cow. Leave them people alone, dem wi get wey a come to dem.' Remember how Port Royal sank in 1692 with all them wicked people just like in the Bible" [Jamaican "folk" language and historical interpretation of Old Testament scriptures].

With that the girls folded their Jippy Jappa hats [Jamaican hats made from the Carlucovica palmate leaf] and put them in their schoolbags and proceeded to chase each other down the Constant Spring Road. It would be many hours before they got home but they were free. Free from school for the day. Free from slavery. They were descended from many cultures but they were one. They were Jamaicans.

Transcultural Caring-Based Learning Approach

Please review the information about the Transcultural Caring Dynamics for Nursing and Health-Care Theory and Model, the assessment tools, the transcultural caring-based learning (TCCBL) approach, and the transcultural caring inquiry information explained in previous chapters of this book, including the relevant literary and Internet information, before dialoguing about this transcultural caring experience. In your small group, apply the TCCBL approach, and all processes in relation to your transcultural caring situation for pattern identification (i.e., pattern seeing, pattern mapping, pattern recognizing, and pattern transforming). Use dimensions of the Transcultural Caring Dynamics in Nursing and Health-Care Model and use the most appropriate assessment tools for transcultural evidence gathering.

Reflections with Questions

Reflect on Florence's story with imagination. Imagine yourself as a nurse, working with children and families who were members of this school-age group in Jamaica, or perhaps as a nurse representative of the Pan American Health Organization (PAHO), or as a Jamaican immigrant yourself caring for, not only, Jamaican immigrants but people of all cultures living in the United States or Canada. Also, in your small group, what transcultural caring thoughts come to your mind initially about this story of the multicultural children of Jamaica in 1963, 1 year after Jamaican independence from Britain and the year that U.S. President Kennedy was shot and killed in Dallas, Texas?

Reflect on the rich history of Jamaica, the intercultural experience and migration patterns among the United States, Canada, and Jamaica and other island nations of the Caribbean. Focus on the rich cultural heritage of Jamaica, including the multiculturalism, public health, food, dress, education, and music. Consider PAHO and the data on Jamaica and its health-care system. What are your responsibilities as a transcultural nurse in understanding the Jamaican culture as well as other Caribbean island cultures and possibly working with nurses from Jamaica who have immigrated to North America?

Transcultural Nursing Reflections

- What are the multicultural images that arise in the narrative? Can you name the diverse cultures in this story that make up the motto, Out of Many, One People?
- What values are the girls portraying? What types of caring actions (i.e., compassion, or noncompassionate behaviors, and justice) were exhibited in this transcultural experience? How do the values of the past influence the way in which these girls understand their own past, present, and future? What values prevailed when the students were given a day off when President Kennedy was shot and killed?
- What history is revealed in the communicative interaction among the students? In the history of Jamaica, what were the migration patterns revealed by the different groups of people coming to Jamaica? Who is the dominant group in Jamaica? Why did the different groups come?
- Who are the Arawak people and where are they from? After the Arawak people migrated to Jamaica, which country laid claim to it next? When did the British take over the country?
- Why was there slavery on the island? Discuss the history of slavery in Jamaica and the Caribbean Islands. When was the island nation emancipated from slavery? What happened in the years after independence from Britain?
- What ideas come to your mind about teachers, the Catholic religion and its traditions, traditions of other Christian faiths, and traditional customs of the descendants of many cultures, including former slaves from Africa? What other religions are represented in the nation?
- What are all the symbols of the culture illuminated in this story, from the school, the bus, the clothes, the food, and the way in which the traditional Christmas holiday is celebrated?
- What is the symbolism of the original name of the country from the Arawak inhabitants and the name of the street, the Constant Spring Road?

- In this island nation, the land of the tropics, what is the major commodity for export? What is the nature of tourism on the island? How does the music of reggae, ska, rock-steady, dub, and dance hall give life to the people, the island, and the world? How do they fuel the economy?
- What is the meaning of the Jamaican Diaspora? What are the migration patterns to and from Jamaica? Why do you think that the people of Jamaica migrate when there seems to be an impressive model of multicultural harmony? Do the same issues that face Jamaica, face, for example, the Virgin Islands, Barbados, Haiti, or Cuba?
- What is the official language of Jamaica? What other languages/dialects are spoken? What does the dialect reflected in the above narrative in 1963, tell us about the country? Are dialects still in use?
- What type of health-care system exists in Jamaica? The girls talked about a Ministry of Health. What is its role in Jamaica? How does it relate to the PAHO? How do the goals of PAHO relate to its mother organization, the World Health Organization?
- The narrative of the young girls addresses issues that occurred in 1963 about dialysis treatment for kidney disease and the shortage of kidney dialysis machines at that time, and the care of the aged, especially those of modest economic means. What is the life expectancy of Jamaicans, in comparison with other island nations and in comparison with Canada and the United States?
- What is the state of access to health care, access to advanced technology for health problems, and for care of the aged in the modern era?
- Discuss the concepts of vulnerability, at-risk populations, and health disparities.
- What is the state of knowledge and attitudes toward risky sexual behaviors and HIV/AIDS among Caribbean African Americans in the Caribbean and the United States and Canada?
- What is the system of nursing education? Are nurses recruited to the United States to fill the shortage of nurses? Compare and contrast the health-care system with the Canadian, United Kingdom, and United States health-care systems.
- What is the political structure of Jamaica? What is the role of Jamaica in the Federation of the British Commonwealth of Nations, the CARICOM [Caribbean Community], and the nations of North and South America? What is Jamaica's role in the United Nations? How does Jamaica compare with other island nations in terms of political structures, economic systems, rules of law, and the advance of technology? Where is the largest Jamaican population in the United States and in Canada?
- What is Jamaica's contribution to entertainment and tourism?

AUTHOR'S REFLECTION

Caribbean nations are important to the United States, especially the southern United States. Caribbean nations are members of the PAHO, headquartered in Washington, DC, and are a division of the World Health Organization. PAHO has been instrumental in developing national and local public health and welfare of the peoples of the Caribbean and the Americas (35 member states with a few other nations as participants and observers). PAHO assists the nations in fighting older diseases, such as tuberculosis; decreasing infant mortality; improving the drinking water and sanitation; increasing attention on HIV/AIDS and especially HIV/AIDS among adolescents, cardiovascular disease, diabetes, and cancer; and reducing the use of tobacco. PAHO also assists with strengthening the learning facilities for the education of health-care professionals.

Select Bibliography

Archibald, C. (2007). Knowledge and attitudes toward HIV/AIDS and risky sexual behaviors among Caribbean African American female adolescents. *Journal of the Association of Nurses in AIDS Care, 18*(4), 64–72.

Archibald, C. (2011). Cultural tailoring for an Afro-Caribbean community: A naturalistic approach. *Journal of Cultural Diversity, 18*(4), 114–119.

Breda, K. (2009). *Nursing and globalization in the Americas: A critical perspective.* Amityville, NY: Baywood Publishing Company.

Long, E. (2003). *The history of Jamaica: Reflections on its situation, settlement, inhabitants, climate, products, commerce, laws, and government.* Montreal, QC: McGill-Queen's University Press.

Monteith, K., & Richards, G. (2002). *Jamaica in slavery and freedom: History, heritage and culture.* Kingston, Jamaica: University of West Indies Press.

Web Listings

Pan American Health Organization, http://www.paho.org

World Health Organization, www.who.int

U.S. Department of Health and Human Services, http://www.dhhs.gov

CHAPTER 14

Cuban American Transcultural Experiences and the Quest for Freedom in the United States: A New Era Beginning

*B*inational partnership and binational crises have dominated the history of Cuba and the United States. Prior to the Cuban revolution in 1959, the island nation was used as a "playground" and vacation spot for many people in the United States. After the Cuban revolution, political relationships between the two countries became strained and contentious because of the alignment of Cuba with the then Soviet Union (now Russia). The prolonged conflict led to invasion of the Bay of Pigs and what followed, the Cuban missile crisis with the Soviet Union (Russia), which was averted by President Kennedy, and the quest for freedom by the Cuban people with the freedom flights, the Mariel Boatlift, and the many escapes by raft over the Florida Straits to Miami, Florida, which continue to this day. Besides freedom from oppression, preservation of the family, education, health, healing, and economic well-being are at the heart of the Cuban people's flight to freedom in the United States.

The Cuban culture, rich with a strong multicultural family heritage, rhythmic music, delicious food, and blended religions, is colorful and interesting and firmly rooted in Miami. After nearly 50 years in power, and experiencing a serious illness, the president of Cuba, Fidel Castro, relinquished power to his brother, Raul Castro, on February 19, 2008. Cuban American relations under the Obama Administration remained hopeful. On December 18, 2014, the United States announced an agreement/policy (negotiated for 18 months and encouraged by Pope Francis and hosted in Canada), whereby full diplomatic relations with Cuba would be restored, including the opening of embassies for the first time in more than 50 years *(www.nytimes/2014/12/18/world/americas/us-cuba-relations.html). In the past, there had been economic reforms and some travel restrictions were lifted that helped Cuba strengthen its international relationships (Council on Foreign Relations, Retrieved from www.cfr.org). A new era is beginning following the announcement of the resumption of diplomatic relations and the lifting of some trade restrictions between the two countries. The trade embargo imposed by the United States in 1960 and further reinforced by the Helms-Burton Act of 1996 will remain, pending Congressional action in the United States (www.nytimes.com). However, some embargo restrictions were lifted in early 2015 (Cuellar, 2015), when the United States Embassy was reopened in Cuba (havana.usembassy.gov). The following is a story of Susana, who is sharing her quest for freedom.*

Susana's Story

I came from Cuba to Miami, Florida when I was 18 years old, with my father, grandmother, two single aunts, and another relative. We came aboard one of the Freedom Flights from Varadero, Cuba on October 2, 1969. These Freedom Flights were established by U.S. President Johnson and were operable from 1966 to 1971. Fidel Castro, the leader of the Cuban Revolution of 1959, who was president and ruler until he relinquished power to his brother, Raul, in 2008, permitted some Cubans to leave the country after relatives who already had made their way to Miami, made out an application. Before leaving Cuba after the revolution, our property was confiscated and many of my family members had to work on the farms—the sugar plantations. Some stayed at home, such as my mother who was ill, and died before we were permitted to leave on the Freedom Flight. I, myself, had no bad memories of the persecution or the Communist government but others in my family did. I had asthma and did not have to go to the farms. I did go to school. After the revolution, my family all lived together in the same apartment. The Cuban Missile Crisis with the United States and the Soviet Union (Russia) in 1962 increased fear of persecution. When we were given permission to leave Cuba, we were told to take only two changes of clothes but no money, pictures, books, or personal belongings.

When on the plane, I recall all of the crying and the screaming in preparation for our landing in Miami. We had a sense that we were going to be free. Cuban American families who already escaped accommodated their relatives or friends when they arrived in Miami. We were legal aliens. Cuban people all lived together so the Cuban American culture was born in Miami and was changing all the time. We were all close. We loved our music, and we loved to prepare our native foods. The food was so plentiful in the United States! When we came to Miami, we rented a little house. We were allowed to work in restaurants and other shops.

To this day, freedom is so important to me. I ponder it all the time. When I see the things happening today, for example, the terrorist movement, I am concerned. I am happy that I am able to think for myself, to have opinions, and be able to communicate thoughts freely. In a free society, you can have desires, hopes and you can also "fight" for what you want (in a good way). In a restricted society, people are put down; they lose their inner desire to create; they lose their initiative; they lose their spirit.

In the Cuban situation, after the Freedom Flights stopped, there were the Mariel Boatlifts under President Carter in 1980. Castro sent people from jails and mental hospitals, so when they came to Miami there was an increase in crime. I have a friend who worked with the Mariel Boatlift people and she thought there was "nothing much to work with" when they had lost their sense of valuing life, culture, and others. Is this what happens when there is no caring for someone and no love?

The history of the migration to Miami is complex. There was something called Operation Peter Pan, boys under 15 who were taken out of the country of Cuba from 1960 to 1962 and sent to the United States alone. Religious organizations took care of them initially and then they were in foster care. Interestingly, a high percentage of them became successful lawyers, doctors, and Congress people. Their biological families came to Miami later. They have a healthy respect for their biological and their foster families. There were the Freedom Flights, of which I was a part. Then there were and are the raft people—people who come at different times on the sea. There is the Wet-Foot/Dry-Foot Policy for Cuban people here in the United States where, if people are intercepted at sea, they are sent back to Cuba, but if they set foot on the land, they can stay here; they are not illegal aliens, and can pursue residency. (The "wet-foot/dry-foot policy" is officially the U.S.–Cuba Migration Policy of 1995, an amendment to the 1966 Cuban Adjustment Act).

Cubans integrated well into American society and have been successful. Many, however, did not learn to speak English. There was and is such a strong community of Cuban Americans speaking only Spanish that they were never forced to learn English.

I went to college and because I didn't speak English at first, I was interested in mathematics. I was interested in medicine but it required English. I studied in Miami, then at the Florida Institute of Technology in biology. I then had a chance to study biomedical engineering in St. Louis. I always loved medicine so I used to go out on EMT (emergency medical technician) visits and also worked with a medical company in orthopedic technologies. I taught physicians about the equipment needed. I then went to Montana where I got my PhD in electrical engineering after studying biological effects of electromagnetic energy fields, such as the effects related to cancer. At that time, I was also with a spiritual community. We were engaged in construction engineering but studying and living New Age and Buddhist principles. I always wanted to be free. I never married. A few years ago, I returned to Miami. My family members were getting ill—my father and two aunts. I was now "head of the house." I was always concerned about the use and abuse of technology at the end of life. I didn't want my family to have their last days on machines or technological equipment. I don't believe in extending life unnecessarily though. I have always respected duty because of love for my family and love for duty. I love when people have freedom to choose. I have decided to stay in Miami. I am now a professor in a university developing online computer engineering courses, which I love.

Transcultural Caring-Based Learning Approach

Please review the information about the Transcultural Caring Dynamics for Nursing and Health-Care Theory and Model, the assessment tools, the transcultural caring-based learning (TCCBL) approach, and the transcultural caring inquiry information explained in previous chapters of this book and any other relevant literary and Internet information before dialoguing about this transcultural caring experience. In your small group, apply the TCCBL approach and other processes in relation to your transcultural caring situation for pattern identification (i.e., pattern seeing, pattern mapping, pattern recognizing, and pattern transforming). Use dimensions of the Transcultural Caring Dynamics in Nursing and Health-Care Model and use the most appropriate assessment tools for transcultural evidence gathering.

Reflections with Questions

Reflect on the concept of freedom and how it has affected Cuban Americans living in Miami, and Cuban political officials who have taken the political reins in the United States. The flight to freedom of Cubans to Miami has been exceptional and has changed the face of Miami, Florida. The Cuban culture—the Spanish language, food, belief systems, political and economic systems—have had a strong effect on the area. Focus attention on Susana's life in relation to the notion of freedom, education, and the role of women, and commitment to family and health care of family members. What are your responsibilities as a transcultural nurse in understanding the Cuban American culture? What are your responsibilities in understanding Hispanic/Latino culture in the United States?

Transcultural Nursing Reflections

Many of the questions that appear in these Transcultural Nursing Reflections are in the process of changing now that the United States has re-established relations with Cuba. Many of the people who fled Cuba during the revolution and beyond to Miami, Florida continue to struggle with the "wounds of the loss of freedom" and mistrust in terms of having to flee their homeland to be free. Contemplation of these questions helps us, as transcultural nurses, to not only understand what the Cuban people have experienced, but also, what all emigres experience. We can contemplate what displacement and the struggle for acceptance and integration mean to all migrants as they seek freedom from ideological conflict, terror, war, and dislocation. Please review the following questions also in light of what is occurring to migrants in so many countries around the world.

- Contemplate the role of Cuban American people and their concerns about what has happened and is happening in Cuba. What changes have occurred with Raul Castro continuing in power, if any? Reflect on the desire of the Cuban Americans to return to their homeland of Cuba someday.
- What ways of understanding freedom versus oppression in the Cuban American experience in the United States are important for the city of Miami and the state of Florida and the United Sates in general?
- Can you identify the special foods of Cuba and how they have changed food preferences of people living in North America?
- What opportunities for education, health, and well-being were available for Susana after she came to Miami?
- What are the drawbacks or difficulties when a culture does not learn the English language when living in the United States?
- What ideas come to your mind about Susana's story, her chosen profession, and her spiritual community in Montana? What may have been the draw of a New Age and Buddhist spiritual community for Susana in a different part of the United States (Montana)?
- Outline the transcultural caring experience of Susana and her family and extended family in Miami. What is Susana, as a Cuban American relative with obligations to family, facing now that she has returned to Miami to care for her aging family?
- In your small group, think of yourself in the role of a gerontological nurse with few Spanish speaking skills. What caring actions (compassion and justice) would you exhibit in this transcultural experience for Susana and her aging family members? What would help you to understand Susana and her Cuban American experience and family?
- What are the kin group structures identified in this story—familial, Cuban American extended family, religious, or spiritual community? How would you do a culturological assessment of aged people with a different set of language skills? Would a culturological assessment for aging people be different? Project what the health needs would be for Susana's family and herself.
- Contemplate end-of-life decisions for the use and/or abuse of technology. What are the ethical implications? What resources would be available for assisted living, palliative care, nursing home care in any large city in the United States, and Miami in particular because of the focus on Cuban Americans? Contemplate the new directive for physician reimbursement with Medicare patients to discuss "end of life" decisions (www.cms.gov). What about physician-assisted "right to die" legislation?
- Cuban history is important to the United States. Determine why Cuba is so important to the United States, and to Cuban Americans. Reflect upon and outline Cuban American history prior to the Cuban revolution, historical developments between the United States and Cuba, and immigration and migration patterns to and from Miami, including Operation Peter Pan, Freedom Flights, Mariel Boatlift, and Wet-Foot/Dry-Foot Policy.

What does this mean to United States? What will more freedom for Cubans in Cuba mean to the United States and other nations?

- What has been the history of Guantanamo and Guantanamo Bay in U.S. policy? What do you think will happen if Cuba's government changes and freedom is declared? How does the lifting of restrictions against Cuba and the restoration of diplomatic relations by the United States in 2015 affect Cuban Americans? What are your thoughts about how Miami and the health-care system will accommodate the change?

- What role has the notion of freedom played in Susana's life? What is the meaning of freedom from Susana's viewpoint? How do *you* view freedom?

- Contemplate what it would be like to be a Cuban and then a Cuban American. What is unique about the Cuban American culture within cultures—Cuban American culture within the culture of Miami and the culture of the United States? Do you think there is a difference between freedom "from" something and freedom "to" something? What is the meaning of freedom in general in American society?

- Think about the knowledge needed for you to care for the Operation Peter Pan people who are reaching old age and may be in the dying process; the Mariel Boatlift people of the past who may have experienced periods in jail or in mental hospitals in Cuba and the United States; and the raft people, who are continually coming to Miami for freedom and resettlement.

- Contemplate the health-care system of Cuba. What do you think the impact on health care will be now that some of the restrictions have been lifted in Cuba in 2015 by the United States? How does one compare and contrast health care between the United States and Cuba? (Cuba is ranked #1 in public health and preventive primary health-care services [Cuellar, 2015].) How many physicians have been educated in Cuba? Is nursing a profession in Cuba? How do the Pan American Health Organization (PAHO) and the Caribbean Community (CARICOM) play a role in Miami, Florida and the United States? In Cuba?

- With the change in leadership in Cuba, contemplate the shift from strictly socialistic practices to more capitalistic practices in 2008, such as the ownership of land by farmers; the capability to hire workers and sell farm products as well as cars and homes; and other changes, such as the ownership of cell phones; and the increase in tourism?

- How does the Cuban American migration experience differ from the Haitian migration experience in the United States and South Florida? What policy differences prevail? What are the circumstances in legal or illegal immigration? What, as a transcultural nurse, would you think is the best term to use, legal or illegal immigrants or documented or undocumented immigrants? What are your thoughts about immigration reform in the United States?

- As you contemplate the historical developments, how would you share your views with people of other Caribbean nations, such as Haitians who may be perplexed about the perceived special rights of Cubans arriving in the United States, and the rights of other people from the Caribbean countries?

- What does it mean now that Cuba has been readmitted May, 3, 2009 to the Organization of American States (OAS)? What does it mean for U.S./Cuba relations now that the U. S. Embassy has reopened in Cuba?

Select Bibliography

Chomsky, A. (2010). *A history of the Cuban revolution*. New York, NY: Wiley-Blackwell.

Cuellar, N. (2015). Cuban embargo restrictions lifted: Impact on health care? *Journal of Transcultural Nursing, 26*(3), 217-218.

Diaz, G. (2007). *The Cuban American experience: Issues, perceptions, and realities*. St. Louis, MO: Reedy Press.

Medicare proposes to pay doctors to have end of life care discussions. Retrieved August 31, 2015 from https://www.washingtonpost.com/national/health-science/medicare-proposes-to-pay-doctors-to-have-end-of-life-care-discussions/2015/07/08/1d7bb436-25a7-11e5-aae2-6c4f59b050aa_story.html

Mendez-Franco, J. (2009). Cuba, USA:OAS says "yes". *Global Voices Online*. Retrieved July 19, 2009, from http://www.globalvoicesonline.org/2009/06/04/cuba-usa-oas-says-yes/

Morley, J. (1997). U.S. Cuba Migration Policy. Frequently asked questions. *The Washington Post*. Retrieved July 19, 2009, from http://www.washingtonpost.com/wp-dyn/content/article/2007/07/27/AR2007072701493.html

Ramonet, I., & Castro, F. (2008). *Fidel Castro: My life: A spoken autobiography*. New York: Scribner.

The Cuban Adjustment Act and Immigration Policies, 1966, Law 89. Retrieved July 19, 2009, from http://www.state.gov/www/regions/wha/cuba/fs_000828-migration-accord.html

U.S.- Cuba Migration Accord, 1995. Retrieved July 19, 2009, from http://www.state.gov/www/regions/wha/cuba/fs_000828-migration-accord.html

CHAPTER 15

Puerto Rican Transcultural and Health Beliefs in a Western New York Community

*B*arbara's story is dedicated to Dr. Barbara Higgins, a former student and colleague who died too early and before many of her research results could be realized. Barbara conducted ethnographic/ethnonursing research in western New York where she studied Puerto Rican families; their cultural beliefs and attitudes; and the influence that the kinship structure, cultural values and lifeways, and family life had on infants, children, and feeding practices. Barbara spent about 1 year "living with the people in the area" observing and participating to begin to understand Puerto Rican culture in western New York. She was interested in migration patterns to and from Puerto Rico, family life, health care of children and the aging, and the desires of the people for a good life. Barbara was interested in bringing to light the late Madeleine Leininger's Culture Care Diversity and Universality Theory of Nursing. Her ultimate goal was to communicate ways in which nurses can provide culturally congruent care to families and children. The following is a scenario that captures Barbara's views of a Puerto Rican American extended family experience.

Barbara's Story

Maria, a 23-year-old woman, and Carlos, her 25-year-old husband, moved from a New York City, Puerto Rican community (where they lived with Maria's family who came from Puerto Rico) to Buffalo, New York. They moved to create a home and to care for Carlos's aging mother. Carlos's father, who had died a few months earlier, had run a small food shop and Carlos's family moved back and forth between Puerto Rico and Buffalo on a regular basis.

Maria and Carlos have two boys, Miguel and Juan, ages 3 and 1, and Maria is 3 months pregnant. Although Maria was scared to move away from her mother—whom she relied upon for help and advice with the children, cooking, and overall love and support—she wanted to help Carlos care for his mother, who was ailing with heart and blood pressure problems.

After arriving in the Puerto Rican community in western New York, they moved in with Christiana (Carlos's mother) in a small duplex. Carlos decided to manage the small grocery store that his father had opened. Right away, Maria had problems in her new home. She was used to living with her own mother and family, and was afraid that her children would upset her mother-in-law in the small quarters if they were too noisy. Christiana spoke little English and Maria was afraid that she would lose her English skills, which were necessary for helping in the grocery store. Maria missed her mother and the Puerto Rican religious practices that she used to ward off evil spirits. Maria also missed her mother's cooking. She did not like to cook and often resorted to junk food. Her boys had gained weight since babyhood; they were big children because of the Puerto Rican belief that "big is beautiful and healthy," especially for babies. Juan, her youngest child, had a problem with anemia when he was a few months old because of feeding practices.

Walking around the community, Maria located a local health clinic for herself and her children. Christiana had been there but did not go regularly for checkups because her husband had been so busy and she did not have additional transportation. Maria found out that Dr. Jorge Padilla and a nurse practitioner, Kelly Dunn (fluent in Spanish), would be taking care of her when she came for her prenatal visits. Maria was hoping that when it was time for her to deliver her baby and go back to the duplex a nurse could come to her home like they did in New York City. She also hoped her mother would come to care for her. Maria learned that the Children's Hospital was 10 minutes by car and that there was another hospital not too far away for the adults. But they did need a car to get there. She wanted Christiana to begin to go to the clinic for regular visits. Maria found a Catholic church that she thought would be a source of comfort for her since she was so lonely for prayer services, family, and friends. Maria also explored the neighborhood for schools for her older child. She found out that he would be able to attend preschool soon, and would then be able to go to the public school close to the duplex for kindergarten and grade school.

The little grocery store where Carlos was managing was a few blocks away. She knew that Carlos may have to go back and forth to Puerto Rico to arrange imports of special foods from the island. Plus, Maria found out at the church that soon a large supermarket chain was going to open a store near their small grocery store, which worried her because of the possible competition and financial implications. Maria was slowly getting adjusted. But, she still called her mother every day on her cell phone and wished she could go back "home."

Transcultural Caring-Based Learning Approach

Please review the information about the Transcultural Caring Dynamics for Nursing and Health-Care Theory and Model, the assessment tools, the transcultural caring-based learning (TCCBL) approach, and the transcultural caring inquiry information explained in previous chapters of this book, and any other relevant literary and Internet information before dialoguing about this transcultural caring experience. In your small group, apply the TCCBL approach in relation to your transcultural caring situation for pattern identification (i.e., pattern seeing, pattern mapping, pattern recognizing, and pattern transforming). Use dimensions of the Transcultural Caring Dynamics in Nursing and Health-Care Model and use the most appropriate assessment tools for transcultural evidence gathering. The Reflections with Questions section that follows is a guide that will assist you individually and collectively in your learning group with dialogue and interpretation of what is happening to Maria and her family who have moved to a city in western New York state from New York City with ties to Puerto Rico.

Reflections with Questions

Reflect on the lifeworld experience of a Puerto Rican American woman and family moving to a new city, moving in with a relative, trying to find health-care facilities for prenatal care, and care for her family and ailing mother-in-law who is a new widow. Puerto Rico has an interesting history with the United States. The migration patterns of a Commonwealth state illuminate the binational partnership between the United States and Puerto Rico. The culture reflects the interaction of two nations. The cultural belief systems, lifeways, kinship structure, Spanish language, food, and nutritional and infant feeding practices have a strong effect on the health and well-being of children and families. What are your responsibilities as a transcultural nurse in understanding the Puerto Rican American lifeways, and migration patterns? As you relate to others in your small group, decide how you would take the role of Kelly, the nurse practitioner who will do a culturological assessment and plan of care in the clinic.

Transcultural Nursing Reflections

- What compassionate and just actions should be exhibited by Kelly in this nursing situation?
- Although Kelly is fluent in Spanish, do you think it is necessary when working in a culturally specific health-care setting to be able to speak the language of the people? Is a professional interpreter necessary if a nurse cannot fully comprehend a transcultural health-care situation?
- What assessment tools should be used for a familial and extended family culturological assessment?
- How would you assess Maria and her family, and her husband's mother, Christiana using a transcultural holistic approach (i.e., physical, emotional, and spiritual)?
- Contemplate the history and culture and health-care system of Puerto Rico, and the intercultural relationship with the United States.
- How could you use Leininger's Culture Care Diversity and Universality Theory (1991; Leininger & McFarland, 2006; McFarland & Wehbe-Alamah, 2015) and Leininger's ethnonursing method (OPR—Observation, Participation, Reflection) (Ray, Morris, & McFarland, 2013) in the story of Maria and her family? What are the philosophy, assumptions, and concepts of the Leininger theory? What does providing culturally congruent care mean? Reflect upon the professional and scientific care differences between Kelly, the nurse practitioner, and Maria and Maria's health beliefs about children in this story. How are they reconciled in transcultural nursing?
- Outline the kinship structure of Maria and her family of Puerto Rican American heritage. What unique components of Puerto Rico culture can be identified in this transcultural caring experience?
- What are the *foundational* cultures of Puerto Rico? What are the diverse cultures of Puerto Rico? What does Afro Caribbean mean? Are there differences of the multicultural heritage between Puerto Rico and the other Caribbean nations?
- As Kelly, the nurse practitioner, what would you recommend to help Maria with her pregnancy, her husband, her children, her relationship with Christiana, and her resettlement to a new area? Contemplate what you would do to provide culturally congruent prenatal care to Maria.
- When contemplating this transcultural nursing situation, what ideas come to your mind about the story of kinship of Maria and Carlos and their immediate family, and with Carlos's mother, Christiana? Are there specific cultural practices for widows in the Puerto Rican culture? What specific gerontological Puerto Rican cultural care would you recommend for Christiana?
- What public health opportunities for health and well-being may be available in this Puerto Rican cultural community in western New York or any other state? Why is health care so different in the distinct geographical areas of the United States?

- What are the unique nutritional patterns of children in a Puerto Rican community? As a nurse practitioner, how would you help Maria with not only her own nutrition during pregnancy, but also, the feeding practices of a new baby and the ongoing culturally aware nutrition of her other two children?
- What does it mean for a baby to wear a bracelet made of gold jet and coral?
- Contemplate the historical role of the Catholic Church in Puerto Rican life. How are values conveyed? What are the spiritual aspects of traditional Puerto Rican culture and the Catholic Church? How are the differences in religious practices blended in Puerto Rican culture?
- Contemplate the experience of multiple generations living together, especially if the head of the household is your mother-in-law, who has cardiac and blood pressure problems. How would you help the families in the transcultural nursing situation? Would there be ways that the social community of the church could help?
- Think about Carlos taking over management of the store and having to import some of his produce and products from Puerto Rico. What specific health and family caring needs do you think he would have as he cares for his mother and family?
- Are there unique health problems in the Commonwealth of Puerto Rico? What type of health-care system exists in Puerto Rico?
- What is the political, economic, and social relationship between the United States and Puerto Rico? What are key historical developments between the United States and Puerto Rico? Why is Puerto Rico so important to the United States?
- What is the meaning of the Commonwealth of Puerto Rico? Has statehood been considered for Puerto Rico? Who is the head of state in Puerto Rico? Is Puerto Rico self-governing? Are Puerto Ricans citizens of the United States?
- Contemplate the unique migration patterns to and from Puerto Rico, and immigration process for Puerto Ricans in the United States.
- What is Puerto Rico's role in the Caribbean Community (CARICOM) and with the Pan American Health Organization (PAHO)?
- Name other commonwealths and territories in the United States. Are they self-governing? What are the specific cultures? Can you describe the health-care systems?

Select Bibliography

Higgins, B. (2000). Puerto Rican cultural beliefs: Influence on infant feeding practices in western New York. *Journal of Transcultural Nursing, 1*(11), 19–30.

Leininger, M. (Ed.). (1991). *Culture care diversity and universality: A theory of nursing.* New York: National League for Nursing Press.

Leininger, M., & McFarland, M. (Eds.). (2006). *Culture care diversity and universality: A worldwide theory of nursing* (2nd ed.). Sudbury, MA: Jones & Bartlett.

McFarland, M., & Webhe-Alamah, H. (2015). *Leininger's culture care diversity and universality: A worldwide nursing theory.* Burlington, MA: Jones & Bartlett Learning.

Melendez, E. (2007). Changes in the characteristics of Puerto Rican migrants to the United States. In M. Montero-Sieburth & E. Melendez (Eds.), *Latinos in a changing society.* Westport, CT: Praeger.

Ray, M., Morris, E., & McFarland, M. (2013). Ethnonursing method of Dr. Madeleine Leininger. In C. Beck (Ed.), *Routledge international handbook of qualitative research.* London: Routledge.

❖
The Nurse Manager in a Cardiovascular Intensive Care Unit and the Organizational Complexity of a Hospital Culture

"*A* *n organization is a system of consciously coordinated activities or forces of two or more people created for specific ends*" (Downs, 1993, p. 24). *A hospital is one example, created to meet the needs of the sick. Organizations have been recognized as cultures since the rise of Japan as an industrial power in the 1960s. Culture includes the values, beliefs, philosophy, attitudes, rituals, and behaviors of groups of people and a culture is transmitted from one group to the other through complex social interactions. Culture is a metaphor for the way in which distinctive groups of people manifest different ways of life—how diverse people construct and cocreate their complex and dynamic social reality through social interaction, especially communication. The organization as a cultural phenomenon reveals the formal structure (including technological, political, economic, and legal dimensions) and informal lifeways. Often the culture of an organization is considered a bureaucracy, a specific organization with a formal structure: rules/policies and a division of labor created to achieve the goals of the organization (the legal), technological specialization (technical resources available for a specific end), and a method of competing for and allocating resources (political and economic). The work-life environment uncovers the complexity of the organizational culture. In the new age of complexity, including social media and networking, organizational cultures and work life are both hierarchical and relational, with motivation to be present, respectful, trustworthy, and compassionate to co-create frameworks for "caring" alliances (Davidson, Ray, & Turkel, 2011; Hoffman, Casnocha, & Yeh, 2014; Ray, 2010a, 2010b, 2010c; Ray & Turkel, 2012) . Not all health care organizations have reached this significant insight; however, with increasing knowledge of the meaning of the network of relationships, concerted efforts are being made to transform health care organizations (Boykin, Schoenhofer, & Valentine, 2014; Coffman, 2014; Ray & Turkel, 2014, 2015). In a hospital, the culture represents the philosophy, values, goals, and objectives of the corporate system, and professional responsibilities for patient care in response to the prevailing health-care system of a nation-state. The corporate culture not only includes the philosophy, policies, procedures, rules, and regulations of the hospital itself but external regulation from other corporate bodies, such as The Joint Commission (TJC) and Occupational Safety & Health Administration (OSHA). The philosophy of a hospital organization includes spiritual-ethical values and the regulatory values for efficiency and effectiveness. A mission of a hospital could be "the provision of quality patient care within a well-managed economic approach." Understanding the hospital organization as a bureaucratic culture and each unit as a subset or part of the organization requires understanding of the organization as an integration of corporate values and professional medical, nursing, and allied health-care values. Thus, in a hospital, work life is a reflection of beliefs and values of the organization but, at the same time, it is a living history of relationships, the beliefs and patterns of relational experience. The following is Cecilia's story as she manages a cardiovascular specialty unit of a Catholic hospital.*

Cecilia's Story

Cecilia is the new nurse manager of the cardiovascular intensive care unit (CVICU) at St. Bonaventure Hospital in a western region of the United States. A religious/spiritual culture has prevailed with a commitment to patient-centered care, patient safety, and maintaining the economic well-being of the hospital. The hospital and CVICU mission statement reflects the value "caring for the heart of the community." The hospital underwent major structural renovations last year to accommodate an increase in total patients with the establishment of a new cardiac care center. Since the renovations in the hospital, a good portion of the budget is now being allocated to accommodating physicians and their requests for newer technologies. Computer documentation is established. Because the hospital administrators and architecture committee started the project before Cecilia became the nurse manager, she did not participate in the planning process. She agreed to take the position if she could have a voice in future leadership and management processes not only with the chief nursing officer (CNO) but also with the physician staff of the CVICU.

The new cardiac care center has two surgery suites, a CVICU, which can house 12 patients, each with a private room and the latest in advanced technological equipment and a 12-bed transitional care unit. The cardiac surgical program was established with a team of medical and nursing specialists. Three new cardiac surgeons were recruited. At the same time, however, the hospital was not able to recruit the number of experienced registered nurses needed to care adequately for the increase in heart surgical patients.

One major issue in the CVICU is the age of the patients having surgery. There are many patients (more men than women) over 80 years of age. Although some of the patients tolerate the surgery quite well, side effects abound. The mortality rate is increasing and these deaths are occurring within the unit. Cecilia is learning in her ongoing assessment of the organization that her nurses are concerned with the changes in morbidity and mortality rates attributed to the age risk, the age of the surgical patients, and their potential health problems. Some older patients do not recover sufficiently well enough under the "burden" of technology, ventilators, and the surgical intervention itself. There are issues for families and the nursing staff regarding decisions for cardiac resuscitation or withdrawal of support: do not resuscitate (DNR) or do not intubate (DNI) orders. The Ethics Committee at the hospital is concerned. The chief cardiac surgeon is involved and Cecilia would like to be on the committee. Cecilia has a belief that some patients should be in palliative care rather than going through the stress of cardiac surgery at such a late stage in life. In some cases, patients' physical health is already compromised by years of cardiovascular diseases, such as hypertension, arrhythmias, congestive heart failure, diabetes, retinopathy, and other problems.

Not only is there a problem with the number of aging people having surgery, but also with infectious diseases (nosocomial), such as methicillin-resistant *Staphylococcus aureus* (MRSA), that are beginning to rise. Cecilia does not know if the MRSA is totally hospital-related or it is community-associated MRSA. Sometimes these patients are being cared for in the CVICU. Cecilia is worried about the ethics of this decision and about patient safety; whether or not these dangerous infections could potentially affect the health and well-being of other surgical patients. She is not sure the extent to which her nurses are educated in and committed to regular hand washing with soap and water or the use of alcohol hand sanitizers. She is very concerned about physicians and their notorious lack of hand washing in hospitals. She is also worried that there have been some medical errors and there is a need for more education about informed consent now initiated by physicians. She has found out that there has been in increase in medication errors in the hospital and an increase in the CVICU. She knows that they have had communication errors in the hospital and on the unit. Cecilia would like to initiate continuing education and a research study on patient safety issues.

To add to these issues, many of the Hispanic or Latino patients have specific cultural needs that are not being met. The CVICU nurses told Cecilia that they cannot deal with so many cultural and language differences without more help. They are concerned with all of the family members who want to visit in large numbers in the CVICU. Staff nurses are weighed down with a low staffing ratio, especially in the 7 p.m. to 7 a.m. shifts. There is a law pending in the state legislature that would protect patients and nurses with respect to staffing ratios. The nurses state that they are overworked and becoming increasingly anxious about fulfilling their responsibilities. Cecilia learned that no staff member has had a course in transcultural nursing, although a few nurses were introduced to the idea of culture, cultural diversity, and cultural competence in some of their university courses and in continuing education courses. The hospital does not have a strong continuing education program to date.

As the new nurse manager, Cecilia reflected upon all that is happening in her new unit. She is not fond of the way that her nurses look; the unironed scrubs and dirty shoes do not reflect well on the management of the unit. She knows that she has to establish a better relationship with the chief nursing officer (CNO). She also knows that she and her group will have to produce a plan of action to begin to solve the problems facing the members of the CVICU and the hospital.

Issues for Analysis

The complexities of the role of a nurse manager as leader and manager of a complex cultural system, such as the CVICU within St. Bonaventure's Hospital, reveal many issues that need to be examined in how to:

- Provide safe patient care
- Improve patient safety standards
- Improve caring relationships among nurses, physicians, administrators, and patients
- Improve staffing
- Meet the cultural and linguistic needs of patients
- Provide transcultural nursing continuing education for the development of culturally competent care
- Increase management of the budget to assist with the advancement of computer and surgical technologies

AUTHOR'S REFLECTION

As a learning group, you can see that a hospital is a complex culture, often more complex than other corporations and businesses. A hospital is a living organization. A hospital exists for the purpose of providing care to patients. Although there are many professions represented in a hospital, for the most part, nursing is the most active in the provision of care. Most physicians are not actual employees of a hospital (with the exception of hospitalists), which makes a hospital more unique than other types of organizations. People *outside of* the organization direct the care within the organization.

* Meet the needs of nurses as a professional group
* Improve relationships among professionals
* Assess gerontological care for an aging population
* Deal with the ethical problems
* Reign in the problem of nosocomial or community-associated infections, such as MRSA in the CVICU
* Initiate continuing education for infection control

Transcultural Caring-Based Learning Approach

Please review the information about the Transcultural Caring Dynamics for Nursing and Health-Care Theory and Model, the assessment tools, the transcultural caring-based learning (TCCBL) approach, and the transcultural caring inquiry information explained in previous chapters of this book, and any other relevant literary and Internet information before dialoguing about this transcultural caring experience. In your small group, apply the TCCBL approach in relation to your transcultural caring situation for pattern identification (i.e., pattern seeing, pattern mapping, pattern recognizing, and pattern transforming). Use dimensions of the Transcultural Caring Dynamics in Nursing and Health-Care Model and use the most appropriate assessment tools for transcultural evidence gathering. The section that follows is a guide that will assist you individually and collectively in your learning group with dialogue and interpretation of the complex dynamics that are occurring in the CVICU that Cecelia is managing.

As Cecelia reflects on her position as nurse manager, she is concerned about so many problems that are facing nursing and patients in the hospital and unit settings. Reflect on the organization as a small culture and on the dimensions of a bureaucracy (i.e., the political, legal, economic, and technological dimensions). Reflect upon human caring not only for patients but also for nurses, physicians, and other professionals.

Transcultural Nursing Reflections and Questions

In this transcultural caring experience, imagine that you are Cecelia and you are charged with responsibility for the CVICU at St. Bonaventure Hospital.

* What transcultural caring thoughts come to your mind about this story of Cecelia?
* What compassionate and just actions are exhibited or should be exhibited in this nursing situation? What are the values, beliefs, attitudes, and behaviors that may be in play in the transcultural caring experience?
* What meaning does the the mission statement of the CVICU have for you as a nurse and/or as a nurse manager or leader?
* As you contemplate this transcultural experience, what do you think about the hospital as a culture, a bureaucracy, a complex system, and a business whose first priority is caring for patients but at the same time has a priority to maintain its economic viability? Is it

living up to its model of caring? Do you think the workplace should be a place to develop small workplace caring communities?

- In your small group, think about and discuss the meaning of a hospital as a bureaucratic culture (i.e., a political, economic, technological, legal and humanistic, spiritual, and ethical culture). How do you feel about using a term such as bureaucracy? What are the controversial elements or what is the opposition to this term? How do you link culture and bureaucracy? Do they have similar or diverse characteristics?

- Reflect on the nature of the intercultural relationships among the health-care professionals, allied health-care personnel, nursing and non-nursing administrators, and others, including volunteers as cultural groups, each with their own sets of values, beliefs, attitudes, opinions, and behaviors.

- Contemplate nursing as a culture. What are its central values? What is the meaning of nursing care, nurse caring, and the nurse-patient relationship? Are there certain rituals that you can identify that point out the meaning of certain practices in nursing? How are the uniform, the scrubs, the stethoscope, and medical language symbols of the nursing culture? What meanings do they convey? Examine the concepts of symbol and ritual (Wolf, 2013), and review Roach's 6Cs of Caring, especially the concept of comportment.

- Do you think that nursing differs from medicine in its central values? If so, how do they differ? What do you think about interprofessional education?

- Contemplate the meaning of hospital bureaucracies classified according to levels in the United States and Canada or other national cultural contexts. Determine what classification system is in place in your city or country. What do levels mean in the context of care, trauma care, preparedness, nurse, physician, and other response systems to emergencies and disasters?

- Are you familiar with triage systems, disaster and bioterrorism preparedness, mass casualties, and surge capacity in the community? Are hospital bureaucracies coordinated with bureaucracies of public health departments; local, regional, and national governments; Department of Homeland Security, global governments; police organizations including International Police Organization (Interpol); and the military?

- After contemplating the meaning of the hospital as a bureaucracy, how would you use Ray's Theory of Bureaucratic Caring as a foundation for evaluation of the CVICU? What does theory-guided practice mean?

- How is the CVICU in part a technological culture? Are using machine technology and computer technology, social media, robotics, components of caring? Reflect on the electronic patient record (EPR), or EHR (electronic health record), and nursing informatics in general.

- How does technology fit with gerontological nursing in a CVICU?

- What end-of-life care processes should be in place in a CVICU?

- What are your thoughts about the use or overuse of technology in a CVICU?

- How would a nurse confront a physician on what he or she may recognize as technological abuse?

- What is a medical durable power of attorney? What is a living will? What is palliative care? Reflect on the value of a palliative care team for patients and their families, clinical nursing specialists, physicians, social workers, and chaplains in the CVICU. What about legal physician-assisted dying and death? How does it differ from palliative care?

- What processes would you use to get a handle on the issues that Cecelia identified within her unit? How would you speak with the CNO if you were Cecelia?

- How do you think Cecelia should solve the problems facing her? What type of meetings should she conduct? Who should she gather together? What does the shortage of nurses contribute in this CVICU? How would you handle nurses' anxiety and concern about overwork?

- From an ethical viewpoint, what concerns come into play in this story? Would evidence-based practices make a difference? Why is transcultural caring ethics so important in a hospital or on a unit?

- What is a hospital's or unit's responsibility when it comes to patient safety, infection control, and placement of patients on units or in isolation?
- Why do you think more and more patients with MRSA may be admitted to intensive care units? What are the ethical issues involved? Why have antibiotic-resistant diseases become so prevalent? Explore the concept of the "new biology" (encoding the genomes of environmental microbes) for infectious diseases. Explore the issue of the H1N1 virus (swine flu) or other viruses.
- Is there an ethical situation to confront in advanced aging populations? What do you think about the "oldest old," people over the age of 85, having cardiac surgery? Are hospital statistics kept regarding patients over the age of 85 years having major surgery, especially cardiac surgery? Explore new nasal treatments for infectious disease prevention, e.g. Nozin (Steed, Costello, Shivangi, Jones, Spannhake, & Nguyen, 2014).
- Why and how do ethics committees play a role in a hospital? What would you as a staff nurse or nurse manager discuss in an ethics committee in age-related care in a CVICU, end-of-life issues, palliative care, and diverse cultural groups represented in your patient population? Should staffing issues be considered an ethical issue for ethics committees?
- How would you handle the cultural and linguistic needs of the cultural groups? What provisions are there in hospitals for "language-line interpreters?"
- How would you deal with an increase in visitors or many people from diverse cultures desiring to visit because of cultural beliefs about a family community?
- What are the main components advanced in this book that contribute to understanding the hospital as a culture and a transcultural experience for Cecilia and her nurses? What about her patients?
- Examine the list of potential presurgical morbidities, such as congestive heart failure, arrhythmias, and diabetes in the United States. What are the root causes of these diseases? Why has cardiac surgery increased in the United States? Is there a relationship between the numbers of specialists and the numbers of surgeries? Compare these figures with World Health Organization's figures or statistics in other Western nations.
- Why is patient safety so important in hospitals and on intensive care units? What organizations in the United States oversee patient safety? Can you describe policies that regulate patient safety in hospitals?
- What are the statistics for infections in hospitals? Name all the major hospital and community-related infections that are prevalent today. Why is this so? How long should one wash hands with soap and water, and how long should one rub with an alcohol sanitizer to be considered safe from passing germs from one person or surface to another?

Select Bibliography

Barnard, A., & Locsin, R. (Eds.). (2007). *Technology and nursing: Practice, concepts, and issues.* United Kingdom: Palgrave.

Bar-Yam, Y. (2004). *Making things work: Solving problems in a complex world.* Boston, MA: Knowledge Press.

Bennet, A. (2004). *Organizational survival in the new world: The intelligent complex adaptive system.* Burlington, MA: Elsevier.

Boykin, A., Schoenhofer, S., & Valentine, K. (2014). *Health care system transformation for nursing and health care leaders.* New York, NY: Springer Publishing Company.

Coffman, S. (2006). Marilyn Anne Ray, theory of bureaucratic caring. In A. Marriner Tomey & M. Alligood (Eds.), *Nursing theorists and their work* (6th ed., pp. 116–139). St. Louis: Mosby Elsevier.

Coffman, S. (2014). Marilyn Anne Ray's theory of bureaucratic caring. In M. Alligood (Ed.), *Nursing theorists and their work* (8th ed., pp. 98–119). St. Louis: Elsevier.

Davidson, A., Ray, M., & Turkel, M. (2011). *Nursing, caring, and complexity science: For human-environment well-being.* New York, NY: Springer Publishing Company.

Downs, A. (1993). *Inside bureaucracy.* Prospect Heights, IL: Waveland Press.

Hoffman, R., Casnocha, B., & Yeh, C. (2014). *The Alliance: Managing talent in the networked age.* Cambridge, MA: Harvard Business Review.

Locsin, R. (2005). *Technological competency as caring in nursing.* Indianapolis, IN: Sigma Theta Tau International.

McCloskey, D. (2008). Nurses' perceptions of research utilization in a corporate health care system. *Journal of Nursing Scholarship, 40*(1), 39–45.

Perrow, C. (1986). *Complex organizations: A critical essay.* New York: McGraw-Hill, Inc.

Ray, M. (2005). The theory of bureaucratic caring. In M. Parker (Ed.), *Nursing theory, nursing practice* (2nd ed., pp. 421–444). Philadelphia: F. A. Davis Company.

Ray, M. (2007). Technological caring as a dynamic of complexity in nursing practice. In A. Barnard & R. Locsin (Eds.), *Technology and nursing: Practice, concepts, and issues.* United Kingdom: Palgrave.

Ray, M. (2010a). *Transcultural caring dynamics in nursing and health care.* Philadelphia: F. A. Davis Company.

Ray, M. (2010b). *A study of caring within the institutional culture: The discovery of the Theory of Bureaucratic Caring.* Germany: Lambert Academic Publishers.

Ray, M. (2010c). Creating caring organizations and cultures through communitarian ethics. *Journal of the World Universities Forum, 3*(5), 41–52.

Ray, M., & Turkel, M. (2012). A transtheoretical evolution of caring science within complex systems. *International Journal for Human Caring, 16*(2), 28–49.

Ray, M., & Turkel, M. (2014). Caring as emancipatory nursing praxis: The theory of Relational Caring Complexity. *Advances in Nursing Science, 37*(2), 132-146).

Ray, M., & Turkel, M. (2015). Marilyn Anne Ray's Theory of Bureaucratic Caring. In M. Smith (Ed.), *Nursing theories and nursing practice* (4th ed.). Philadelphia: F. A. Davis Company.

Sherman, R., Bishop, M., Eggenberger, T., & Karden, R. (2007). Development of a leadership competency model from insights shared by nurse managers. *Journal of Nursing Administration, 37*(2), 85–94.

Smith, M., Turkel, M., & Wolf, Z. (2013). *Caring in nursing classics: An essential resource.* New York, NY: Springer Publishing Company.

Steed, L., Costello, J., Shivangi, L., Jones, T., Spannhake, E., & Nguyen, S. (2014). Reduction of nasal Staphylococcus aureus carriage in health care professionals by treatment with nonantibiotic alcohol-based nasal antiseptic. *American Journal of Infection Control.* http://dx.doi.org/10.1016/j.ajic.2014.04.008.

Turkel, M., & Ray, M. (2004). Creating a caring practice environment through self-renewal. *Nursing Administration Quarterly, 28*(4), 259–254.

Wolf, Z. (2014). *Exploring rituals in nursing: Joining art and science.* New York, NY: Springer Publishing Company.

Wu, C.J., & Ray, M. (2016, in press). Technological caring for healthcare complexities of patients with cardiac disease comorbid with diabetes. *International Journal for Human Caring.*

Web Listings

Centers for Disease Control and Prevention, http://www.cdc.gov

Occupational Safety & Health Administration, http://www.osha.gov

The Joint Commission, http://www.jointcommission.org

United States Department of Homeland Security, www.dhs.gov

World Health Organization, http://www.who.int

CHAPTER 17

Haitian Family's Health Experience and the Public School System

*T*he story of Haiti and the Haitian people is a complex picture of discovery, exploration, wealth, tragedy, violence, abuse, bloodshed, and the devastating earthquake of 2010, including hope within political and economic transition. Discovered by Christopher Columbus and named Hispaniola, the island of palm trees and colorful flowers was inhabited by the Arawak Indians, who referred to their home as "Hayti" for the mountainous land. The Arawak Indians were decimated by the Spaniards. Because of its location in the Caribbean, the land was sought after by many colonists and finally was colonized by France in the mid-17th century. Haiti shares the island with the Dominican Republic. The French elite relied on the slave trade to develop Haiti's economic base of cocoa, cotton, sugarcane, and coffee. The religion was a blend of Catholic and Vodou, an animistic faith from West Africa where objects and natural phenomena are believed to possess holy significance to possess a soul. French and Creole are the two languages. Haitian Creole is a pidgin French spoken by 90% of people and is considered by some to be the language of the poor. Creole was not a written language until the later years of the 20th century.

Haiti (the north of the island) became the first independent black republic in the world in 1804 and was fully negotiated with the French in 1820. Over the course of the next 100 years, the country was ravaged by wars and disputes. The United States invaded in 1915 and left in 1934. The infrastructure and economy improved under the Americans, but they were opposed by the Haitians. In the course of the next 70 years, Haitian elitists came to power but regimes collapsed because of the hunger for power manned by gangs, corrupt police and international forces, and authoritarian practices. The transition to democracy has been

267

tumultuous. Many Haitians tried to leave the island for the United States or Canada, where they could begin a life free from the fear of annihilation.

A minimalist democracy is now in place and struggling to rebuild from within and with the help of the world community, especially after the earthquake of 2010. The following is Charlotte's story of a family who has come to the United States to begin a new life. Reflect on the struggle with family life, language, and engaging with the public school and the school nurse.

Charlotte's Story

Henri recently started school after he and his family arrived from Haiti about 3 months ago. He was enrolled in the fourth grade of a local public school, but because of language differences (he spoke Creole and a little French), he was having difficulty with some subjects. He did try to speak English slowly with the help of a language facilitator. One day, a short time after he was enrolled in school, he wanted to talk with the school nurse to ask her to help his family. Charlotte, a school nurse practitioner, listened to the student with the help of the school language facilitator from the school board who was hired to assist Haitian students. After the visit, Charlotte decided to gather together administrators for a meeting, including the migrant educator and the school language facilitator. They decided to make a home visit to meet the family. A day was selected with his mother's approval. The team set out for the visit.

Henri's mother, Claudette, welcomed them into their home. Following introductions, Claudette shared the family's story by means of the language facilitator. Henri's father, Jacques, worked for 8 years in the agriculture business in Haiti to save enough money to bring his whole family to the United States. The family was granted legal immigration status. Henri and his parents knew that many of the people of their country tried to come to the United States illegally by boat, mostly because of political and economic crises in Haiti. Some of Claudette's and Jacques's family members immigrated to Montreal, Quebec, Canada where they were given refugee status because of political and economic circumstances. Although in the United States for about 3 months, the family is beginning to settle into a modest home and their new life. Henri's father, Jacques, got a job in agriculture, in a produce farm close to their home where other people from Haiti work. He makes a little more than the minimum wage. Henri is the only child enrolled in the school. The mother, Claudette is at home with Henri's two sisters, Angela and Evangeline, and their cousin, Renee, a 19-year-old who lives with them, whom they brought with them from Haiti to help with the children. She attended only a few years of school in Haiti. Claudette prays many times a day for help for her family. The family is Catholic but sometimes Claudette practices Vodou by maintaining a strong belief in the spirit world through different ritual practices. Claudette does not go out much because she cannot speak English. She does go grocery shopping but always asks Henri for help with speaking in public.

Henri's 10-year-old sister Angela had meningitis as an infant and is unable to walk. She is confined to a wheelchair that Social Services provided. She is able to get herself in and out of the chair where she can propel herself across the floor. She never attended school in Haiti. His sister Evangeline is 20 months old and does not walk but crawls in a pattern similar to the movements of Angela. Claudette is 3 months pregnant. Henri said that after school he has tried to help his mother with cleaning the house and with Angela and Evangeline. He does get along with Renee and follows her instructions.

Henri is having some difficulty in school, especially in the subjects of English, history, and social sciences. He is good at mathematics and likes physical education. He wants to learn to speak English better so he can do better in his studies, and play soccer after school. But because he has to help take care of his sisters, he does not know if he will be able to play after school. He was hoping that he could be on the soccer team. He has a dream of being on a football team when he gets to high school.

Transcultural Caring-Based Learning Approach

Please review the information about the Transcultural Caring Dynamics for Nursing and Health-Care Theory and Model, the assessment tools, the transcultural caring-based learning (TCCBL) approach, and the transcultural caring inquiry information explained in previous chapters of this book, and any other relevant literary and Internet information before dialoguing about this transcultural caring experience. In your small group, apply the TCCBL approach in relation to your transcultural caring situation for pattern identification (i.e., pattern seeing, pattern mapping, pattern recognizing, and pattern transforming). Use dimensions of the Transcultural Caring Dynamics in Nursing and Health-Care Model and use the most appropriate assessment tools for transcultural evidence gathering. The Reflections with Questions section that follows is a guide that will assist you individually and collectively in your learning group with dialogue and interpretation of the Haitian family's experience in the United States.

Reflections with Questions

Reflect on the history of Haiti and the meaning of leaving one's homeland to come to the highly technologically developed United States or Canada. Even though this family story illuminated legal immigration, the flight to freedom of Haitians is often illegal, and the rules for Haitians or Haitian Americans are unlike the Wet-Foot/Dry-Foot Policy and legal immigration status of people within the Cuban American culture. Reflect on the policy differences between Haiti and the United States, and Cuba and the United States. As a unique Franco-Afro-Caribbean culture and because of a tumultuous history, Haitians have been deprived of opportunities for securing a progressive education and jobs for their economic well-being. They desire the opportunities that are available in the United States and Canada. In the United States, the Haitian-American Nurses Association is contributing to the social, health care, and financial welfare of the people of Haiti.

Focus attention on Charlotte's story of the immigration of the Haitian family to the United States, the family's commitment to family, and to the well-being of the family. They are very worried about learning English. They hope that Henri's difficulties in the school system will not inhibit him too much. What are your responsibilities as a transcultural nurse in understanding the Haitian American culture and integration into the school system? Contemplate your role as a school nurse practitioner developing a program for Henri and his family with members of the administrative school team.

Transcultural Nursing Reflections

- Since Henri is the school-age child and the school system has initiated an in-home assessment at the request of Henri, how would you provide for Henri and his family—including, Claudette, Jacques, Angela, Evangeline, and Renee?
- What is the role of a school nurse in a transcultural situation within the public or private school system? What is the role of the school board in support or nonsupport given to school nurses or school nurse practitioners for children from a diverse culture within the public school systems?
- In your region, what is the role of nursing in school systems? Is there or should there be a policy of a "nurse in every school"? Does the school have responsibility for the child's social-cultural needs beyond the school?
- Are there immigration issues in your community that may affect families?
- What resources would be available through the public health system or private health system for prenatal care for Claudette and care for the children, Henri, Angela, Evangeline, and cousin Renee? Is health-care insurance available for new immigrants in your state or province; what type may be available?
- What health-care and learning resources are available for physically challenged or handicapped people? Is there transportation available?

- Overall, what may be the short-term and long-term prospects for health care for this family?
- What educational opportunities are there for learning English in your community or school system? How prominent are English as a second language (ESL) courses in the community?
- To understand the Haitian American family, contemplate what has occurred in Haiti throughout its history. What are the population and economic and geopolitical structures of Haiti? What is the political structure of Haiti, the military and peacekeeping presence in Haiti? What has happened to Haiti since the 2010 earthquake?
- What is the nature of poverty, health, health care, sanitation, and education in Haiti? What are the health beliefs and practices in Haiti? What is the nature of maternal-child care and what is the health of children and life expectancy of the Haitian people? What is the nutritional status of the people of Haiti?
- What are the spiritual beliefs and religions of Haiti? What is Vodou spiritualism and spirituality?
- What is the literacy level? Describe the languages that are spoken in Haiti and their derivation. What are the educational levels?
- How do elements within the population of Haiti compare with elements of health, public health, health-care access, and human safety in the population in the United States, Canada, and standards of the Pan American Health Organization (World Health Organization)?
- What are missionary groups contributing in Haiti?
- What are the migration patterns of Haitian people? What is the meaning of crime and insecurity and how do they play a role in the feelings of safety within Haiti and for people immigrating to other countries? What is the meaning of freedom and risk of migration?
- How does Haiti's economy and political structure compare with other nations in the Caribbean Community (CARICOM), in the United States, and Canada? Are there similar kinds of poverty, illiteracy, educational problems, crime, and health-care problems in the United States? How do Canada and the United States differ in these areas?
- What are the differences in immigration policy between Canada and the United States for political and economic refugees?

Select Bibliography

Barry, C., & Gordon, S. (2006). Theories and models of school nursing. In J. Selekman (Ed.), *Comprehensive textbook of school nursing*. Scarborough, ME: National Association of School Nursing.

Barry, C., & Gordon, S. (2006). Caring for students in school using a community nursing practice model. *International Journal for Human Caring, 9*(3), 38–42.

Barry, C., King, B., Goodman, R., Gullet, D. & Grumme, V. (2015). Coming to know a community: A community assessment in Rural Haiti. In M. Ray, Transcultural caring dynamics in nursing and health care (2nd ed.). Philadelphia, PA: F. A. Davis Company.

Center for Haitian Studies. http://www.med.miami.ed/news/center-for-haitian-studies/

Cianelli, R., Wilkinson, O., Mitchell, E., Anglade, D., Nicolas, G., Mitrani, V.. & Peragallo, N. (2013). Mental health training experiences among Haitian healthcare workers post-earthquake 2010. *International Nursing Review, 60*(4), 528–535.

De Santis, L., & Ugarriza, D. (1995). Potential for intergenerational conflict in Cuban and Haitian immigrant families. *Archives of Psychiatric Nursing, 9*, 102–107.

Dupuy, A. (2007). *Jean-Bertrand Aristide, the international community, and Haiti*. Lanham: Rowman & Littlefield Publishers, Inc.

Global Studies/School of Nursing and Health Studies, University of Miami, Miami, Florida.

http://www.miami.edu/sonhs/index.php/sonhs/academics/global_studies/hait-1/

Schantz, S., Charron, S., & Folden, S. (2003). Health seeking behavior of Haitian families. *Journal of Cultural Diversity, 10*, 62–68.

CHAPTER 18

Elderly Native American Navajo's Health Experience in the Nursing Home Culture

*T*he Native Indian, Aboriginal, Indigenous, or First People of North America and around the world are an ever-changing and complex assembly. They range from the first natives themselves, the Inuit, to the northernmost native people who had contact with the Vikings around 984 A.D., to the first native Navy commander, a Chickasaw astronaut, traveling in the space shuttle Endeavor to outer space in 2002 (McMaster & Trafzer, 2004). Many stories shed light on the beginning of the First People. The most widely accepted explanation of how Indians, Inuit (formerly Eskimos), and Aleut (Alaska Natives) people arrived in North America is that nomadic tribes from Asia crossed the Bering Strait and moved throughout the continent some 12,000 to 60,000 years ago. When the Spanish explorers came upon the New World about 1492, there were 110 million indigenous Indians in the Americas. The name Indian comes from explorers who believed that they had landed in India. The name survived even though names, such as "First People(s) or First Nations People (Aboriginal of North America, particularly noted in Canada), Aboriginal, or indigenous" are becoming more common (Hill, 2002). There are many native tribes in North America and Central and South America. Native Indians number about 2.5 million people, with about 1.6 million people who consider themselves to be of Native heritage in the United States (Hill, 2002), and about 1 million people in Canada (Davidhizar & Giger, 1998; Hill, 2002). There are 40 million indigenous people living in Latin America and the Caribbean, of which about 12.6% are indigenous (600 tribes), with 40% of the aboriginals living in rural settings (www.iwgia.org).

This transcultural story highlights a Navajo elder. The Navajo, called the "Diné or the people" (a similar term, Dené, represents the aboriginal group of First Nations primarily in Canada), live on the largest reservation in the United States. According to the 2000 U.S. census, there are about 174,987 Navajos within the borders of the Navajo Nation, and about 298,215 Navajos living throughout the United States. The Navajo nation is more than 16 million acres located over three states, New Mexico, Arizona, and Utah. The reservation surrounds the Hopi Indian Reservation. The Navajo nation preserves its land, kinship, language and religion and the right to govern itself. On the Navajo reservation, traditions are strong. Hogans (traditional homes) face the rising sun. The mountains surrounding the reservation are sacred and storytellers illuminate ancient myths about the journeys from the first to the fourth world. Many stories give honor to the earth and each other; some speak of fear, starvation, warfare, and other dangers. The mountains that serve as boundaries on the reservation represent symbols of the different worlds and are identified in narrative with colors—white, blue, yellow, and black.

Many elders still wear traditional dress; medicine men perform healing rituals, and the Navajo language is spoken and considered special. "Navajo Code Talkers" helped to win the war in the Pacific during World War II. Weaving is elevated to an art form highlighting very old and contemporary art. Other cultural activities, such as the pipe ceremony, and Native symbolism of the circle, show respect for family, kin, ancestors, and guests. The survival of Indian ceremonies is not easy in today's pressured world but the annual powwow (the word meaning sacred) honors many Native populations who celebrate their religions and warrior status by bringing together the voices of all Indians in North America. Ceremonial rituals, native foods, drum music, songs and dances, headdresses of feathers of the eagle and other birds, breastplates, skirts, and shoes are expressions of spiritual beliefs and overall community fidelity of the diverse tribes. The following is a transcultural experience of an elderly Navajo man, Bill Silversmith, who is now living in a nursing home. Bill participated in the diverse realities of historical and contemporary Native American life.

Bill Silversmith's Story

Bill Silversmith, a Navajo from the Navajo Nation, is in his twilight years and resides in a nursing home in New Mexico administered by the order of Catholic Sisters for the Poor and Aging (a pseudonym). Very frail from general old age, dementia, type 2 diabetes (12 times the national average in the Indian population), and some effects of drinking alcohol, Bill wanted to go to the Catholic Sisters for the Poor and Aging nursing home, where the sisters created a loving and caring home for aging Native American people. Bill got to meet the sisters when they provided nursing care and midwifery services on the Navajo reservation. Bill had had some care provided by the Veterans' Administration (VA) part of the time; there was no VA nursing home available in the area. The Catholic Sisters for the Poor and Aging nursing home has been a godsend for Bill because most of his immediate family has already died. His granddaughter Miranda, however, is dedicated to him and visits him every week. Miranda likes to tell stories of her grandfather. Bill was a great silversmith on the reservation after learning how to make jewelry and belt buckles from his own grandmother as a little boy. He is proud of his name, Bill Silversmith.

Bill also was one of the original Navajo Indian Code Talkers who served in the Pacific during World War II. The Navajo Code Talkers, through their special success in relaying military messages using the Navajo language as a secret code, were able to foil the advance of the enemy against the United States after the attack on Pearl Harbor. They saved thousands of lives. Only a few of the original 29 Navajo Code Talkers are still living.

Over the years, Bill told his granddaughter that he always hoped there would be some recognition for the veteran Navajo Code Talkers' service to the United States. In 2001, Bill's dream came true. They were honored by President George Bush with a Congressional Medal of

Honor in 2001, and in 2005, the State of New Mexico and the city of Gallup, New Mexico began to make progress to establish a National Code Talkers' Museum to honor the Navajo men who gave so much to their country.

While living on the reservation, Bill and his late wife and three children did not have amenities like a large home with good sewer and septic systems that he would have had if he lived off the reservation, but he enjoyed the life because he was with his people. After his experience in World War II, Bill worked for the local telephone company and put in some phone lines on the reservation (there were not too many in those days).

Luckily for Bill, he didn't develop severe kidney disease or neuropathy from the diabetes like so many of his friends. But he finally had to take insulin to control his diabetes. He also has atrial fibrillation, high cholesterol, and high blood pressure, which are controlled with warfarin (Coumadin, blood thinner) and Caduet (antihypertensive and anticholesterol) medications. Bill takes Aricept (Donepezil HCl) and Namenda (memantine HCl) medications to help control the advance of his dementia. He loves to go outside and enjoy nature if the weather permits. Bill likes to talk about old customs and Miranda often records some of his stories. Miranda spoke for him at the monthly residents' appreciation day at the nursing home. Bill's increasing dementia interferes with his own ability to speak with clarity. Miranda talked about Bill as a Code Talker during World War II. She also spoke of his enjoyment over the years of their annual trip to Window Rock, Arizona where Bill and the family attended the Navajo Nation Fair. The fair featured a lot of his favorite things, many customs, rituals, and symbols of the Native Indians. They loved to talk within a circle and share stories of old from their rich heritage.

Bill did miss his life on the reservation when he came to the nursing home. He used to tell Miranda that he always hoped that she would be able to contribute to life on the reservation through her social work, and her dedication to the National Code Talkers' Museum. Bill's other legacy was encouraging his children and grandchildren to go to school. He knew that if they were educated, they would have more to give back to the Navajo Nation and all Native people.

There are a few nuns who minister spiritually to the residents/patients. They are dedicated to their patients and take joy in meeting their needs as older Indian residents. They take into consideration the spiritual rituals of the Navajo. One key way that they honor the Navajo is by incorporating cultural activities and calling upon the elders in the Navajo Nation to assist. Medicine men and their rituals are important to the Navajo culture and the Sisters have one of the Medicine Men from the community come to the nursing home once a week. Participation in Residents' Appreciation Day each month features two residents who share their memories from "days of old." In this environment, the spiritual needs of the patient are oriented to Native American wisdom—everything in a circle, everything round, and part of the environment. They incorporate wisdom about the soil, hogans, mesas, pueblos, mountains, and deserts, and the sun, moon, and sky.

Transcultural Caring-Based Learning Approach

Please review the information about the Transcultural Caring Dynamics for Nursing and Health-Care Model, the assessment tools, the transcultural caring-based learning (TCCBL) approach, and the transcultural caring inquiry information explained in previous chapters of this book, and any other relevant literary and Internet information before dialoguing about this transcultural caring experience. In your small group, apply the TCCBL approach in relation to your transcultural caring situation for pattern identification (i.e., pattern seeing, pattern mapping, pattern recognizing, and pattern transforming). Use dimensions of the Transcultural Caring Dynamics in Nursing and Health-Care Theory and Model and use the most appropriate assessment tools for transcultural evidence gathering. The Reflections with Questions section that follows is a guide that will assist you individually and collectively in your learning group with dialogue and interpretation of a Native American man's traditional and modern life.

AUTHOR'S REFLECTION

In this transcultural caring experience, we are reminded of the relationship between the individual as a culture and in his sociocultural heritage and context. The context of Bill Silversmith's life is very complex—the family, the environment, the Navajo Nation, the Navajo Reservation, the American Indian experience, the United States nation, the world in serving in the military in the Pacific during World War II, the military, the U.S. Army, the National Code Talkers service group, the Veterans' Administration for health-care services, the telephone company for work, the nursing home for aged care, and also an important and unique museum that honors his service to the nation. Also important to Bill are the customs, rituals, and symbols of his ancient culture experienced holistically in annual powwows. As an honored member of the National Code Talkers, Bill has become a legend in his own time. It is now a part of his spiritual nature.

Reflections with Questions

The story of Bill shows the rich and diverse realities of the life experiences of a Native American. What are your responsibilities as a transcultural nurse in understanding the culture of the Navajo Indian culture and the culture of a nursing home?

Imagine yourself as a young graduate Caucasian nurse caring for an aging Navajo, Native American man in the nursing home in New Mexico. You have recently graduated from the University of Arizona and have come back to work as a nurse in New Mexico where you grew up. Although you have lived in "Indian country" your whole life and studied in Arizona where many different tribal groups are represented, you have never had a lot of contact with the Native Indian/First Nations' or aboriginal people of North America. You have decided that the two areas that you needed to experience were caring for the North American Indians and caring for the aged. You are trying to understand yourself as a "multicultural being" in addition to the Indian people as "multicultural beings" with a unique history. You also are trying to understand more about the history of U.S. expansion and early aggression toward the Indians. At the University of Arizona, School of Nursing, you had a course on transcultural nursing and two courses on gerontological nursing. So you feel quite prepared.

At the nursing home, because you have a bachelor of science in nursing, the administration would like you to be more involved with a nursing leadership role, but you have asked to do general nursing to gain experience directly with the residents and gain experience in caring for aging Navajo people. You are committed to the culture and want to learn more about it. The sisters who are in possession of the nursing home are amenable to you doing direct care but asked if you could also consider taking on the nurse manager role as soon as possible. In nursing homes, usually licensed practical nurses, nursing assistants, aides and recreation and physical therapists assist with the patient care, and recreation. Registered nurses generally are the nurse managers.

Transcultural Nursing Reflections

As a new graduate RN, consider how you would develop a transculturally sensitive plan of care that would incorporate a holistic view of scientific and Indian health practices into nursing care (i.e., body, mind, spirit, and culture). Nursing constructs in a Native American culture include the following seven dimensions: caring, traditions, respect, connection, holism, trust, and spirituality (Lowe & Nichols, 2014).

- What type of cultural care would you design?
- How would you care for Bill relative to his type 2 diabetes, cardiovascular problems, dementia, and frailty?
- Would you be asking Bill about any other health problems, such as alcohol intake or tobacco use over the years?

- What side effects may affect Bill?
- What signs and symptoms will you have to be prepared to care for and also teach the assistants to be aware of?
- How would you incorporate the Navajo beliefs into his care? How would the rituals, symbols, and customs of the culture play a role in the care of Bill? What is meant by the "talking circle"?
- How would you coordinate Bill's care with the other members of the team and the Sisters?
- In the Native population, and on reservations, how significant are health or social dilemmas, such as HIV/AIDS; drug use; hepatitis A, B, and C; alcoholism; sexually transmitted diseases; cancer; and chronic obstructive pulmonary disease from tobacco use? How widespread is teenage pregnancy or single-parent families?
- What is the total population of Native peoples in North America, in the United States? What border restrictions are there between Canada and the United States and the United States and Canada for Native peoples?
- Examine the ways in which the countries of North America name and transculturally integrate their original citizens (e.g., Indians, Natives, North American Indians, First Nations' People, Aboriginals, Inuit, Mestizoes (European and Native American ancestry in Latin America), and Frontierizos (Borderland Hispanic Texans).
- Consider the creation of reservations, the geopolitical nature of reservation cultures of North America, and the effect of reservations on the Native people.
- Compare and contrast Native/Aboriginal peoples of the United States and Canada. Why are the terms aboriginal, indigenous, and First Peoples used more in Canada and Australia than in the United States?
- Compare and contrast these cultural historical perspectives with the Gypsy lifeworld in the European Union, and tribal emergence and evolution in the African Union.
- What is the role of gambling casinos on reservations in the United States? State the purposes, goals, and also the problems associated with legalized gambling and its impact on health and well-being.

Select Bibliography

Davidhizar, R., & Giger, J. (1998). *Canadian transcultural nursing: Assessment and intervention.* St. Louis: Mosby.

Definition of Frontierizos. Retrieved July 20, 2009, from *Texana: Ethnic heritage*, http://www.miscybrarian.com/archives/texana/ethnicheritage.shtml

Definition of Mestizo/Mestizoes. Retrieved July 20, 2009, from the *Free online dictionary*, http://www.the freedictionary.com/mestizo

Edwards, K., & Patchell, B. (2009). State of the science: A cultural view of Native Americans and diabetes prevention. *Journal of Cultural Diversity, 15*(1), 32–35.

Hain, D., Touhy, T., Sparks-Compton, D., & Engstrom, G. (2014). Using narratives of individuals and couples living with early stage dementia to guide practice. *Journal of Practice Applications and Reviews of Research, 4*(2), 82–93.

Hill, L. (2002). *American Indians.* New York: Workman Publishing.

Hodge, F., Pasque, A., Marquez, C., & Gershirt-Cantrell, B. (2002). Utilizing traditional storytelling to promote wellness in American Indian communities. *Journal of Transcultural Nursing, 13*, 6–11.

Lauderdale, J., Nichols, L., Tom-Orme, L., & Strickland, C. (2005). Respecting tribal traditions in research and publications: Voices of five Native American nurse scholars. *Journal of Transcultural Nursing, 16*, 193–201.

Lowe, J. (2002). Balance and harmony through connectedness. *Holistic Nursing Practice, 16*(4), 4–11.

Lowe, J. (2007). The need for historically grounded HIV/AIDS prevention research among Native Americans. *Journal of the Association of Nurses in AIDS Care, 18*(2), 15–17.

Lowe, J., Liang, H., Riggs, C., & Henson, J. (2012). Community partnership to affect substance abuse among Native American adolescents. *The American Journal of Drug and Alcohol Abuse, 38*(5), 450–455.

Lowe, J., & Nichols, L. (2014). Utilisation [Utilization] of native American nursing conceptual framework: Implications for practice and research. *Australian Journal of Advanced Nursing, 31*(2), 13–210.

McMaster, G., & Trafzer, C. (Eds.). (2004). *Native universe.* Washington, DC: National Museum of the American Indian.

Newhouse, D., Voyageur, C., & Beavon, D. (2005). *Hidden in plain sight: Contributions of Aboriginal peoples to Canadian identity and culture* (Vol. I). Toronto: University of Toronto Press.

Ordonez, M., & Hain, D. (2014). Healthy transitions from hospital to skilled nursing facility post-CABG. *Journal of Practice Applications & Reviews of Research, 4*(2), 123–134.

Tom-Orme, L. (2006). Research and American/Alaska Native health: A nursing perspective. *Journal of Transcultural Nursing, 17,* 261–265.

Touhy, T., & Jett, K. (2011). *Ebersole & Hess' gerontological nursing and healthy aging* (4th ed.). St. Louis: Mosby.

Touhy, T., & Williams, C. (2008). Communicating with older adults. In C. Williams, *Therapeutic interaction in nursing* (2nd ed.). Sudbury, MA: Jones & Bartlett.

CHAPTER 19

The Transcultural Caring Experience of a Haitian Girl and a Nurse Practitioner in an Adolescent Correctional Facility

*orrectional facilities or prisons represent a specific culture or, in some cases, multiple cultures based upon diverse values, beliefs, attitudes, and behaviors that are transmitted from one group to another (i.e., the penal system administrators, correctional officers, and the inmates themselves). The overarching culture is the criminal justice system whereby the goals are punishment (under the law) for conviction of crimes against humanity or society and, in some cases, rehabilitation and return to the society. Correctional facilities are institutions that confine individuals in terms of their security risk, which has a classification system ranging from minimum to maximum security risk. Maximum security risk inmates are housed in institutions with small cells surrounded by fences and barbed wire, and are under the strict supervision of prison guards. Minimum security risk inmates often are in open rooms similar to dormitories, and can be placed in work camps, work release centers, or road prisons (Campbell, 2007; Schmalleger, 2009; Schmalleger & Smykla, 2008)). Juvenile incarceration in correctional facilities has increased due in part to changes in values, lack of loving and effective parenting, low incomes, culturally specific discrimination, increase in violence in the home, physical and sexual abuse, drug addiction or abuse (including prescription drugs), and alcohol abuse. In addition, other issues, such as prostitution and human trafficking, are coming to the fore. Often, HIV/AIDS is a result. The contemporary literature reports that there is a lack of appropriate prevention, diversion, treatment alternatives, and victims' advocacy, though there is an *increase in probation and parole field services with more resources. There are less gender-specific programs based upon a review of women's pathways into crime. Task forces and different organizations, especially in southeast Florida, have been created to try to rectify the problems associated with crime in general and juvenile crime and juvenile justice in particular (Campbell, 2007; Ryder, 2005; Van Wormer & Bartollas, 2007). Health care in correctional facilities is an accepted practice and often nurse practitioners fulfill the need to assist the victims of crime or assault, perpetrators, or the prison population of inmates with their health problems (Gibson, 2008; Weiss, 2007).*

The following is a transcultural caring experience of a nurse practitioner who is assigned to care for an adolescent girl who is charged with a felony and in an adolescent correctional facility.

Josie's Story

"Working with incarcerated adolescents can be challenging. The girls in this facility, whose ages range from 10 to 18 years, often touch my heart. Many are estranged from their parents due to neglect, abuse, crime, violence, illness, or sometimes death from AIDS. The constant turnover of medical/nursing staff in this wilderness rehabilitation facility is clear evidence of the difficulty of the job working with struggling adolescents; staff members cannot tolerate it. At times, the girls and the bureaucratic system are so frustrating that I wonder why I continue in this 1-day-per-week position.

As an advanced practice nurse, my job is to ensure the health of each female admitted by performing a complete physical examination, and providing care for those who are infirmed. Sometimes I need to be reminded to treat these girls with the individualized care and concern that they deserve without regard to the choices (drugs or criminal acts) that brought them here to the facility. One particular experience has left a lasting impression on me. After a particularly difficult day where there was a great deal of yelling and unkindness exhibited by the staff outside my clinic door, a young girl came in for her initial visit. As she sat on my examination table, this quiet Haitian American child began to cry. She missed her family and could not understand the anger of the staff. As I wrapped my arms around her, encouraging her to be strong while she was incarcerated, she quietly began to recite *Psalm 27*. As she sat there, her sad story tumbled forth. She spoke of waiting outside her boyfriend's door for hours only to learn that he was inside with another girl. During the fight that followed, she lost the tiny infant that had just begun to grow in her womb. I, too, mourned the losses that she had sustained in her short life. But I realized the strength that she had been given in a culture far different from mine as she spoke the words of the *Psalm*. (Being unfamiliar with this scripture, I sought out the text that evening and realized that these verses speak of being brave in times of trouble.) Her mother had equipped her to persevere during this difficult time in ways foreign to many people in American culture.

As I recall that incident I am reminded once again of the richness that nursing allows. As nurses, our patients trust us with their lives and we have great opportunities for good or harm. When we are too busy or self-absorbed and fail to appreciate the unique qualities of each person, we, as well as our patients, are short changed. This child touched my life as I, too, now think of *Psalm 27* in times of trouble or insomnia. Sometimes I wonder, as I provide health care to these girls in juvenile detention, if I am really providing what they need in the most culturally appropriate ways. I also wonder how often the essence of my nursing care remains after my name and face are only a blur."

Transcultural Caring-Based Learning Approach

Please review the information about the Transcultural Caring Dynamics for Nursing and Health-Care Model, the assessment tools, the transcultural caring-based learning (TCCBL) approach, and the transcultural caring inquiry information and any other relevant literary and Internet information before dialoguing about this transcultural caring experience. In your small group, apply the TCCBL approach, in relation to your transcultural caring situation for pattern identification (i.e., pattern seeing, pattern mapping, pattern recognizing, and pattern transforming). Use dimensions of the Transcultural Caring Dynamics in Nursing and Health-Care Theory and Model and use the most appropriate assessment tools for transcultural evidence gathering to what is happening in the relationship between Josie, the nurse practitioner, and the Haitian American girl in the correctional facility.

Reflections with Questions

Focus attention on Josie's story in her reflections on the type of nursing (forensic nursing) in which she is engaged, the culture of adolescence, the Haitian American culture, incarceration of juveniles, and correctional facilities. What are your responsibilities as a transcultural nurse in understanding nursing in the juvenile justice system, adolescent culture, the Haitian American culture, adolescent pregnancy, the care of an adolescent girl who was pregnant and now coming to terms with the outcomes of a miscarriage due to violence, and the meaning of spirituality and courage in the face of bewilderment and fear? Contemplate the American prison system as a culture and the paradox between incarceration and rehabilitation of young people. What transcultural caring processes of compassion and justice come to your mind in Josie's story?

Transcultural Nursing Reflections

Nursing scholars state that caring is compassion and right action and seeking understanding of the meaning of suffering to facilitate health and healing for the patient. In this transcultural caring experience, imagine that you are the nurse practitioner.

* Reflect on the meaning of trust and the relationship that was established in this story. What is the role of a nurse practitioner in an adolescent correctional facility? Given the examples of the nurse-patient relationship in this story, describe how transcultural caring was established. What may be the cultural differences and cultural customs of a Haitian American girl that may need to be bridged?
* Using the pattern-identification process, the Transcultural Caring in Nursing and Health-Care Theory and Model, and any of the assessment tools, think about and discuss the meaning of a correctional facility or prison system as a culture. What values, beliefs, attitudes, and behaviors do you see exhibited in this transcultural caring experience?
* Reflect on the role of a nurse or nurse practitioner in a correctional facility (Panosky & Shalton, 2015). What is the meaning of compassion in relationship to justice?
* Reflect on the physical examination that must be conducted in the correctional facility. What type of trust also is needed when conducting a vaginal examination for miscarriage? What type of interview is identified, if any? Are there different types of interviews that are allowed in a forensic case or correctional facility for age and sex? How would *you* speak with the young Haitian American girl about the procedure that you are performing? Would there be any differences if it were a rape case? What is a rape kit?
* What is legal caring?
* What is the meaning of a correctional facility as a culture, a bureaucracy? How could Ray's Theory of Bureaucratic Caring fit into this transcultural nursing experience?
* How were the adolescent and the nurse transformed by the recitation of *Psalm 27* and the experience of the relationship that followed? What is the meaning of "reciprocity in interaction or transpersonal caring" (see Watson, 1988)? What is the role of prayer or prayer support in nursing?
* What transcultural caring thoughts come to your mind about this story of the young girl? What ethical concerns come to mind when you think about a juvenile correctional facility

AUTHOR'S REFLECTION

The experience of prison life becomes a learning process. People incarcerated learn the culture of prison life, the values, attitudes, and belief systems that are transmitted from one group to the other. Often, the lifeworld for adolescents or any other inmate soon becomes a "normative" system. Is it possible for a prison to be a restorative and healing environment rather than a punitive environment? Is it possible for positive transformative behavioral (i.e., mental, emotional, and spiritual) change once a person is incarcerated? Can a transcultural caring nurse change an entrenched system?

and the staff? How would you, as the nurse practitioner, teach the staff about the cultural differences, and the meaning of being a young girl in the correctional facility?

- How would you deal with staff anger or frustration that builds up over time? Do you think prison system personnel have to exhibit anger? Why do they lose control?
- How would you construct a different type of community?
- What concerns come to your mind for adolescent culture, the Haitian American culture, or any other cultural group that could be represented within the correctional facility?
- Contemplate all the issues facing adolescents both in the general culture and in the juvenile justice system and the correctional facility.
- What does it mean to ensure prisoners' or inmates' rights? Should inmates who have been rehabilitated wait for any period of time for the right to vote?
- What is the meaning of correction? What is the meaning of distributive justice? Why is there so much recidivism? What is the meaning of rehabilitation and restoration back to life in the community? How can people be integrated back into the community after living in a correctional facility? Can a caring system be integrated into a prison?
- What is the role of transcultural caring ethics in a correctional facility? Do you think values of evil overtake the compassion of nurses when working with the "not so picture perfect person"? Is it difficult to be caring in systems that are there to punish crimes against people or society?
- Overall, is it possible to change cultures, the juvenile justice system, and people who work in a correctional facility? What role does nursing have?
- Examine the role of a forensic nurse. How can caring be integrated into forensic nursing?

Select Bibliography

Campbell, D. (2007). *Juvenile justice case processing: The impact of gender and ethnicity on the adjudication and disposition states of juvenile justice court cases in Broward County, Florida.* Bloomington, IN: Xlibris Corp.

Coffman S. (2006). Marilyn Anne Ray, theory of bureaucratic caring. In A. Marriner Tomey & M. Alligood (Eds.), *Nursing theorists and their work* (6th ed., pp. 116–139). St. Louis: Mosby.

Dubois, L. (2012). *Haiti: The aftershocks of history.* New York: Metropolitan Books, Henry Holt Company.

Gibson, S. (2008). Legal caring: Preventing re-traumatization of abused children through the caring nursing interview using Roach's six C's. *International Journal for Human Caring, 12*(4), 32–37.

Lynch, V. (2005). *Forensic nursing.* St. Louis: Mosby.

Miller, J., Leininger, M., Leuning, C., Pacquiao, D., Ludwig-Beymer, P., & Papadopoulos, I. (2008). Transcultural Nursing Society position statement on human rights. *Journal of Transcultural Nursing, 19*(1), 5–7.

O'Brien, E. (2002). *Prayer in nursing: The spirituality of compassionate caregiving.* Burlington, MA: Jones & Bartlett Learning.

Panosky, D., & Shelton, D. (2015). Evaluating an adolescent behavior program: Leadership, education, achievement and development for adolescent female offenders in corrections. *Journal of Forensic Nursing, 11*(3), 144-153.

Ray, M. (2005). The theory of bureaucratic caring. In M. Parker (Ed.), *Nursing theories and nursing practice* (2nd ed., pp. 421–444). Philadelphia: F. A. Davis Company.

Ryder, R. (2005). *Juvenile justice: A social, historical and legal perspective* (2nd ed.). Sudbury, MA: Jones and Bartlett.

Schmalleger, F. (2009). *Criminal justice: A brief introduction* (8th ed.). Upper Saddle River, NJ: Prentice-Hall.

Schmalleger, F., & Smykla, J. (2008). *Corrections in the 21st century* (4th ed.). New York: McGraw-Hill Humanities/Social Sciences/Languages.

Sherman, F. (2007). Access to community healthcare in the juvenile justice system: Initial lessons from Massachusetts health passport project. *Women, Girls, and Criminal Justice, 8*(6), 81–82, 87–91.

The Book of Psalms. (1993). New York: Dover Publications.

Turkel, M., & Ray, M. (2009). Caring for "not so picture perfect patients": Ethical caring in the moral community of nursing. In R. Locsin & M. Purnell (Eds.), *A contemporary nursing process: The (un)bearable weight of knowing persons* (pp. 225–249). New York: Springer Publishing Company.

Van Wormer, K., & Bartollas, C. (2007). *Women and the criminal justice system.* (2nd ed.). Needham Heights, MA: Allyn & Bacon.

Van Wormer, K. (2008). *Restorative justice across the East & West.* Manchester, UK: Case Verde Publishing.

Voorhis, P., & Salisbury, E. (2014). *Correctional counseling and rehabilitation* (8th ed.). New York: Elsevier.

Watson, J. (1988). *Nursing: Human science and human care: A theory of nursing.* New York: National League for Nursing Press.

Weiss, J. (2007). Let's talk about it: Safe adolescent sexual decision making. *Journal of the American Academy of Nurse Practitioners, 19*, 450–458.

CHAPTER 20

The Heart of Suffering, Mourning, and Healing in the Jewish Spiritual Culture: A Mother's Story

Introduction to Jewish Traditions

"In order to understand my story of personal tragedy it requires that I share with you some traditions of the Jewish faith regarding the death and mourning of a beloved individual. When a person is born, there is both a physical presence and, as I believe, a spiritual presence. When a person dies, one's physical presence is returned to whence it came but the spirit of the deceased is forever present. The Jewish tradition dictates very set practices to observe, practices that allow the bereaved to live the days and months of mourning in a manner honoring the loved one who died and relieve the bereaved from decision making. When the death of a loved one occurs, traditional acts of honoring the deceased begin. Preparation of the deceased begins for burial (i.e., the washing of the body, the dressing of the deceased in simple white garments [shroud], the placing of the deceased in a simple pine coffin [made without nails, only wooden pegs]). These acts are followed by the honor of having Psalms read in the room where the deceased lies, never leaving him or her alone until the actual burial takes place. The traditions that follow after the actual burial has taken place are also ways for the mourners to honor and respect the deceased while at the same time live and experience their grief. Shiva, the first 7 days of mourning, begins immediately after the burial.

This personal and more private time of mourning takes place in the home of the mourner. This is a time when friends and community members come to comfort the mourner, to share in the special stories of the deceased, and to be there for them in ways that respect the needs *of the mourner. This special, personal time of mourning ends at the end of 7 days and is marked by a walk around the block by the mourner(s) to bring them back into the community of others.*

After Shiva, begins a period of mourning called Shloshim, the 30-day period of mourning where prayers of mourning are usually said at daily services at the synagogue. Return to work, to one's responsibilities thus begins, but revelry (joyfully participating in life) is more reserved. After the end of the 30 days, mourners return to their normal life as fully as before the death of the deceased, but they continue for a year to recite the Mourner's Kaddish *(the prayer for the dead). The custom at the end of the official year of mourning is an "unveiling" of a memorial plaque placed at the gravesite of the deceased, with a special prayer service held to honor the loved one. All these traditions have variations within the different practices of the Jewish religion. What I have shared with you is from the perspective of a Conservative Jew, one who honors the Bible and its writings, with a perspective within today's changing world.*

Anita's Story

My story continues by sharing the sudden, unforeseen happening of my youngest son's death. Simply stated, he took his own life: suicide. To begin that sharing, I ask you to read the letter I wrote just a month before the death of my son, a letter that was written to each of my five children, hoping to help them when—in what I always felt was the normal cycle of life events—my husband and I would die. This is my letter written to my children shortly before Lawrence's death.

Dear Lawrence,

The purpose of this letter is to be both informative and reflective. On the informative side, Dad and I want you to have some knowledge of what we have recently done regarding what we want to happen when we die, which we don't see as tomorrow or next month, or very soon. But it was important to us to relieve any additional stress on our children that occurs when a parent dies. For that reason, last week we purchased two cemetery plots at the Eternal Cemetery near our home. The total costs of all the charges incurred with the purchase have been taken care of by us.

As far as service arrangements, we will leave it to be done when needed, but we do have very specific requests for what we both want. Israel Chapel, right outside of our community, is where services would be held. It is hoped that our children and perhaps grandchildren would want to lead the services. Hiring a Rabbi whom we do not have any connection to is not our preference. I, Mom, would like some poetry read such as the poem, "If I Had My Life to Live Over, I Would Plant More Daisies." I would also like some music played, such as Four Seasons *by Vivaldi; something not usually done, but then again, I seem to at times do things that shouldn't be done. Dad doesn't want music, but there are other ways to share who he is. We want our day of leaving to be a celebration of who we were and not a day of sadness.*

On some more specifics, Dad and I both want a kosher casket, with no lining. We want the traditional body preparation, with wrapping in cotton, and not being left alone until burial. So that is it.

On an individual personal note, we need to say how sorry we are for not always being there for you, like when you had to have surgery on your head and Ethel took you. It should have been your Mother who was there for you. We also wish we had attended more of your gymnastic meets, had attended your college graduation, and spent more time talking with each other, knowing each other better. You have done well in your life, married now to someone who loves you very much and whom you love very much. Dad and I only wish you both a long life together, in good health, with happiness surrounding you.

My Dedication to Lawrence at His Burial

Dear Lawrence,

Everyone calls you Larry in your professional life, but your family only knows you as Lawrence. Not that we felt you were so formal but that from the time of your arrival on this earth some 47 years ago, you were always Lawrence, no nickname, no shortened name, just Lawrence.

As I stand here today, trying so hard to be quiet in my mind but certainly not in my heart, I find it somewhat ironic that it is you whom we have come together to say good-bye to.

Just a month ago, your father and I sat down to write each of your siblings and you a letter informing them of our preferences when we died. We wanted a traditional Jewish burial, simple, but dignified, although I stated in the letter that I wanted a particular poem read and a special song played. I wanted my death to be a celebration of my life, which until today I thought was pretty good. A number of bumps in the road but with the love of my family, my children, we all got through it. At the end of each letter to all of you, I wrote a personal note, apologizing for things not done, not said, but also told each how special they are. To you Lawrence my personal note told you how proud we are of you, how we knew that you married Michelle who loved you very much and whom you loved very much. The letter ended with saying Dad and I only wish you both a long life together, in good health, with happiness surrounding you.

Your response to the letter was: *"Mom, you are more than welcome to send me as many letters as you want. But please know that you and Dad have nothing to apologize about during my 47 years of life. You both were and are great parents. Most people could not have raised five, what I think are pretty good children, when both of you were so young. So the only thing you should be doing is looking back on life and celebrate your success in raising a great family . . . that would be a good letter. Talk to you soon,*

Love, Lawrence (and Michelle)."

That letter was written just 4 weeks ago and now I am standing here saying good-bye to you my youngest child, who was loved so much by all of his family and who will forever be missed. My heart is full with that love and when I hear your voice answering on your cell phone "Larry Beckerman" my heart breaks. I have played your voice message over and over since we received the call. It brings to mind those who died on 9/11 and left messages on loved ones' cell phones saying good-bye.

I need to say something about the suffering of my son these last years, keeping it to himself, feeling ashamed that he who was so successful in his career was not able to overcome this disease. As his mother, deep down I can't help feeling that I missed something important, that I wasn't listening. Everyone tries to tell me that you hid your intense overpowering suffering so well. Michelle took care of you after your heart attack 3 years ago and was always there for you. Just these last weeks it seemed that you sought help and seemed to be feeling better. But it just wasn't meant to be.

Rabbi Small [pseudonym] said to me yesterday that the demons in your head just took over and I truly believe that you were thinking of others and the grief of your illness, so for me your death became courageous, not cowardly. You were trying to protect others from what you considered a shameful illness but we know it is a horrendous illness that can overpower the most strong and most bright.

Lawrence, I promised myself that I do not want you to be remembered only by your illness, so I am sharing some things about you that speak of you as a whole person, successful, happy, and fun to be with. You will always be in my heart as a son who cared about others, being with family to celebrate many joyous occasions. You were the one who volunteered to be the sibling that would accompany me to my first chemotherapy treatment in January 1999. When you walked into the house, you said that you had done all your crying and that we had some serious work to do. As I was getting my chemo you just hovered over me, helping me to the restroom, making sure I was comfortable when I sat in the chair. You were so afraid of what was happening to me, but your presence made me less afraid. You were also the one who came to Florida to take me to the hospital in 2002 when I had back surgery. You made sure that Dad and I were O.K. before you went back home. When you had your heart attack and couldn't attend Mayaan's Bat Mitzvah the following week, David and I were there with you and a videotape was made of you talking to Mayaan, congratulating and sending her your love. You wanted so badly to be there, but the doctor said no.

But there were also fun times we had together. You loved golf and played it as often as you could and you were good, but I remember when we lived at Gleneagles and I went out with you in the golf cart. I watched you hit and once made a comment how good you hit the ball. You politely told me that my comments weren't correct or wanted. You were hard on yourself with golf and that is what made you a very good golfer.

I think that this pursuit of perfection was seen in many aspects of your life, your career in the field of management information systems, which when you were registered at the State University of New York at Binghamton in the MIS tract, it was truly a mystery to Dad and me as to what this career specialty was, but we soon found out. In your first job at Anderson Consulting; you were able to get us the first IBM PC. When you installed it in our home in New York, you quietly informed us that food and drink were not allowed in the computer room and you were serious about this.

On my visit alone with you in May of this year, when you came to spend some time with me in Oxnard at the beach house of David and David, it was very special. We had a wonderful time, talking, eating great food, which included the Passover sweet loaded with ginger and honey that only you and I enjoyed. We drank great wine, and had a very special day when we went whale watching. I saw you turn into a little boy loose in a toy store who couldn't stop taking pictures of the whales, and we saw many that day. I am sure Michelle remembers the many calls you made to her from the boat to share with her your joy of the day, telling her that she would just love it, that they would have to come to the beach house again very soon and do this boat trip. You laughed a lot. You were fun to be with. This was the last time I saw you.

I also remember you as a teenager, a state star in gymnastics, on the rings and the parallel bars. When we went to see you participate in a meet, and you were doing your routines, sometimes I had to go out of the hall because I was so afraid you would fall and hurt yourself. But you did well and loved it and because of your success in this sport, you received more than one college scholarship. But when your computer career tract started at Binghamton, you found something else to excel in and that you did.

Lawrence loved animals and his home has many—two dogs, one quite huge but lovable, a Weimer and a Golden Retriever who had diabetes and needed insulin, which you, Lawrence, injected very lovingly. Those animals gave love and received love and I am thankful for them being there for you.

How does a mother say good-bye to her child? In the scheme of life, it is the parents who the children say good-bye to, but forces in life don't always follow this road. So I am not going to say good-bye because you will be forever in my heart and in my mind. I will try very hard to focus on the good times of your life and times we were together. I will cry often for I know the void your death has left in your father's and my life, and in our family; but I will also be thankful that you are at peace, your courageous fight over.

Shalom Bayit—wishing you peace in your home away from home.

Love, Mommy and Daddy

The Unveiling Ceremony

One year passed since the untimely death of my son Lawrence and as Jewish tradition dictates, it is the time to mark the grave with a tombstone, bringing reality to the death. Before the tombstone was placed, there was a surreal feeling that was experienced when visiting the gravesite. There was a small temporary marker with Lawrence's name and date of death.

When the permanent grave marker was placed, the reality took hold. What the heart said couldn't be was now confronted with the brain saying yes, Lawrence is dead and the marker says it for all to see.

The date of the unveiling was a day of gathering of the family both to honor Lawrence and to celebrate his life. The honoring took place at the cemetery, with special prayers and readings. A book of remembrance, with prayers, readings, poetry, and pictures, was created by Lawrence's sister, Ruth. The service of the unveiling began with the traditional prayer of the Shema,

"Hear O' Israel, the Lord our G-d, the Lord is one. Blessed be G-d's glorious name forever and ever."

This prayer is an affirmation of our belief in G-d [In Conservative and Reform Judaism, some Jews observe the custom of spelling God as G-d, which honors the sacredness of the divine name], said even in the most tortuous times (as when concentration camp inmates walked into the ovens to be killed) as well as in good times.

Following the Shema, those assembled were led in the reading of the *23rd Psalm, The Lord is my Shepherd*, a prayer that honors G-d, the living and the deceased, telling us that G-d helps us to ". . . walk through the valley of the shadow of death," fearing no evil, knowing that G-d will comfort each of us. Other readings were led by family and those present at the unveiling.

The prayer of the Kaddish, a prayer honoring those who died but which has no mention of death in the prayer, is said by the family, followed by the chanting of the prayer, *El Maley Rachameem*, a prayer for the soul of the departed. The service of the unveiling concluded with the singing of *Havenu Shalom Aleichum*, "We have brought peace unto you."

At the conclusion of the unveiling ceremony, small rocks are given to all those present to place on the grave marker to signify to others that they were there. This is a tradition that is carried out whenever one visits the grave of a loved one.

Before leaving the cemetery, water is poured over one's hands (3 times for each hand) so as not to bring the sadness of death into one's home.

It was said that the unveiling ceremony both honors and celebrates the life of the deceased. The celebration of Lawrence's life took place in our home, surrounded by family sharing stories of Lawrence, looking at pictures of him and family, singing songs that reminded one of good times together, all activities that celebrated life and Lawrence, while at the same time making the unreal a reality of life.

Epilogue

How one continues to live one's life after the loss of a beloved child, my son Lawrence, is very difficult to even think about. But Jewish custom proscribes some helpful ways to "walk through the Valley of the Shadow of Death" in a way that the mourning becomes more internal, but never sadder, but wants and desires one to return to life.

My life is right now, like a roller coaster, or rather more like the waves of an ocean, overwhelming and calm at the same time. Tears are a constant. Triggers I had never thought of bring me right back to the moment of my son's death. Right outside the community where I live is the chapel where the funeral services for Lawrence took place. When we moved into our community, that chapel for me was new, was there, but not for me in the immediate present. Yes, it would be there for the services for my husband and me but not for my son. So now, I work to find alternate ways of bypassing the chapel in order to get home. Will this trigger always be there—that I don't know, but right now my response to it has to be what is right for me.

I have also found myself needing to visit the cemetery where my son is buried, reading to him from the book *Marley and Me*, which is a story of a lover of animals and especially dogs. I feel that he would approve of me doing this. There are some persons who are afraid of me doing this, making this a ritual, but isn't ritual what life is all about? I have found that I need to do right now what is right for me. Will it be right months from now; time will only tell.

Time is also another facet of loss that has so many different meanings. People in their caring tell you that time will heal. What I find time doing for me is making the happening of my son's death a reality, not a nightmare.

There are also other ways to travel this road of intense grief. I attend counseling sessions weekly, not for the purpose of someone solving my problems, but this time and space allows me the expression of intense grief without guilt or embarrassment.

So that is my story, sharing my feelings and emotions as a mother who has lost a shining person in her life, but is trying in a traditional way, with support from a wonderful family, (and my goal right now) is to attempt to focus on what I know that Lawrence would have wanted me to do—to go on living and give love to those who are still with us. Maybe I will succeed, and maybe I won't, but I certainly will try."

Anita Beckerman Dr. Anita Beckerman passed away December 21, 2013, with her loving family present and engaging in the beautiful Jewish rituals of preparation for eternal life.

Transcultural Caring-Based Learning Approach

Please review the information about the Transcultural Caring Dynamics for Nursing and Health-Care Model, the assessment tools, the transcultural caring-based learning (TCCBL) approach, and the transcultural caring inquiry information explained in previous chapters of this book, and any other relevant literary and Internet information before dialoguing about this transcultural caring experience. In your small group, apply the TCCBL approach in relation to your transcultural caring situation for pattern identification (i.e., pattern seeing, pattern mapping, pattern recognizing, and pattern transforming). Use dimensions of the Transcultural Caring Dynamics in Nursing and Health-Care Theory and Model and use the most appropriate assessment tools for transcultural evidence gathering. The Reflections with Questions section that follows is a guide that will assist you individually and collectively in your learning group with dialogue and interpretation of the spiritual traditions of the Jews at the time of death, burial, mourning, and unveiling the grave marker.

Reflections with Questions

Reflect on the story of Anita. The story illuminates the foundation of a consciousness of love for a beloved son, and a duty to honor him in the most referential way through Jewish custom, tradition, ritual, and spirituality. Reflect on the words of Anita, on the life of Lawrence expressed through the written words. Focus attention on the mourning process, on the faith, and Jewish religious practices for the dead. What are your responsibilities as a transcultural nurse in understanding the love of a mother for a child who has died, the Jewish culture, the different forms of Judaism, the mourning process, Jewish spirituality and rituals, and the after-care of a mother who has experienced a child with depression and the taking of his own life?

Transcultural Nursing Reflections

- What transcultural caring compassionate experiences come to mind both as a person and as a nurse when you reflect upon Anita's story?
- What is the meaning of suffering and grief to you as you read Anita's story?
- What is the meaning of faith, spiritual practices, and rituals in this story? What do they mean to you as you contemplate your own life and death? What spiritual rituals are you familiar with within your own religious traditions?
- What are the signs and symptoms of depression? What procedures are used in the diagnosis and treatment of depression? What medications are used in the treatment of depression? What are the differences between a psychologist, psychiatrist, and a psychiatric nurse practitioner in the care of the depressed patient? Is there a difference between a young person and an older adult with depression?

- The death of a child no matter how old, is a tragedy to a mother, father, and family. What does this situation mean to you personally and as a professional nurse?
- What are **your** definitions of health and illness, and of mental health or disease?
- How can we best understand the sorrow and grief that surrounds illness or the problems of the human condition that lead to illness, genetic, social, cultural, and religious, and so forth?
- What are the Web sites available to assist you and the group with understanding depression and suicide?
- How would you begin to seek understanding of what is happening to Anita and her family? What would be your first step? How would you develop a professional program (i.e., spiritually and culturally appropriate nursing care plan) to assist Anita with her grief and mourning? Are there professional tools or questionnaires available that you could use to identify the issues? How would you integrate religious beliefs into the group counseling sessions?
- How do you begin to frame illness, death, burial rites, and mourning within a cultural framework? What are the various religious practices between the different traditions (i.e., Orthodox, Conservatism, and Reform) of Judaism and the dynamic view of Judaism in the world? Are the Orthodox Jewish customs different? Are there different needs for those who may have experienced or listened to the stories of relatives in the Holocaust? What bearing does the state of Israel have on suffering? Are there differences between countries in the rituals that are practiced, such as between Israel and the United States?
- In the Jewish tradition, there are varying beliefs about suicide. What are they? What division in Judaism represents the diverse beliefs? What are the religious dimensions of the Jewish faith that you will need to know to understand depression and suicide as a cultural phenomenon and as an illness or disease?
- What are the percentages of people in the U.S. Jewish population and in the general U.S. population who are diagnosed with depression?
- Anita pointed out the rituals for mourning and burial. Are there additional ones that you would need to know if you were beginning a support group in a hospital or community health center?
- Compare and contrast rituals of the cultures of illness, death, burial, mourning, and grief in Christianity and Islam. Is the meaning of death different in the different religious cultures? What are the death rituals of the Catholic and Protestant Christian traditions? What are the death and mourning rituals of Islam?
- Explore the meaning of animals and pet therapy in health care and nursing. How do pets care for human beings? How do pets provide a source of comfort and peace to people? How do pets sense the needs of their masters, and sense dying and death? Explore when pets may not heal.

AUTHOR'S REFLECTION

Depression is an insidious disease. It is often overlooked due to denial and fear. It is estimated that a good portion of Americans suffer from depressive disorders. Depression affects all age groups, from children to the elderly, and can range in severity from very mild to a very serious psychosis. Bipolar disease or the old-fashioned way of saying it, manic-depressive disorder, seems to be becoming more common. Perhaps it is because it is being reported and can be treated. Many people avoid treatment or attempt to self-medicate, often with drugs and alcohol, to block out the symptoms of the disease. Professionally prescribed medications can offset or alleviate the symptoms.

Select Bibliography

Arnold, J. (2011). *Through a dog's eyes: Understanding our dogs.* New York: Spiegel & Grau.

Becker, M. (2002). *The healing power of pets.* New York: Hyperion.

Blum, C. (2006). 'Til Death Do Us Part?' The nurse's role in the care of the dead, A historical perspective: 1850–2004. *Geriatric Nursing, 27*(1), 58–63.

Eriksson, K. (2006). *The suffering human being.* Chicago: Nordic Studies Press.

Greenberg, I. (2005). *Dignity beyond death: The Jewish preparation for burial.* Jerusalem: Urim Publications.

Heschel, A. (1976). *Man is not alone: A philosophy of religion.* New York: Farrar, Straus and Giroux.

Heschel, A., & Heschel, S. (1976). *God in search of man: A philosophy of Judaism.* New York: Farrar, Straus and Giroux. (Original work published 1955)

Lamm, M. (2000). *The Jewish way in death and mourning.* New York: Jonathan David Publishers.

Leffler, W., & Jones, P. (2005). *The structure of religion: Judaism and Christianity.* Boulder: University Press of America, Inc.

Martin, G. (1985/2014). *The holocaust: The human tragedy.* New York: Henry Holt & Company.

Raus, H., & Pysh, G. (2011). *Ben: The very best furry friend—a children's book about a therapy dog and the friends he makes at the library and nursing homes.* Atlanta, GA: Pylon Publishing Company.

The book of Psalms. (1993). New York: Dover Publications.

Townsend, M. (2006). *Psychiatric mental health nursing: Concepts of care.* Philadelphia: F. A. Davis Company.

Wenger, B. (2007). *The Jewish Americans.* New York: Doubleday.

CHAPTER 21

The American Chinese Transcultural Maternal-Child and Family Experience in China

he culture of China evolved over the past 5,000 years. Its ancient and modern history; art; Confucian, Tao, and Buddhist philosophies; diverse cultures; commanding military; fascinating politics ranging from imperial dynasties to a Communist political system; and now emerging as a new global market-driven economic power has made China one of the most complex societies in the world. The ruling dynasties of the past were powerful and provided a rich backdrop for the philosophies, art, architecture, technology, and commerce that emerged. A large country geographically with a population of well over 1 billion, the family remains, despite rigorous population control, as one of the strongholds of Chinese culture. Ninety-two percent are Han, the largest ethnic group in the world. The Chinese language, what now is called the family of many languages (diverse dialects), is unified by the written Chinese language, one of the last of its kind that survives as a major language in the contemporary world. English as a second language (ESL) taught by North Americans is becoming a dominant trend. In the recent history of the last century, communism, fueled by the Cultural Revolution led by Mao Zedong from 1966–1976, emerged as a political, economic, and social way of life. Many commonalities such as a central government and dress (a blue uniform) existed because of the socialist system. In the 21st century, however, the Cultural Revolution has been replaced by the economic revolution with the beginning of a new social, political, and economic organization. Economically, China has entered the global market, and has become a primary manufacturer around the world. As the economy improves and manufacturing increases, China is facing increased environmental challenges.

While the quest for modernity continues, governmental control still prevails. There is a concern that the stringent population control measures in force, "the-one-child-per-family" policy, is leading to serious problems for the future related to the number of women available for marriage and reproduction. China also has the most rapidly growing aging population the world (www.cia.gov/library/publications/theworld-factbook.geos/ch.html#, Retrieved April 15, 2008).

The family as a cultural norm and the availability of people, especially women, to care for the aged is challenged further by the migration of people to work in the major cities of China and abroad. The opening of China to the West and the Olympic summer games brought China into the spotlight. Many people travel not only for tourism but also for education. The exchange of engineers and scientists, including nursing educators and academics, over the past decade is phenomenal. The following is a transcultural caring experience bringing together two people in Beijing—one from the United States teaching ESL in China and a woman from China. Their love relationships grew over time, leading to the birth of a son of Jewish American and Chinese heritage.

Abe and Liu's Story

Abraham was born in New York City and educated at New York University, and he first became a biologist and then a lawyer. Abe, as he likes to be called, came from a prominent Jewish family. He had been married once to another lawyer but the marriage was not successful. They had no children. Abe was anxious to contribute to the world. He loved education and was very committed to American educational philosophers, such as John Dewey, because he thought that they were in touch with ideas about the importance of the creation of community through education and how we ought to live in a complex society. Abe wanted to teach, but not chemistry or law. Soon, he was seeking out a place to teach. He decided to go to Beijing in the People's Republic of China (PRC), where he had the opportunity to be a teacher of English as a second language (ESL). He really did not know how to speak Chinese but felt he would have the best chance to learn Chinese with students who, at first, did not speak English. Abe was worried about the Chinese language characters and how he would have to learn to be more artistic when writing in Chinese.

Many of the "expatriates" from different countries who taught at different institutions lived in an apartment house fairly close to the school. After a slow start and a period of adjusting, Abe soon became interested in a culture that is changing rapidly from revolutionary Communist values of power and government control to the new modernism of economics and economic advancement. Most of all, he was fascinated with the ancient beliefs and dynasties that influenced Chinese culture for more than 5,000 years, the theory of opposites and balance with the yin-and-yang philosophy and hot-and-cold theory, the spiritual teaching of harmony of the Buddhist way of life, and the principles of Confucianism and Taoism. Spirituality and religion, including Christianity, now are becoming a force in China despite their suppression during the Cultural Revolution. What has remained strong throughout history has been the role of relationships, especially the family. Over the years, the Chinese have always been defined by hierarchical relationships with others. There are five basic social relationships in Chinese culture: father and son, sovereign and subject, husband and wife, elder brother and younger brother, and friend and friend (Yu-Lan, 1948, p. 21).

Because of Abe's interest in philosophy and ethics, he became more and more oriented to Chinese values but not at the risk of losing his Jewish heritage. He spent time trying to come to a common ground between the two sets of values and beliefs. One day, in an Internet café, Abe met Liu. He noticed how beautiful she was sitting at the computer. He was so smitten that he immediately found a way to talk with her. He tried to speak Mandarin but she spoke in broken English. Liu told him that she worked downtown in an accounting office but came from a rural community about 60 kilometers from Beijing. After seeing each other for a short time, they fell in love. Liu had not taken Abe home to her father and mother though. Her parents lived rather simply because of their orientation to communal farm living during the revolution. Liu was worried about whether or not her father would approve of their relationship. Both Abe and Liu wanted to marry and have a family and Liu became pregnant. She finally told her family and they were not happy with the decision she'd made. Liu's father was ready to disown her. While Liu and her family did not practice a religion, they were immersed in the ethical principles of Confucianism.

In the maternity hospital in Beijing, Liu had a baby boy, Cheung Jacob. It was a Western-type hospital but it carried out traditional Chinese medical practices. Abe shared pictures and a little story with his friends in the West over the Internet after the delivery. Abe was overjoyed. Abe was allowed to be in the delivery room with Liu and she had the baby with her immediately after the birth. He said that the doctors were not oriented to money as he thinks they are in the United States. They seemed more attentive. The delivery room was fairly well equipped and had emergency supplies, such as oxygen for use if necessary. The doctors and nurses assisted Liu during the labor and delivery process and tried to calm her. Although she had to have a small episiotomy during the birthing process, one of the doctors gave her acupuncture beforehand to help with the final stages of labor. Tired after a long labor of 18 hours, Liu was given some herbal tea and a massage to keep her balanced. Cheung Jacob was a handsome baby, with Asian and Caucasian features. Liu knew that Abe would help her at home but she longed for her mother to be with her when she was learning how to breast-feed and care for her baby. She was worried about who would help her at home. She did not know if any nurses or assistants would come to their apartment. Liu wanted to see her mother so Abe got up his courage and called her family.

Transcultural Caring-Based Learning Approach

Please review the information about the Transcultural Caring Dynamics for Nursing and Health-Care Model, the assessment tools, the transcultural caring-based learning (TCCBL) approach, and the transcultural caring inquiry information, and any other relevant literary and Internet information before dialoguing about the transcultural caring experience. In your small group, apply the TCCBL approach in relation to your transcultural caring situation for pattern identification (i.e., pattern seeing, pattern mapping, pattern recognizing, and pattern transforming). Use dimensions of the Transcultural Caring Dynamics in Nursing and Health-Care Theory and Model and use the most appropriate assessment tools for transcultural evidence gathering for what is happening in the lifeworld of Abe and Liu in Beijing.

Reflections with Questions

Abe and Liu's story reveals how people of diverse cultures, Jewish American and rural Chinese, come together in a global world, and in a transcultural caring experience. The story reveals the essence of their relationship, the birth of their son. What are your responsibilities as a transcultural nurse in understanding the history and culture of China, the Asian culture, the culture of an American in China, the relationship between China and the United States, the issue of intermarriage in China, birthing practices in China, the different types of hospitals in the larger Chinese cities, the culture, the lineage, and the structure of the family in China?

Transcultural Nursing Reflections

As a group of nursing students, contemplate the story of Abe and Liu and their relationship in the complex culture of both Beijing and rural China. Reflect on the story of their relationship. They wanted to marry and raise a family.

- What does intermarriage mean to the family structure and lineage in China? How are ideas changing about intermarriage between an Asian woman and Caucasian man? Are there family rules about having a baby out of wedlock? What is the meaning of an inter-racial baby in Asian culture?

- What does this story tell you about China, the culture in the present era, the past and immediate past culture, and hope for the future? What does this story tell you about Chinese health and maternity care, baby care, and human relationships?
- What is the role of the family in China? What is the role of respect for family in China?
- What is the effect of diverse cultural changes on a traditional people who respect authority, especially the authority of the family?
- How do you think that Liu's family will be affected by Liu's decision to have a baby with-out family support and marriage? What do you think will be the effect on Liu and her new family, Abe and their baby boy? If Liu had delivered a baby girl, what may be the impact of a one-child-per-family policy on her and Abe?
- Identify the significant birthing practices of Chinese women in China. Identify what roles medical and nursing personnel play in Chinese health care. Are the health and maternal-child practices different in rural communities and urban environments? Compare and contrast these practices with birthing practices of China and North America (Canada and the United States). Compare and contrast these family and birthing practices of Chinese North Americans. Are there differences, for example, between Canada, the United States, and Europe?
- In the maternity hospital, examine the differences between the Western medical system and the traditional Chinese system of practice in China. What is the role of the midwife? Are midwives nurses? What are the significant practices in Chinese medicine? Who can practice Chinese medicine—in China and in North America? What are the primary herbs of China? How do they play a role in healing and health?
- What are the significant maternal-child birthing practices in Chinese hospitals? How are they exemplified in this transcultural experience?
- What are the nursing care practices of mothers, children, and families? In hospitals, what is the significance of the registered nurse? Are there professional nurses in the community? Do they make home visits?
- Health care is an important service in China. And, East is meeting West and West is meeting East. There are traditional hospitals where Eastern medicine is practiced, and there are contemporary hospitals where both Eastern and Western medicine and care are practiced. Explain the health-care system in China. Compare and contrast Eastern and Western health-care systems.
- What is the educational role of North American nursing in China and vice versa? What are the changes coming forward in nursing and medical education in China?
- What are the nutrition practices of China for mothers and children? Do mothers prefer breastfeeding over bottle feeding?
- What type of care is extended to visitors or "expatriates" in China? How do dominant Chinese maternal-child birthing practices compare with other Asian nations, such as Taiwan, Korea (North and South), Japan, Thailand, Malaysia, Vietnam, Laos, Cambodia, and Myanmar?
- What is China's relationship with the World Health Organization?
- Why is there a diaspora from China to different parts of the world?
- The educational system in China has changed since the Cultural Revolution. What is the educational system in China? What is the relationship among the academic com-munity in the United States, Canada, and China? Why are many North Americans invited to China to teach a variety of subjects, such as nursing or ESL or to consult on curricula?
- How is the Communist system adapting to the reality of the global community?
- How powerful is the Chinese influence on the United States and the rest of the world?

- How has Hong Kong unfolded since it was returned to China from the United Kingdom?
- How does China view Taiwan? What is the relationship of Taiwan to China?
- What is China's influence with its neighbors, Taiwan, Japan, North and South Korea, Vietnam, Thailand, and so forth? Although Tibet is considered part of China, what is the relationship? What is its relationship with the Uyghurs?
- Given the strength of Abe's Jewish heritage, do you imagine any effect on the way that Cheung Jacob might be raised? Would there be discrimination of mixed heritages (Asian and Caucasian American) in China itself? How does that compare with mixed heritages (races) in North America? Discuss how Jewish traditions may be integrated with the "philosophy of balance," the five phases and the values of Buddhism, and the ethical ways and path of Confucianism and Taoism in Liu and Abe's new family. What are the other religions prevalent in China? Is there freedom of religion?
- The social, political, and economic structures are changing rapidly in modern China. Identify the changes that occurred in the social, political, and economic structures in the 20th and early 21st centuries and especially the economic and political structures during the Communist Cultural Revolution and compare them with changes in the United States. What new ethnic policies are being considered?
- Contemplate China as the second largest consumer population in the world next to the United States.
- Contemplate the resources that China will need for its people and economic growth. How would they compare with the United States, Japan, Taiwan, Indonesia, Malaysia, India, and other developing nations, such as Thailand, Myanmar, Laos, Cambodia, Vietnam, and so forth?
- Contemplate China as the country that has the largest greenhouse gas problem in the world. Contemplate the resources that China will need for its people, economic growth, and control of the environment.
- What environmental health problems are advancing because of cigarette smoking and air pollution? How do they compare with the United States or Canada? What are the morbidity and mortality rates in China? How do they compare with the United States and Canada, and with other developed countries?
- What are the statistics and what is the nature of the aging population in China? How is the aging population cared for? What changes are the Chinese encountering as the population and the social picture change?
- How would you compare and contrast the social, economic, and health-care development of China with other Asian countries, such as Japan?

Select Bibliography

Economy, E., & Levi, M. (2014). *By all means necessary: How China's resource quest is changing the world.* Oxford: Oxford University Press.

Fung, Y. (1948). *A short history of Chinese philosophy.* New York: The Free Press.

Hoobler, D., & Hoobler, T. (2004). *Confucianism.* New York: Facts on File, Inc.

Huang, W., & Qun, A. (2003). *Chinese language and culture.* Hong Kong: The Chinese University Press.

Kalishch, B., & Liu, Y. (2009). Comparison of nursing: China and the United States. *Nursing Economics, 27*(5), 322–331.

Koblinsky, M. (Ed.). (2003). *Reducing maternal mortality: Learning from Bolivia, China, Egypt, Honduras, Indonesia, Jamaica and Zimbabwe.* Washington, DC: The International Bank for Reconstruction and Development/The World Bank.

Liu, Y. (2007). Inpatient satisfaction with nursing care and factors influencing satisfaction in a teaching hospital in China. *Journal of Nursing Care Quality, 22*(3), 266–271.

Lu, S. (2007). *Chinese modernity and global biopolitics*. Honolulu: University of Hawaii Press.

Morton, W., & Lewis, C. (2004). *China: Its history and culture* (4th ed.). New York: McGraw-Hill.

Wan, H., Yu, F., & Kolanowski, K. (2008). Caring for aging Chinese: Lessons learned from the United States. *Journal of Transcultural Nursing, 19*(2), 114–120.

Yu-Lan, F. (1948). *A short history of Chinese philosophy*. (Ed. by D. Bodde). New York: The Free Press.

Web Listing

Facts about China. Retrieved April 15, 2008, from: https://www.cia.gov/library/publications/the-world-factbook/geos/ch.html

CHAPTER 22

Extending Understanding: Transcultural Caring for Muslims in the United States

*I slamic/Muslim culture is the story of the ancient world interfacing with the contempo-
rary world. The Middle East, from where this culture and religion emerged in the 7th century A.D., was first settled by migrants of Mesopotamia (the land around modern Iraq). Severe climate change with disappearing river systems caused these nomadic people to move
from arid lands to more fertile mountainous valleys and oases for survival. The land and
coastal trade routes of Arabia connected Mesopotamia, ancient Europe, and the southern Arabian lands (modern-day Yemen) with trade routes to the Far East. Saudi Arabia is the heart-
land of the Muslim faith, one of the largest monotheistic religions. After 610 A.D., the
Prophet Muhammad established Islam as the religion of the Arabian Peninsula, and others after him extended its influence beyond North Africa and parts of Spain, India, and China and,
in modern times, around the world.*

*In the western region of Saudi Arabia, the holy cities of Mecca and Medina are the two
most important religious sites in the Muslim world. Islam's central shrine is in Mecca, and
the tomb of the Prophet Mohammed and his mosque are in Medina. Islamic solidarity is
preserved through the symbols and rituals of the pilgrims visiting these holy sites. The Hajj,*

a pilgrimage to the city of Mecca, is an obligation for all Muslims, whose numbers are more than 1 billion—one in six people—worldwide. Islam is one of the world's fastest growing religions; Islam means total submission and obedience to the will of Allah (Al-Shahri, 2002). Islam and Islamic law, called Sharia, provides guidance on personal, social, political, economic, moral, and spiritual affairs for the life of the individual and society. There are two major divisions in Islam, Sunni and Shi'a; devout Muslims incorporate religion into all aspects of their lives (Esposition, 2010) The concept of tawheed, meaning "the Oneness of Allah" or "unification," means maintaining Allah's unity in all human actions, spiritually, intellectually, and practically (Rassool, 2000). There is no separation of the body from the spiritual dimension—a mind-body-spiritual unity (Luna, 1998).

Muslims presently live in many countries across the world and over the centuries have faced the challenges and rewards of migration and acculturation. Since the events of September 11, 2001 ("9/11"), Muslims have been subject to racism, suspicion, scrutiny, and prejudice about their culture, values, beliefs, and behaviors in the United States and other Western nations (Sheridan, 2006). Muslims are often feared, and according to the Pew Forum on Religious and Public Life (2009), Muslims have encountered discrimination more than any other religious groups in the United States since 9/11. Peek (2011) attested that the events of this day initiated national and international analysis of the people responsible for this attack, which resulted in a backlash against Arabs and Muslims. Additionally, a lack of understanding about distinctions between Arabs and Muslims and other religious groups prevailed. Muslims are followers of the religion Islam; Arabs are a heterogeneous ethnic group from 22 Arabic-speaking nations across the Middle East and northern Africa that comprises Christians, Muslims, and other religions (Peek, 2011).

The Muslim population in the United States is speculated to be 2 to 7 million (U.S. Department of State, 2009); the U.S. Census does not track religion. Of all Muslim Americans, 65% are foreign born, 35% have been born in the United States, and approximately 20% are African Americans (Pew Forum on Religious and Public Life, 2008). Of Muslim Americans who are foreign born, 25% are Arab immigrants from the Middle East; the rest include immigrants from South Asia (including Pakistan, India, and Bangladesh), Turkey, Iran, Malaysia, Indonesia, Nigeria, Somalia, Liberia, Kenya, and Senegal (U.S. Department of State, 2009). The number of mosques in the United States has increased from 19 in 1939 to 2,106 in 2011 (Bagby, 2011). As in any religion, observance among followers of Islam varies, especially regarding mosque attendance, use of Muslim clothing, and adherence to the tenets of the faith.

Muslim Americans live mainly in the states of California, New York, Illinois, New Jersey, Indiana, Michigan, Virginia, Texas, Ohio, and Maryland and in the cities of New York, Los Angeles, Chicago, and Detroit/Dearborn (U.S. Department of State, 2009). Most Muslim Americans are highly educated, are fluent in English, are politically astute, and hold a similar economic status to the main population; most are employed, one-fourth hold bachelor degrees, and one-fourth live in households with incomes of $75,000 per year or more (Read, 2008). Languages spoken among Muslim Americans reflect their countries of origin and may include English, Arabic, Urdu, Farsi, Turkish, and Indonesian and African languages; however, non-Arab Muslims must know Arabic to recite the Qur'an as the original revelatory language of Islam (Denny, 2011). Devout Muslim Americans profess their faith by adhering to the five pillars of Islam, which provide a foundation for the behaviors of believers: (1) the profession of faith, shahada (belief in one God and that Mohamed is his prophet); (2) daily prayers (performed facing Mecca five times a day before which there is ritual cleansing); (3) fasting during the holy lunar month of Ramadan, wherein Muslims refrain from food, drinking, and sexual activity from sunrise to sunset; (4) zakat, giving alms to the poor; and (5) the pilgrimage to the holy city of Mecca, Saudi Arabia (the Hajj), once during a lifetime (Denny, 2011).

The following story relates to the query and research of Dr. Mary Brigid Martin, who wanted to explore perceptions of Muslim Americans living in the United States and their health-care needs. Significant national and international events over the 20th and 21st centuries have influenced the long-standing negative perceptions of Muslims, such as ongoing Middle East conflict since Israeli statehood in 1948, the American-Iran hostage crisis and the American Marine barracks attack in Beirut in the 1980s, the World Trade Center bombing in the 1990s, the momentous event of 9/11/2001, radical Islamic terrorism in many parts of the world, and the Boston Marathon bombings in the United States in 2013 (Preston & Mackey, 2013).

Mary's Story

The above-mentioned sociopolitical and sociocultural phenomena and the predicament of Muslim Americans moved me to inquire about the crossover of anti-Muslim discrimination from society to the health-care setting, a problem that, if not addressed, has detrimental outcomes for this patient population. Anti-Muslim discrimination leads to disparity in health care by negatively affecting the health and quality of care for Muslim families and their children (Laird, Amer, Barnett, & Barnes, 2007). Muslim Americans, an underserved, understudied minority of ethnic and racial diversity, pose challenges for health-care providers unfamiliar with Islam and its influences on health care (Padela, Gunter, Killawi, & Heisler, 2012). Three main concerns that promoted the need to address the problem of anti-Muslim discrimination included (1) discrimination as a health care disparity, (2) discrimination and its impact on mental health and well-being, and (3) discrimination related to lack of knowledge about culturally congruent care.

Laying the Groundwork for Research About Muslim Americans

Research related to health-care disparities can inform ways to improve care for vulnerable and minority groups by bridging the knowledge and practice gap on this subject and improving patient outcomes in the health-care setting (U.S. Department of Health and Human Services, 2011). Although research has been conducted on discrimination against Muslims in the employment and educational segments of society, more studies are needed that quantify the extent and type of discrimination faced by this group in the health-care setting. There is growing concern about the discrimination faced by Muslims and its impact on mental health (Ahmed & Reddy, 2007). Research evidence indicates a positive link between discrimination and poor mental health in minority groups (Williams, Neighbors, & Jackson, 2003). The paucity of studies specifically about anti-Muslim religious discrimination, as opposed to racial or ethnic discrimination, makes it difficult to investigate types, incidences, and contributing factors of anti-Muslim discrimination related to religious practice—hence the need to pursue this study with a focus on religious practices. Cultural competence entails the knowledge, abilities, and skills to provide care that is consistent with cultural beliefs and practices (Purnell & Paulanka, 2012). Muslim patients may have expectations in the health-care setting that, if not met by health-care staff, may generate feelings of discrimination or poor clinical experiences (Padela et al, 2012).

After contemplating the disparities, vulnerability, and potential poor delivery of health care to Muslim Americans, the objective of my research was to discover the extent of perceived anti-Muslim discrimination in the United States, the extent of perceived anti-Muslim discrimination in American health-care settings, and the types of discriminatory behaviors Muslims report in health-care settings in the United States. Additionally, I attempted to uncover care preferences among Muslim Americans that may inform culturally congruent care practices.

Perceived Discrimination of Muslims in Health Care in the United States

MY RESEARCH STUDY

In my research study (Martin, 2013), I employed an established perceived discrimination scale that measures anti-Muslim discrimination in society adapted by Rippy and Newman (2008). I created a tool to measure occurrences of anti-Muslim discrimination in health care that also elicited information about culturally congruent care practices based on principles of cultural safety (Ramsden & Papps, 1996) within the nurse-patient relationship and the cultural care beliefs of the Muslim patient/family (Wehbe-Alamah, 2008). Ray's *Transcultural Caring Dynamics in Nursing and Health Care* (2010) served as a framework for this quantitative, univariate, descriptive, cross-sectional design because Ray's model emphasized the relatedness of the human-environment connection, particularly with respect to the disparaging social context within which this group has dwelled in the United States since 9/11.

A nation-wide convenience sample of 227 ethnically diverse, native and foreign-born adults (older than 18 years) who reside in the United States and who report Islam as their religion, either by birth or by conversion, participated in this investigation. An electronic questionnaire created with Survey Monkey (2013) was sent to Muslim organizations across the United States using e-mail and Facebook (2013). Snowball sampling was employed among participants who agreed to send the link to friends and acquaintances. Demographic characteristics of the sample were consistent with the general description of Muslim Americans as highly educated, with one-fourth holding bachelor degrees, and employed, with one-fourth of annual household incomes of $75,000 or greater (Read, 2008).

Findings revealed that nearly one-third of subjects perceived they were discriminated against in the health-care setting in the United States. Being excluded or ignored was the most frequently indicated type of discrimination, followed by problems related to the use of Muslim clothing; offensive or insensitive verbal remarks; and problems related to Islamic holidays, prayer rituals, and physical assault. Age was positively correlated with perceived anti-Muslim discrimination in society. Education was negatively correlated with perceived discrimination in society and the health-care setting. Findings revealed that three out of five individuals surveyed reported that they wear Muslim clothing, the most frequently reported of which was the *hijab*. Participants who wore Muslim clothing, especially women, reported more anti-Muslim discrimination than participants who did not. Scores for self-reported perceived anti-Muslim discrimination were found to be higher after the Boston Marathon bombings, April 15, 2013, an act perpetrated by Muslims that occurred during the time of data collection. The number one Muslim care preference reported was same-gender caregiver followed by respect for modesty, prayer rituals, respect for privacy, family involvement in care, and dietary concerns.

MY REFLECTION ON RESULTS OF RESEARCH

Ray's (2010) theory and model provided a guide to address Islamic influences on caring, spirituality, ethics, and the social and political context for Muslim Americans. This work served as an effective means to discern culturally congruent care practices based on mutual decision making and choice between provider and patient. These issues included preference for same-gender caregiver, respect for modesty, prayer ritual accommodations, privacy, family involvement, and dietary needs.

The most frequently reported type of discrimination reported, being excluded and ignored, affirms the imperative to consider the concept of "cultural other" (Ray, 2010, p. xi), wherein the quality, or lack thereof, of relationship with Muslims exists. Other forms of discrimination reported, such as wearing the *hijab* and Islamic dress, and prayer rituals, characteristically Muslim, reinforce a distinct identification of Muslims as a religious minority amid a dominant culture. Islamic identifiers such as clothing, prayer rituals, and holidays, which serve as symbols of Islam, are explained by Ray (2010) as symbols and expressions of behavior that hold meaning at many levels.

Findings of this investigation suggest that anti-Muslim discrimination in the United States carries over to the health-care setting. Nearly one out of three Muslims reported a perception of being discriminated against in the health-care setting in the United States. The verbal remarks, offensive comments, and physical assaults reveal the harm imposed on Muslims, which implores attention from health-care providers. The relationship between the Boston Marathon bombings, which occurred during the time of data collection, and subsequent higher scores for perceived anti-Muslim discrimination reinforce Ray's (2010) emphasis on the significance of sociopolitical and sociocultural contextual influences on health and well-being.

APPLICATION OF RAY'S THEORY AND MODEL TO MUSLIM AMERICANS

The dimensions of Ray's theory and model published in 2010 and presented again in this edition of the book guided this research about Muslim Americans, with consideration for the provision of care that is culturally appropriate. The use of this work facilitated gaining an Islamic perspective of the identified dimensions of the model in terms of meanings and expressions of caring, transcultural ethics, cultural context, and universal source (spirituality/religion), which supported mutual awareness, understanding, and choice in health care for this population.

Dimension 1 of Ray's Model: The Essence of Caring and Its Application to Muslim Americans

Muslims Americans may demonstrate caring behaviors for loved ones in many ways. The concept of caring among Muslims is "embedded in the theological framework of Islam" (Rassool, 2000, p. 1481). Muslims traditionally show that they care about each other by frequent contact, conversation, social gatherings, and shared rituals. Nurses may notice a strong family presence as a source of security and support in times of sickness. Caring for family during illness is a moral and religious obligation in Islam (Nigosian, 2004). Visitation is traditionally encouraged and expected, a responsibility that conveys love and concern for family needs.

Nurses may demonstrate care of Muslim Americans by listening to patient needs and respecting the critical role of family in the care of the sick patient. Accommodating frequent visitation from relatives and friends and perhaps the request by a member to remain around the clock in the room with the patient supports family involvement. The caring nurse patiently interviews and conducts a history and physical examination and in doing so elicits patient needs and preferences. Attentive presence, nonjudgment, and self-reflection are key in gaining trust. Care preferences should be accommodated as much as possible. These preferences may include a same-gender caregiver, if requested, and *halal* food (Padela et al, 2012), a diet free of pork and one in which meat is slaughtered in a specified manner (Riaz & Chaudry, 2003). If the latter is unavailable, the omission of pork and pork products may suffice. For Muslim women, the *hijab* may serve to assert Muslim identity, prompt modest behavior, achieve respect, and prevent sexual objectification (Droogsma, 2007). If a patient wears a *hijab*, or head cover, nurses should ensure that other staff maintain this choice—for example, ensure head covering in the operating room and diagnostic procedures.

Although illness and death of a loved one are deeply sad and emotional, acceptance of the will of God is above all for Muslims. Hospital staff may show compassion to the family and anticipate that burial takes place within 24 hours, followed by 3 days of mourning, usually at the family home whereby friends and relations pay their respect by visitation and assisting the bereaved in the home as needed (Wehbe-Alamah, 2008).

Dimension 2 of Ray's Model: Transcultural Caring Ethics and Its Application to Muslim Americans

Islamic ethics are guided by Qur'anic scripture and steeped in acceptance of the will of God, and its principles share much common ground with secular ethics (Kyriakides-Yeldham, 2005), for example, support for equality and human rights (Esposito, 2010). In Islam, health promotion and disease prevention are highly valued (Rathor, Rani, Shah, Leman, Akter, & Omar, 2011). Rassool (2000) adapted an Islamic code of ethics from the work of Athar (1996), which detailed these priorities of patient care: involvement of the family and patient in decision making, interpretation of the Qur'an as related to patient concerns, consolation of patient and family to pray for acceptance of God's will regarding health status, and attention to the needs of the family after death has occurred.

Nurses convey respect for Islamic ethical values by advocating for involvement of the Muslim family in health-care decisions for and with the patient; prayer as a means of comfort; and hope for wellness, recovery from illness, and a peaceful death and family support after peaceful end of life. Open discussion with the family about after-death procedures is necessary. After death, ritual cleansing of the body is required. Because there is preference in Islam that the body of a deceased Muslim be touched only by a same-gender Muslim (Wehbe-Alamah, 2008), arrangements for this must be conferred with the family, who may engage relatives, mosque personnel, or funeral home personnel to do so.

The four universal ethical principles of respect for autonomy, beneficence, nonmaleficence, and justice may assist nurses in analyzing ethical dilemmas but require cultural considerations of all patients including Muslims. In individualistic oriented Western bioethics, patient autonomy takes absolute precedence over all aspects of social and personal life, which may be unacceptable in cultures that are more collectivist oriented, such as Islam, and consideration must be given to the role of faith in an increasingly multicultural society (Rathor et al, 2011).

The non-Muslim nurse must be aware of concepts of autonomy and nonmalfeasance within Islam and the belief that life and death are decided by God (Allah). For example, withdrawing life-sustaining treatment of a Muslim patient and family may be debated, as may be the case with non-Muslim patients and families. Culturally astute nurses would ask Muslim patients and family about comfort measures and views about resuscitation as they would any patient. Patient and family education about advanced directives is crucial to promote clarity for the course of treatment, while respecting acceptance of the will of God.

Specifics about Islamic ethical choices in health care are critical for health-care staff to understand. Broadly speaking, in Islam, reversible contraception and in vitro fertilization (using only husband and wife as sources) are acceptable, as is abortion, but only for medical reasons; permanent sterilization and embryonic experimentation are unacceptable. Muslim fetuses who die in utero and are more than 120 days old are named and buried (Charles & Daroszewski, 2012). Euthanasia, assisted suicide, and cloning are unacceptable, and prolonged life support is discouraged; however, genetic engineering to cure disease, blood transfusion, organ transplantation, and the use of a living will are acceptable practices (Rassool, 2000). Some families may withhold a diagnosis or prognosis from a loved one as a means of protection from emotional distress; however, there is no Islamic basis for this behavior.

Although the principles of Islam are unchanging, in health care, scientific judgments that are made may change over time, and practitioners must realize that there are differing views in bioethical matters among Muslims (Kyriakides-Yeldham, 2005). Respect for individual choice among a population as ethnically and culturally diverse as Muslim Americans must be taken into account.

Dimension 3 of Ray's Model: Transcultural Context and Its Application for Muslim Americans

The experience of Muslims in the United States varies widely depending on their social, cultural, economic, and educational background and factors such as migration and degrees of acculturation. It is essential for nurses to comprehend the social context by which their lives may be impacted. The phenomenon facing this group after the 9/11 attacks has been compared with the treatment of Japanese Americans following Pearl Harbor when the Japanese Imperial Air Force struck and demolished the American naval base at Pearl Harbor in Hawaii on December 7, 1941 (Kaplan, 2006). President Roosevelt then signed an executive order that led to the internment of approximately 120,000 citizens and legal residents in the United States, of whom 75% were Japanese Americans; however, only 2,000 were charged with a crime (Sundquist, 1988). After 9/11, President Bush passed the Patriot Act, which eased restrictions on government authorities to interrogate and arrest individuals (U.S. Government Printing Office, 2001). At least 100,000 Arabs and Muslims in the United States were subject to Immigration and Customs Enforcement property seizures, raids, wiretappings, deportations, detentions, and home and workplace visits (Murray, 2004).

The reactions and actions by the U.S. government to these two distinct attacks by employing internment camps and legislation such as the Patriot Act not only shaped American history but also impacted the social context for Japanese and Muslims living in the United States. Although Muslims face challenges related to discrimination because of past actions in the United States, this group values the social principles of this country. Huda (2006) explained that Muslim Americans do not view any conflict between democracy and Islam in the United States; Islamic organizations call for greater community involvement, education, and self-scrutiny of their larger heritage to advance combining religious values with the American experience to promote mutual understanding.

Long-standing suspicion of Muslims has been instigated by decades of events worldwide in which Muslims are central. Potential ongoing discrimination is faced by this group today (Ahmed & Reddy, 2007). As stated previously, since September 11, 2001, Muslim Americans have encountered discrimination more than any other religious group in the United States (Pew Forum on Religious and Public Life, 2009), including verbal and physical assaults and hate crimes (Peek, 2011). There is evidence of anti-Muslim discrimination in the health-care setting in the United States related to being excluded or ignored, followed by problems related to the use of Muslim clothing; offensive or insensitive verbal remarks; and problems related to Islamic holidays, prayer rituals, and physical assault (Martin, 2013). Although the American Civil Rights Act of 1964 (Office of the Clerk, U.S. House of Representatives, 1964) outlaws discrimination against race, ethnicity, national and religious minorities, and women, anti-Muslim bigotry in the United States persists. By way of knowledge of transcultural caring, nurses may advocate for fair and just treatment of Muslim American patients and maintain a keen awareness of potentially discriminatory behaviors against this group. Support for patient, civil, and human rights in the clinical setting is paramount, in accordance with American Nurses Association (2015) position statement about discrimination and racism in health care.

Dimension 4 of Ray's Model: Universal Sources (Spirituality/Religion) and Its Application to Muslim Americans

Islam offers its believers not only a theology but also a way of life, a united worldview, belief in salvation, an afterlife, the meaning of acceptable deeds, and specific tenets to adhere to in life. Nasr (2003) explained that the Muslim soul is connected to Qur'anic expressions such as *Insha'Allah* ("if God wills"), *al-humdu li'Llah* ("thanks be to God"), and *bismi'Llah* ("in the name of God"). These expressions may be frequently used in daily life among religious Muslims. Teachings of Islam are based on the original and unchanging Quranic text that was relayed through the Angel Gabriel in Arabic to the prophet Mohammed and hadiths, or teachings of the prophet (Iqbal, 2007). To belong to Islam is to be part of a community of Muslim brothers and sisters who share deep connections to this faith. This principle of connectedness in Ray's (2010) theory and model applies to this sense of unison in Islam and highlights the value of spiritual unity among Muslims. An example of this powerful relatedness is that

Islamic prayer and fasting rituals are grounded in the universal recognition of the lunar calendar (Iqbal, 2007).

Illness may be seen as a time to reflect on one's faith and spiritual growth for Muslims (Rassool, 2000). Observant Muslim Americans profess their faith by adhering to the five pillars of Islam. During birth and death, the nurse may expect that the declaration of faith prayer in Arabic may be whispered in the ear of the child or dying loved one by a relative or *imam*, a Muslim cleric, and allow a quiet space for this revered act. Nurses may locate which direction is east (toward Mecca) so that patients know which direction to pray. Religious items such as prayer beads, prayer mat, and the *Qur'an* should be handled respectfully and should not be placed in an unclean place such as the bathroom or floor. Patients who fast require attention to dietary needs and may need their medication administration routine adjusted. Male and female Muslims who have completed the pilgrimage may be referred to as *Hajj* and *Hajji*, respectively, as a gesture of respect and acknowledgment of this pious act.

The Center of Ray's Model: Application of Understanding, Awareness, and Choice for Muslim Americans

Implications for culturally congruent care responsive to researched and prioritized preferences increase awareness, understanding, and choice for Muslim American patients. Important caregiver actions, such as initiation of same-gender caregiver, respect for modesty, prayer ritual accommodations, privacy, family involvement, and dietary needs may be addressed in considerate, simplistic ways (Martin, 2013). A request for a same-gender caregiver should be accommodated if possible; the presence of a family member to stay with the patient may be requested. Privacy and modesty may be respected by a simple knock on the door before entering the room of a female patient to give time for a woman to place her *hijab* or scarf properly. This is a courtesy that is likely to be appreciated by any patient, not just a Muslim. Because male and female patients who wear Muslim clothing might be at risk for discriminatory behaviors in the health-care setting, increased vigilance is needed for patients who wear Islamic dress to be treated with the same respect and equity as other patients.

If a Muslim patient is admitted to a private room, facing the bed east to Mecca accommodates prayer rituals. If the patient is ambulatory, they may be oriented to the east by placing a paper indicator on the wall that conveys easterly direction, toward Mecca, for prayer. Staff should ensure a clean space for prayer where the patient may lay a prayer mat; no one should walk in front of a person while praying. Although Muslim diet prohibits pork and alcohol, diets vary among Muslim Americans and may reflect the ethnic backgrounds of this group, including, but not limited to, Arab, Persian, Pakistani, Asian, African, European, and African Americans. Dietary accommodations that are free from pork and pork products are accommodated easily in most hospitals today. During the period of Ramadan, patients may desire to fast, though it is not required during illness; nurses may discuss with patients ways to accommodate this ritual.

Gaining knowledge about Islam, not only as a religion but also as a way of life, can assist in planning and guiding care that is consistent with cultural needs. Health-care providers who attempt to accommodate and advocate for Muslims to have *choices* convey appreciation and respect for Islamic values and support patient satisfaction.

Transcultural Caring-Based Learning Approach

Please review the Transcultural Caring Dynamics in Nursing and Health Care Theory and Model, the assessment tool, the transcultural caring–based learning (TCCBL) approach, and the critical caring inquiry information and access other relevant resources. In your small group, apply the TCCBL approach while using the dimensions of the Transcultural Caring Dynamics in Nursing and Health Care Model outlined in this chapter. Select the most appropriate assessment tools, including the Culture-Value Conflict tool for transcultural evidence gathering. The Reflections with Questions section that follows is a guide that will assist you individually and collectively in your learning group with dialogue and interpretation of the transcultural caring, ethical, contextual, and spiritual foundational experience of a Muslim American nursing situation.

Reflections with Questions

Reflect on Mary's story, a nurse who sought to discern the crossover of anti-Muslim discrimination in society to nursing and health care through research. What does her work suggest about the role of the nurse in supporting human and civil rights? What aspects of Ray's theory and model address justice and support for human rights? Consider how findings from Mary's research apply to your nursing practice. What aspect of Ray's theory serves to promote culturally congruent practice? How are you personally influenced by media portrayals of Muslims? What is your reaction to one who wears the *hijab*? What are the similarities and differences between Islam and other monotheistic religions? Consider other groups who face adversity in society, not only in the United States but also in other countries. How may the issues discussed in this exemplar be compared, contrasted, and applied?

Transcultural Nursing Reflections

- Reflect on your spiritual beliefs, and compare and contrast them to Islamic beliefs.
- Reflect on how 9/11 and other conflicts or incidents involving Muslims around the world affect your views.
- Consider how American media, including television and cinema, portray Muslims.
- Read the Patriot Act, and consider how this legislation impacted the rights of Americans.
- Look up on the Internet incidents about surveillance, arrests, and unfair treatment of Muslims since 9/11 and the Boston Marathon bombings.
- Read the Civil Rights Act of 1964, and consider how can you uphold this landmark legislation in your nursing practice.
- Read about the *National Standards for Culturally and Linguistically Appropriate Services in Health and Health Care* (Office of Minority Health, 2013) and Standards from the Transcultural Nursing Society, and reflect on how these standards are followed in your practice setting.
- Describe the difference between translation and interpretation, and reflect on interpreter services in your practice setting that would affect Muslim Americans or any other culture group.

Select Bibliography

Ahmed, S., & Reddy, L. (2007). Understanding the mental health needs of American Muslims: Recommendations and considerations for practice. *Journal of Multicultural Counseling and Development, 35*, 207–218.

Ali, D., & Spencer, R. (2003). *Inside Islam: A guide for Catholics.* London: Ascension Press.

Al-Shahri, M. (2002). Culturally sensitive caring for Saudi patients. *Journal of Transcultural Nursing, 13*(2), 133–138.

American Nurses Association. (2015). *Discrimination and racism in health care.* Retrieved from

http://www.nursingworld.org/MainMenuCategories/Policy-Advocacy/Positions-and-Resolutions/ANAPositionStatements/Position-Statements-Alphabetically/Copy-of-prtetdisrac14448.html

Athar, S. (1996). Islamic perspectives in medical ethics. In S. Athar (Ed.), *Islamic perspectives in medicine: A survey of Islamic medicine: Achievements and contemporary issues* (pp. 187–194). Chicago, IL: Kazi Publications.

Atighetchi, D. (2007). *Islamic bioethics: Problems and perspectives*. Dordrecht, The Netherlands: Springer.

Bagby, I. (2011). *The American Mosque 2011*. Retrieved from http://faithcommunitiestoday.org/sites/faithcommunitiestoday.org/files/The%20American%20Mosque%202011%20web.pdf

Begara, J., & Tashjian, J. (2006). End-of-life practices at a Lebanese hospital: Courage or knowledge? *Journal of Transcultural Nursing, 17*(4), 381–388.

Charles, C., & Daroszewski, E. (2012). Culturally competent nursing care of the Muslim patient. *Issues in Mental Health Nursing, 33*(1), 61–63.

Droogsma, R.A. (2007). Redefining hijab: American Muslim women's standpoint on veiling. *Journal of Applied Communication Research, 35*(3), 294–319.

Esposito, J. (2010). *Islam: The straight path*. New York, NY: Oxford University Press.

Facebook. (2013). *Welcome to Facebook*. Retrieved from https://www.facebook.com

Huda, Q. (2006). *The diversity of Muslims in the United States: Views as Americans*. Retrieved from http://www.usip.org/publications/diversity-muslims-united-states-views-americans

Iqbal, M. (2007). *Science and Islam*. Westport, CT: Greenwood Press.

Kaplan, J. (2006). Islamophobia in America? September 11 and Islamophobic hate crime. *Terrorism and Political Violence, 18*(1), 1–33.

Kyriakides-Yeldham, A. (2005). Islamic medical ethics and the straight path of God. *Islam and Christian-Muslim Relations, 16*(3), 213–225.

Laird, L., Amer, M., Barnett, E., & Barnes, L. (2007). Muslim patients and health disparities in the U.K and the U.S. *Archives of Diseases in Childhood, 92*, 922–926.

Luna, L. (1998). Culturally competent health care: A challenge for nurses in Saudi Arabia, *Journal of Transcultural Nursing, 9*, 8–14.

Martin, M.B. (2013). *Perceived discrimination of Muslims in health care in the United States*. Retrieved from http://search.proquest.com/docview/1508821207?accountid=131239

McFarland, M., & Webhe-Alamah, H. (2015). *Leininger's culture care diversity and universality: A worldwide nursing theory* (4th ed.). Burlington, MA: Jones & Bartlett Learning.

Murray, N. (2004). Profiled: Arabs, Muslims, and the post-9/11 hunt for the enemy within. In E.C. Hagopian (Ed.), *Civil rights in peril: The targeting of Arabs and Muslims* (pp. 27–70). Chicago, IL: Haymarket Books.

Nasr, S. (2003). *Islam: Religion, history, and civilization*. New York, NY: Harper Collins.

Nigosian, S. (2004). *Islam: Its history, teaching, and practices*. Bloomington, IN: Indiana University Press.

Office of the Clerk, U.S. House of Representatives. (1964). Civil Rights Act of 1964. Retrieved from http://library.clerk.house.gov/reference-files/PPL_CivilRightsAct_1964.pdf

Office of Minority Health. (2013). *National standards for culturally and linguistically appropriate services*. Retrieved from https://www.thinkculturalhealth.hhs.gov/Content/clas.asp

Padela, A., Gunter, K., Killawi, A., & Heisler, M. (2012). Religious values and healthcare accommodations: Voices from the American Muslim community. *Journal of General Internal Medicine, 27*(6), 708–715.

Patel, E. (2009). *Being Muslim in America*. Washington, DC: Bureau of International Information on Programs. United States Department of State. Retrieved from http://photos.state.gov/libraries/korea/49271/dwoa_122709/being-muslim-in-america.pdf

Peek, L. (2011). *Behind the backlash: Muslim Americans after 9/11*. Philadelphia, PA: Temple University Press.

Pew Forum on Religious and Public Life. (2008). *U.S. religious landscape survey*. Retrieved from http://www.umsl.edu/~keelr/010/Pew_Report_on_Religion/report-religious-landscape-study-full.pdf

Pew Forum on Religious and Public Life. (2009). *Views of religious similarities and differences: Muslims widely seen as facing discrimination.* Retrieved from http://www.pewforum.org/uploadedfiles/Topics/Religious_Affiliation/Muslim/survey0909.pdf

Preston, J., & Mackey, R. (2013, April 15). April 15 updates on explosions at the Boston Marathon. *The New York Times.* Retrieved from http://thelede.blogs.nytimes.com/2013/04/15/live-updates-explosion-at-boston-marathon/?_r=0

Purnell, L., & Paulanka, B. (2012). *Transcultural health care: A culturally competent approach.* Philadelphia, PA: F.A. Davis.

Ramsden, I., & Papps, E. (1996). Cultural safety in nursing: The New Zealand experience. *International Journal for Quality in Healthcare, 8*(5), 491–497.

Rassool, G. (2000). The crescent and Islam: Healing, nursing and the spiritual dimension. Some considerations towards an understanding of the Islamic perspectives on caring. *Journal of Advanced Nursing, 32*(6), 1476–1484.

Rathor, M., Rani, M., Shah, A., Leman, W., Akter, S., & Omar, A. (2011). The principle of autonomy as related to personal decision making concerning health and research from an 'Islamic viewpoint'. *Journal of the Islamic Medical Association of North America, 43*(1).

Ray, M. (1994). Transcultural nursing ethics: A framework and model for transcultural ethical analysis. *Journal of Holistic Nursing, 12*(3), 251–264.

Ray, M. (2010). *Transcultural caring dynamics in nursing and health care.* Philadelphia, PA: F.A. Davis.

Read, J. (2008). Muslims in America. *Contexts, 7,* 39–43.

Riaz, M.N., & Chaudry, M.M. (2003). *Halal food production.* Boca Raton, FL: CRC Press.

Rippy, A., & Newman, E. (2008). Adaptation of a scale of race-related stress for use with Muslim Americans. *Journal of Muslim Mental Health, 3,* 53–68. Retrieved from http://assets.paleycenter.org/assets/media-council/Documents/Media-and-the-Muslim-World-Paley-Center-Report.pdf

Sundquist, E. (1988). The Japanese-American internment: A reappraisal. *The American Scholar, 57*(4), 529–547.

Survey Monkey. (2013). *About.* Retrieved from http://www.surveymonkey.com/mp/aboutus/

United States Department of Health and Human Services. (2011). *HHS action plan to reduce racial and ethnic health disparities.* Retrieved from http://minorityhealth.hhs.gov/npa/files/Plans/HHS/HHS_Plan_complete.pdf

United States Government Printing Office. (2001). *The Patriot Act.* Retrieved from http://www.gpo.gov/fdsys/pkg/PLAW-107publ56/pdf/PLAW-107publ56.pdf

Wehbe-Alamah, H. (2008). Bridging generic and professional care practices for Muslim patients through use of Leininger's culture care modes. *Contemporary Nurse, 28*(1–2), 83–97.

Williams, D., Neighbors, H., & Jackson, J. (2003). Racial/ethnic discrimination and health: Findings from community studies. *American Journal of Public Health, 93*(2), 200–208.

CHAPTER 23

American Nurses and the Native People of Ecuador: The Transcultural Experience of Shamanism

History and Background of Native People of Ecuador

"I was privileged to take a group of students, faculty, and health-care colleagues to Ecuador in May of 2007. Visiting Ecuador was both an opportunity and an adventure that will forever affect the lives of individuals in our group. My interest in Ecuador started when I was teaching a course entitled Praxis: Therapies of Imagination at the University. I was put in touch with two Shamans: Raphael Yamberla (now living in Santa Fe) and his cousin Raphael Cascal, both from Ecuador. Both came to my class and shared their wisdom as Quechua healers/shamans, performing healings using carnations, liquor, tobacco, and eggs. Their stories of Ecuador and the lives of their people sparked an interest in me and led me to assemble a group of faculty, students, and family members to journey to Ecuador. This journey put us in contact with a variety of indigenous (indigenas) Quechua healers referred to as Shamans and Yachajs."

Mary's Story

The journey began the weekend before Memorial Day in 2007. After several hours on a plane, we arrived first in Miami and then took a connecting flight to Quito, Ecuador. We spent the first night outside of Quito in one of the oldest haciendas (farms) in Ecuador, providing us with our first of many wonderful experiences with the Ecuadorian people. We arrived late in the evening, all travel weary and ready for sleep. The next day we toured the *hacienda* and surrounding farm complete with horses, pigs, and cattle. The group was served a nutritional breakfast of eggs, toast, orange juice, fruit, and coffee, along with informative conversation about the history of the *hacienda*. After breakfast we were off to experience the equator and our first of several meetings with Shamans.

Otovalo is a small community outside of Quito where many of the local Shamans are located. Raphael Cascal was the first Shaman the group met. We realized on arrival that he was unable to meet with us, but directed us to Maria Juana Yamberla, one of the few female Shamans/Yachajs in Ecuador. She was a very petite woman who was dressed in traditional Ecuadorian clothing and a headdress made of select bird feathers that identify her as a bird person (a special symbol of the traditional *native* culture). Over the next few hours she performed several healings with individuals, including myself. Each healing took about a half an hour and involved ceremony, flowers, nettle leaves, alcohol, and chanting. The alcohol was used as a way to cleanse and purify the flowers for healing and we drank tea after the healing and the chanting. The ceremony was a spiritual way of experiencing the healing power of the Shaman/Yachaj. Maria shared with each of us her sensing of us and what she felt we should work on. She was a phenomenal women and her energy quite healing.

After the healings we traveled to another *hacienda* nearby and spent the night. The next day we returned to Raphael Cascal's home and experienced a group healing. He too used flowers, liquor, and nettles to purify and energize, and the flowers and fire to heal. He also performed select healings with group members and even performed a marriage ceremony for a couple who were engaged on the trip. We later would find out that virtually every Ecuadorian community has a healer, most of them male. These individuals know the healing properties of various plants and are able to diagnose and treat by correcting spiritual imbalances in the individual. The healers are known by various names. In the Quichua communities, they are called *yachaj mamas* or *yachaj taitas* (knowledgeable mothers and fathers). There are also midwives who are known as *parteras*.

After a good night's rest at a second *hacienda*, we were off for a shopping spree at a local market area in Otovalo. Many of the people within the market were there to sell weavings, artwork, musical instruments, hats, and garments. We all had the opportunity to barter and experience the locals and their talents. After a day of shopping and more eating, we moved on to a local hotel for the night in preparation for our visit to either a school or clinic.

The next day the group split and half went to a local school and the other half to the community clinic. Those at the school were shown the classrooms and spent time with the children. Those of us who went to the clinic experienced the healing practices of Yachajs and midwives. The Yachajs at the clinic were performing a healing on a child with diarrhea. It was there that the Yachaj shared how guinea pigs are used in some healings to assess the illnesses and are euthanized by the Yachaj and analyzed to discover the organs that have bad energy. In essence, they say the guinea pig pulls the bad energy out of the ill person. We also spoke with the midwife who provides the maternity care for the local women. There was also a dentist at the clinic.

Day three began with another traditional breakfast; we were off to another market in Otovalo to purchase rubber boots, a necessary item to wear for the hike into the rain forest. Once outfitted with the boots we were taken to the river, boarded motorized canoes and taken to the other side where we would hike for 4 and one-half hours into the rain forest. The trek was physically exhaustive and really separated the young and fit from the elders. The younger group made the trek in about 3 hours; the elders took 4 and one-half hours. At the end of the trek, we arrived at a set of grass huts and met Augustine, a Yachaj and one of the most profound healers I have ever experienced. I had developed a migraine during the trek. Augustine made a tea for me, instructed me to lie down, and within an hour the headache was completely gone. After naps, we met for the first of a number of sessions with Augustine, learning about his skills with herbs, Iawaska (a powerful hallucinogen), and healing. His family lives there with him and he introduced us to 10 of his 12 children, six boys and six girls. His wife was in the local town with one of his children, who had been hit by a car and was recovering. His older son was with his mother as a helper. Clever, one of his sons was introduced to us and was the son chosen from infancy to follow his father as a Yachaj. After dinner that night, Augustine talked about his life as a Yachaj. He was born to parents who were in bondage for a debt and taken to Peru to work off the debt through physical labor. They were working on a sugarcane plantation and during their bondage; both parents died and left him as an orphan. At the age of eight he traveled from Peru back to Otovalo, Ecuador to return to his grandparents. The journey took a long time according to Augustine. He states that from childhood he was identified as a healer and over time was taken in by the community where he now lives. He is a recognized leader within this community, particularly because he is the Yachaj.

Yachajs are indigenous healers who are recognized for their ability to heal both through ceremony and herbs and often become leaders within the community. They are truly herbalists.

Over the next day, Augustine prepared the group for the Iawaska, the powerful hallucinogenic root that is used in some healings. Augustine and his sons showed us how they prepare Iawaska root that had been harvested. Some individuals chose this healing modality while others chose to observe. As a leader, I felt the need to be an observer. Iawaska is a hallucinogen that aids people in discovering personal healing through visions. All of us attended a personal healing with Augustine the following morning after the Iawaska ceremony. Augustine met with each of us and interpreted the visions of the Iawaska for those who experienced it and his insights about each of us who had not.

That evening, Augustine introduced us to some of the community representatives who performed a native dance and shared a meal with us. We were also asked to share our talents of singing, guitar playing, and dance. The next morning we toured his garden, and on the walking tour of his herb garden, he shared how he uses herbs in his healings; it was a very informative lecture.

On our last evening we sat around with Augustine's family and shared stories and a meal. The following morning we left to trek out of the rain forest and continue our journey to the town where Maria, Augustine's wife, was staying. We met Maria and the child who was recovering. We left Augustine there, waved good-bye and made our journey to a spa resort where we had a massage, steam bath, and just experienced the warm water spas. Our last night in Ecuador was spent in Quito in a large hotel. The following day we returned to the United States.

It is difficult to capture all of the experiences and knowledge I gained about these gentle people living a simple life. Ecuador is about the size of Colorado. Five different tribes inhabit Ecuador, but the Quichoa people are the tribe from which most Shamans emerge. Ecuador, for a long period, was controlled by the Spanish and therefore both Spanish and the native language of Quichua are spoken. Our tour guide spoke both the Spanish language and Quichua. The religion of Ecuador is predominately Christian, with 95% of this population of people Catholic and 5% Protestant. Many of the communities are made up of skilled laborers, a few teachers, and a healer, often a Yachaj or a Shaman. Quichua believe in an inner and outer body, which must be kept in balance. The Yachaj or Shaman is there to help one maintain that balance.

The Ecuadorian diet is simple, comprising lots of fruits, vegetables, legumes, beans, fish, chicken, and occasional beef. Clinics exist in larger cities and midwives assist with the birthing of the children. I saw very little obesity; in fact, the people are very trim, short, and athletic. The Quichoa people are very family centered. Each member supports other members and contributes to the health of the family.

The larger cities like Quito have formalized educational institutions. In fact Clever, Augustine's son, was a student in Quito at the college. Most village families exist on small plots of land, growing their own food. Families in the larger cities are involved in industry or the markets. Many of the Quichoa men have long braids and wear Panama hats. Women are dressed in brightly colored garments. Many of the locals are weavers, wood-carvers, and painters. These were people whom we met at the markets.

There is a value in this indigenous society of reciprocity and a collective work effort. There is a great respect for the land, the air, and rain. Mother Earth (*Pacha Mama*) feeds the people by producing crops, so the people think she should be thanked and she is fed the last drops of alcohol that are used to celebrate the harvest. These compassionate people welcomed us, cared for us, provided healings, and left us with great memories.

Transcultural Caring-Based Learning Approach

Please review the information about: Transcultural Caring Dynamics for Nursing and Health-Care Theory and Model, the assessment tools, the transcultural caring-based learning (TCCBL) approach, and the critical caring inquiry information, and accessing other relevant literary and Internet resources. In your small group, apply the TCCBL approach, while using dimensions of the Transcultural Caring Dynamics in Nursing and Health-Care Model and the most appropriate assessment tools for transcultural evidence gathering. The Reflections with Questions section that follows is a guide that will assist you individually and collectively in your learning group with dialogue and interpretation of the Ecuadorian native people's transcultural experience.

Reflections with Questions

As Mary reflects on the experience of the transcultural interaction with indigenous people, what values come to mind in their families, the role of Shamans (Yachajs), and the holistic healing practices? Reflect on how the villagers desire to and preserve their culture by sharing with others in the developed world. Reflect on how the changes in Ecuador as a country will affect indigenous people and their languages. What are your responsibilities as a transcultural nurse in understanding indigenous people in the Ecuadorian culture and their preservation around the world?

Transcultural Nursing Reflections

• Reflect on yourselves as student nurses journeying to Ecuador to experience the culture, and engage with the indigenous people in their values, beliefs, attitudes, opinions, and lifeworld practices. How would you prepare yourself? (See Andrews & Boyle, 2016; McFarland & Wehbe-Alamah, 2015.)

- Reflect upon the meaning of holistic nursing. How would you prepare to engage in cross-cultural comparison and contrasting for the purposes of education and learning about another culture?
- Reflect on the Ecuadorian culture, the people described in Mary's story, the culture of the healer (Shamans/Yachajs), and the indigenous healing practices in Ecuador and how they were demonstrated by Augustine, the Shaman or Yachaj.
- How do the people live? What are their lifeways, family values, and kinship system? What is their religion? Compare and contrast the native people of Ecuador in this story with, for example, the Navajo people or any other tribe of North America.
- How have indigenous practices affected holistic nursing and the subdiscipline of holistic nursing in the United States and Canada and around the Western world? How does this exchange of people enhance opportunities to learn, communicate, and begin to know another culture that may have diverse practices from one's own?
- Reflect upon indigenous languages and whether or not these languages will be preserved as people interact together. How are some universities with Social Science Departments preserving native languages?
- The health and healing of the native people depends on their beliefs and the herbs that have been demonstrated to have healing properties. What are the practices of the indigenous people in health and healing advanced in Mary's story? What is their purpose? When the people participated in the Shaman's experience, what practices could be identified? Why do you think special dress, chanting, flowers, alcohol, and tea were used in the healing ceremony? How can the healing ceremony be compared with healing ceremonies in North America? What is the unique blend of Catholicism and indigenous spirituality? Is there conflict?
- What does an herbalist mean? What do you think about the use of alcohol, and Iawaska, the hallucinogenic root, in personal healing? What are your thoughts of the inducement of visions? In a transcultural experience, such as the healing ceremony, would you have any ethical concerns based upon your own view of health and healing? What would they be if you did? Are there differences between what may be used in psychiatric care, such as hypnosis in North American health-care facilities in relation to healing?
- Identify the history of Ecuador and its place in the continent of South America. What is its form of government? What is its economic base? What are the Galapagos Islands? How are they financed? What is its relationship with other Latin American countries? Are there disputes about multinational oil? Are there disputes about making and exporting coca? What is Ecuador's relationship with the United States and other Western nations? How many Ecuadorians live in the United States?
- What is the essence of holistic nursing? Describe the major tenets and the standards of practice. How do the tenets compare with the philosophy of caring? How do they compare with the tenets of transcultural nursing?

Select Bibliography

Andres, M., & Boyle, J. (2016). *Transcultural concepts in nursing care* (7th ed.). Philadelphia, PA: Wolters Kluwer.

Cuellar, N. (2006). *Conversations in complementary and alternative medicine.* Sudbury, MA: Jones & Bartlett Publishers.

Dossey, B., & Keegan, L. (2013). *Holistic nursing: A handbook for practice* (6th ed.). Burlington, MA: Jones & Bartlett Learning.

Frisch, N., Dossey, B., Guzzetta, C., & Quinn, J. (Eds.). (2000). *AHNA Standards of holistic nursing practice: Guidelines for caring and healing.* Sudbury, MA: Jones & Bartlett.

Dossey, B., Keagan, L., & Guzzetta, C. (Eds.). (2008). *Holistic nursing: A handbook for practice* (5th ed.) Sudbury, MA: Jones & Bartlett.

McFarland, M., & Webhe-Alamah, H. (2015). *Leininger's culture care diversity and universality: A worldwide theory of nursing* (3rd. ed.). Burlington, MA: Jones & Bartlett Learning.

Palmerlee, D., McCarthy, C., & Grosberg, M. (Eds.). (2006). *Lonely planet Ecuador and the Galapagos Islands.* Victoria, Australia: Lonely Planet Publications.

Reyes-Ortiz, C., Rodriquez, M., & Markides, K. (2009). The role of spirituality healing with perceptions of the medical encounter among Latinos. *Journal of General Internal Medicine, 24,* 542–547.

Sawyer, S. (2004). *Crude chronicles: Indigenous politics, multinational oil, and neoliberalism in Ecuador*: Durham, NC: Duke University Press.

Titus, S. (2014). Seeking and utilizing a Curandero in the United States: A literature review. *Journal of Holistic Nursing, 32*(3), 189–201.

Watson, J. (2005). *Caring science as sacred science.* Philadelphia: F. A. Davis Company.

CHAPTER 24

The Culture of Physical, Mental, Spiritual, and Political/Sociocultural Illness: Healing Through Education and Love

*T*he following story is about Amanda. She suffered from abuse, bipolar disease, homelessness, prostitution, drug addiction, incarceration, HIV, and tuberculosis (TB). One
can barely believe that one person could endure so much. The life of Amanda is a challenge
to nurses who must be compassionate in the wake of a society that often prefers to "throw
people away" when they become really sick and enter the universe of suffering, a type of
dying but where despair and hope meet. Caring from the heart and what motivates caring for
nurses is ". . . about the human being's infinite potential and the all-embracing communion
of love that unites human beings around the world . . .; where love and suffering meet, true
compassion and true caring emerge" (Eriksson, 2006, vi–viii).

    Nurses engage in holistic care; the integration of body, mind, and spirit is a central con-
struct of nursing. Physical, mental, and spiritual illness, even political/sociocultural illness is
based upon various levels of challenges and possibilities of holism: our state of being, the
makeup and function of the sociocultural environment including the health-care system, and
our ability to find meaning in and reconcile suffering through caring (Ray, 1998, 2007). "To
live is to suffer, thus, suffering is a part of human life"(Eriksson, 2006, pp. 28–29). As human
beings and as health-care professionals, "we are forced to reflect and make ourselves responsible for an answer" (p. 29) to the question: Why do we and especially our patients suffer?
As transcultural caring nurses, we come to the answer after contemplating holism and the

313

frailties of human life, that is, "only love [compassion and justice or right action, Ray, 1989] can give meaning to suffering . . . the greatest of all is love" (St. Paul to the Romans, 8:28 in Eriksson, 2006, p. 39). The wounds of illness, pain, helplessness, abandonment, and loss offer a window to the seeds of understanding. Victor Frankl (2006) reminds us about giving meaning to suffering from his experiences in the death camps during the Holocaust. When we give meaning to pain and suffering, as human beings we become more sensitive. If we run away from pain, we lose our vitality, our energy, our strength, and our ability to feel, and even love (such as the pain, suffering, and healing reflected in Amanda's story). The meaning in suffering as love is expressed inwardly and outwardly. It is, first of all, understood as the love of God or a higher power that helps us to reconcile the feelings of hopelessness and helplessness in hope from the pain of abuse, abandonment, loss, and despair. Second, it facilitates seeking increased understanding of the meaning in suffering in culture and society, in the health-care system, in the political and societal structures. Through this understanding as health-care professionals, we make possible the choices for health and healing for our patients.

Thus, making a choice to find hope and meaning in suffering is a process of emergence, and inner and outer healing. Inner and outer healing is relational (Scanlan, 1974). "Inner healing is the healing of the inner man. By inner man we mean the intellectual, volitional and affective areas commonly referred to as mind, will and heart but including such other areas as related to emotions, psyche, soul and spirit. Outer healing is distinguished from inner healing; it is commonly called physical healing, a living process known only to the cells themselves that are involved both independent of and dependent on human relationships such as professionals providing medical and pharmacologic treatment" (Scanlan, 1974, pp. 7–9). With participatory reaching out and help, there can be an integral mental, spiritual, and physical emergence—a change, a transformation toward feelings of self-worth and well-being, not only in the person suffering but also for the person caring. Hope and love direct adherence to recovery, a treatment process that integrates physical, mental, spiritual, and sociocultural care. Hope is faith in the "compassionate we" (Ray, 1991, 2013). The following transcultural experience is a story of darkness of body, mind, and spirit and the awakening of Amanda to life's purpose through human love and professional caring. It is the story of a person who suffered the grief and loss of self-worth through abuse, homelessness, prostitution, drug addiction, incarceration, disease—tuberculosis, the retrovirus HIV (human immunodeficiency virus) and AIDS (acquired immunodeficiency syndrome), and mental illness (bipolar disorder)—and the hope revealed through human, professional, and spiritual caring relationships.

Amanda's Story

Amanda, a 48-year-old woman, lived her life on the streets working as a commercial sex worker for a number of years after leaving her parents' home at a young age. During her time on the streets she endured many arrests for prostitution and drug use. Without access to television or newspapers, her knowledge of HIV and AIDS was sparse and essentially nonexistent. Amanda's pimp did not provide a safe environment and only rewarded her and his other workers with drugs when they met their quota of sexual encounters. He punished them with physical abuse when they did not. This incredible challenge to self-worth in addition to the pain of being raised in an alcoholic family contributed to Amanda's inability to recognize the consequences of her life choices, which finally resulted in the diagnosis of HIV in her 20s. (See Andrews & Boyle, 2016 regarding HIV among American women.)

The diagnosis of HIV came during an arrest and incarceration, leaving her feeling that she had a death sentence. Her reaction was hopelessness and, back to the streets, a disregard for herself and others. When her body continued to weaken with HIV, she eventually developed TB. Amanda was forced into a local TB hospital by authorities where her life would forever change. During an angry outburst in the confined space of the TB hospital, Amanda decided to imitate having a seizure, hoping that this action would provide her with medicine to calm her nerves and give her the high she missed from the street drugs. Instead of her desired response, the nurse clinician recognized the false seizure and offered some advice to help her to become "grounded in reality." Only through Amanda's truthfulness about her illnesses and addiction would she be able to move forward in her life. Following more angry interactions and positive reactions from her therapists, Amanda started to see herself in a new way. Ultimately, meeting a special man in a support group, Amanda accepted her diagnosis and made the choice to move forward into recovery.

During her treatment for TB, Amanda also received mental health care for the bipolar diagnosis (manic-depressive mental illness) and physical care (medical treatment) for her HIV, neither of which she fully understood. The special member of her HIV-support group became the one person (who later became her significant other) who helped to convince her that she had self-worth and could be happy in life after all.

The road to improved health and well-being was, at the very least, challenging. Living her life primarily independent of any sort of a caring environment, Amanda resisted many of the interventions and efforts of health-care professionals. Moving through different regimens of antiretroviral therapy, it was only when her HIV became advanced that Amanda realized that *she* had the ability to partner in care with her health-care providers. She chose to be authentically a part of the decision making in a positive way. Through much effort and several providers, Amanda finally recognized the need for patient education instead of relying only on what information she received in her short visits with the infectious disease physician. In addition, she found that going to the "lunch and learn" program allowed her to share her experience and learn from others about her disease and its treatments.

The cocreation of Amanda's "extended family," including her partner and the community of HIV-positive patients she bonded with, allowed her to move into a more nurturing environment. She realized that it was more than she could have ever imagined. After being HIV positive for 18 years, Amanda now acknowledges her disease as a formidable challenge that requires her full attention to treatment and "care of the soul" (Moore, 1992) every day. The reality that confronts someone when they are forced to deal with a serious illness can often provide the opportunity for the beginning of a change in their life. Amanda, fortunate enough to have been forced to face such a realization, became able to confront the "demons" that would continue to surface during her recovery. The acknowledgment eventually helped her to embrace adherence to a treatment regimen. Before this time, anger, fear, financial problems, literacy, disease-specific issues, and trust challenged her and her health-care providers. Every day they influenced her self-worth and her ability to adhere to treatments. Despite the challenges to adherence, Amanda remains committed to maintaining a good quality of life. Adherence to a plan of care is the perpetual trial but expectant hope for healing for all HIV patients.

Transcultural Caring-Based Learning Approach

Please review the information about: Transcultural Caring Dynamics for Nursing and Health-Care Theory and Model, the assessment tools, the transcultural caring-based learning (TCCBL) approach, and the transcultural caring inquiry information, and accessing the Internet and other relevant literary and Internet resources. In your small group, apply the TCCBL approach, while using dimensions of the Transcultural Caring Dynamics in Nursing and Health-Care Model and the most appropriate assessment tools for transcultural evidence gathering. The Reflections with Questions section that follows is a guide that will assist you individually and collectively in your learning group with dialogue and interpretation of Amanda's story of severe illness, despair, and hope for recovery and transformation.

Reflections with Questions

Reflect on the story of Amanda, who has faced and is facing physical, mental, spiritual, and political challenges in her life. The story of Amanda illuminates a life of illness. Amanda has had to face what happens with abuse; homelessness; prostitution; drug addiction; physical, mental, and spiritual illness in a ruthless sociocultural environment. Focus on the inner paralysis of Amanda to caring.

Transcultural Nursing Reflections

- What transcultural caring compassionate understanding comes to your mind both as a person and as a nurse when you reflect upon Amanda's story?
- What happened to Amanda in the disintegration of body, mind, and spirit?
- What is the meaning of being present to a person who has been a victim of the culture of "darkness": abuse, homelessness, drug addiction, and prostitution?
- How would you relate in a caring and just way in the physical, mental, spiritual, and sociocultural trauma that Amanda endured?
- What is the nature of loss of self-worth that leads to the culture of poverty of body, mind, and spirit? What are actual sources of Amanda's suffering?
- How did Amanda finally come to the source of healing inside herself (i.e., reintegration of body, mind, and spirit, and the healing of her response to the power of the sociocultural environment)? What are the sources of the gift of healing for her? Focus on adherence to a protocol or regimen of care for physical and mental illness.
- What does adherence mean to you? What are your responsibilities as a transcultural nurse in understanding adherence or compliance with a treatment regimen?
- Does adherence interfere with the patient's right to choose? How do you as a nurse deal with transcultural nursing competency in the wake of trying to help a patient adhere to a regimen of care, especially with drug and alcohol addiction, and other diseases that affect the body, mind, and spirit? Although this experience deals more with suffering, illness, and poverty, what are experiences of people of means who are addicted to Internet, Internet gaming, potentially legal marijuana, and so forth, that may affect their well-being and livelihood? How can transcultural mental health nurses come to their aid?
- What is the state of mental health care and mental health nursing in the United States? Is there a regimen of care for spiritual and political illness (i.e., social, sexual, gender, and technological and health-care issues in a society)? Refer to the DSM-5 for assistance with mental health categories.
- Does caring produce suffering in the caregiver in the "compassionate we relationship"?
- What is your view of compassion and justice or fairness in transcultural nursing? What does caring mean to you in the context of this transcultural caring experience of Amanda?

Note on Holism

The following reflections in part facilitate our understanding of *holism* (the whole). A person-in-relationship is holographic. The "whole is in the part and the part is in the whole"—the whole is reflected in each part (i.e., physical, mental, spiritual and sociocultural/political) and each of the parts (i.e., physical, mental, spiritual, and sociocultural/political) is the whole person (Ray 2006). Every part secures its meaning from each of the parts, which are then considered wholes. Everything is interconnected. Each disease, disorder, or social issue affects the whole community, and the world community at the same time the disease, disorder, or social issue affects a person's body, mind, and spirit. Nursing is committed to holistic caring, caring for the body, mind, and spirit in a compassionate way and a "compassionate we" relationship. Nurses are committed to understanding the social and cultural situations that lead to health, healing, and well-being or the destruction of the human body, mind, and spirit by nonresponse to suffering and inhumane transcultural care (Ray, 2015).

- How do you view holistic nursing, your role as a transcultural nurse at the interpersonal and intercommunity, and political levels?
- What is the role of public health nurses/community health nurses as transcultural nurses in seeking understanding of the social, public health, and cultural arenas of a community?
- Express your views of cultural competence. What ethical caring responsibilities do you as a transcultural caring nurse have toward people like Amanda and toward seeking understanding of the general health and cultural care and human rights issues facing in your community?
- Pulmonary TB is a contagious bacterial infection caused by *Mycobacterium tuberculosis* (*M. tuberculosis*). How are the lungs involved and invaded by this bacterium? How does the disease spread? How does it spread to other organs? What central medications are used to hold this disease "in check"? *M. tuberculosis* is a cross-cultural disease. Why is it resurfacing in the United States and Canada when it was considered essentially "cured" with medication? How is the disease spreading across cultures?
- HIV/AIDS infects lymphocytes and results in destruction of the entire immune system. HIV and AIDS are affecting more than 1 million people in the United States. HIV (retrovirus) is attracted to T lymphocytes in the cells because of their CD4 receptors. The CD4 T cells are part of the white blood cells (WBC) that fight infection. Once HIV is inside these cells, the HIV produces abnormal DNA and when fused with normal DNA takes over the cells' operation. How is the whole patient affected?
- What is the pathophysiology/disease development of HIV? What is the disease progression? What are the AIDS-defining illnesses, TB, hepatitis C, sexually transmitted diseases (STDs), and so forth? What are the risk factors? What other serious STDs are manifest with HIV/AIDS? How can the disease be prevented? What tests are used to diagnose HIV infection? What are the treatments/pharmacotherapeutics for HIV/AIDS? How is this disease manifest worldwide? How are people who have no health-care insurance, or no access to health-care affected by this disease? How does a patient live with HIV/AIDS? How does the HIV/AIDS virus affect the well-being of the patient? What is the grief-response to the trauma of HIV/AIDS? What is the life expectancy associated with HIV/AIDS?
- How are diverse culture groups affected by this disease? How are the gay, lesbian, and bisexual communities and the heterosexual community affected by this disease? Are different culture groups affected more by this disease? Besides the physical, mental, and spiritual trauma related to HIV/AIDS, name some of the diverse ethical, and religious views associated with this disease. What does adherence to a treatment protocol or regimen mean? How does a transcultural nurse cocreate a compassionate response and environment to help the patient with the issue of choice and participation in decision making?
- Bipolar disorder (known previously as manic depressive disorder) is a complex and dangerous disease characterized by extreme changes in moods, from one pole (mania) to the other (depression), and between these mood swings the person experiences "normal" behavior. Mania is described as experiencing restlessness, talkativeness, and recklessness with periods of euphoria within which the person may have lavish spending sprees or become involved in risky sexual behavior. Depression is described as the opposite of mania where the person is very sad, has a lack of energy, cries, feels worthless, has sleep problems, and could become suicidal. The disorder wreaks havoc on families and others (Frisch & Frisch, 2005; Bipolar Disorder, 2009). Is bipolar disorder inherited or acquired? How does this disorder potentially coincide with the social situation, where a woman, Amanda, is driven to hopelessness and helplessness by virtue of homelessness, prostitution, drug abuse, incarceration, and physical illness?
- Psychotherapy and psychopharmacologic intervention are critical for bipolar disease. What are the treatment protocols for this disorder? Does a person have to be on medications in both the manic and depressive mood swings and the periods of "normal" behavior? Is there a danger of suicide with this disorder? How does a health professional know that a person's depression could lead to suicide? Are there any side effects with the medications in

treatment for HIV/AIDS? Do psychopharmacological drugs interfere with HIV/AIDS medications? How are the family and the community affected by a person suffering from this disorder?

- What is spirituality to you? What does *spiritual illness* mean to you? What is the meaning of suffering to you?
- How do the wounds of physical, mental, and sociocultural illness offer a window to the soul (spirituality)?
- What happens to the inner soul of a person who is experiencing trauma?
- What is the grieving process? (Examine Kübler-Ross' stages of grief and grieving [Kübler-Ross & Kessler, 2007.) How do you think Amanda dealt with her grief?
- How did the process of soul and body restoration take place for Amanda?
- What occurred at the TB hospital that alerted her health-care professional that something was wrong? How did he help her?
- What is the meaning of trust in relationship?
- How do you think Amanda developed trust in her health-care professional to adhere to a treatment regimen of attending a support group and taking medication for her health-care problems? What are your views of health care professionals personally involved with patients (as in this story)? Are there ethical considerations?
- Is depression or any other health-care problem ever a gift?
- Overall, how does spirituality play a role in living? In living with HIV and TB?
- What is your view of the sociocultural environment in your area, in your country? What is social justice in your view? Do transcultural nurses have a responsibility for human rights and social justice? (See *Transcultural Nursing Society Position Statement on Human Rights*, Miller et al, 2008; see Update by Douglas et al., 2011.)
- How much of a role should the public sphere have in protecting and caring for people? Compare and contrast the protection of the society in neglect and incarceration. What are your views about incarceration for homelessness, prostitution, and drug addiction? What is the role of the criminal justice system in your community?
- What is the meaning of homelessness to you? What are the parameters of homelessness? How does homelessness happen in adolescence, in middle age, in the aged, and with veterans? Is homelessness the same or different in the United States in comparison with other parts of the world? How does helplessness ensue when there is homelessness?
- Does the lack of access to health care have a bearing on homelessness? Also, consider how a politician would deal with homelessness in a community. What or how should the community deal with homelessness, with drug or alcohol addiction? Should people be fed and clothed and offered counseling or spiritual help? Should apartments be secured for the homeless? Should city or county parks be secured for the homeless? Should people be housed against their will?
- What are your views about prostitution, the sex trade, and sex trafficking both within local communities and around the world? What is the role of a pimp?
- Is prostitution considered a health problem, a public health issue? How are some communities, such as the city of San Francisco, California, examining sex trafficking as a public health issue?
- What is the role of public health in the diagnosis and treatment of TB in HIV/AIDS? How does a person get admitted to a hospital for TB?
- Compare and contrast major public health problems, such as HIV/AIDS and TB, around the world. Which countries have the most difficulties? Why?

Select Bibliography

American Psychiatric Association (2013). *Diagnostic and Statistical Manual of Psychiatric Disorders, 5th ed.* (DSM-5). Arlington, VA: American Psychiatric Association.

Andrews, M., & Boyle, J. (2016). *Transcultural concepts in nursing care* (7th ed.). Philadelphia, PA: Wolters Kluwer.

Bartlett, J., & Finkbeiner, A. (2006). *A guide to living with HIV infection.* Baltimore: Johns Hopkins University Press.

Bipolar disorder. Retrieved July 21, 2009, from www.webmd.com/bipolar-disorder/default.htm

Centers for Disease Control and Prevention. (2006). *Intimate partner violence: Fact sheet.* Retrieved April, 2006, from http://www.cdc.gov/nicpe/factsheets/ipvfacts.htm

Cowling, W. R. (2008). An essay on women, despair, and healing: A personal narrative. *Advances in Nursing Science, 31*(3), 249–258.

Davidson, A., Ray, M., & Turkel, M. (2011). *Nursing, caring, and complexity science: For human-environment well-being.* New York: Springer Publishing Company.

Dossey, B., & Keegan, L. (2013). *Holistic nursing: A handbook for practice* (6th ed.). Burlington, MA: Jones & Bartlett Learning.

Douglas, M., Uhl-Pierce, J., Rosenkoetter, M., et al. (2011). Standards of practice for culturally competent care: 2011 Update. *Journal of Transcultural Nursing, 22*(4), 317–333.

Eriksson, K. (2006). *The suffering human being.* Chicago: Nordic Studies Press.

Farley, M. (Ed.). (2003). *Prostitution, trafficking, and traumatic stress.* Binghamton, NY: The Haworth Maltreatment & Traumatic Press.

Frankl, V. (2006). *Man's search for meaning.* Boston: Beacon Press.

Frisch, N., & Frisch, L. (2005). *Psychiatric mental health nursing* (3rd ed.). Florence, KY: Delmar Cengage Learning.

Hunter, S. (2006). *AIDS in America.* United Kingdom: Palgrave Macmillan.

Jencks, C. (2005). *The homeless.* Cambridge: Harvard University Press.

Kaufmann, S., & Britton, W. (Eds.). (2008). *Handbook of tuberculosis: Immunology and cell biology.* New York: Wiley-VCH.

Kübler-Ross, E., & Kessler, D. (2007). *On grief and grieving: Finding the meaning of grief through the five stages of loss.* New York: Scribner.

Lather, P., & Smithies, C. (1997). *Troubling the angels: Women living with HIV/AIDS.* Boulder, CO: Westview Press.

May, R. (1972). *Power and innocence.* Stockholm, Sweden: Bonnier Fakta.

Miller, J., Leininger, M., Leuning, C., Pacquiao, D., Andrews, M., Ludwig-Beymer, P., & Papadopoulos, I. (2008). Transcultural Nursing Society position statement on human rights. *Journal of Transcultural Nursing, 19*(1), 5–7.

Moore, T. (1992). *Care of the soul* (1st ed.). New York: HarperCollins Publishers.

Ray, M. (1991). Caring inquiry: The esthetic process in the way of compassion. *Caring: The compassionate healer* (pp. 181–189). New York: National League for Nursing Press.

Ray, M. (1998). The interface of caring and technology: A new reflexive ethics in intermediate care. *Holistic Nursing Practice, 12*(4), 71–79.

Ray, M. (2007). Technological caring as a dynamic of complexity in nursing practice. In A. Barnard & R. Locsin (Eds.), *Technology and nursing: Practice, concepts and issues* (pp. 174–190). New York: Palgrave Macmillan.

Ray, M. (2013). Caring inquiry: The esthetic process in the way of compassion. In M. Smith, M. Turkel, & Z. Wolf (Eds.), *Caring in nursing classics: An essential resource.* New York: Springer Publishing Company.

Ray, M. (2015). Rootedness in holistic nursing: The ontologic mystery and structure of caring. *Beginnings, 35*(2), 12–14.

Ray, M. & Turkel, M. (2015). Marilyn Anne Ray's theory of bureaucratic caring. In M. Parker & M. Smith (Eds.). *Nursing theories and nursing practice* (4th ed.). Philadelphia: F. A. Davis Company.

Scanlan, M. (1974). *Inner healing.* New York: Paulist Press.

CHAPTER 25

The Political-Legal Culture of Multiculturalism and Interculturality: The Story of Canada

*T*he name Canada is from the Iroquois Natives, meaning *settlement*. From the period of 20,000 years ago, the Aboriginal or First People migrated followed by people of diverse cultures to the country of Canada and settled into communities and enclaves more than a 10-million square kilometer wide land mass. Widely diverse in climate and geography ranging from the 49th parallel (the border with the United States) to the far North, the Arctic Circle, Canada is divided into 10 provinces and three northern territories, with a most recent one chartered in 1999, Nunavut, for the Inuit (formerly Eskimo) people who call it "our land" (Davidhizar & Giger, 1998). With a population of more than 34 million (Statistics Canada), the first settler from Europe was John Cabot, an Italian in the service of the British arriving in Newfoundland in 1497, followed by French settlers who came to New France, now Quebec, in 1532. The land was taken for France by the French explorer Jacques Cartier in 1534 (Reidy & Taggart, 1998). After the British conquest of New France in 1763, Canada began to be more populated by people from England, Americans at the time of the Revolutionary War, followed by other Europeans, then Asians and others who shared different ways of life, kinship systems, religions, languages, politics, customs, in essence multiple diverse cultures, some universal values and behaviors, some very different (French & Emed, 2009; Leininger & McFarland, 2006). Both before and after Canadian Confederation of the provinces in 1867, there existed intercultural challenges between aboriginals, French Canadians, and "English" Canadians; the French Canadians, predominantly Francophone, mainly settled in the province of Quebec, and the Anglophone population settled from the Atlantic to the Pacific Oceans. When Canada was *implementing its democracy and throughout its history, it developed a relatively strong partnership with the United States, especially since the War of 1812 to 1814. The U.S.-Canadian border was established with the Anglo-American Convention of 1818 and the Oregon Treaty of 1846, and has been peaceful since that time despite different struggles or misunderstandings of immigration, trade, and security coming from both sides of the border.*

Canada now is considered a mosaic with racial and ethnic differences, a fact of modern society beginning with the long history of the struggle for recognition of French Canadian and Aboriginal identities to the political and legal recognition of all cultural groups immigrating to Canada. In 1971, Canada advanced the concept of multiculturalism (a term coined in Canada) into an official policy. It was the first country in the world to do so with The Multiculturalism Policy of Canada (1971), which gave recognition first to the idea of biculturalism, created by the government of Canada to honor equally both French and Anglo Canadians; second, to developing a new respect for the voice of Aboriginals and black Canadians; and third, to acknowledging the numbers of ethnically diverse people immigrating to Canada. After the enactment of The Canada Act and the Constitution Act of 1982 in which the new Canadian Charter of Rights and Freedoms was legislated, April 17, 1982 for all people of Canada, the late Prime Minister of Canada, Pierre Elliot Trudeau stated the following:

> *"It is my deepest hope that Canada will match its new legal maturity with that degree of political maturity which will allow us to make a total commitment to the Canadian ideal. I speak of a Canada where men and women of Aboriginal ancestry, of French and British heritage, of the diverse cultures of the world, demonstrate the will to share this land in peace, in justice, and with mutual respect"* (Select Remarks from the First Among Equals Speech at the Constitution of Canada Proclamation Ceremony, April, 17, 1982).

The commitment to biculturalism followed by multiculturalism prompted policy legislation, The Multiculturalism Act by the Government of Canada in 1987, and was adopted in 1988. Ministries of Multiculturalism have been established in all provinces. The spirit of multiculturalism continues to this day and has initiated what Taylor (1993) calls the "politics of recognition" where issues of identity and recognition are debated. Canada has been a model in seeking, understanding, and cocreating political recognition of diverse cultures based upon living history and human dignity, the most recent action after the election of Prime Minister Justin Trudeau on October 19, 2015, the resettlement of 25,000 Syrian refugees (McCray, 2015). Multiculturalism is about social justice, inclusiveness, and empowerment. "Multiculturalism [thus] is a relationship between Canada and the Canadian people." (Department of Canadian Heritage, 2009).

Seeking answers to questions of the moral ideal of relational diversity (hearing the voices of all peoples), equal recognition, tolerance, dialogue, and effective choice making within a democracy are ongoing. As a leader in the choice toward multicultural understanding, Canada is an example to other democracies that are challenged to embrace the reality of multiculturalism and beyond, the politics of recognition of individual cultural identities coexistent with nationhood, and anticipating the emergence of panethnicities and cultural pluralism in a globalizing world. On the other side of the border, while making progress to deal with the cultural diversity in the United States, the tragic events of September 11, 2001 challenged multicultural progress and facilitated marked mistrust and fear of what may happen when some groups bend toward political violence and religious radicalism. In Canada, ethical and legal inquiry into the questions of cultural identity and respect for equal recognition continues to be at the forefront of discourse. How diverse human beings maintain trust and respect for others is shaped by dialogue in a healthy democratic society (Taylor, 1993).

In Canada, there is "a willingness to weigh the importance of certain forms of uniform treatment against the importance of cultural survival and opt sometimes in favor of the latter . . . judgments in which the integrity of cultures has an important place" (Taylor, 1993, p. 61). Focusing on the preservation of cultures (multiculturalism) within a collective dialogical process is a form and process of cultural dynamics, moving toward a concept of interculturality or multiculturalism without culture (Phillips, 2007; and described in Chapter 4: Transcultural Context for Transcultural Nursing). Despite some rupture in the mosaic in recent years (Swan, 2007), the politics of equal respect foster appreciation, compassion, and important dialogue and evaluation within the law in an intercultural society. Most people recognize in the politics and ethics of recognition that as people learn together, they stay together through the struggles and challenges of communicating and cocreating a living history. This perspective also will be important to all societies and nations dealing with different cultural groups emerging all over the world. Transcultural nursing, with its focus on transcultural relationships, the dynamics of ethical and spiritual caring and cultural competence, and ethical accountability and responsibility, will be a main contributor in the public sphere (De Vries & Sullivan, 2006).

Michael's Story

Michael, a former politician in Canada, was a Member of Parliament (Provincial) (MPP) during the different phases of the development of multiculturalism and after the enactment of the Multicultural Act of 1987/1988 in Canada and during the movement toward interculturality/transculturality. He was first a high school teacher in a small community north of Lake Superior, then a lawyer in Windsor, Ontario practicing family law. Windsor borders Detroit, Michigan. The two cities have deep ties to each other, especially because of the shared business and challenges of the North American auto industry and the trade policies developed after the passage of the North American Free Trade Agreement (NAFTA, 1994, see SICE Trade Agreements). Michael loved his role as a politician. He loved to help people and met with many groups of citizens from different walks of life and different cultures. His constituency encompassed young and old, rich and poor, diverse cultural groups and seasoned Canadians, auto workers, health-care professionals and patients seeking health care, and legal and illegal immigrants. He said that he tried to see two sides of the story, even between the Jews and the Arabs, both having large populations in the city of Windsor. One thing that he knew was that one cultural group always had to give up something for the other and vice versa. No one group could have something at the expense of the other, part of the cultural balance and unity. It was an awesome job to him, one that often kept him up at night. Michael appreciated where he lived in Windsor, Ontario because of its close proximity to the United States, where he had many relatives and friends. He studied political science and economics prior to law school and had a good grasp of constitutional law in Canada and the United States.

In his political role, Michael had a keen interest in health care and the environment. In the Canadian health-care system, by 1961, all provinces in Canada had adopted a universal health-care system. In 1966, the federal government passed the Medical Care Act for a universal hospital insurance system supporting principles of portability, public administration, universality, comprehensiveness, and accessibility. Since 1971, in Canada, all Canadian citizens, regardless of income, employment, or health, have access to basic health care whether it is provided in a hospital, clinic, or home. The Canadian health-care system is a single-payer, nonprofit primary, secondary, and tertiary care delivery model with a focus on primary care, prevention, and health promotion. Physicians provide medical care on a "fee-for-service" basis but the bill is sent to the government (provincial) rather than hundreds of insurance companies. Today, to meet the health-care needs of the diverse citizenry of each province, the Canadian health-care system is decentralized to each of the 10 provinces and fiscally managed regionally with about 20% cost-sharing with the federal governments. Above the 60th parallel, in the circumpolar North, the Arctic region, the federal government continues to manage the system. The citizens, for the most part, are grateful for the universal health-care system, but budgets, costs, and quality of care often plague the system. Provincial governments initiate health-care reforms on a regular basis to deal with issues of longer wait times for surgery, the need for additional medical technologies, lack of hospital beds, nurse and specialty physician shortages, hospital- and nonhospital-induced infections, and overall quality-of-care issues. Cost control while still trying to maintain high standards of care is a major component of health-care reform (Canada Health Act, 1981, 1985). According to recent statistics, the Canadian universal plan is slightly over 10% of the gross domestic product (GDP) in comparison with the United States health-care system. Despite persistent issues related to cost, quality, and shortages, the principles of universality, portability, public administration, comprehensibility, and accessibility outlined in the federal Medical Care Act remain sacred to the citizens of Canada.

Michael worked on challenges of the day, multiculturalism and integration to balance diversity within a unity of purpose. He was successful in improving nursing home legislation and dealing with environmental challenges, especially in his legislative constituency.

Michael was faithful in working with the Michigan and Ontario Harbor Commission to improve the state of the Detroit River that fed into some of the Great Lakes. He maintained a working relationship with legislators in the state of Michigan. One thing that Michael reinforced was that "every political decision is a moral decision." A politician has a responsibility, not only in how to govern but also how to govern with a moral compass. Michael stated that the making of political decisions always had to be tempered with ethical appraisals, "what is the right thing to do" when evaluating two sides for competing needs and desires of diverse citizens. His goal was fairness in all transactions.

After public life, Michael continued to work in family law in the provincial government as a director to evaluate fathers who were not supporting their children financially (colloquially, dealing with "deadbeat dads"). After retirement, he then chose to become involved in health care once again by participation as a board chairperson of a major hospital in his city. In this role, Michael uses his political skills of presenting proposals, ethical evaluation, negotiation, compromise, and participatory decision making. Participating with the chief executive office, he has sought out medical, nursing, and administrative consultants and the views of board members so as to provide the best knowledge and information for dealing with health-care problems in the Canadian health-care and the hospital systems. His major responsibilities as a coparticipant with other professionals include: working with a major university educating nurses and other professionals, and meeting the cultural health-care needs of citizens. Other responsibilities entail: running an efficient and effective hospital, economic/fiscal leadership and management, professional and patient relationships, inpatient care, end-of-life (palliative) care, multicultural health-care delivery, primary and urgent/emergency care in the emergency department, implementation of a rape center, 16-hour or better technological use of x-ray, computed tomography (CT), and magnetic resonance imaging (MRI) equipment, the electronic health record, technological improvements, potentially seeking magnet status (i.e., excellence in nursing and hospital care), nursing clinical placements, local clinical placements for education of physicians, and the planning of a new medical school at the city university. One of the interesting developments that Michael has initiated is working with universities, health sciences centers, and hospitals in Ontario and Michigan. Michigan health sciences need additional clinical space for the education of physicians, thus, they are engaging in care in the Canadian hospital. Also, Michael is working with professionals to determine if and when patients who need specialized care can receive it in Michigan hospitals. This initiative is not only a clinical improvement measure in the provision of care and dealing with wait times in the Canadian health-care system, but also an economic measure whereby patients, rather than having to be flown to specialty centers in Toronto, for example, can be taken by ambulance 5 miles over the border for care. The sharing of professional, educational, research, and economic resources on the part of Canada and the United States illuminates the commitment that professionals of both countries have to multicultural and multinational friendship and cooperation in health care, education, policies, and the law.

Transcultural Caring-Based Learning Approach

Please review the information about the Transcultural Caring Dynamics for Nursing and Health-Care Theory and Model, the assessment tools, the transcultural caring-based learning (TCCBL) approach, and the transcultural caring inquiry information and any other relevant literary and Internet information before dialoguing about this transcultural caring experience. In your small group, apply the TCCBL approach in relation to your transcultural caring situation for pattern identification (i.e., pattern seeing, pattern mapping, pattern recognizing, and pattern transforming). Use dimensions of the Transcultural Caring Dynamics in Nursing and Health-Care Model and use the most appropriate assessment tools for transcultural evidence gathering of what is happening in multiculturalism, binationalism, and universal health care in Canada.

Reflections with Questions

Reflect on the story of Michael and what he has done and is doing to improve health care, nursing care, and medical education using his past experience as a lawyer and legal educator. The story of Michael illuminates a life of service to his country, to the principles of multiculturalism to the Canadian health-care principles, and to a continuing partnership with professionals in Canada and the United States. Michael believes that the "politics of identity and recognition" need to be constantly at work so that as the world shrinks, people can count on politicians and people in leadership roles to make ethical decisions and practice the meaning of "intellectual charity" (Pope Benedict XVI, 2008).

Focus attention on two elements in these stories: (1) settlement and the advance of migration, biculturalism, and multiculturalism in Canada, and (2) the story of Michael and his commitment to public service, multiculturalism, and then initiating partnership with the state of Michigan and city of Detroit for improved education and health-care delivery.

Transcultural Nursing Reflections

- Examine what it means to be multicultural. Examine how laws can facilitate multicultural developments. Examine the need for public discourse, ethical questions, and analysis.
- What does it mean to institute a health-care system that cares for its citizens without reference to pre-existing conditions and tries to provide a high standard of care—despite problems of cost controls—to meet the health-care needs of all citizens? Compare and contrast the Canadian Health Care System with the new Patient Protection and Affordable Care Act (PPACA) in the United States.
- What are your responsibilities as a transcultural nurse in understanding multiculturalism, the politics of recognition, and working toward improving the health-care system of one's country?
- Consider the Canadian example of multiculturalism and yourself as a political assistant to a politician who is dealing with multicultural and multinational issues. How do you define multiculturalism? What do you think about resettlement increases of African and Middle Eastern refugees in North America? Are there concerns between the United States and Canada?
- What is public service to you? What is a critical communicative spiritual-ethical caring; critical social theory (for example, Sumner's theory of communicative caring action)? What is the U.S. philosophy of global communicative action? How does it fit into the meaning of social justice to you? Is social justice a part of caring in nursing? How would you be challenged with multicultural issues where there is a movement toward appreciation and compassion for cultural diversity rather than "a melting-pot" view? How would you handle what could be perceived as racism or prejudice? How would you deal with the culturally dynamic paradox of the politics of identity, the politics of recognition (the multicultural mosaic), and the politics of the melting pot? Is there a breach of a harmonious relationship in the multicultural mosaic in Canada?

- What is "compassion fatigue" toward immigrants and immigration?
- What would you do if there are requests or demands for recognition while at the same time there is a demand to maintain the status quo? Are you familiar with the Constitution and rules of law in your country? What laws govern cultural diversity? How are immigration issues being addressed in your country? How do they compare with other nations, especially in the Western Hemisphere? How would you encourage dialogue? How would you gather data to present to groups of people who all *want* something different? What do shared ethics (communitarian ethics) mean to you? What do you think the economics would dictate? Do you think compromise is a bad thing? How would you argue or agree to balance diversity with unity?
- How do you think the issues associated with multiculturalism and transculturality/interculturality will evolve in the United States?
- Consider the issue of language or language preference. What does language diversity mean? What does Anglophone, English only, bilingualism, or allophonic mean to you? Do you think that English literacy is necessary in a North American multicultural society? Should there be a single language in a country? What is/are the language(s) of diplomacy, the language(s) of the United Nations?
- How would you incorporate into your lexicon the different voices and understandings of the past history of your country of place or community, such as constitutional documents, legislation regarding policies on Native and Aboriginal rights, slavery, human rights, civil rights, the stories of war, bombings, and the Jewish Holocaust during World War II, the Palestinian issue, and so forth?
- What is your view of healing past injustices? How could this type of reconciliation happen? How would you teach if you were a professional, parent, or teacher about what should be said in the wake of prejudice and discrimination? What type of multicultural education is appropriate at the elementary, high school, and college levels? Can the Holocaust, Rwanda, or Darfur, or even police brutality or sectarian hostilities, be used as examples of prejudice in the local and world communities? What is the state of affairs regarding Islamic terrorism in Nigeria? How do you think one maintains respect when teaching about issues of prejudice and extermination of some groups of people? What progress has been made in Europe and around the world regarding human rights and dealing with living memories, past hurts, and hope in the future? Compare and contrast the state of or patterns of migration in the Middle East and Europe with the migratory patterning in the United States, especially from Mexico and Central America.
- Do you think that social justice is a health issue? What are our national, international, and global responsibilities as transcultural nurses in a globalizing world? Choose *some* of the following countries to compare and contrast multicultural differences and policies, such as, the United States, Canada, Australia, the United Kingdom, Europe, and South Africa and other African countries. What about Central, South American, and Caribbean countries? Reflect on the Asian countries, such as Japan, China, Korea, Taiwan, Philippines, Thailand, Indonesia, and so forth.
- Consider yourself as a staff nurse in a hospital where new organizational ideas for the future of nursing care and health-care delivery are being discussed. What leadership role should you take as a staff nurse, as a transcultural caring nurse? What does it mean to participate with others in the debate about patient and professional care and costs, technology, and new developments in hospitals and community health centers?
- What is your life's purpose in nursing? What is your role as a transcultural caring nurse? How would you encourage compassionate spiritual-ethical caring and justice in your hospital or health-care clinic, or public health department? How would you teach about cultural understanding and competence in nursing—to your colleagues, to an organization, and to the public? What is your role in the global health-care arena?

- What new ideas do you have as you contemplate nursing and health care, and health-care systems? What would you think about having a nursing program dedicated to graduate study in Foresight (Futures Studies) toward coming to understand the world that is culturally dynamic, practical, and empowering? How do nursing programs engage in international relations, education, research, and practice? What would you do to improve the practice of caring in nursing? Compare and contrast two or more health-care systems in different countries according to the principles that Canada has defined: universality, comprehensibility, portability, public administration, and accessibility. How does the Canadian health-care policy compare with the other countries of the Commonwealth of Nations and the United States? Are there other concepts that should be added given your own views of health-care systems or what have been defined in your own country? Do you think that you could begin to draft a health-care system or improve the health-care system that you are currently experiencing in your own country? How do you think citizens should pay for a health-care system?
- What is a system (bureaucracy/organization)? How can systems maintain quality of care when they are dynamic, culturally diverse, and bureaucratic? Are there issues of workplace violence, bullying, or discrimination in the workplace because of cultural diversity of the staff? What is the meaning of human rights, social justice, and social suffering in the health-care system or in a hospital system? How does Ray's Theory of Bureaucratic Caring help to understand and reconcile human caring and ethical-spiritual dimensionss in bureaucratic systems (socio-cultural, political, economic, technological, and legal dimensions), such as hospitals, educational facilities, Veterans' Administration, the military organizations, and so forth? What do human rights and social justice mean in hospital systems (See Ray and Turkel, 2014).
- Focus on the environment. Why is the environment, including the air and water, a public health issue? What international principles, laws, or agreements are in place to protect the environment, and the animals and other creatures that inhabit the earth? What is the role of the United Nations in environmental protection? What does sustainability mean? Identify the principles of the U.N. Decade of Education for Sustainable Development (DESD). What is the Kyoto Protocol? What has the United Nations Climate Change Summit in Paris 2015 achieved? Is the agreement still in effect? Are views changing about environmental protection around the world? What is the state of "water" in the world, the lakes, rivers, oceans, and the access to clean drinking water for the citizens of the world? What is the state of sanitation in different countries, especially in developing countries? What are the role of politicians and the World Health Organization and the United Nations in those enterprises? What could be the role for nurses, especially transcultural nurses?

Select Bibliography

Canada Health Act R.S.C., c.c.-6 (1984, 1985; Current version in force since April 1, 1999). Retrieved July 21, 2009, from http://www.canlii.org/en/ca/laws/stat/rsc-1985-c-c-6/latest

Canadian multiculturalism: An inclusive citizenship. (1971). Government of Canada. Retrieved July 21, 2009, from http://www.cic.gc.ca/multi/inclusv-eng.asp

Coffman, S. (2014). Marilyn Anne Ray: The theory of bureaucratic caring. In M. Alligood (Ed.), *Nursing theorists and their work* (8th ed.). St Louis: Mosby.

Davidhizar, R., & Giger, J. (Eds.). (1998). *Canadian transcultural nursing.* St. Louis: Mosby.

Department of Canadian Heritage. (2009). *Cultural Diversity: A Canadian perspective.* Retrieved July 21, 2009, from http://www.pch.gc.ca/index-eng.cfm

De Vries, H., & Sullivan, L. (2006). *Political theologies: Public religions in a post-secular world.* New York: Fordham University Press.

French, S., & Emed, J. (2009). Nursing in Canada. In K. Breda (Ed.), Nursing and globalization in the Americas: A critical perspective. Amityville, NY: Baywood Publishing Company, Inc.

Gunew, S. (2008). *Multicultural differences: Canada, USA, Australia.* Retrieved April, 24, 2008, from http://faculty.srts.ubc.ca/sgunew/MCMULTI.HTM

Gutmann, A. (Ed.). (1993). *Multiculturalism: Examining the politics of recognition*. Princeton: Princeton University Press.

Kyoto Protocol. Retrieved April, 24, 2008, from http://www.Canadaonline.about.com/od/environment/i/kyotoprotocol.htm

Leininger, M., & McFarland, M. (Eds.). (2006). *Culture care diversity and universality: A worldwide theory of nursing* (2nd ed.). Sudbury, MA: Jones and Bartlett.

McCray R. (October 20, 2015). Canada's new prime minister to open doors for Syrian refugees. http://www.takepart.com/article/2015/10/20/trudeau-refugees.

Phillips, A. (2007). *Multiculturalism without culture*. Princeton: Princeton University Press.

Policy and Legislation Concerning Multiculturalism. (1971). Retrieved July 21, 2009, from http://cic.gc.ca/multi/pol/framework-eng.asp

Pope Benedict XVI. (2008). [Text of Pope Benedict XVI's talk with Catholic educators.] Retrieved April 26, 2008 from http://www.thefloridacatholic.org/pope_usa/pope_articles/20080417-daily-educators-

Postero, N. (2007). *Now we are citizens*. Stanford: Stanford University Press.

Ray, M. (2010). Creating caring organizations and cultures through communitarian ethics. *Journal of the World Universities Forum, 3*(5), 41–52.

Ray, M., & Turkel, M. (2014). Caring as emancipatory nursing praxis: The theory of Relational Caring Complexity. *Advances in Nursing Science, 37*(2), 132–146.

Ray, M., & Turkel, M. (2015). The theory of bureaucratic caring. In M. Parker & M. Smith (Eds.), *Nursing theories & nursing practice* (4th ed.). Philadelphia: F. A. Davis Company.

Reidy, M., & Taggart, M. (1998). French Canadians of Quebec origin. In R. Davidhizar & J. Giger (Eds.), *Canadian transcultural nursing* (pp. 155–178). St Louis: Mosby.

Reitz, J., & Breton, R. (1994). *The illusion of difference: Realities of ethnicity in Canada and the United States*. Toronto: CD Howe Institute.

Remarks [Select] by Prime Minister Pierre Elliot Trudeau, "First Among Equals" speech at the Proclamation Ceremony, April 17, 1982 [The Constitution of Canada]. Retrieved July 21, 2009, from http://www.collectionscanada.gc.ca/primeministers/h4-4024-e.html

Robinson, A. (2007). *Multiculturalism and the foundations of meaningful life*. Vancouver, BC: UBC Press.

SICE (Foreign Trade Information System of the Organization of American States). Trade Agreements: *North American Free Trade Agreement*. Retrieved July 21, 2009, from http://www.sice.org.oas.nafta/naftatce.asp

Statistics Canada: Canada's National Statistical Agency, Retrieved July 21, 2009, from http://www.statcan.gc.ca/start-debut.eng.html

Stein, J., Robertson, D., Cameron, J., Kymlicka, W., Meisei, J., Haroon, S., & Valpy, M. (2007). *Uneasy partners: Multiculturalism and rights in Canada*. Ottawa: Wilfrid Laurier University Press.

Sumner, J. (2008). *The moral construct of caring in nursing as communicative action*. Saarbrücken, Germany: VDM Verlag Dr. Müller.

Swan, M. (2007). *The rupture of Canada's multicultural mosaic*. Retrieved July 21, 2009, from http://www.catholicregister.org/content/view/1103/858/-38k

Taylor, C. (1993). *The politics of recognition*. In A. Gutmann (Ed.), Multiculturalism (pp. 25–73). Princeton: Princeton University Press.

University of Houston/Technology/Master of Science in Foresight. http://www.uh.edu/technology/programs/graduate/foresight/

Walcott, R. (2000). *Black like who: Writing black Canada* (2nd ed.). Toronto: Insomniac Press.

World Futures Society. Retrieved from www.wfs.org/futurist update.htm

CHAPTER 26

Transcultural Nursing and Ethnonursing for Japanese Graduate Students at Red Cross College of Nursing, Toyko, Japan

*T*he following is a description of the historical evolution of nursing education in Japan (see graphs in Box 26-1) and the initiation of the discipline of transcultural nursing founded by the late Dr. Madeleine Leininger into Japanese nursing. Dr. Leininger claimed "caring as the essence of nursing" in 1977. She not only originated the Transcultural Nursing Society but also established the International Association for Human Caring. Leininger's earliest research on caring and culture emerged when she studied anthropology for her Doctor *of Philosophy degree revealing the caring knowledge and practices of the Gadsup people of the Eastern Highlands of New Guinea in the late 1950s. In conjunction with the development of transcultural nursing disciplinary knowledge, Leininger created the Ethnonursing Qualitative Research Methodology to study human caring in diverse cultures. Leininger's theory Culture Care Diversity and Universality: A Worldwide Theory of Nursing was translated into Japanese by the author of this chapter, Dr. Mayumi Tsutsui (see Figures 26-1 and 26-2), dean of the Graduate School of Japanese Red Cross College of Nursing, Tokyo, Japan, and is used extensively in Japanese colleges of nursing. Using the ethnonursing method, 50 theses in Japanese nursing have been written (see titles in Box 26-2). In 2014, in Kyoto, Japanese scholars coordinated by Drs. Naohiro Hohashi and Junko Honda (see Figures 26-3 and 26-4) and Marian Turkel and others in the United States hosted the 35th International Association for Human Caring Conference, "The Universality of Caring," and a Special Interest Group on Transcultural Nursing and Caring honoring the legacy of Dr. Leininger, the "mother" of transcultural nursing in Japan. Dr. Leininger led the way for additional culture theories to be implemented in Japan, such as the Theory of Bureaucratic Caring (2013) of Marilyn Ray and the Transcultural Caring Dynamics in Nursing and Health-Care Theory and Model created in the first edition of this book (Ray, 2010). Photos of Dr. Honda and her family along with other members of Kobe University and their families can be seen in Figures 26-5 to 26-16.*

Education of Master's Students for Qualitative Research

In the first year of the Master's program, students take classes in Nursing Research Methods, including quantitative and qualitative research. Eight classes in qualitative research are taken, including Ethnographic Research, Ethnonursing, Grounded Theory Research, Phenomenological Research, Narrative Research, and Action Research. Students in International/Disaster Nursing, Child and Family Nursing, and Psychiatric Mental Health Nursing most commonly pursue ethnographic research and ethnonursing.

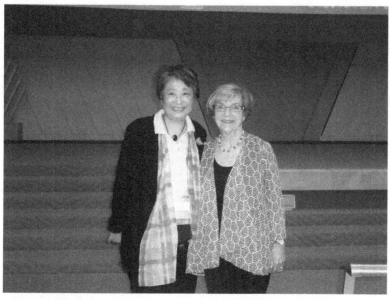

Figure 26–1: Drs. Mayumi Tsutsui, Dean and Professor, Red Cross University, College of Nursing, Tokyo, and Marilyn Ray, Professor Emeritus, Florida Atlantic University.

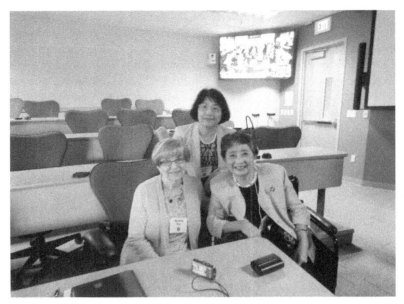

Figure 26–2: Left to right, Dr. Marilyn Ray; Dr. Fusako Sato, Professor Emeritus, Aichi University; and Dr. MaymeTsutsu in Kyoto, Japan.

Figure 26–3: From left to right, Dr. Junko Honda, University of Kobe, Japan; Dr. Marilyn Ray; and Dr. Naohiro Hohashi, University of Kobe, Japan, at the Award Ceremony of the Transcultural Nursing Society Scholars where Dr. Hohashi was awarded Transcultural Nursing Scholar, October 2014. *Photo courtesy of Dr. Junko Honda.*

Figure 26–4: Dr. Naohiro Hohashi, Satoshi Takatani, Miyuki Ono, Yuko Hiratani, and Dr. Marilyn Ray teaching via Skype (in background) to students and Dr. Junko Honda at Kobe University, Japan. *Photo courtesy of Dr. Junko Honda.*

Figure 26–5: Miyuki Ono, Yuko Hiratani, Satoshi Takatani, Dr. Junko Honda, Dr. Naohiro Hohashi, and Dr. Marilyn Ray, teaching via Skype (in background) at Kobe University, Japan. *Photo courtesy of Dr. Junko Honda.*

Japanese Red Cross College of Nursing

Nursing education started at the Japanese Red Cross Hospital in 1890. The Japanese Red Cross Practical College of Nursing was established in 1946, and the Japanese Red Cross Junior College was established in 1954. In 1986, a 4-year curriculum was established at the Japanese Red Cross College. The Master's program was developed in 1993, followed by the Doctoral program in 1995. Master's program courses are offered in Fundamentals of Nursing Science, Child and Family Nursing, Adult Health Nursing, Gerontological Nursing, Psychiatric Mental Health Nursing, Community Health Nursing, Nursing Education, Nursing Management, International/Disaster Nursing, Cancer Nursing, Chronic Care Nursing, Critical Care Nursing, and International Health and Midwifery.

In 2013, 87 students were enrolled in the Master's program, and 23 were enrolled in the Doctoral program. As of 2012, 436 people had completed the Master's program, and 57 had completed the Doctoral program.

For additional information on nursing in Japan, see Box 26-1.

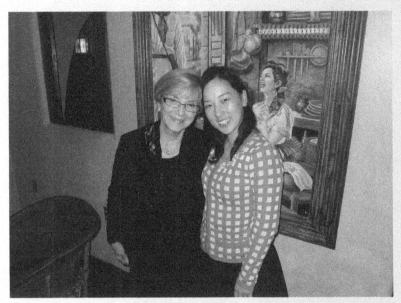

Figure 26–6: Drs. Marilyn Ray and Junko Honda at Transcultural Nursing Society Conference, October 2014. *Photo courtesy of Dr. Junko Honda.*

BOX 26–1 ❖ Nursing Education in Japan

The following are excerpts from the Japanese Nursing Association leaflet, "Nursing in Japan" (2011) (http://www.nurse.or.jp/jna/english/nursing/).

1. Basic Nursing Education
There are several courses of basic nursing education in Japan. In the main courses, basic nursing education is provided at 4-year colleges/universities, 3-year junior colleges, or 3-year training schools after graduation from high school to take a national examination to obtain the national license.

Main Basic Nursing Education Courses
1. Nursing university/colleges provide public health nursing course or midwifery course in 4-year education; graduates could get qualification to sit for national examination for public health nurse or midwife in addition to nurse.
2. To obtain public health nursing/midwifery license, it is required to hold a nursing license.
3. Assistant nurse courses are omitted.

BOX 26–1 ❖ **Nursing Education in Japan**

2. Development of University Nursing Education

The first nursing university was inaugurated in 1952. There were just 11 nursing colleges/universities until 1992, when they sharply increased with flexible curriculum organization in accordance with the university establishment standards outlined in 1991 and basic principles concerning nursing college/university establishment prescribed in the Act on Assurance of Work Forces of Nurses and Other Medical Experts, enacted in 1992. In addition, lower birth rates and increasing rates of students advancing to college or university encourage schools to launch training for nursing personnel in high social demand from the perspective of ensuring students. As a result, nursing colleges/universities numbered 193 as of 2010, and Master's programs are provided at 121 graduate schools, and doctoral programs are provided at 61 graduate schools.

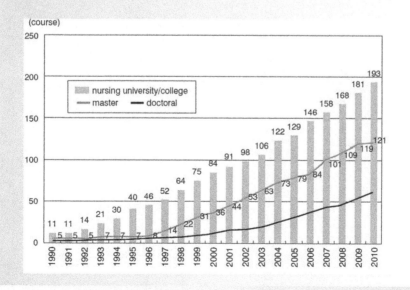

> ### BOX 26–1 ❖ Nursing Education in Japan—cont'd
>
> #### 3. Employment Status of Nursing Personnel
> The demand for nursing personnel is exceeding the supply because of advanced health care and an increasingly severely ill and aging population. Japan has been experiencing a chronic shortage of nurses in terms of both quality and quantity. Approximately 60% of nursing personnel work at hospitals. However, the ratio has decreased year after year, which shows the diversification of nurses' workplaces.
>
> #### Reference
> Ministry of Education, Culture, Sports, Science and Technology.
>
> Statistical Data on Nursing. (2010). Tokyo: Japanese Nursing Association Publishing Company.
>
> Service in Japan. (2009). Tokyo: Japanese Nursing Association Publishing Company.
>
> Nursing in Japan. (2011). Tokyo: Japanese Nursing Association.

Students who studied ethnonursing and used it later as a research method in their thesis are limited (as of 2014) to students in the Child and Family Nursing course that I teach as a professor. The reason for that is given later on.

DR. MADELEINE LEININGER AND MASTER'S STUDENTS' THESES

In 1993, undergraduate students in International Nursing had a study tour to Wayne State University in Detroit, Michigan, where the late Dr. Madeleine Leininger, the founder of transcultural nursing and the ethnonursing methodology was a professor. They listened to a

Figure 26–7: Dr. Junko Honda and her grandfather. *Photo courtesy of Dr. Junko Honda.*

Figure 26–8: Dr. Junko Honda's grandparents. *Photo courtesy of Dr. Junko Honda.*

lecture in transcultural nursing by Dr. Leininger. This encounter led to my joining a team of four people to translate her book into Japanese, *Culture Care Diversity and Universality: A Theory of Nursing*, published by the National League for Nursing Press, New York, in 1991. The Japanese-language version was published in 1995 by Igaku-Shoin Ltd.

The student who enrolled in the school's first Master's program in 1993 (the inaugural class) in the Child and Family Nursing course used ethnonursing and completed her Master's degree in March 1995. Another student in the 1994 (second) class in the Child and Family Nursing course also used ethnonursing. Dr. Leininger came to Japan in August 1995; at Igaku-Shoin, the company that published her book, she gave guidance directly to the student who had enrolled in 1993 and had completed her thesis based on ethnonursing and to the student who had enrolled in 1994 and who was still working on her thesis. In 1997, their theses were published by Igaku-Shoin in the journal *Nursing Research.*

Later I continued to receive guidance from Dr. Leininger by letter. I also had the opportunity to receive her guidance directly at conferences in the United States. In a letter from 2002, Dr. Leininger wrote: "I first want to congratulate you and your students for using the theory and method, which is most encouraging. I am glad it has become most meaningful and relevant to you during the past decades."

After receiving this letter, I felt that I no longer needed guidance from Dr. Leininger. In her letter, Dr. Leininger recommended that I translate into Japanese *Transcultural Nursing: Concepts, Theories, Research and Practice* (2002), but I became busy and was unable to do so.

TITLES OF MASTER'S STUDENTS' THESES

Almost 60 students in the Master's program have completed the Child and Family Nursing course at the present time, with close to 50 using ethnonursing for their thesis. At present, five students are working on their thesis. Titles of Master's students' theses as of the end of the last academic year are listed in Box 26-2.

In the Child and Family Nursing course, informants include children, families, nurses, and others. Because children have not yet developed extensive language capabilities, it is important to observe them closely in the field. It is also important to understand the environment and culture that children are in, so using ethnonursing as a research method is appropriate for the Master's program students.

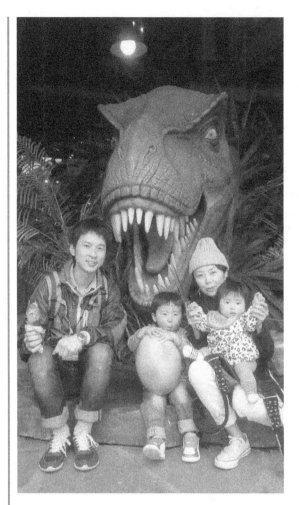

Figure 26–9: Dr. Junko Honda's brother, Masatoshi Ohta, with his wife, Satoko, and their children, Yusuke and Shiho. *Photo courtesy of Dr. Junko Honda.*

Figure 26–10: The Ohta family. *Photo courtesy of Dr. Junko Honda.*

BOX 26-2 ❖ Titles of Master Students' Theses

"Feelings of Mothers Who Are Accompanying Hospitalized Children"

"Consideration for the Experiences of Children With Congenital Heart Disease"

"State of Late-Stage Preschoolers Following Minor Surgery"

"Position of Nurses in Relations With Mothers of Hospitalized Children"

"Response of Preschoolers With Movement Restrictions Following Surgery"

"Approach of Preschoolers Receiving Painful Medical Procedures"

"Experiences of Hospitalized School-Age Children With Restricted Physical Activity"

"Response Toward Meals of Preschoolers With Gastrointestinal Disease Obliged to Fast"

"Feelings of Nurses Caring for School-Age Children Experiencing Nausea and Vomiting Associated With Chemotherapy"

"Response of Children in Late-Stage Preschoolers Repeatedly Experiencing the Discharge of Other Infants From the Hospital"

"Involvement of Nurses With Fathers of Children Hospitalized in the NICU"

"Care of Nurses for Children With Progressive Muscular Dystrophy"

"Difficulties Faced by Nurses Working in Mixed Wards of Adults and Children"

"Experiences of School-Age Children With Pain Following Adenoidectomy and Tonsillectomy"

"Experiences of Mothers With Infants Transferred to the Pediatric Ward From the NICU"

"Complicated Feelings of Nurses Working in the Pediatric Intensive Care Unit (PICU)"

"Involvement of Nurses With Children Who Have Extremely Severe Disabilities and Are Virtually Non-responsive"

"Various Aspects in the Care of Nurses for Preschoolers Who Were Immediately Hospitalized"

"Experience of Parents Who Are at Home With Their Child Up Until the Radical Surgery After the Creation of an Artificial Anus"

"Behavior of Preschoolers Toward the Unfamiliar Environment of the Pediatric Ward"

"Experience of Nurses Transferred to a Pediatric Ward"

"Involvement of Nurses Given to Infants and Preschoolers and Their Parents in the Emergency Outpatient Waiting Room of an Emergency Medical Service Secondary-Care Facility"

"Behavior of Taking Medicine by Hospitalized Late-Stage Preschoolers"

"Experience of Preschoolers Receiving Radiographic Imaging Examination During Hospital Stay"

"Care of Nurses for Short-Term Hospitalized Children and Their Families in Pediatric Ward of Community Hospital"

"Nurse Involvement With Long-Term Hospitalized Children Receiving Frequent Medical Care in One Room of Acute-Stage Pediatric Ward"

"Things Adolescents Hospitalized in a Pediatric Ward Want From Nurses"

"Experience of Breathing Difficulty in School-Age Children With Bronchial Asthma"

Continued

BOX 26–2 ❖ Titles of Master Students' Theses—cont'd

"Outpatient Nurse and Ward Nurse Care Related to Infants and Preschoolers Hospitalized on Day of Outpatient Visit"

"Experiences of School-Age Children Required to Rest in Bed in Short-Term Hospitalization"

"Nurse Involvement With Mothers of Short-Term Hospitalized Infants and Preschoolers"

"Nurse Care for Children Who Have a Childhood Neoplastic Disorder and Their Families"

"Care of Nurses for Crying Toddlers in Short-Term Hospitalization"

"Decision of Nurses on Clinical Condition in the Holding of Infants and Preschoolers With Congenital Heart Disease and Aspects Thereof"

"Care of Nurses for Short-Term Hospitalized Preschoolers Receiving Oxygen for Respiratory Symptoms"

"Nurse-Based Confirmation of the Condition of Infants With Severe Motor and Intellectual Disabilities in At-Home Respite Care"

"Involvement of Nurses in the Feeding of Short-Term Hospitalized Toddlers With Respiratory Disease"

"Involvement of Nurses in the Activities of Daily Living of School-Age and Adolescent Children With Cerebral Palsy"

"Nurses' Awareness of the Vital Sign Values of and Care for Children With Severe Motor and Intellectual Disabilities Hospitalized in a Pediatric Ward"

"Care of Nurses With School-Age Children Who Have Developmental Disorders and Cannot Be Mentally and Physically Left Alone"

"Care of Nurses for Adolescents Hospitalized for Inflammatory Bowel Disease"

"Care of Nurses for Preschool Children Who Have Food Allergies Who Undergo the Food Challenge as Day Cases and Their Families"

Figure 26–11: Masatoshi and Satoko Ohta and family members. *Photo courtesy of Dr. Junko Honda.*

Figure 26–12: Dr. Junko Honda with the Ohtas. *Photo courtesy of Dr. Junko Honda.*

POST-MASTER'S STUDENTS

At the present time, 15 students who have completed the Master's program are actively working in the field as clinical nurse specialists, whereas others are working as generalists, administrators, or faculty members. Ethnonursing has taught these individuals many things that help them to understand and support children, families, and medical staff.

Figure 26–13: Masatoshi and Satoko Ohta. *Photo courtesy of Dr. Junko Honda.*

I am grateful that I was able to learn ethnonursing through Dr. Leininger's kind support. Although I regret that I was unable to translate the book as she had asked, I feel that the students who received Dr. Leininger's guidance are working hard to improve the health of children and their families. In addition, Dr. Leininger's ideas are being communicated in Japan through individuals who learned ethnonursing as a research method in the Master's program.

Figure 26–14: Yasuyo Nishimoto, Associate Professor at Kobe University, and Hiroshige Nishimoto and their children, Rin and Ryunosuke. *Photo courtesy of Yasuyo Nishimoto.*

Figure 26–15: Hiroshige, Rin, and Ryunosuke Nishimoto. *Photo courtesy of Yasuyo Nishimoto.*

Figure 26–16: Hiroshige, Rin, and Ryunosuke Nishimoto. *Photo courtesy of Yasuyo Nishimoto.*

References

Honda, J., Ray, M. & Hohashi, N. (2013). Ray's theory of bureaucratic caring and nursing organization management. *Health Care, 55*(12), 819–825.

Imai, M. (1997). Kodomono nyuinni tukisou hahaoyani kansuru kenkyu. *Kangokenkyu, 30*(2), 119–131.

Leininger, M. (1977). The phenomenon of caring: Caring, the essence and central focus of nursing. *American Nurses' Foundation*, March 2 and 14, 1977.

Leininger, M. M. (1991). *Culture care diversity and university: A theory of nursing.* New York: National League for Nursing Press.

Leininger, M. M. (1991), in Inaoka, F. (1997). *Reininga-kangoron.* Tokyo: Igaku-Shoin.

Leininger, M.M. (1997), in Tsutsui, M. (1997). Reininga-kangoron to kenkyu houhou. *Kangokenkyu, 30*(2), 93–105.

Leininger, M. (2002). *Transcultural nursing: Concepts, theories, research and practice* (3rd ed.). New York, NY: McGraw-Hill Inc.

Masumori, K. (1997). Senten seishin shikkan no kodomono taiken ni kansuru kenkyu. *Kangokenkyu, 30*(3), 233–244.

Ray, M. (2010). *Transcultural caring dynamics in nursing and health care.* Philadelphia: F. A. Davis Company.

CHAPTER 27

Transcultural Caring for Buddhists and Muslims in Thailand

*T*hailand is located in Southeast Asia and is known as "a land of smiles," which represents the friendliness of Thai people. The total population in Thailand in 2013 was 64,621,302 (Ministry of Public Health, 2013). Buddhism is the official religion of Thailand, and Islam is the next largest religion. Most Thai people are Buddhists (94.6%), followed by Muslims (4.6%), and Christians (0.7%) (National Statistic Organization, Ministry of Information and Communication Technology, 2011). Thailand has five regions—central, north, north east, east, and south—each of which has a unique culture. Religion and culture strongly influence the beliefs of Thai people in regard to living and dying and have a relationship to their health behaviors. Nursing has an impact on a person's health from birth until death. Understanding the religious or spiritual and cultural beliefs of persons being nursed is necessary to deliver appropriate nursing interventions to improve their health status and promote a peaceful death. This chapter presents the experiences of transcultural caring for Buddhists and Muslims in Thailand. This chapter comprises two stories. The first is about spiritual and cultural beliefs influencing the well-being of Thai Buddhists. The second story reveals the belief of some Thai Muslims that health conditions are destined by God.

342

Spiritual and Cultural Beliefs Influencing Thai Buddhists' Well-Being

The following story of the author's experience in nursing practice in a hospital in the south of Thailand is an exemplar of Thai Buddhists' spiritual and cultural beliefs as related to illness and wellness.

Thongkam's Story

Thongkam was an 80-year-old Buddhist man. He was admitted to the hospital with an infected diabetic foot that had turned to sepsis. At home, Thongkam used some herbals to control his blood sugar and treat his foot ulcer himself with knowledge that was transferred from his ancestors. He denied taking medicines prescribed by the physician. Thongkam had a strong belief in Buddhism and practiced chanting and meditation every night. However, he could not manage his food intake and blood sugar or take care of his personal hygiene well because of his old age.

During his hospital stay, Thongkam was conscious. His left foot ulcer was severely inflamed, pus-filled, and caused him severe pain. His temperature was 38°C. He received antibiotic injections and pain relief medication. His infected wound was cleaned twice a day. Thongkam could not eat well or sleep well. He was restless with a high respiratory rate and high pulse rate at night. The doctor thought that Thongkam had delirium or acute confusion from his old age and side effects of some medicines. However, Thongkam's family believed that spirits of the dead patients in the hospital ward made him fearful and unable to sleep. The family went to the temple. They asked the monk to give a "holy thread" to be worn on Thongkam's arm (Figure 27-1). A holy thread is made of white or other color thread that has been blessed in a ritual performed by the respected Buddhist monks; it is believed that the holy thread will protect the patient

Figure 27–1: Holy thread on the patient's arm. *Photo courtesy of Supattra Uppanisakorn.*

from the bad souls or ghosts that would do harm to the patient and take the patient's soul out of his/her body. Thongkam's family also put a small image of Buddha/respected Buddhist monk/"talisman" (Figure 27-2) on Thongkam's pillow. Commonly in Thai hospitals, Thai Buddhists will put a small image of Buddha/respected Buddhist monk/talisman on the patient's pillow or on the patient's bed. It is believed that the spiritual power of these sacred images will protect the patient from the souls of dead persons or ghosts on the ward. Thongkam's family believed that the holy thread and Buddha image/talisman had spiritual power and could protect Thongkam from the bad souls or ghosts that might do harm and cause him to die.

Figure 27–2: Small Buddha image/Buddhist monk image/talisman in a bag. *Photo courtesy of Supattra Uppanisakorn.*

It is common in Thai hospitals to promote spiritual and cultural care. Most ward units arrange the shelf (Figure 27-3), and some units dedicate a small area (Figure 27-4) to respected Buddhist monk images for patients and families to pray and ask for protection and cure of the patients. In addition, there is a spirit house in each hospital for angels to stay (Figure 27-5). Thongkam's family asked the angels of the hospital to protect Thongkam and help him to recover from his illness. They also brought offerings, such as yellow ropes and foods, dedicated to Buddhist monks. Thai Buddhists believe that sickness and bad conditions are the results of bad karmas (actions) in the past. Making offerings dedicated to Buddhist monks is making merit or doing good karma (action) in the present. Thongkam's family hoped the present merit would liberate Thongkam's bad karma in the past and would help him to recover from his illness.

Thongkam's agitation during the night concerned a Buddhist nurse caring for him. She witnessed that Thongkam attempted to turn his body very often. The nurse was at his bedside and compassionately talked to him while touching his chest to calm him. Thongkam

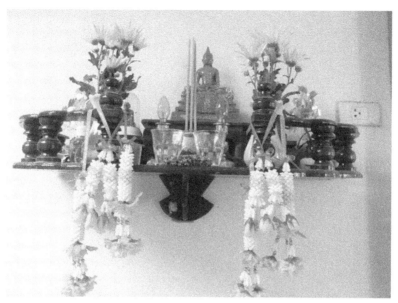

Figure 27–3: Buddha image/respected Buddhist monk image on the shelf. Most hospital wards arrange Buddha images and respected Buddhist monk images on the shelf or tables. *Photo courtesy of Orapan Chaipetch.*

Figure 27–4: Buddha image/respected Buddhist monk image on the tables. Frequently, the patient's family members bring flowers and garlands to show respect to the images and ask for protecting and saving the patient's life with their spiritual power. *Photo courtesy of Supattra Uppanisakorn.*

Figure 27–5: An example of a spiritual house for angels. Most Thai Buddhists have the spiritual house outside and near the entrance of their houses and institutes, including hospitals. Angels are invited to stay in the spiritual houses to protect persons' houses/institutes/hospitals as well as persons' well-being. *Photo courtesy of Waraporn Kongsuwan.*

trusted the nurse and told the nurse that he felt uncomfortable breathing and felt like he was dying because the head of his bed was directed to the west, which was the direction for the deceased. The direction of the head at death is a cultural belief of most Thai Buddhists: When Thai Buddhists die, the position of their heads is directed to the west. The nurse understood this belief and informed the other nurses on the team to move him to another bed. After Thongkam laid down on the bed that faced his head to the east, he could sleep and did not experience restlessness during the night again. The nurse also encouraged Thongkam and the other patients who practiced chanting and meditation to do these together on the ward. Some wards foster group activity of practicing chanting and meditation every week.

Thongkam's condition improved daily, and his infected foot healed. On the day that he was discharged home, his family brought gold leaf to stick at Thongkam's bed (Figure 27-6). Some patients or family members will bring gold leaf to stick at the patients' beds or on the wall above the patients' beds or at the Buddha/respected Buddhist monk image to show respect and gratitude to the angels and the Buddha or the respected Buddhist monks for their help and protection of the patients. The patients or family members do this when the patients' conditions are improved or on the day that the patients are discharged from the hospital. The family did this following their prayer to the angels and the respected Buddhist monks to protect Thongkam, which was effective.

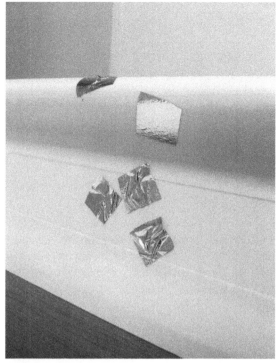

Figure 27–6: Gold leaf at the patient's bed. *Photo courtesy of Supattra Uppanisakorn.*

AUTHOR'S REFLECTION ON THONGKAM'S STORY

This story is an example of transcultural caring for Thai Buddhists in an acute care setting or in a hospital in Thailand. Thai hospitals and Thai nurses support patients and their family members to preserve their own cultural traditions and religious practicing. The nurse in Thongkam's story exhibited her cultural competency in caring for Thongkam under the complexity of physician's perspective, spiritual and cultural beliefs of patient and family members, and physical environment of ward unit (beds' positions). The nurse's intentions in regard to caring, forming a trusting relationship, compassionate knowing of the patient as a whole person, and appreciating spiritual and cultural beliefs were imperative in transcultural caring and providing successful interventions that promoted the patient's well-being during hospitalization.

The essences of transcultural caring communication for patient care in Thongkam's story can be reflected through Ray's Transcultural Communicative Spiritual-Ethical CARING tool (Ray, 2010, p. 47), as follows:

C: Compassion

- The nurse responded in authentic presence in person by opening her mind and heart to Thongkam.
- The nurse acted ethically by providing care to Thongkam to decrease his spiritual fear and promote sleeping well and being well during hospitalization.

Continued

AUTHOR'S REFLECTION ON THONGKAM'S STORY—cont'd

A: Advocacy

• The nurse discovered and explained Thongkam's worldviews about the direction of his bed and death and practicing chanting and meditation to the nursing team for mutual understanding.

R: Respect

• The nurse respected the cultures of Thongkam and the dynamics of the transcultural relationship of the patient and family members.

I: Interaction

• The nurse acted competently by touching, listening, talking, and manifesting transcultural knowledge and skill.

N: Negotiation

• The nurse recognized Thongkam's belief about bed direction and allowed and fostered the change of Thongkam's bed to the appropriate direction. In addition, the nurse recognized Thongkam's practice of chanting and meditation and promoted group activity of chanting and meditation on the ward.

G: Guidance

• The nurse advised and encouraged Thongkam to do chanting and meditation on the ward.

Thai Muslims' Belief That Health Conditions Are Destined by God

This story is derived from the author's experience in clinical practice in a hospital located in the South of Thailand where many Muslims live.

Ali's Story

Ali, a 12-year-old Muslim boy, was in a motorcycle accident and was admitted to the male orthopedic ward. He sustained a comminuted open fracture of the right femur and was scheduled for emergency surgery. To save his life, the doctor decided to amputate Ali's right leg because his bone was broken into small pieces and blood vessels were damaged beyond repair. However, the operation was postponed because Ali's father refused to sign a consent form. He did not want his son's leg to be amputated. The health care team carefully explained to the father about his son's condition and the quality of his life after removing the leg. The father still refused the amputation. He allowed the health care team to perform every procedure or treatment on his son including a wet dressing, antibiotic injection, and analgesic drugs except amputating his leg. Many relatives and people living in the same village came to visit Ali continuously (Figure 27-7).

Ali experienced severe pain 2 days later. He requested an analgesic drug injection every 2 hours. His wound became gangrenous with a bad smell. The mother did not want to see her son suffering, and she pleaded with her husband to change his mind and allow his son to have the surgery. However, the father would not change his mind.

Ali's father, who practiced the Islam religion, believed that the human body came directly from God. Every organ or part of the body we have from birth is created by God. After we die, we must go back to meet God in the same condition as at birth. The father believed that

Figure 27–7: Thai Muslims visiting the patient. In Thai Muslims' culture, there is a belief that visiting the sick patient is making merit. Muslim family members, relatives, and people in their community or village will come to see the patient and pray for him.

amputating his son's leg was a sin because his son was born with all completed organs. When he dies, he will meet God in a different condition.

The nurse who was the head of the ward and was Buddhist had talked to Ali's father many times to gain consent for Ali to have the amputation, but his father still did not consent. The head nurse understood the father's belief of removing the leg was doing wrong to God and this sin would belong to his son. The head nurse asked a Muslim pediatrician to talk to Ali's father. The pediatrician explained to the father that in this case, amputation could be performed because the purpose was to save his son's life. It was not an offense. Nonetheless, the father did not change his mind. He gave as his reason that it was not mentioned in "The Noble Qur'an" as the pediatrician stated it.

The head nurse went to the patient's village to meet the Islamic headman (*imam* or *dtó i-màam*) of the village. She asked the Islamic headman to talk to the father. The Islamic headman said that the amputation could be done and should be performed because it would save his son's life. The headman instructed the father to bury the leg at a Muslim cemetery (Gu Bohr) after the amputation. When his son died, his dead body could be taken to be buried at the same place with his leg, and he would meet God in the same condition as at his birth. However, the father did not change his mind. He said that these statements made by the *imam* were not written clearly in "The Noble Qur'an."

Ali's doctor explained to the father that if he did not allow Ali to have a surgery, there was no treatment that would lead to his recovery. Ali would ultimately die of sepsis. The father decided to take Ali back home. The head nurse did not wish Ali to be suffer at home. She requested the doctor to prescribe wound dressing sets, antibiotic injections, and pain relief medicines for Ali. She went to the community hospital near Ali's house and asked the nurses to care for Ali's wound and inject the medicines according to the scheduled time and received their cooperation.

After staying at home for about 2 weeks, Ali died in a loving and comfortable environment surrounded by his family members and relatives. His completed dead body in the same condition as at his birth was buried in the Muslim cemetery in his village (Figures 27-8 and 27-9).

Figure 27–8: Burial ceremony of Thai Muslims.

Figure 27–9: Muslim cemetery (Gu Bohr)

According to Muslim practice, the dead body was transferred to the tomb of Muslim (Gu Bohr) for burial 24 hours after death. Before burying, the religion leader, families, and neighbors prayed for the dead body. In Thai Muslim culture, the families go to the cemetery to pray for and visit the dead body every day for a week.

AUTHOR'S REFLECTION ON ALI'S STORY

Knowledge and understanding of values and beliefs of patients and families and skill in nursing that emphasizes culture are important and necessary for nurses, especially nurses who practice in areas that have cultural diversity. The head nurse in Ali's story performed compassionate care even though the father of the patient had a different view from the health-care team and did not agree on the treatment that the health-care team had agreed was the only treatment beneficial to the patient. The head nurse performed an ethical role by being a patient advocate and a collaborative role with the others who were involved in the case, ensuring an understanding between the different parties and not creating any conflict.

Because the head nurse's role is a preliminary nursing administrator, her performance can be a good role model of ethical behavior to the other nurses in the ward to implement in their practice to provide the most benefit to patients and families. Also, adhering to ethical behavior can assist nurses to avoid psychological distress when they care for patients from different cultures and result in nursing professionals being accepted by society.

According to Ray's Model on Transcultural Caring Ethics (Ray, 2010), the head ward nurse exhibited behaviors involving transcultural ethical caring. The transcultural ethical caring behaviors respected the patient's father who had a different religion, values, and beliefs from the head ward nurse and refined the differences in values and beliefs through dialogue and communicative action. In addition, the transcultural ethical caring behaviors included commitment in doing beneficence to the patient in relieving his suffering, thinking critically with an informed conscience, acting justly through a mutual understanding between the health-care providers and the patient's father, and facilitating reasoned decision making for the patient's father in regard to his son's life.

References

Ministry of Public Health. (2013). Heath Information. Retrieved from http://bps.ops.moph.go.th/Healthinformation/index.htm

National Statistic Organization, Ministry of Information and Communication Technology. (2011). Report of Surveying Social and Cultural Status in the year 2011. Retrieved from http://service.nso.go.th/nso/nsopublish/themes/files/soc-culPocket.pdf

Ray, M. A. (2010). *Transcultural caring dynamics in nursing and health care.* Philadelphia: F. A. Davis Company.

CHAPTER 28

"Like a Moth to a Flame": Ebola and the Culture of Caregiving in Sub-Saharan Africa

"*Like a moth to a flame*"—*the attraction and the consequence. In days past, stories told by the elderly in villages included how moths would be attracted to light at night. In their search for their mates, moths fly into the night spraying the night air with their pheromones to attract a mate. Attracted to the light, moths gather near oil lamps and in doing so frequently scorch themselves and eventually die. Such is the metaphorical behavior that commonly characterizes the actions of persons who care for patients exposed to Ebola. Eventually, their proximity leads to possible direct contact with the contagious patients with Ebola. Like fire, bodily fluids transmit the deadly virus. Ebola is spread without the individual knowingly contaminating others. The caregiver is like the moth—before it knows what has happened, its wings get singed and are scorched, leading to its death.*

"Playing with Fire"—The Nursing Assistant Who Unknowingly Cared for Patients with Ebola Hemorrhagic Fever

Mary's Story

I did not know there was an Ebola outbreak until I fell sick and was admitted to the hospital in an isolation ward, where I was later told that I had been infected with Ebola. A few days before being brought to the hospital, I had a fever that was persistent. One morning, as I was preparing to go to see a doctor because of the unrelenting fever, I suddenly saw people arriving in an ambulance to my compound; the people were covered head to toe. One of them called out asking where I was. When they saw me, they handed a thermometer to me and asked me to take my temperature, which I did. Then they asked me about the history of my sickness. I told them how it all started. Then they told me, "Pack your things to go to the hospital!" I packed my things and I boarded the ambulance. I traveled to the hospital without knowing there were rumors of a possible Ebola outbreak. When I reached the hospital, I saw that part of the hospital had been cordoned off and was now serving as an isolation ward (Figure 28-1). They took me straight to the isolation ward, where I found only one patient.

In the isolation ward, I learned of the death of a health worker that had occurred a few days earlier under unclear circumstances. The following day, I had a spontaneous abortion [miscarriage]. I was bleeding profusely. There was nobody to help me. I was all alone, without any attendant. The fetus came out, but the placenta remained in me. I tried to remove the placenta, but it broke. I tried to pull, but the placenta still failed to come. The *basawo* [health workers] feared me; they wouldn't touch my blood. When they saw I was bleeding a lot, they would say that it was Ebola, and they would retreat. The bleeding continued. I collapsed and became unconscious. A few days later, when I regained consciousness, I realized the placenta

Figure 28–1: The far ground of Kagadi Hospital where the isolation facility was situated for treating patients.

was still in me. The *basawo* would come and give me treatment and would return outside. I continued to bleed because the placenta was still retained. I even requested a fellow patient to phone my husband, so that he could come and plead with the *basawo* to give me proper treatment. I felt they were not assisting me, until my condition got worse.

One day, as I lay helplessly, having fallen off the bed, one of the doctors came toward me with other *basawo*; they surrounded me and put me back to bed. They told me they wanted to remove the placenta. When they removed the placenta, the bleeding decreased. They then gave me a tablet to stop the bleeding, which they told me to insert in the birth canal, and then the bleeding was minimal. Subsequently, they gave me treatment for diarrhoea, Ringer's solution, and other IV fluids.

As I got better, I realized that I was not thinking well. I was still weak, but I was not fearful. I did not fear death. Although I had been told that I had Ebola, I did not think I was going to die. I was firm in this belief despite being unable to lift myself from the bed for some days. I don't know why! Even before all this, at home when they took me away, I did not fear as such. I remember I called a priest when I fell sick to give me the sacrament for the sick because my fever was not disappearing despite treatment at home. Then after that I was firm in my belief.

Some days later, when the *basawo* said I was going to be discharged after the most recent viral load test results, I wondered, am I the one going to survive? Is Ebola what I have survived? I could not believe it. I kept thanking God, praying that indeed I should survive. Counselors and nurses came and encouraged me to continue eating and drinking as I waited for my results before I could be sent home.

I spent almost a month in the hospital before I was discharged home. Something very striking that happened as I was being discharged is the level of worry I saw in the community. When I reached home I found the locals were extremely worried and scared about Ebola, much more than the patients in the ward. They couldn't eat. They even stopped carrying out their chores and ran away from their duties. The population was greatly affected. They even closed the open air market. People could not move about freely. In banks, tellers wore latex gloves. Things changed a lot. In the hospital, everywhere you would step in Jik (Clorox). At home, Jik was everywhere! There were stories that some people were considering drinking Jik.

When I arrived home, I found very many people waiting for me. Surprisingly, my local community did not run away from me; instead, they were happy I had survived. They welcomed me warmly. Although in other places people run away from survivors, people did not run away from me; neighbors even came to see me. The community showed me love and made me feel comfortable. Even now, they still come to visit! My neighbors tell me that I survived Ebola because of the "good things I did to them." They even told me that when I was admitted to the hospital, people prayed hard for me; Catholics performed novena, [special Catholic prayers] and Muslims performed dua [special prayer for the sick] for me.

These days when I think that people thought I survived because of my actions before Ebola, I feel good and strong. I praise God because in the situation I passed through, God really helped me. My survival has made me love my job even more. These days when I see patients, especially patients who need quick attention, I like to help them. When I see patients helpless, I like to help them because when I remember my experience in the ward, it was not easy. Whenever I needed help, I was alone with no one to help me. I had to help myself. Surviving Ebola has made me learn that when someone is suffering, they need to be helped. I have also learned to love God. When you love God or when you pray, God can answer your prayers. Finally, as a health worker, I have learned that you also have to protect yourself when dealing with patients.

Culture and Its Influences on Health and Illness

The concept of "culture" according to Donini-Lenhoff and Hedrick (2000) is an integrated pattern of learned beliefs and behaviors that are shared among groups. These include, but are not limited to, thoughts, styles of communicating, patterns of interaction, views of roles and relationships, values, practices, and customs. Culture is central in human life, consisting of rules that have been handed down from generation to generation that guide how individuals, families, and groups live as well as how they make important decisions (Mio, Barker-Hackett, & Tumambing, 2009; Wyatt, Williams, Gupta, & Malebranche, 2012).

In view of the complex nature of human relationships, especially how we are influenced by our backgrounds, culture is the inherited "lens" that shapes our perception and understanding of the world in which we live. It is the pathway through which we experience the world emotionally and socially, including how we behave toward others, toward supernatural forces, and toward the natural environment, further demonstrating the supremacy of culture in our lives (Ariff & Beng, 2006; Helman, 2007). Understanding the sociocultural dimensions that underlie people's health values, beliefs, and behaviors is vital in ensuring positive patient outcomes during devastating illnesses such as Ebola.

The link between culture and patient outcomes has been demonstrated through various studies. It has been shown that cultural beliefs and practices affect patients' attitudes about medical care and their ability to understand, manage, and cope with the course of an illness, the meaning of a diagnosis, and the consequences of medical treatment (Ariff & Beng, 2006; Carteret, 2011; McLaughlin & Braun, 1998). Another linkage between culture and patient outcomes is the assertion that cultural beliefs and practices influence patients' perceptions of symptoms, the impact of the illness, where to seek health care, and how to communicate the symptoms to caregivers. Moreover, Flores (2000) and Selim (2010) declared that one's culture to a larger or lesser degree influences how one understands disease management strategies including expectations of care as well as the requisite measures for adherence to preventive measures and medications. Furthermore, McLaughlin and Braun (1998) stated that cultural values also influence patient roles and expectations, in particular, the manner in which they seek and use information about illness and treatment and, importantly, how they perceive notions of death, dying, and bereavement.

A critical aspect of cultural beliefs and practices, which has positive and negative consequences on health behaviors, is the fact that they are tightly held by patients, families, and community members. The central role culture plays in the life of people implies that it profoundly affects health care, in particular, how people behave toward one another during illness, how they react to disease and illness, and how they deal with the consequences of illness. These culturally linked health beliefs and practices are so crucial that, depending on how deeply they are held, they can significantly impede preventive efforts, delay or complicate health care, and result in the use of remedies that can benefit or harm affected individuals, families, and communities (Carteret, 2011). These positive or negative consequences of people's beliefs and practices related to diseases arise from their culturally linked understandings about the cause, mode of transmission, and disease management protocols of various illnesses.

African Cultural Beliefs and Practices Related to Human Disease

In most parts of Africa south of the Sahara, the concept of disease and illness is frequently associated with the world of "spirits" that come to the fore through agents of worship, intercession, misfortune, or witchcraft or the acts and spells of sorcerers (Essien, 2013; Giles, 1995). Spirits are central proponents in the realm of health and illness and are believed to be either "good" or "bad," depending on how they affect humans (Appiah & Gates, 1999;

Essien, 2013; Giles, 1995). Across Africa, south of the Sahara, it is widely conceived that the "good" spirits protect against physical harm, misfortune, or illness. In contrast, "bad" spirits are implicated in causing human and animal disease, misfortune, or various forms of suffering (Essien, 2013; Oraegbunam, 2010).

This belief system is structured around the notion that protection from the spirits is directed at individuals who respect social, cultural, and religious rituals and practices (Giles, 1995; Irele & Jeyifo, 2010; Uchem, 2001). This notion implies that individuals who do not fall into line with the expectations of these practices risk being deserted by "good" spirits, further exposing them to harmful spirits. Individuals, families, and community members who fail to adhere to the "must do's" risk being branded and ostracized should calamity such as illness strike them (Giles, 1995; Oraegbunam, 2010). In such circumstances, affected persons and their families experience alienation reinforced by the belief that their suffering is a result of their own bad deed toward others or the ancestors, as witnessed during the Ebola epidemics in East, Central, and West Africa (Mason, 2008; Matua, 2014; Misha, 2014).

In the Ebola outbreaks in East, Central, and West Africa, such alienation and ostracism triggered by cultural beliefs and the fear of the disease itself played out as strict sociocultural sanctioning during the 2000/2001 Ebola outbreak in northern Uganda (Hewlett & Amola, 2003; Matua & Locsin, 2005), during the outbreak in the Democratic Republic of the Congo and Republic of Congo (Hewlett & Hewlett, 2005), and during the current outbreak in West Africa (Davtyan, Brown, & Folayan, 2014; Misha, 2014). In the case of the 2000/2001 outbreak in Gulu, northern Uganda, Hewlett and Amola (2003), similar to Al Safi (2007), reported that when the locals classified the Ebola outbreak as *gemo*, which means "a killer epidemic," a very stringent form of sociocultural sanctioning was applied to affected patients, families, and community members even before the health ministry's epidemic management protocol began. This social sanctioning compelled affected families to isolate persons suspected to be affected by the strange disease (before Ebola diagnosis) in houses no less than 100 m from all other houses, with no visitors permitted except elderly adults, who were the only sanctioned caregivers for them. The sanction also required obvious labeling of the house where the sick people were isolated and generally restricted the free movement of people across homes and villages (Al Safi, 2007; Matua & Locsin, 2005). This culturally instituted protocol further forbade villagers from dancing, engaging in any sexual relations, and eating meat from animals that died of strange symptoms, including banishing the eating of food cooked outside of one's homestead. The protocol obliged survivors of this strange illness, which eventually became Ebola, to remain in isolation for 4 weeks before they could be allowed to move freely in the villages. Finally, whenever death occurred, the deceased could be buried only at the edge of the village by survivors of the *gemo* or people known to have cared for other sick patients without becoming ill (Hewlett & Amola, 2003).

In Uganda, similar socioculturally inspired practices resurfaced during the 2007 Ebola Bundibugyo outbreak in Western Uganda, where incidences of social sanctioning occurred. Mugisa, Businge, Mugisha, Kisakye, Nzinjah, and Thawite (2007) stated that, as the epidemic spread, sociocultural sanctioning in the form of stigma and ostracism became more frequent. The impetus for such community action characterized by widespread fear and panic could have been fueled by the community's perception of the strange disease and their cultural beliefs related to strange illnesses (Mugisa, Tumusiime, & Kajubu, 2007). Similar incidences of sociocultural sanctioning appeared again during the July 2012 Ebola outbreak in Kibale in western Uganda (Figure 28-2). As the outbreak peaked, fear and the associated stigma and ostracism increased to unprecedented levels to such an extent that the Ugandan president had to appeal for calm and sensibility after survivors and others involved in the care of the sick were experiencing extreme sanctioning (Matua, 2014; Mugerwa & Ayebazibwe, 2012).

Figure 28–2: This is the homestead of the index patient traced by the surveillance team members. The index patient was a 1-year-old baby whose mother later became ill but survived; however, the child's father died. This is also the home of the patient from whom Mary, the nursing assistant in "Mary's Story," most likely contracted Ebola infection after caring for a patient who later died.

Explanatory Models of Disease in Sub-Saharan Africa

Globally, explanatory models are used to understand disease causation. The various models and the accompanying belief systems tend to vary widely, from witchcraft and soul loss to germs, weak immunity, or bad air (Carteret, 2011; Eisenberg, Kessler, Foster, Norlock, Calkins, & Delbanco, 1993). In Western cultures, the human body is perceived as an intricate machine that must be kept in good working order; informed by this perspective, illness is considered as a breakdown of the machine. In contrast, most traditional African and Eastern cultures do not generally subscribe to this belief system about disease causation. Instead, they traditionally have a more a "holistic" view about health and illness encompassing spiritual aspects of disease causation as well as biological and psychosocial aspects (Carteret, 2011; Essien, 2013; Tirodkar, Baker, Makoul, Khurana, Paracha, & Kandula, 2011). Dominant themes related to health and illnesses are linked to concepts such as spirits, witchcraft, negative thought, bad eye, misfortune, stress, or bad food (Appiah & Gates, 1999; Ariff & Beng, 2006; Carteret, 2011; Giles, 1995; Tirodkar et al, 2011).

In line with these widely held holistic views of disease causation, some communities in sub-Saharan Africa have built explanatory frameworks to illuminate the etiology of different diseases. The biological or physical aspects of these models portray disease as resulting from internal imbalance in the body, whereas the spiritual or psychosocial aspects may arise from negative external influences related to actions of bad people, bad spirits, wizards, witches, or deities. Broadly speaking, although small variations may exist across the different cultural groupings in sub-Saharan Africa, disease causation in sub-Saharan Africa may also be explained from two major frameworks: "naturalistic category," which relates to natural causes, and "personalistic category," which is related to external causes, among them supernatural factors (Carteret, 2011; Foster, 1976/2009; Foster & Anderson, 1978).

Within the naturalistic category, illness and health are explained in terms of impersonal, natural forces, conditions, and inert elements in the human body, such as water, salts, humors, heat, and cold. Informed by this view, a person is believed to be healthy when there is equilibrium within the body, when all these elements are in perfect balance. Health manifests when the body's humors and energies are balanced as expected for a person's age and condition in a given time. In contrast, disease results when the delicate balance between these elements is upset (Foster, 1976/2009; Foster & Anderson, 1978; Matua, 2014). In most communities, the naturalistic framework is used to explain simple and clearly discernible illnesses such as aches, fevers, and colds (Al Safi, 2007). When a particular illness falls within the naturalistic realm, the sick patient and his or her close family members are expected to seek treatment from specific healers. These healers often use various locally established remedies such as herbs, foods, dietary restrictions, massage, poultices, and enemas to correct such "imbalances" and ailments (Foster, 1976/2009; Iwu, 2014; Johns, Kokwaro, & Kimanani, 1990).

In the personalistic framework, disease causation is associated with an active and purposeful intervention of an external "agent" who, as Foster (1976/2009) and Alland (1964/2012) described, may be a supernatural being, such as a deity; a lesser nonhuman being, such as a spirit; or a human being, in the form of a wizard, witch, or sorcerer. In this framework, the sick person is primarily considered a victim of aggression or punishment by the "other." Appiah and Gates (1999) in agreement with Foster and Anderson (1978) emphasized that most cultures in sub-Saharan Africa believe that individuals often become prone to illness if they do not conform to certain personal or social standards or if they misbehave or breach taboos, customs, and traditions expected of them or their parents because of "loss of protection from ancestors."

The social implication of this perspective is that people who become afflicted by serious diseases may be treated unfairly by community members, bolstered by the belief that such affliction is "self-made" and may be "worthy punishment" for their failure to abide by norms, leading to their undue ostracism and neglect. When a disease arises from the personalistic perspective, the affected person or close family members are expected to seek help from specific curers known to have supernatural and magical skills not only to treat the illness but to also to identify the responsible "agent" and to establish why the person might have been targeted (Foster, 1976/2009; Matua, 2014). These "curers" are believed to have supernatural powers to connect with the world of spirits as well as to invoke magical powers to find out who was responsible for the disease and why the victim was afflicted. This diagnostic process is followed by an appropriate treatment, which may include prescribed rituals.

Furthermore, in regard to the naturalistic and personalistic views of causation, Grove (1919) and Mumo (2012) posited that a third framework commonly encountered in sub-Saharan Africa relates to "misfortune." Misfortune may significantly influence a person's life, including the person's proneness to good health, ill health, or untimely death, and it usually comes from "displeased" ancestors because of their kin's failure to fulfill cultural obligations or by doing something intentionally and engaging in vice including taking false oaths (Foster, 1978; Grove, 1919; Osemwenkha, 2000). Misfortune may also come from evil influences of a person who has supernatural powers, such as sorcerers or witches, being subjected onto a vulnerable person who lacks protection from "good" spirits (Giles, 1995; Osemwenkha, 2000). The concept of misfortune as a causative agent of disease, particularly the linkage with "displeased" ancestors, means that, similar to the personalistic perspectives, individuals who often become sick through an act of misfortune risk being perceived as "serving deserved sentences" for wrongful acts committed by them or their parents, leading to undue ostracism and alienation.

However, regardless of whether the illness is related to naturalistic causes, personalistic causes, or simply misfortune, the response of most communities depends on the severity. If the illness is serious, rigorous actions are considered, and when the illness is seen to have low risk, a less aggressive response follows (Hewlett & Hewlett, 2005; Hewlett & Amola, 2003). For instance, among the Acholi peoples of northern Uganda, illness is classified as either *yat* or *gemo* depending on its severity. An illness is categorized as *yat* if it is strange and mysterious and is associated with a charm or poison placed on a person or hidden in their vicinity, leading them to become ill (Hewlett & Amola, 2003; Matua & Locsin, 2005). The remedy of *yat* involves a traditional healer locating and removing the *yat* through a prescribed ritual, which may include animal sacrifice to invoke the protection of ancestral spirits and to chase away any evil spirits. A *gemo* classification is reserved for illness that is more severe than *yat*, that appears suddenly, and causes numerous deaths in a short time. The Acholi link *gemo* to acts of witchcraft, charm, or unhappy spirits (Hewlett & Amola, 2003).

When *gemo* is suspected, affected persons and sometimes their close family members are required to be isolated to prevent them from mixing with other members of the village. This practice of culturally instituted social exclusion guards against the perceived contagious nature of *gemo*. When a person afflicted by *gemo* dies, no one is permitted to touch the body except designated caregivers only, usually survivors of the *gemo* or elderly members of the community (Hewlett & Amola, 2003). Although these measures prevent massive deaths, application of such *gemo*-related principles during serious epidemics has had negative consequences on affected individuals and families, leading to their alienation and often banishment from their homes by spouses and relatives (Hewlett & Amola, 2003; Matua, 2014; Matua & Locsin, 2005; Sensasi, 2012). Such occurrences during and after epidemics support the argument that deep-rooted sociocultural perspectives strongly influence a community's reaction toward afflicted persons and their families.

Cultural Influences on Caregiving During Illness in Sub-Saharan Africa

In sub-Saharan Africa, caring for persons in need is considered part of an invaluable social support system that every member is expected to cherish. Integral in this expectation is the concept of *ubuntu*, (humanity or communtarianism), which espouses the idea that every member of the community needs to work toward the good of the other (Chaplin, 2010; Poovan, Du Toit, & Engelbrecht, 2006). This philosophy of humanism firmly links the individual to the community as well as to other individuals through the concept of "brotherhood" or "sisterhood" (Chaplin, 2010; Swanson, 2008). The *ubuntu* philosophy, which is widely practiced in most African communities, emphasizes that every member of the community should be human and cherish the good of the community above self-interest. This community spirit requires members of the community to consciously strive to help others. It further requires that service to others, including caring for others, should be done in a respectful, honest, and trustworthy manner, emphasizing fairness, compassion, and respect for human dignity and collective good always (Cezula, 2013; Chaplin, 2010; Poovan, et al, 2006).

In effect, the philosophy of *ubuntu* makes caring for sick, wounded, and suffering persons an integral part of an ethical-moral code of conduct that every member of the community is mandated to follow. In fulfilling this expectation, caregivers working within this ethical framework are expected to cherish community well-being (Chaplin, 2010; Kasoma, 1996; Swanson, 2008), which translates to looking after the well-being of individual members of the community as well as the well-being of the community as a whole. It follows that when a member of the community is unwell, caring for him or her becomes the caregivers' moral responsibility as enshrined and firmly rooted in the concept of *ubuntu,* which emphasizes good human relations that foster meaningful human life (Chaplin, 2010; Poovan et al, 2006). Individuals who care for others are respected and regarded with high esteem, whereas individuals perceived as uncaring are considered as morally lacking and often rebuked, drawing from the humane approach to life espoused by the African moral thinking, which hinges on the *ubuntu* philosophy (Cezula, 2013; Chaplin, 2010; Kasoma, 1996).

A central guiding principle that influences the community's individual and collective action to support sick and suffering persons stems from the belief that sick persons deserve to be assisted to help them meet their human needs as part of the community's social obligation to afford every member respect and dignity (Cezula, 2013; Swanson, 2008). In view of this, caregivers may act on behalf of the local "community" to meet the needs of the sick or injured. Another cultural perspective that grounds caregiving in sub-Saharan African societies is the concept of "relatedness of one person with others." In these communities, there is traditionally an underlying belief that a "person is what they are because of their community" (Cezula, 2013; Chaplin, 2010), effectively linking each and every one directly to his or her community. This relatedness with members of one's community sustains caring behaviors toward the sick. The welfare of sick members of a community becomes the responsibility of the community, beginning with members of their immediate family.

As an integral part of the community, caregiving during illness is preferably provided by an experienced person so that outcomes are better. Most caregivers are female because of the community's perception that females are more experienced and more suited to care for the sick (Ravi & Gauldin, 2014; World Health Organization, 2007). As a result of this cultural belief, research evidence shows in sub-Saharan Africa that mostly women are involved in direct care of the sick of their families (Bunting, 2001; Mushonga, 2001; Ogunmefun, Gilbert, & Schatz, 2011; Songwathana, 2001). In circumstances where an illness is considered to be very serious, the caregiving protocol exempts the young and the vulnerable, usually children and pregnant women and breastfeeding mothers, from caregiving roles (Matua & Locsin, 2005).

In such circumstances, the caregiving role becomes a preserve of mainly elderly adults and individuals known to have survived similar illnesses (Hewlett & Amola, 2003). This is what happened in Gulu in northern Uganda during the 2000/2001 Ebola outbreak, where persons infected by the hitherto unknown disease, which eventually became known as Ebola, were cared for by elderly adults and survivors and in some cases by individuals known to be resistant to illnesses. This epidemic control "protocol" existed long before the strange illness was declared to be Ebola. In tandem with the *ubuntu* ethic, such protocols help guide caring actions of caregivers and serve to preserve the well-being of the community, especially to safeguard the survival of weak, sick, and other vulnerable members of the community, all offshoots of the communitarian thought.

Ebola Outbreaks and Influences on Caregivers in Saharan Africa

Since its discovery in 1976, the relatively frequent outbreaks of Ebola have continued to threaten the *ubuntu* spirit in East, Central, and West Africa in the various communities where the epidemics have emerged (De Wit, Feldmann, & Munster, 2011; Fauci, 2014). In most of these outbreaks, a defining and often enduring feature has been that of panic, hysteria, and antisocial behavior associated with these outbreaks. Consequently, despite the *ubuntu* spirit, Ebola outbreaks have through their power eroded community resilience and induced fear and caused caregivers to be subjected to unfair discrimination and eventually ostracism, causing them to feel downtrodden and depressed (Locsin & Matua, 2002; Matua, 2014). In a way, these Ebola outbreaks have inadvertently caused caregivers, despite their good and kind intentions, to suffer social, psychological, and economic consequences.

The social consequences of caring for Ebola patients include social isolation, rejection, discrimination, and widespread stigmatization. De Roo, Ado, Rose, Guimard, Fonck, and Colebunders (1998) and Mason (2008) as well as Hewlett and Amola (2003) reported that across epidemics in East, Central, and West Africa, professional and lay caregivers continued to experience "untoward" suffering because of their association with Ebola. In Uganda during the 2007/2008 outbreak in the Bundibugyo district, where the fourth Ebola virus species, *Bundibugyo ebolavirus,* was first discovered, caregivers, similar to Ebola patients, were quarantined by the local community, sometimes to the point of using threats of violence to stop them from leaving their homes (Mason, 2008; Matua, 2014). These incidences of social isolation and rejection permeated throughout the outbreak and sometimes extended well into the aftermath of these epidemics.

Caregivers, similar to survivors and their close family members, in addition to social consequences, experienced psychological difficulties as a result of the intensely negative social realities to which they were subjected, including the lingering fear of the unknown—whether or not they would contract and succumb to the deadly Ebola virus (Locsin, Barnard, Matua, & Bongomin, 2003; Matua, 2014; Matua & Locsin, 2005). The negative psychological reactions included despair, anxiety, sleeplessness, paralysis, helplessness, and stress (Hewlett & Hewlett, 2007; Locsin & Matua, 2002; Wolz, 2014).

In addition to experiencing social and psychological consequences, individuals who offered to help Ebola patients in outbreaks in East, Central, and West Africa continued to experience serious economic implications. The economic difficulty arises in part from inability of caregivers to participate fully in any significant economic activity because of the constant "cloud" of fear inspired from stigmatization in the community, let alone the compulsory 21-day quarantine for every case of exposure imposed by health authorities and local community members (Frieden, Damon, Bell, Kenyon, & Nichol, 2014; Hewlett & Amola, 2003; Mason, 2008). Reports from Uganda, Democratic Republic of the Congo, Republic of the Congo, and West Africa all further confirm that some of the economic challenges are directly related to the actions of epidemic response teams including burning and spraying of personal belongings of suspects and patients believed to have become contaminated. The loss of personal effects is compounded by the diminished possibility of finding work, especially in the immediate term when fear and hysteria are high in the affected communities (Frieden et al, 2014; Hewlett & Amola, 2003; Hewlett & Hewlett, 2005).

Using Ray's Conceptual Model to Understand Caregivers' Experiences

Ray's (2010) conceptual model is an excellent tool that can be used to illuminate the actions of caregivers during the various Ebola outbreaks in East, Central, and West Africa. The model provides a platform from which readers can gain a deeper awareness about how professional and lay caregivers operate in sub-Saharan Africa to understand their experiences better. The actions of the caregivers are discussed in line with principles within the five domains of the model: (1) "essence of caring"; (2) "transcultural caring ethics"; (3) "transcultural context"; (4) "universal sources"; and (5) "transcultural caring inquiry: awareness, understanding, and choice." The actions, choices, and practices in which various caregivers engaged during outbreaks are discussed in line with the tenets of the model.

DIMENSION 1: ESSENCE OF CARING AND ITS APPLICATION TO CAREGIVERS

The concept of caring among caregivers of patients in general and of Ebola patients in particular is grounded on the African ethic of *ubuntu*, where every member of the family and community has a responsibility toward the other (Cezula, 2013; Chaplin, 2010; Kasoma, 1996; Swanson, 2008). As enshrined in the *ubuntu* ethic, caregivers as members of a given community are expected to care about others, particularly persons in need, through acts of authentic physical presence; supportive communication; and sharing in socioculturally prized events and rituals such as funerals, weddings, and birthdays. Caring for the sick, whether a family member or a patient, is considered a morally befitting act that is worthy of praise and rewarded by the community (Cezula, 2013; Chaplin, 2010; Kasoma, 1996).

This ethic and moral expectation drives caregivers, whether professionals or lay individuals, to care for people who became infected with Ebola. In line with the expectations of Ray's (2010) domain of "essence of caring," caregivers in sub-Saharan Africa during various Ebola outbreaks have continued to uphold the moral imperative of showing concern for the other. By choosing to care for Ebola patients, despite the associated risks, as evidenced in various studies, professional and lay caregivers continue to demonstrate undying love, compassion, and moral uprightness as espoused within the ubuntu framework (Hewlett & Hewlett, 2005; Locsin & Matua, 2002; Matua, 2014; Matua & Locsin, 2005; Wolz, 2014).

DIMENSION 2: TRANSCULTURAL CARING ETHICS AND ITS APPLICATION TO CAREGIVERS

African moral thought is guided by the *ubuntu* philosophy (Cezula, 2013; Chaplin, 2010; Kasoma, 1996). This widely cherished moral imperative emphasizes that everyone, whether acting alone or within a group, should engage in actions and conduct that builds their community rather than destroys it. After all, the *ubuntu* ethic emphasis is "I am a person through other people and my humanity is tied to yours" (Connolly, 2012), signifying that "people can only be people through other people" (Chaplin, 2010). This spirit of mutual support and respect is what motivates others to provide for the well-being of patients including patients with Ebola (Cezula, 2013; Chaplin, 2010). The genesis of the mutual respect in the *ubuntu* philosophical thought is that it teaches that each individual's humanity is expressed through a cordial relationship with others, further underscoring the centrality of the other. Similarly, when viewed from the perspective of the larger society, the *ubuntu* ethic acknowledges that every citizen has the right and the responsibility to promote individual and societal well-being, signifying the critical role of individual and collective responsibility toward others (Cezula, 2013; Chaplin, 2010; Kasoma, 1996).

The main ethical framework that may be used to contextualize the actions of caregivers during Ebola outbreaks is the *ubuntu* ethics as well as the "Western" ethical principles, among them beneficence and autonomy. According to the *ubuntu* ethical framework, caring for a sick person is a moral obligation, and all able members of the community are expected to undertake this obligation should there be need (Cezula, 2013). The *ubuntu* ethical and moral framework is respected across sub-Saharan Africa and is arguably the main motivation for caregivers risking their lives to care for others (Hewlett & Hewlett, 2007; Matua, 2014).

Another ethical principle that may be used to explain the actions of caregivers during the Ebola crisis is beneficence, which means doing good to others. In the heat of an Ebola crisis, "doing good to others" has a wide range of applications. It may mean meeting patients' needs for their survival, or it may imply isolating or quarantining patients to limit infection transmission to their family and the community (Matua, 2014; Wolz, 2014). Although the practice of isolation may go against a patient's autonomy, which refers to a patient's right to make his or her own decisions, given the heat of an Ebola epidemic, the patient's right to freedom of choice is waived to protect the larger community (Bryan, Call, & Elliott, 2007; Kass, 2004; Olick, 2004). In such cases, caregivers' actions of enforcing surveillance protocols, including quarantine, maximize "good" consequences for the community, while undermining the patient's personal freedom. In the sociocultural contexts in which these outbreaks occur, such seemingly "harsh" disease control protocols enforced by caregivers are often encouraged by local custom (Hewlett & Hewlett, 2005; Matua & Locsin, 2005) because it helps to contain serious disease outbreaks such as Ebola (Allaranga, Kone, Formenty, Libama, Boumandouki, Woodfill, Sow, Duale, Alemu, & Yada, 2010; Borchert, Mutyaba, Van Kerkhove, Lutwama, Luwaga, Bisoborwa, Turyagaruka, Pirard, Ndayimirije, Roddy, & Van Der Stuyft, 2011; Farrar & Piot, 2014).

This practice of surveillance and disease control, which is an aspect of beneficence, go well with the ethical theory of consequentialism (also utilitarianism), which asserts that an act is morally right when the act causes "the greatest happiness for the greatest number" (Bryan, et al, 2007; Kass, 2004; Sinnott-Armstrong, 2014). The justification for such surveillance actions is the fact that an act of patient isolation, for instance, while being "uncomfortable" to a patient, when seen from the context of community well-being is "benefitting and beneficial" because such actions help in protecting others from further infection (Bryan et al, 2007; Haas, 2014; Olick, 2004).

These actions that exemplify caring ethics that surrounds caregiving during Ebola outbreaks demonstrate that caregivers appear to prioritize the well-being of the larger community over the needs of individual patients. This prioritization seems to indicate that the culture of promoting communitarian or *ubuntu* spirit is deeply entrenched in the actions of caregivers during Ebola outbreaks. This well-established sociocultural expectation guides the activities of caregivers because they feel personally responsible for promoting the well-being of their communities by caring for the vulnerable other, in this case Ebola patients.

DIMENSION 3: TRANSCULTURAL CONTEXT AND ITS APPLICATION TO CAREGIVERS

The actions of caregivers during Ebola outbreaks in sub-Saharan Africa to a large extent have been influenced by the culture in the local area in which the outbreak occurs as well as whether or not the caregivers are related to the patient. In most cases, the actions of the caregivers have been influenced to a large extent by the sociocultural ethic of *ubuntu*, which as previously articulated promotes the idea of enhancing community well-being (Cezula, 2013; Chaplin, 2010). This communitarian spirit has continued to encourage caregivers such as Mary (Figure 28-3) to sacrifice their lives by choosing to care for Ebola patients despite the associated dangers.

In some affected communities, such as the Acholi of Northern Uganda, where the 2000/2001 Ebola outbreak occurred, "cultural epidemic protocols" exist as part of the local culture (Hewlett & Amola, 2003). For instance, among the Acholi people, when there is an outbreak of serious illness, it is classified either as *yat* or *gemo* depending on the severity of

Figure 28–3: Co-author Dr. Gerald Amandu Matua, right, with one of the survivors from the index homestead who contracted Ebola and survived after caring for sick relatives during the 2012 epidemic in Kibale, Uganda. She is one of the few members of the index family to have survived after nine others perished.

the illness. Special caregivers, usually elderly adults, are designated to care for the sick. When there are no elderly members of the community, survivors of the illness or people with strong immunity are called on by the village or community leaders to care for the sick. In all cases, the cultural protocol emphasizes caring for persons in need to uphold the well-being of the community. In essence, such cultural protocols influence caregivers' actions, whether they are professionals or lay members of the community.

Another cultural context from which the actions of caregivers of Ebola patients can be understood is when a particular caregiver is related to the patients. In sub-Saharan Africa, there is a general practice that family members are obliged by cultural norms to care for the needs of their family members, especially in cases of sickness (Kipp, Tindyebwa, Rubaale, Karamagi, & Bajenja, 2007; MacNeil, 1996; Olenja, 1999). If a husband becomes ill, it is expected that the wife will take care of him and vice versa. Similarly, if a child is sick, his or her mother is expected to care for him or her regardless of the health condition present (Hewlett & Hewlett, 2005; Hewlett & Amola, 2002; Kipp, Tindyebwa, Karamagi, & Rubaale, 2006). Such sociocultural norms have played a key role in family members continuing to care for Ebola patients, despite the risk. The apparent difficulty experienced by Ebola response teams in sometimes "extracting" the sick from their homes for hospitalization is the strong underlying notion of "if I do not care for 'XX,' who will?" as well as "I cannot let 'XX' suffer as if they do not have relatives." Such beliefs are widely held across traditional African communities and are probably one of the strongest reasons why relatives often hide suspected Ebola patients from health workers, often considered strangers, preferring to care for the patients themselves. This concept of "inseparability" has translated in family members caring for Ebola patients without knowing what infection their relative is suffering from, consequently leading to many of them, especially the female relatives, to contract Ebola (Francesconi, Yoti, Declich, Onek, Fabiani, Olango, Andraghetti, Rollin, Opira, Greco, & Salmaso, 2003; Hewlett & Hewlett, 2007; Sadek, Khan, Stevens, Peters, Ksiazek, 1999).

A critical aspect of this cultural norm of "family caregiving" protocol is the central role played by female family members (wives, mothers, mothers-in-law, and grandmothers). The traditional African cultural norm considers female family members as the principal caregivers during illness (Kipp et al, 2007; MacNeil, 1996; Olenja, 1999). As a result, a disproportionately higher number of women compared with men have contracted and died of Ebola infection as a direct consequence of caring for sick family members (Dowell, Mukunu, Ksiazek, Khan, Rollin, & Peters, 1999; Hewlett & Hewlett, 2007; Hogan, 2014). In sub-Saharan Africa, when a family member falls ill, a female member of the family commonly cooks and serves food to the sick person and provides for their personal hygiene including washing their stained clothes. This close proximity exposes women to a greater risk of contracting the Ebola virus compared with men. This disproportionate exposure of women to Ebola resurfaced during the current outbreak in Liberia, Guinea, and Sierra Leone, where the rate of infection among women is significantly higher—55% to 60% more than among men—because women are the main caregivers, both as lay family caregivers and as emergency workers, nurses, and midwives (Golberg, 2014; Hogan, 2014; United Nations Children's Fund, 2014).

Although women in general are disproportionately affected by Ebola compared with men, older women are even more prone to contract Ebola and die. An important cultural norm that contributes to this situation is the designation of the caring role during illness to elderly women including mothers, aunts, grandmothers, and mothers-in-law. This culturally assigned role includes preparing the body of the deceased as part of burial rituals and for the afterlife as dictated by various cultural norms (Hewlett & Hewlett, 2005; Hogan, 2014; MacNeil, Farnon, Wamala, Okware, Cannon, Reed, Towner, Tappero, Lutwama, Downing, Nichol, Ksiazek, & Rollin, 2010). These cultural contexts in which caregivers operate as professional and lay care workers inform their "caring" practices during illness, including during Ebola outbreaks, as it has played out in sub-Saharan Africa.

DIMENSION 4: UNIVERSAL SOURCES AND APPLICATION TO CAREGIVERS

African spiritual heritage is deeply religious and consists of myriad spiritual expressions, referred to as indigenous African religions; some are vastly different, whereas some are closely related to each other depending on geopolitical differences because religious practices in traditional African societies tend to be linked to the spirituality of a particular people (Essien, 2013; Irele & Jeyifo, 2010; Lawson, 1998; Mbiti, 1970/2011). As far back as the period before the colonial era until today, a strong sense of belief in God exists among the indigenous African peoples across ethnic or cultural groups, underscoring the central role of spirituality or religion in defining African identity. Key and widely shared themes within Africa spirituality include the belief in a supreme deity, the same as the God figure of modern religions, who is far greater than "lesser gods or semi-divine figures," comparable to the prophets, miracle workers, or apostles of today (Bomki, 2011; Lawson, 1998; Mbiti, 1970/2011); belief in ancestral spirits and their power and intercession ability (Kirwen, 2005; Nyamiti, 2005; Orobator, 2008; Ukpong, 1983/2010); the role of sacrifice as a way to ensure divine protection and generosity (Kasooha, 2009; Pew Research Center, 2010; Salisbury & Roberts, 2012); and the central role different stages of life play in human transition from childhood to adulthood and from life to death (Baum, 2013; Lawson, 1998; Pew Research Center, 2010).

Just as there are many ethnically and culturally distinct groups in the African continent, religious (spiritual) forms are equally varying because each indigenous African cultural or ethnic group relates to a particular form of spirituality (van Binsbergen, 2003; Mbiti 1970/2011). Many indigenous African religions are inseparable from the ethnic identity and culture in which they existed, implying, for example, that the religion of the Masai of Kenya, East Africa, constitutes a deep part of the Masai related to cultural identity including social life (Lawson, 1998; Mbiti, 1970/2011). Contrary to the belief that the African continent is uniform in terms of religious beliefs and practices, differences exist across the continent; some are minor, whereas others are major (Bomki, 2011; Baum, 2013). Compared with modern times, some of the religious beliefs and practices are closely related to the practices of Seventh Day Adventists, which are similar to that of Jehovah's Witnesses. In other instances, some of the differences are major, similar to how far apart the beliefs and practices are of today's evangelical Christians, which differ from that of today's Muslims (Lawson, 1998; Mbiti 1970/2011; Nyamiti, 2005; van Binsbergen, 2003).

In the context of indigenous African religions, the differences in spiritual expressions are partly a reflection of how close the various cultural groupings are related in terms of kinship and geographic distance and how much influence non-African powers have had on the groups (Baum, 2013; Bomki, 2011; Lawson, 1998). In precolonial Africa, when communities existed as separate ethnic groupings, groups that settled and lived in geographic areas adjacent to each other tended to share spiritual beliefs and practices as part of sociocultural integration, whereas groups that lived far apart with little socioeconomic contact tended to differ significantly (Baum, 2013; Mbiti, 1970/2011; Nyamiti, 2005; Ukpong, 1983/2010).

In view of this reality, the concept of "spirituality" in the context of African communities is best considered as a political category, which defines a "local spirituality"—that is, the spiritual practices of a particular political unit (e.g., the Akan of West Africa, the Zulu of South Africa, the Igbo of Nigeria, the Acholi of Uganda) (Bomki, 2011; Hewlett & Amola, 2003; van Binsbergen, 2003). Within these communities, spiritual expressions related to "universal concepts" of spirit, prayer, death, and sacrifice and rituals that endow meaning and order to members of the various ethnic groups are interpreted similarly or differently depending on the specific ethnic grouping (Baum, 2013; Bomki, 2011; Mbiti,1970/2011; Nyamiti, 2005).

Furthermore, as previously stated, in addition to the differences and similarities that exist among the spiritual practices of various groups for geopolitical reasons, an important factor that has altered the religious landscape in the African continent is the influence of trade and colonization (Udeze, 2009; van Binsbergen, 2003). The advent of trade and colonization brought Europeans and Arabs in close contact, which influenced the spiritual beliefs and practices of many African communities. In the end, as a result of either natural assimilation or coercion, many of these culturally distinct African communities adopted "foreign" religious beliefs and practices such as Hinduism, Buddhism, Judaism, Islam, and Christianity that have their origins outside the continent (Bomki, 2011; Udeze, 2009). However, what is key is that the level of assimilation differed, with some communities abandoning the traditional African spiritual practices completely, and some integrating aspects of these "non-African" religious practices into their "traditional" practices. A third group has remained impervious to these non-African religious practices and continues to follow their "traditional" spiritual practices that prevailed before the advent of colonization (Udeze, 2009; van Binsbergen, 2010).

Consequently, in addressing the question of African spirituality that influences the actions of caregivers, it is important to recognize that three lines of spirituality exist: first, followers of modern-day world religions with most following Islam and Christianity; second, followers of an integrated mix of modern and traditional African religious practices; and third, followers of various traditional African religions. However, despite these differences in spiritual orientations in Africa, certain values tend to cut across these three main religious divides. As a result of these interactions, the key spiritual element that is widely found throughout sub-Saharan Africa includes belief in a supreme, unique, and transcendent God similar to the concept in modern-day religions. There is also a high reverence for worship and prayer; sacred places, persons, and objects; and times that are usually followed and celebrated, making religion an integral aspect of African community life (Bomki, 2011; Lawson, 1998; van Binsbergen, 1991). Another important aspect of African spirituality that compares well with modern faiths is the existence of the afterlife giving rise to a world of spirits including ancestors to whom sacrifices are often offered for appeasement to seek protection from harm, including from disease, further underscoring the centrality of religion in the lives of most African people (Kirwen, 2005; Ukpong, 1983/2010).

As a consequence of the centrality of spirituality in peoples' lives, the effect of religion on sociocultural interactions in these communities is very evident. Traditionally, hospitality is highly regarded and valued, requiring every member of the community to treat others with respect and humility. A strong bond may also exist between people of the same clan characterized by a strong sense of belongingness, sharing, and solidarity; providing for the needs of the vulnerable members of their community, taking care of the poor, the sick, widows, and orphans is highly regarded and cherished as evidenced by the actions of caregivers during the Ebola outbreaks (Udeze, 2009; van Binsbergen, 2010).

These and other tightly knit sociocultural and religious principles continue to motivate caregivers to look after the sick, including during outbreaks of disease such as Ebola, as part of the religious expectation of respect for life and the belief in the sacredness of human life as well as connectedness among families and clans. This principle of connectedness as similarly espoused in Ray's (2010) model fits well within the tenets of traditional African spirituality and sociocultural belief systems, at the center of which are issues of preservation of human life, through meaningful caring for the other, including the sick, and preserving human dignity among others. In essence, by caring for the sick and the vulnerable during illness such as Ebola outbreaks, caregivers are meeting their sociocultural and religious obligations toward their family and society.

DIMENSION 5: TRANSCULTURAL CARING INQUIRY AND ITS APPLICATION TO CAREGIVERS

The centerpiece of Ray's (2010) model, the domain of "Transcultural Caring Inquiry: Awareness, Understanding, and Choice," along with the other four dimensions of the model, provides a quintessential tool to help nurses and other health-care workers to engage in meaningful inquiry that reveals experiences such as that of caregivers in sub-Saharan Africa to become more aware of human realities that lie hidden in poorly understood "cultural cocoons." In effect, by engaging in such inquiry, nurses and other health-care workers can become more aware of caring dynamics in distant "lands," including the roles spirituality and culture play in the conceptualization of "caring" in those communities.

Thoughtfully visualizing the actions of caregivers through the "lens" of Ray's (2010) model allows nurses and other health-care workers to understand better what it means to care for patients within various sociocultural contexts. The actions of the caregivers as seen from the perspectives of the model also enable nurses and other health-care workers to understand better the challenges and opportunities associated with caring under such conditions. With a clearer understanding, nurses and others can better critique the choices caregivers have made in their quest to save the lives of Ebola patients, in light of how these choices may affect their own health and well-being. In the end, such deeper understanding and awareness that emanate from thoughtful immersion into the real-life experiences of caregivers such as Mary open our often "closed" eyes and hearts to new realities that every nurse or health worker may encounter in their own practice as they nurture and facilitate the health, well-being, and wholeness of patients, communities, and nations in a culturally congruent manner.

Cultural awareness gained through in-depth understanding and conceptualization of such unique human experiences, in this case that of caregivers of Ebola, enables us to be constantly aware of the need to plan and guide care in a manner that is consistent with the cultural needs of our clientele, whether they belong to a cultural group similar to or distant from us (Ray, 2010; Saha, Komaromy, Koepsell, & Bindman, 1999; Schim, Doorenbos, Benkert, & Miller, 2007). As an ethical call, such cultural astuteness enables nurses and health-care workers to accommodate the needs and preferences of "vulnerable" consumers of health services by advocating for choices that convey respect and acceptance, which promote patient satisfaction, resulting in better outcomes for the nurse and the nursed (Beach, Sugarman, Johnson, Arbelaez, Duggan, & Cooper, 2005; Ray, 2010; Saha et al, 1999; Schim et al, 2007).

Reflections with Questions

Reflect on Mary, a caregiver who provided nursing care to patients unaware that some of the patients would later infect her with the Ebola virus. She continued to work until she became indisposed through sickness. What lessons do we learn from Mary's story? What may have been Mary's greatest motivation to care? What does her work suggest about the role of caregivers in Africa and globally? What aspects of Ray's (2010) model can you use to explain Mary's actions? What aspect of Ray's theory would help you promote culturally congruent practice if you were Mary? If you encountered situations comparable to Mary's situation, how would it affect your practice? What are the similarities and differences between the sociocultural and moral standards that relate to the "other" in sub-Saharan Africa and the rest of the world? How has this exemplar influenced you in terms of caring for others who are different from you socially and culturally?

Transcultural Nursing Reflections

- Reflect on your opinion about African belief systems, especially the Ubuntu ethic.
- Reflect on how Africa and African beliefs and practices are perceived in the West.
- Reflect on what your first reaction would be if you were asked by a reputable charity organization to go on a medical mission to sub-Saharan Africa.
- Reflect on your responsibility in terms of providing care that is culturally consistent with existing national and international standards in your home country.

AUTHORS' REFLECTIONS

Patients are commonly treated in a socially, culturally, and linguistically inappropriate manner in health-care institutions globally. Patients and their family members who are considered to be inferior or different usually experience this maltreatment. As a result of such unfair and sometimes inhumane treatment, the well-being and quality of life of vulnerable individuals, families, and communities are negatively affected in an unprecedented manner.

Cognizant of such unfair practices, the transcultural movement continues to advocate for deliberate efforts to ensure that persons in government and in the private sector provide services including health-care services in a manner that respects and accommodates individuality of people, including their sociocultural beliefs and practices. As globalization and technology, particularly technology that enhances human travel and communication, continue to develop, it is hoped that the social, cultural, and political differences that divided us in the past will vanish. Every one of us will, more often than not, encounter another person, family, or cultural group that is different from us. Health-care workers in general and nurses in particular encounter this cultural diversity because of the nature of their job. A serious reorientation of the thoughts and practices of all nurses and health-care workers is needed. In our view, the model and theory presented in *Transcultural Caring Dynamics in Nursing and Health Care* provide an excellent foundation on which the nursing profession and other human sciences can build evidence-based knowledge that fosters the well-being and wholeness of persons, families, and members of culturally distinct communities across the world.

References

Alland, A. (1964/2012). Division of anthropology: Native therapists and Western medical practitioners among the Abron of the Ivory Coast. *Transactions of the New York Academy of Sciences*, 26 (6 Series II), 714–725.

Allaranga, Y., Kone, M.L., Formenty, P., Libama, F., Boumandouki, P., Woodfill, C.J., Sow, I., Duale, S., Alemu, W., & Yada, A. (2010). Lessons learned during active epidemiological surveillance of Ebola and Marburg viral hemorrhagic fever epidemics in Africa. *East African Journal of Public Health*, 7(1), 30–36.

Al Safi, A. (2007). *Traditional Sudanese medicine: A primer for health care providers, researchers and students*. Khartoum: Dar al-Azza Publishers.

Appiah, K.A., & Gates Jr., H.A. (Eds.). (1999). *Encarta Africana: The encyclopaedia of the African and African American experience*. [CD-ROM]. Richmond, WA: Microsoft Corporation.

Ariff, K.M., & Beng, K.S. (2006). Cultural health beliefs in a rural family practice: A Malaysian perspective. *Australian Journal of Rural Health*, 14(1), 2–8.

Baum, R.M. (2013). Indigenous African religions. In J. Parker & R. Reid (Eds.), *The Oxford handbook of modern African history* (pp. 281–297). London: Oxford University Press.

Beach, M.C., Sugarman, J., Johnson, R.L., Arbelaez, J.J., Duggan, P.S., & Cooper, L.A. (2005). Do patients treated with dignity report higher satisfaction, adherence, and receipt of preventive care? *The Annals of Family Medicine*, 3(4), 331–338.

Bomki, L.M. (2011). Ancestral cult in African traditional religious belief systems and its theological relevance today. *International Journal of African Catholicism*, 2(1), 1–11.

Borchert, M., Mutyaba, I., van Kerkhove, M.D., Lutwama, J., Luwaga, H., Bisoborwa, G., Turyagaruka, J., Pirard, P., Ndayimirije, N., Roddy, P., & van der Stuyft, P. (2011). Ebola haemorrhagic fever outbreak in Masindi District, Uganda: Outbreak description and lessons learned. *BMC Infectious Diseases*, 11(1), 1–17.

Bryan, C.S., Call, T.J., & Elliott, K.C. (2007). The ethics of infection control: Philosophical frameworks. *Ethics*, 28(9), 1077–1084.

Bunting, S. (2001). Sustaining the relationship: Women's caregiving in the context of caregivers. *Journal of Transcultural Nursing*, 7(2), 14–20.

Carteret, M. (2011). *Cultural based beliefs about illness causation*. Retrieved from http://www.dimensions ofculture.com/2011/02/culturally-based-beliefs-about-illness-causation/

Cezula, N.S. (2013). *Identity formation and community solidarity: Second Temple historiographies in discourse with (South) African theologies of reconstruction*. Doctoral thesis. Stellenbosch University. Retrieved from http://hdl.handle.net/10019.1/91298

Chaplin, K. (2010). *The Ubuntu spirit in African communities*. Retrieved from http://www.coe.int/t/ dg4/cultureheritage/culture/Cities/Publication/BookCoE20-Chaplin.pdf

Connolly, A.M. (2012). *The spirit of Ubuntu*. Retrieved from https://www.clintonfoundation.org/main/ clinton-foundation-blog.html/2012/07/16/the-spirit-of-ubuntu

Davtyan, M., Brown, B., & Folayan, M. (2014). Addressing Ebola-related stigma: Lessons learned from HIV/AIDS. *Global Health Action*, 7(26058), 1–4.

De Roo, A., Ado, B., Rose, B., Guimard, Y., Fonck, K., & Colebunders, R. (1998). Survey among survivors of the 1995 Ebola epidemic in Kikwit, Democratic Republic of Congo: Their feelings and experiences. *Tropical Medicine & International Health*, 3(11), 883–885.

De Wit, E., Feldmann, H., & Munster, V.J. (2011). Tackling Ebola: New insights into prophylactic and therapeutic intervention strategies. *Genome Medicine*, 3(5), 1–10.

Donini-Lenhoff, F.G., & Hedrick, H.L. (2000). Increasing awareness and implementation of cultural competence principles in health professions education. *Journal of Allied Health*, 29(4), 241–245.

Dowell, S.F., Mukunu, R., Ksiazek, T.G., Khan, A.S., Rollin, P.E., & Peters, C.J. (1999). Transmission of Ebola hemorrhagic fever: A study of risk factors in family members, Kikwit, Democratic Republic of the Congo, 1995. *Journal of Infectious Diseases*, 179(Supplement 1), S87–S91.

Eisenberg, D.M., Kessler, R.C., Foster, C., Norlock, F.E., Calkins, D.R., & Delbanco, T.L. (1993). Unconventional medicine in the United States—prevalence, costs, and patterns of use. *New England Journal of Medicine*, 328(4), 246–252.

Essien, E.D. (2013). Notions of healing and transcendence in the trajectory of African traditional religion: Paradigm and strategies. *International Review of Mission*, 102(2), 236–248.

Farrar, J.J., & Piot, P. (2014). The Ebola emergency-immediate action, ongoing strategy. *New England Journal of Medicine*, 371(16), 1545–1546.

Fauci, A.S. (2014). Ebola—underscoring the global disparities in health care resources. *New England Journal of Medicine*, 371(12), 1084–1086.

Flores, G. (2000). Culture and the patient-physician relationship: Achieving cultural competency in health care. *Journal of Pediatrics*, 36 (1), 14–23.

Foster, G., & Anderson, B. (1978). *Medical anthropology*. New York: John Wiley.

Foster, G.M. (1976/2009). Disease aetiologies in non_western medical systems. *American Anthropologist*, 78(4), 773–782.

Francesconi, P., Yoti, Z., Declich, S., Onek, P.A., Fabiani, M., Olango, J., Andraghetti, R., Rollin, P.E., Opira, C., Greco, D., & Salmaso, S. (2003). Ebola hemorrhagic fever transmission and risk factors of contacts, Uganda. *Emerging Infectious Diseases*, 9(11), 1430–1437.

Frieden, T.R., Damon, I., Bell, B.P., Kenyon, T., & Nichol, S. (2014). Ebola 2014—new challenges, new global response and responsibility. *New England Journal of Medicine*, 371(13), 1177–1180.

Giles, L.L. (1995). Sociocultural change and spirit possession on the Swahili coast of East Africa. *Anthropological Quarterly*, 89–106.

Golberg, E. (2014, August 29). More women than men are dying from Ebola. *The Huffington Post*. Retrieved from http://www.huffingtonpost.com/2014/08/29/ebola-women-deaths_n_5738294.html

Grove, E.T.N. (1919). Customs of the Acholi. *Sudan Notes and Records*, 2(2), 157–182.

Haas, C.N. (2014). On the quarantine period for Ebola virus. *PLoS Current Outbreaks*, October 14, 6.

Helman, C.G. (2007). *Culture, Health and Illness* (5th ed.). London: Hodder Arnold Publication.

Hewlett, B.L., & Hewlett, B.S. (2005). Providing care and facing death: Nursing during Ebola outbreaks in central Africa. *Journal of Transcultural Nursing*, 16(4), 289–297.

Hewlett, B.S., & Amola, R.P. (2003). Cultural contexts of Ebola in Northern Uganda. *Emerging Infectious Diseases*, 9(2), 1242–1248.

Hewlett, B.S., & Hewlett, B.L. (2007). *Ebola, culture and politics: The anthropology of an emerging disease*. Belmont, CA: Thomson Wadsworth Publishers.

Hogan, C. (2014, August 14). Ebola striking women more frequently than men. *The Washington Post*. Retrieved from http://www.washingtonpost.com/national/health-science/2014/08/14/3e08d0c8-2312-11e4-8593-da634b334390_story.html

Irele, A., & Jeyifo, B. (Eds.). (2010). *The Oxford encyclopedia of African thought* (Vol. 1). London: Oxford University Press.

Iwu, M.M. (2014). *Handbook of African medicinal plants* (2nd ed.). Boca Raton, FL: Taylor & Francis.

Johns, T., Kokwaro, J.O., & Kimanani, E.K. (1990). Herbal remedies of the Luo of Siaya District, Kenya: Establishing quantitative criteria for consensus. *Economic Botany*, 44(3), 369–381.

Kasoma, F.P. (1996). The foundations of African ethics (Afriethics) and the professional practice of journalism: The case for society-centred media morality. *Africa Media Review*, 10, 93–116.

Kasooha, I., (2009, February 24). Girl beheaded in ritual murder. *The New Vision*. Retrieved from http://business.highbeam.com/3548/article-1G1-194307053/girl-beheaded-ritual-murder

Kass, N.E. (2004). Public health ethics from foundations and frameworks to justice and global public health. *The Journal of Law, Medicine & Ethics*, 32(2), 232–242.

Kipp, W., Tindyebwa, D., Karamagi, E., & Rubaale, T. (2013). Family caregiving to AIDS patients: The role of gender in caregiver burden in Uganda. *Journal of International Women's Studies*, 7(4), 1–13.

Kipp, W., Tindyebwa, D., Rubaale, T., Karamagi, E., & Bajenja, E. (2007). Family caregivers in rural Uganda: The hidden reality. *Health Care for Women International*, 28(10), 856–871.

Kirwen, M.C. (2005). *African cultural knowledge, themes and embodied beliefs*. Nairobi: Mias Books.

Lawson, E.T. (1998). *Religions of Africa: Traditions in transformation*. San Francisco: Harper & Row.

Locsin, R.C., Barnard, A., Matua, A.G., & Bongomin, B. (2003). Surviving Ebola: Understanding experience through artistic expression. *International Nursing Review*, 50(3), 156–166.

Locsin, R.C., & Matua, A.G. (2002). The lived experience of waiting_to_know: Ebola at Mbarara, Uganda—hoping for life, anticipating death. *Journal of Advanced Nursing*, 37(2), 173–181.

MacNeil, A., Farnon, E.C., Wamala, J., Okware, S., Cannon, D.L., Reed, Z., Towner, J.S., Tappero, J.W., Lutwama, J., Downing, R., Nichol, S.T., Ksiazek, T.G., & Rollin, P.E. (2010). Proportion of deaths and clinical features in Bundibugyo Ebola virus infection, Uganda. *Emerging Infectious Diseases*, 16(12), 1969–1972.

MacNeil, J.M. (1996). Use of culture care theory with Baganda women as AIDS caregivers. *Journal of Transcultural Nursing*, 7(2), 14–20.

Mason, C. (2008, February 22). Coping with Ebola stigma. *The Daily Monitor*, p. 1.

Matua, A.G. (2014). *Living under the threat of Ebola: A phenomenological study*. Doctoral thesis. University of South Africa. Retrieved from http://hdl.handle.net/10500/13822

Matua, A.G., & Locsin, R.C. (2005). Conquering death from Ebola: Living the experience of surviving a life-threatening illness. In A.V. Lee (Ed.). *Coping with Disease* (pp. 121-173). New York: Nova Science.

Mbiti, J.S. (1970/2011). Christianity and traditional religions in Africa. *International Review of Mission*, *59*(236), 430–440.

McLaughlin, L., & Braun, K. (1998). Asian and Pacific Islander cultural values: Considerations for health care decision-making. *Health & Social Work*, *23*(2), 116–126.

Mio, J.S., Barker-Hackett, L., & Tumambing, J. (2009). *Multicultural psychology: Understanding our diverse communities* (2nd ed.). Boston: McGraw-Hill.

Misha, H. (2014, April 8). Guinea's first Ebola survivors return to family, stigma remains. *Reuters News Agency*. Retrieved from http://www.reuters.com/article/2014/04/08/us-guinea-ebola-survivors-idUSBREA370WP20140408

Mugerwa F, Ayebazibwe A. (2012, July 31). Be calm, says Museveni as Ebola cases rise to 25. *The Daily Monitor*, p. 4.

Mugisa, A., Businge, C., Mugisha, M., Kisakye, B., Nzinjah, B., & Thawite, J. (2007, December 3). Ebola strikes more nurses. *The New Vision*, pp. 1–3.

Mugisa, A., Tumusiime, C., & Kajubu, E. (2007, December 12). Museveni speaks to Ebola survivor. *The New Vision*, pp. 1–3.

Mumo, P.M. (2012). Holistic healing: An analytical review of medicine-men in African societies. *Thought and Practice: A Journal of the Philosophical Association of Kenya*, *4*(1), 111–122.

Mushonga, R.P. (2001). *Social support, coping and perceived burden of female caregivers of HIV/ AIDS patients in rural Zimbabwe*. Unpublished doctoral dissertation. Case Western Reserve University.

Nyamiti, C. (2005). *Jesus Christ, the ancestor of humankind: Methodological and trinitarian foundations* (Vol. 1). Nairobi: Catholic University of Eastern Africa Publications.

Ogunmefun, C., Gilbert, L., & Schatz, E. (2011). Older female caregivers and HIV/AIDS-related secondary stigma in rural South Africa. *Journal of Cross-Cultural Gerontology*, *26*(1), 85–102.

Olenja, J.M. (1999). Assessing community attitude towards home-based care for people with AIDS (PWAs) in Kenya. *Journal of Community Health*, *24*(3), 187–199.

Olick, R.S. (2004). Ethics, epidemics, and the duty to treat. *Journal of Public Health Management and Practice*, *10*(4), 366–367.

Oraegbunam, I.K. (2010). Crime and punishment in Igbo customary law: The challenge of Nigerian criminal jurisprudence. *OGIRISI: A New Journal of African Studies*, *7*(1), 1–31

Orobator, A.E. (2008). *Theology brewed in an African pot*. New York: Orbis Books.

Osemwenkha, S. (2000). Disease aetiology in traditional African society. *Africa*, *55*(4), 583–590.

Pew Research Center. (2010). Traditional African religious beliefs and practices. In *Tolerance and tension: Islam and Christianity in sub-Saharan Africa*. Washington, D.C: Pew Research Center. Retrieved from http://www.pewforum.org/files/2010/04/sub-saharan-africa-full-report.pdf

Poovan, N., Du Toit, M.K., & Engelbrecht, A.S. (2006). The effect of the social values of Ubuntu on team effectiveness. *South African Journal of Business Management*, *37*(3), 17–27.

Ravi, S.J., & Gauldin, E.M. (2014). Sociocultural dimensions of the Ebola virus disease outbreak in Liberia. *Biosecurity and Bioterrorism: Biodefense Strategy, Practice, and Science*, *12*(6).

Ray, M.A. (2010). *Transcultural caring dynamics in nursing and health care*. Philadelphia: F. A. Davis.

Sadek, R.F., Khan, A.S., Stevens, G., Peters, C.J., & Ksiazek, T.G. (1999). Ebola hemorrhagic fever, Democratic Republic of the Congo, 1995: Determinants of survival. *Journal of Infectious Diseases, 179*(Supplement 1), S24–S27.

Saha, S., Komaromy, M., Koepsell, T.D., & Bindman, A.B. (1999). Patient-physician racial concordance and the perceived quality and use of health care. *Archives of Internal Medicine, 159*(9), 997–1004.

Salisbury, S., & Roberts, L. (2012). *The Practice of Ritual Killings and Human Sacrifice in Africa.* Retrieved from http://hrbrief.org/2012/09/the-practice-of-ritual-killings-and-human-sacrifice-in-africa/

Schim, S.M., Doorenbos, A., Benkert, R., & Miller, J. (2007). Culturally congruent care putting the puzzle together. *Journal of Transcultural Nursing, 18*(2), 103–110.

Selim, N. (2010). Cultural dimensions of depression in Bangladesh: A qualitative study in two villages of Matlab. *Journal of Health, Population and Nutrition, 28*(1), 95–106.

Sensasi, B. (2012, October 12). A tale and plight of three Ebola survivors in Kibale district. *WHO News Feature,* pp. 1–6. Retrieved from http://www.afro.who.int/en/uganda/press-materials/item/5029-a-tale-and-plight-of-three-ebola-survivors-in-kibaale-district.html

Sinnott-Armstrong, W. (2014).Consequentialism. In E.N Zalta (Ed.), *The Stanford Encyclopedia of Philosophy.* Spring 2014 Edition. Retrieved from http://plato.stanford.edu/archives/spr2014/entries/consequentialism/

Songwathana, P. (2001). Women and AIDS caregiving: Women's work? *Health Care for Women International, 22,* 263–279.

Swanson, D.M. (2008). Ubuntu: An African contribution to (re)search for/with a 'humble togetherness.' *Journal of Contemporary Issues in Education, 2*(2), 53–67.

Tirodkar, M.A., Baker, D.W., Makoul, G.T., Khurana, N., Paracha, M.W., & Kandula, N.R. (2011). Explanatory models of health and disease among South Asian immigrants in Chicago. *Journal of Immigrant and Minority Health, 13*(2), 385–394.

Uchem, R.N. (2001). *Overcoming women's subordination in the Igbo African culture and in the Catholic church: Envisioning an inclusive theology with reference to women.* Boca Raton, FL: Universal Publishers.

Udeze, B. (2009). *Why Africa? A Continent in a dilemma of unanswered questions.* Bloomington, IN: Xlibris Corporation.

Ukpong, J.S. (1983/2010). The problem of God and sacrifice in African traditional religion. *Journal of Religion in Africa,* 187–203.

United Nations Children's Fund (2014, July 30). *UNICEF: Women most affected Ebola outbreak in W. Africa.* Retrieved from http://www.unmultimedia.org/radio/english/2014/07/unicef-women-most-affected-ebola-outbreak-in-w-africa/#.VGIfvfmUctP

van Binsbergen, W.M.J. (1991). Becoming a sangoma: Religious anthropological field-work in Francistown, Botswana. *Journal of Religion in Africa, 21*(4), 309–344.

van Binsbergen, W.M.J. (2003). *African spirituality: An approach from intercultural philosophy.* Forum for Intercultural Philosophy. Retrieved from http://them.polylog.org/4/fbw-en.htm

van Binsbergen, W.M.J. (2010). The continuity of African and Eurasian mythologies: General theoretical models and detailed comparative discussion of the case of Nkoya mythology from Zambia, South Central Africa (pp. 143–223). In *New Perspectives on Myth: Proceedings of the Second Annual Conference of the International Association for Comparative Mythology,* Ravenstein (the Netherlands), 19–21 August, 2008. Papers in Intercultural Philosophy and Transcontinental Comparative Studies. Haarlem, Netherlands: Shikanda Press.

Wolz, A. (2014). Face to face with Ebola—an emergency care center in Sierra Leone. *New England Journal of Medicine, 371*(12), 1081–1083.

World Health Organization. (2007). *Addressing sex and gender in epidemic-prone infectious diseases.* Geneva, Switzerland: WHO. Retrieved from http://www.who.int/csr/resources/publications/SexGenderInfectDis.pdf

Wyatt, G.E., Williams, J.K., Gupta, A., & Malebranche, D. (2012). Are cultural values and beliefs included in US based HIV interventions? *Preventive Medicine, 55*(5), 362–370.

CHAPTER 29

A Danish/Norwegian Culture Nursing Care Model: An Ethical Demand

*T*he aim of this chapter is to describe a nursing care model from a Danish/Norwegian *cultural perspective. The development of the model is based on an intertwined approach between a philosophy of care and empirical research from a patient perspective in clinical nursing practice.*

The chapter uses different philosophical and research sources. First is the phenomenological philosophy of care of Norwegian Doctor of Philosophy and Nurse Kari Martinsen (Delmar, 2013a). For the past 35 years, Dr. Martinsen has advocated that care is and should be a prerequisite for good nursing. The philosophy of the late Danish philosopher K. E. Løgstrup, whose work has been a companion to Martinsen's and my own philosophical work, is the underlying ontology (Løgstrup, 1956/1986, 1997). Last but not least, my own empirical nursing research that I have conducted over the last 20 years also forms an essential part of the model.

With a purpose to give an overall picture, I first present the entire nursing care model. Subsequently, I emphasize the following keywords: relationships, trust and power, and life phenomena. At the same time, I provide a demonstration of how the keywords form nursing actions in a concrete clinical practice.

Nursing Care Model from a Danish/Norwegian Perspective

In the course of their illness, patients go through many phases. They are variously disheartened or hopeful, frightened or courageous. They are sometimes beside themselves—their thoughts and actions are unpredictable; moreover, each patient and situation presents a new challenge for caregivers. There are no prescribed ways of practicing good, wise, and right clinical nursing. The challenge to the nurse's ethical and intentional mindfulness lies in the concrete situation (Delmar, 2008).

It may seem like a paradox that we want to proceed systematically on a foundation of a prescribed model because caring ethics does not fit into a formula or even a definition. However, in this world of change, it can be a relief to simplify such complex issues. A prescribed model also gives nurses a basis for discussing what went well and what did not turn out as well in their work. It is important to clarify from the beginning that it is not a question of observing a number of rules in our practice, but rather the model, shown in Box 29-1, is a "thinking horizon" that comes into play only in the specific situation as an ethical demand.

Keyword Relationships

Care ethics is the basis of all human relationships and founded on a relational view of the other. In the words of Løgstrup (1956/1986, 1997), interdependence, or the fact that we are fundamentally dependent on each other, means that we cannot meet each other without being in a mutual relationship, where we mutually hand ourselves to each other. In *The Ethical Demand* (Løgstrup, 1956/1986, 1997), Løgstrup, especially in the first chapter, presented a phenomenological analysis of the origin of the ethical demand, which is precisely that a person has his or her reality with other people and that we give each other reality. Thus, the individual belongs in the world, where he or she has something of the other person's life in his or her power.

Our life-conducive possibilities depend on how other people interact with us. In other words, the meeting between people is essential. If we reflect for a moment on some of those

---

BOX 29–1 ❖ Danish/Norwegian Nursing Care Model—An Ethical Demand

1. A care ethics is based on a relational philosophy of life (Delmar, 1999, 2013a; Martinsen, 1993, 2006).
2. A care ethics is expressed in a moral practice (Delmar, 1999, 2013a; Martinsen, 1993, 2006).
3. A care ethics concerns trust and power (Delmar, 1999, 2012).
4. A care ethics concerns the way in which power is shaped so that trust in relations is maintained (Delmar, 1999, 2012).
5. A care ethics involves helping without infringing (Delmar, 1999, 2012, 2013a; Martinsen, 1993, 2006).
6. A care ethics involves attending to the other so that his life courage is supported and his opportunities for expression and life-conducive possibilities are expanded (Delmar, 1999, 2012, 2013a; Martinsen, 1993).
7. A care ethics involves an attention toward life phenomena and acting on this (Delmar 1999, 2013b; Delmar et al, 2005, 2006).
8. A care ethics presupposes the development of sensuous contextual attention (Delmar, 1999, 2004, 2008).
9. A care ethics presupposes professionalism in nursing (Delmar, 1999; Martinsen, 1993).

encounters of our own lives, I'm sure we all are able to recall meetings with people who expanded our room for action, but we also remember people who constricted our room for action.

Because the aim of nursing is to support life-conducive possibilities for the patient, it is important to reflect on the challenges when people depend on each other. In many societies, and especially in Europe and the United States, the relational view of people is under threat because the prevailing values are based on a liberalist view of the human being (Delmar, Alenius-Karlsson, & Mikkelsen, 2011). These values carry such labels as "independence," "autonomy," "self-management," "freedom of individual choice," and "responsibility for one's life and own learning." The refrain goes: "It's up to you to make a choice and do what you want." Interdependence and dependence are negative values in Western societies grounded in an individual perception. The problem is that in some Western health care institutions and societies the liberalistic values have become so accepted that many people feel as if they were surrounded by a chorus chanting: "Pull yourself together, get with it, do your own thing. You—you alone—are the architect of your own life."

Empirical nursing research documents that there is a tendency to let the liberalistic values dominate and determine lives with a negative outcome for patients. It is not an attempt to deny that those values are in many ways life-conducive ones. Let me offer some examples where self-management is a powerful choice. The two examples are taken from a qualitative research project in nursing. I quote two patients, the latter of whom was a diabetic:

"... you've made some decisions along the way ... made your own choices, you know. And I do think that it gives you something positive, some positive energy and power ... "
(Delmar, Bøje, Dylmer, Forup, Jakobsen, Møller, Sønder, & Pedersen, 2006).

"I must admit I can get fed up with people who worry too much about what I eat. I mean, if I want an ice cream, I can have it ... after all, it's my own responsibility what I do. It's annoying when people treat you as if you're a child by asking, 'Should you really be eating such a big ice cream?'" (Delmar et al, 2006).

Although values concerning the freedom of individual choice and own responsibility are vital to our modern way of life, those values and the responsibility that come with them may also bring a sense of burdensome guilt if something goes wrong in the patient's life. The following quotations are from three different patients and call attention to the life phenomenon of guilt:

"You do stop and think every time [a complication occurs], don't you. If you've squeezed into a pair of shoes that are a bit too small .... You're thinking, maybe I've ruined something for myself ... " (Delmar et al, 2006).

"Say you're feeling really fine and go and do something that maybe isn't too smart. You're wondering whether you have to pay for it 10 years down the line" (Delmar et al, 2006).

". . . well, my position is that if you suffer [late consequences of the disease], you do have to take a little bit of the blame yourself . . ." (Delmar et al, 2006).

If the liberalist view (independence, self-management, etc.) determines the nurse's values and actions, there is a great risk of leaving patients to their own devices where individual choices and own responsibility are concerned—the nurse will leave the patient alone with his or her sense of guilt. It can easily become the patient's own problem to solve different tasks related to his or her condition. If the purpose of nursing is defined as self-management, the danger lurks in unjustified rejection of the patient's plea for help. In such cases, nurses are not offering care. From the conception that fundamentally a person wants to strive to be self-managed, it could easily become an individual perception that everyone has to be self-managed. What could seem unbearable without the help of others can become bearable with the care of others.

The traditional idea of care placed the professional nurse in the expert role and the patient in the role of the passive recipient of treatment. It was a reaction to these roles that brought forward the idea of an active and independent patient who is capable of making his or her own choices from a number of options. Nurses have learned—and are still being taught, at least in Denmark and Norway—the advantages of the self-care models. These models prescribe that patients' responsibility and self-management should not be taken away from them. This is in many ways an animating way of thinking, but it is also underlying a political and economic argument: "We don't have enough money. We don't have enough people to take care of the growing elderly population. You have to learn to take care of yourself."

Nurses may ask if there is a risk that founding nursing on values such as self-management and independence could inspire a conception of patients as being *always* active and self-managing—*always* capable of making the right choices if they are presented with a number of alternatives (Delmar et al, 2011). What about the weakest patients? What about patients with very limited resources (such as fragile elderly patients, patients with a severe mental illness, patients addicted to narcotics and alcohol)? What about jobless persons with a diagnosis of a serious disease? What about their self-management and freedom to choose among the alternatives?

In acknowledging that we all are engaged in relations of dependence, each specific situation requires that the professional nurse, by applying her moral mindfulness, judges how individual values and self-management may be voiced in the specific situation and context and whether it is a life-conducive approach in which those values actually serve to enhance inviolable phenomena such as life courage, hope, trust, and compassion of the individual patient (Delmar, 2004, 2012).

The message is clear. We can pay due respect to the inviolability of autonomy as a life-giving value and as an integral part of living in today's culture and society only if the professional nurse's values are rooted in a care ethics philosophy and real relational view of human beings with an impact on helping the patient and family in different contexts and situations and under different conditions. It requires development of the nurse's ethical and intentional mindfulness, sensitive attention, and good moral judgment in each specific situation. The nursing care model can support discussions of individual patient cases in practice and keep in mind the relevance of the ethical demand as an important framework for good nursing actions.

Trust and Power—The Asymmetry of Power

A care ethics offers support without infringing on the other's domain. This perspective represents a moral practice that concerns the administration of trust and power as fundamental phenomena in every relationship (Delmar, 1999, 2012, 2013a).

As mentioned earlier, my own and Martinsen's ontological care ethics is strongly influenced by Løgstrup's interpretation of existence, and this influence also applies to the phenomena of trust and power. For Løgstrup, trust is a relation-based life phenomenon, a so-called life manifestation, and as such it cannot be created but is a given in our lives. However, trust is vulnerable, and we may undermine it, with the result that, in the worst case, mistrust takes its place (Løgstrup, 1956/1986, 1997; Martinsen, 1993). In our mutual dependence and in the act of surrendering ourselves to one another, power will always be in play along with trust. A receptive attitude may expand the other's room for action by making the other's world wide, light, diverse, and safe. A rejecting attitude reflects a conquering and domineering way of thinking, which can destroy the other by rendering his world narrow, dark, tedious, and menacing. A morally responsible exercise of power is to act in such a way that the other's room for action is expanded. In the trusting relation, there is an expectation that the other receives the trust proffered and responds to it. However, the risk of rejection is always present. In human relationships, we are always subject to power as it plays a role in the way we express ourselves, and it should not be seen as evil (Løgstrup, 1956/1986, 1997). The crux of the matter is how power is exercised. How can we act in such a way that the other is as comfortable as possible? How do we avoid a harmful exercise of power? When do closeness and distance become mutually exclusive?

Because there is no recipe for care as a moral practice, the intention is to communicate a picture of what may be involved when nurses—despite knowledge and descriptions of what good nursing is—are sometimes incapable of maintaining the trustful relation. Instead of acting in a morally responsible way, nurses may end up in positions where they restrict the patient's room for action, with the result that care degenerates into overprotection or even patronizing.

Basically, my goal is that the hidden, more or less unconscious, handling of power in the relationship is made visible, to protect the essential trust, care, and presence in the meeting. An example concerns the matter of keeping one's word where time is involved. A quotation follows of what a young female patient said in an interview:

"They [the staff] shouldn't promise too much—I'd rather they said too little than too much. If they promise this and that and never stick to anything, I get frustrated. Sometimes they'll say, 'It's coming in a minute ... we'll fix that for you ...,' and then it takes half an hour, or an hour, or even more ... " (Delmar, 1999, p. 145, 2008).

This is a typical example from the busy world of hospitals where the staff may not always reflect on how important what they say to patients is. If "It'll be here in a minute" becomes the routine answer, the patient's trust in the nurse can be undermined. Behind our backs, the power vested in the professional may prevail, and this leads to an unproductive situation as the nurse becomes blind to the patient's concrete situation. The essential thing is to protect the confidence that nurses enjoy and to be able to see what is at stake for the patient. Trust and power are essential in every relationship.

Being a Burden

On further reflection in relation to the aforementioned view of trust and power, one can think of how, for example, the nurse's authority is vested in his or her position, uniform, various badges and medals, professional knowledge, and personal demeanor. If the nurse deploys his or her authority in a peremptory manner, it is not a morally responsible exercise of power but an abuse of power. One is left in no doubt about the uneven distribution of power in nurse-patient collaboration. One also needs to think of the hospital as a place of powerlessness where patients come because the state of their health is beyond their control and where they are divested of all tokens of the role that gives them identity in their everyday lives. They have to surrender their rear ends to thermometers and washcloths and give up control over their bedtimes and when to be available for ward rounds and examinations. Even with this knowledge, I have been surprised by research results showing the degree to which not only older patients, who were brought up to bow down to authority, but also younger patients experience that they are being a burden. In adapting to the authoritarian world of the hospital, patients use different coping strategies. Some patients become powerless and just give up. One patient expressed his experience in the following way: "Look, you're trapped here and it might be taken out on you if you say there's something you don't like (. . .) it makes no difference, just keep your mouth shut—you'll be out of here someday anyway" (Delmar, 1999, p. 97). In using the metaphor of being trapped, the patient expressed her sense of helplessness and her feeling that because of her illness she was forced to stay in the hospital, unable to get away. The patient felt trapped and dependent on the nurses, on whose help she would have to rely if she has to go back to the hospital in the future.

Other patients adopt the role of the "easy" patient who is polite and friendly and never complains—maybe because they feel a debt of gratitude to the nurses, who stood by during the period of illness. In contrast to the "difficult" patient who constantly demands the nurse's attention, the "easy" patient is one of the nurses' favorites among the cooperative patients because the relationship is on the nurse's terms. The "easy" patient avoids causing trouble and quietly adapts to the nurse. Some patients use humor and become more extroverted and adaptable to get closer to the nurse.

All in all, the balance of power will always tip to the nurse's advantage. The patient's sense of being a burden may be expressed in many ways. To avoid the excesses of care, the nurse should bear this in mind. The unequal distribution of power is an unavoidable aspect of the relationship, and the nurse needs to acknowledge this fact to maintain trust.

Doing Only What Is Absolutely Necessary

From this preliminary acknowledgment of the asymmetry of power, I shall now approach an aspect that may create distance between people, that can make care a simple question of technique and restrict the patient's room for action. Based on Danish and Norwegian nursing colleges' curricula, with their foundation in a holistic philosophy that aims at training nurses to understand their fellow human beings in a multifaceted context, research with interviewed patients showed that patients had not spoken with a nurse about what had preoccupied them in connection with their illness. I am referring here to life phenomena such as anxiety, grief, hope, loneliness, and worries about the future (Delmar, 2006). This was clearly indicated by a patient when he said to me as a researcher: "I have not spoken about this to anybody in the way that I'm saying it now" (Delmar, 1999, p. 107). Also, patient testimony indicates that it does mean something to patients that the nurse also takes an interest in the life phenomena that are connected with their illness. I use the term "instrumental-technologically oriented" to describe nurses who overlook or disregard patients' suffering and the life phenomena that everyone knows about and that become more prominent in the course of an illness. Among nurses themselves and their patients, it is common to use the phrase "they only do what's absolutely necessary" to describe such nurses. An example expressed by a nurse follows:

> "... sometimes I'm thinking that there are some nurses who are a bit superficial—doing only the necessary ... what has to be done, without getting down to the [patients'] problems. Like washing them, and then perhaps giving them something to drink—and that's bad nursing ..." (Delmar, 1999, p. 111).

This is not an attempt to generalize, but it does make a difference what the orientation is. If the nurse takes care of only the patient's basic needs and overlooks the real problems, there is a risk of creating a distance that may restrict the patient's room for action. To illustrate this kind of work and what it means for the patient, I shall give a picture, however incomplete, of different conceptions of instrumental-technological nursing activities. It may be expressed by the nurse's giving priority to her role as the doctor's right hand—by being more preoccupied with examination reports and treatment routines—rather than to the patient's immediate welfare. Likewise, nursing routines, such as the changing of bandages, may become a question of pure technique when the same procedure is used in all situations or if wound treatment attracts professional interest to the point where it becomes the sole focus of attention, and nursing care is not considered at all. It may also be the nurse's inclination to spend most of her time writing in the nursing station or to ignore the patient—the language used will often reveal this when she instructs the patient to do what she thinks should be done. Also, the nurse neither accepts nor allows the patient the time to participate in collaboration but rather tries to get things done as quickly as possible. The same is true for the nurse who relies on quantifiable documentation methodology and allows measurements and standards to take the place of caring. These are all factors that may involve a risk that the patient's suffering is ignored (Delmar, 1999, pp. 111–118).

This information is meant as an invitation to discuss what should characterize the professional good nurse, taking into consideration that priorities must be made in relation to time and nursing assignments. Because the nursing culture may stimulate an instrumental-technologically oriented nursing, whether the care ethics is to have first priority depends on the nurses' willingness to take a different route, backed up by mutual support.

Paternalism and Overprotectiveness

I have given some illustrative examples of how the patient's room for action many be constrained. I shall now present what is essential in relation to the theme of the asymmetry of power and the nurse's movement between closeness and distance in the asymmetrical power relationship.

One example (Delmar, 1999, pp. 122–131) shows that the nurse, despite her effort to escape the traditional paternalism, finds herself caught up in practicing paternalism by cultivating a value set based on the self-care models, prescribing that patients' responsibility and self-management should not be taken away from them. The description shows that the patient expects a professionally trained, competent nurse who knows what to do when a patient is in pain. In contrast, the nurse expects a patient who is capable of making an independent choice based on a number of suggestions for pain relief. It is bound to go wrong as the patient does not live up to the nurse's expectations concerning his or her ability to make a choice on the basis of a number of possibilities; the nurse perceives the patient as uncooperative, and this is mirrored by the patient's experience of a paternalistic nurse. The distance in the asymmetrical power relation has gained the upper hand.

It is not that the nurse is unaware that her nursing professional training gives her an expertise that the patient does not have. Rather, the case could be that the nurse is stuck in a self-care theory that rests on ideas about individual self-determination and the right to a free choice. The individual, that is, the patient, should naturally be considered as a self-managing and independent master of his or her own existence, a person who strives to be self-dependent and make his or her own choices. I would encourage nursing practitioners to discuss reasons for a poor outcome of the asymmetrical power relationship and to be open toward an understanding of what and how much should be left to the patient's own choice and responsibility in the individual concrete situation. This should also be taken as a recommendation to the nurse to consider carefully why patients may sometimes be uncooperative and difficult and why self-reliant patients with no immediate need of help become "easy" patients. Just like the "difficult" patients, they bear the risk of being let down.

Similar to paternalism, an overprotective administration of power can restrict the patient's room for action. So what may be afoot when, despite her personal and emotional involvement, the nurse does not succeed in giving good care?

In navigating between closeness and distance in the asymmetric power relation, emotions may get the better of the nurse. Nursing care may fossilize and result in sentimental overprotectiveness if the nurse becomes so emotionally affected by the situation that the care and the patient take second place in relation to her own concerns. This could also be the case if, for impenetrable reasons of a psychological nature, the nurse becomes so self-sacrificing, overly considerate, and self-effacing that nursing care fossilizes into overemotional involvement and intimacy. The result is that closeness has taken the upper hand in the asymmetrical power relation.

If the emotions tinge the situation with sentimentality or intimacy, care is at risk. If, in contrast, personal presence and emotional involvement are applied with sensitivity—in other words, as a sensuous contextual attention—this will contribute to preventing closeness from standing alone, and this may result in a true care ethics.

To meet the ethical demand and to preserve the vulnerable trust that is essential in cooperating with the patient, the nurse has to risk himself or herself because there is no recipe for this moral practice. It is in the concrete, specific case that the hard questions have to be lived through and expressed. Being able to see what is at stake, what it really means to the patient—that is, to understand what is going on in a moral sense—is a tightrope walk between being either close to or distancing yourself in relation to the patient. If the nurse is bound by rules, principles, standards, or self-sacrificing emotions rather than sound, professional judgment, the risk grows that the cooperation becomes morally irresponsible (that is, on the part of the nurse). The power of the nurse may, despite the best of intentions, get the upper hand, and the nurse will become blind to the patient's real situation, such as it is.

In such situations, the nursing care model can help the nurse remember that care is about helping without infringing on the patient's integrity and remember the need to keep in mind constantly the need to visualize and discuss with colleagues how trust and power should be managed in the widely differing patient situations.

Life Phenomena

A care ethics involves attention toward life phenomena and taking appropriate actions. "Life phenomena" is a general term for the various relational-ethical and individual-existential phenomena that are a given in our lives (Delmar, 2013b). Following are a few examples:

- Ethical life phenomena (relationship-based): Trust, interpersonal power, hope, compassion, charity, guilt, universally human vulnerability.
- Existential life-conducive life phenomena (based on the individual): Life courage, joy of life, hope, longing, security, harmony, happiness.
- Existential life-constraining life phenomena (based on the individual): Hopelessness, loneliness, powerlessness, longing, despair, shame, vulnerability.

Based on the Danish/Norwegian and German life philosophical tradition, some phenomena are regarded as being of a more ethical nature, some are existentially life-conducive, and others are existentially life-constraining. Ethical and existential life phenomena are both essential life phenomena in their own right and of separate value, but it is the combination of the two phenomena (ethical and existential) that creates the whole person.

You will have noticed that some of the life phenomena were mentioned under more than one heading. This is because it is not a categorical division or a checklist. Whether a life phenomenon such as longing is life-conducive or life-constraining depends on the circumstances and the specific situation in which that longing is expressed. The same may be said about human vulnerability as an ethical phenomenon, which can be life-constraining in certain situations (Delmar, 2013b).

What matters for patients is that nurses support the ethically dignified and existentially life-conducive phenomena. By linking to patients' individual experiences of their suffering and the way the suffering interferes with the existential qualities of life, I shall demonstrate the implications of life phenomena.

When a person becomes ill, everyday life phenomena such as hope, doubt, life courage, fear, pain, powerlessness, and loneliness become more evident for that person; of course, this does not happen all at once, and many things depend on the individual person who becomes ill and on the illness and diagnosis. However, life phenomena become more pronounced when a person's life situation changes with the intrusion of illness on the whole person.

Research from the Nordic countries shows that patients want nurses who are trained in helping ill and vulnerable people with their despair, insecurity, hope, and suffering (Delmar Bøje, Dylmer, Forup, Jakobsen, Møller, Sønder, & Pedersen, 2005, 2006; Delmar, Rasmussen, & Dolmer, 2009). However, it seems to be true that the most basic phenomena of life are those that nurses become aware of only late in the caring process and with the greatest difficulty. To ensure that expressions of these essential life phenomena by patients are not ignored by personnel working with health, illness, and suffering, a conscious effort to focus on them is needed.

Theories of needs, such as the theories of Henderson and Maslow, are well known to health-care providers, not least in documentation and care systems, which often base their work on need theory. Although this knowledge is essential for understanding and helping the patient, it is insufficient by itself (Delmar, 2013b). The development of theory on life phenomena is a supplement to the existing nursing theories—not a replacement, but a new and important supplement that goes beyond the human activity: the drive to satisfy needs in the context of health care and nursing.

This new heuristic insight to the complex field of health-care ethics has been a long time coming. Over more than 10 years, working papers have been added to, changed, and structured on the basis of life philosophy. Within a care ethical frame of understanding, empirical patient-centered research in life phenomena has further contributed to giving voice to the ways in which daily life influences suffering and illness and to what matters in the course of an illness.

The meanings and nuances in the life phenomena of hope, doubt, and life courage can be exemplified by reference to qualitative interviews with chronic sufferers (Delmar et al, 2005, 2006). The study shows how the patients constantly fluctuate between hope, doubt, and hopelessness—in particular in connection with visits to the outpatient clinic. There were periodical swings between self-control and loss of control, and these swings bring uncertainty, frustration, and difficult choices in a process where patients eventually experience a collapse of meaning. After some time, patients may find a new way of living, and a new meaning in life. Contracting a chronic disease is a shattering experience, and the life phenomena are awakened and come to expression.

Hope, doubt, and hopelessness are universally human life phenomena that become more evident when one's life situation changes. Life phenomena are not static, but in constant movement. In moving toward hope, one's life courage also grows, but doubts can come to the fore and shake the hope, setting in motion a swing toward hopelessness and despair. Because hopelessness and despair are not conducive to the patient's healing and rehabilitation process, it is essential for nurses to learn more about how hope and life courage impact on the patient's efforts to take the changes that have occurred in the patient's life into account.

In interviews, several of the patients expressed their hopes and wishes for the future: hope for healing, hope that the disease would pass, hope that a new medicine or technology would appear, hope of living a "normal" life again. Hope enables people to cope with difficult situations in life such as loss and suffering. Hope and life courage are closely knit, and it is one of the nurse's primary tasks to further the patient's life courage amid the suffering.

Where there is hope, life courage can blossom. Hope supplies the energy for life courage and self-realization to grow. Hope looks to the future and entails the wish that one's life situation can change, which gives an experience of feeling a sense of freedom and of having control over one's life—a control that was momentarily lost.

There is no precise definition of hope, and it is important to be aware that hope is expressed in many ways—for example, the readiness to do just about anything to get well again. Two quotes from patients in research projects expressed it as follows:

"I am open-minded towards alternative treatment—when you're at rock bottom, you're willing to try whatever there is" (Delmar et al, 2005, 2006).

"When you're ill, and want to get over it, there isn't a thing you wouldn't do" (Delmar et al, 2005, 2006).

Retaining hope may also come across as naive or purely wishful thinking, which can be mistaken for a repression of reality:

"I pretend to myself that when I enter menopause—and I think I will soon—then it will stop" (Delmar et al, 2005, 2006).

"[I have] this naive belief that I can stop taking the pills at some time, so that I won't be reminded of it every day" (Delmar et al, 2005, 2006).

Repression of the facts may also appear in the form of a belief that it's not you, but "the people next door" who will be affected:

". . . you know, I tend to think that all those things you hear about late complications . . . they won't affect me" (Delmar et al, 2005, 2006).

Denial as a psychological defense mechanism can help the patient through difficult times. However, repression can also appear as a kind of self-deception, with the result that recognition of the suffering and illness fails, and the patient does not achieve harmony with self and the new situation. It is important for the nurse to be aware that it is not always a case of psychological repression. "Forgetting" and pushing away the fear of, say, late complications can help the patient edge back to gaining life courage—one of the life-conducive life phenomena. What at first glance may appear to be a psychological defense mechanism may have the effect of giving relief and supporting the retention of the hope that is absolutely decisive for the patient's life courage and for the opportunities that appear along the road through life with the chronic illness. So the message to the nurse is: Be aware of the various expressions that hope can take, and examine closely if this is a case of a psychological defense mechanism or an expression of relief and the existential life-conducive phenomenon—hope.

Where there is hope, there is also room for doubt. Two quotes express the doubt that is always the companion of hope:

"My father learned to live with a pacemaker, so I suppose I can also learn to live with this" (Delmar et al, 2005, 2006).

". . . [my wife] has always accepted that this is the way it is. So I must say that things have run smoothly, no doubt about it. Of course, you can't take that for granted" (Delmar et al, 2005, 2006).

Hope and doubt are inconstant companions, and to help the patient in the battle between the two, it is the nurse's task to be aware that the patient may swing between hope and doubt—for example, in connection with visits to the outpatient clinic, readmission, or when the patient is confronted with the fact that the illness is chronic. It is important to be aware of the existential qualities in patients who are suffering because life-conducive phenomena enable patients to cope with difficult situations. Life-conducive phenomena are connected with the vitality that is expressed in a vital urge for action in which the patient's ability to come to terms with new life conditions will improve.

However, there is a risk that the biomedical explanation model and theories about needs will dominate the nursing offered. An example concerns a 40-year-old father, who had a blood clot in the heart and completed a rehabilitation program (Delmar et al, 2005, 2006). The rehabilitation program was based in particular on health professionals' knowledge and ideas on patients' general needs for information about the effects of smoking, diet, and exercise and anatomical and physiological information on blood clots in the heart—in other words, general information about the disease. The physiological needs were given special attention, and the patient no longer *had* a blood clot in the heart—he no longer *had* the diagnosed illness. That belonged to the past. But every day, the patient was thinking of life and death as interwoven with the fear that it would happen again. He was constantly pondering the question of what it means to *be* a man, a spouse, and a father. There was a constant, lurking fear, which could become a life-constraining life phenomenon that would disturb his ability to achieve harmony with himself and his new life situation.

Nursing care of patients who have had a blood clot in the heart needs to be concerned not only with smoking, diet, and exercise; nurses also need to give attention to life phenomena in daily clinical practice and in nursing research and science. There is a need to know the nuances and multiple ways that a life phenomenon such as fear can influence patients' lives. Life and in particular *being* a person with an illness takes more than meeting some—in this case—general needs for information concerning lifestyle changes. When nursing is solely driven to satisfy physical needs, there is a risk that the life phenomena become invisible to the nurses whose job is to help a sick and suffering person accustom himself to his new situation. Because sick people are gripped by despair and suffering, sick people are beside themselves, and they are unpredictable.

What is the future challenge for care ethics focusing on life phenomena? The development of theory on life phenomena and some new heuristic insights to the complex field of nursing theory goes beyond the human activity, the drive to satisfy needs. To add a deeper understanding of the existential meaning of being a person with an illness, I present some different human dimensions concerning life phenomena and needs. The focus is on essential distinctions in relation to needs.

Gratification

Needs seek gratification, whether they are bodily, physiological, or cultural. Their fluctuation creates inner tensions that strive for release. Needs rise and seek gratification. Their expression is rhythmical—intensifying until satisfaction, and then a new cycle begins (Pahuus, 1995).

An example is the need for food. You get more and more hungry until you get food, and then it starts all over again. However, existence also embraces phenomena that have nothing to do with needs and gratification. Life phenomena do not have such rhythms. They do not have phases, they are not cyclical, but rather fluctuate between opposite poles, such as hope and doubt (Delmar, 2013b).

Rationalization and Reproduction

Technology and industrial production make a business of gratifying human needs. Needs can be refined, further developed, and diversified (Pahuus, 1995). For example, the need for food can be varied by the gastronome, and the need for a roof above our heads can be refined by aesthetics and subjected to the architect's whim. We see that needs are perfected, and there is a risk of appealing to human desire and greed. Some say that the gratification of insatiable needs is the greatest challenge of the Western world. For if satisfying one's needs becomes the most important thing for a person, it is bound to happen at the expense of other people or of things that are of greater significance to the individual. For instance, there is a risk that developments in health technology may create a vicious circle where the need for ever more advanced methods capable of accomplishing more and more will only stimulate the growth of further needs for more and more technology. Or it could happen at the expense of others' needs, such as needs of the homeless, the mentally ill, the elderly, and underprivileged patients, or at the expense of the individual's lifeworld.

Life phenomena are not a question of the inexhaustible satisfaction of growing individual needs in a constant process of refinement. A life phenomenon is either present or absent, and life phenomena cannot be refined and diversified, although they become more evident when illness intrudes. Life phenomena have their origin outside the realm of technological and industrial solutions. They are not about solving problems but about embracing the existential. Helping the patient in such matters means helping him or her to understand the various expressions of life phenomena to make space for the life phenomena that are ethical and life-conducive rather than life-constraining (Delmar, 2013b).

Consciousness and Attention

Needs that are conscious registered as the experience of want, and the longer gratification is deferred, the stronger the experience of need becomes. The more vital a need is, for example, thirst and hunger, the stronger is our awareness of it, and we direct our attention toward fulfilling the need through goal-directed activity (Pahuus, 1995). In general, needs can be gratified only through directed activity, such as providing food and drink, or dedicating a large part of existence to work—something that does not necessarily entail self-actualization, but whose only merit is to provide the means for acquiring things and material possessions to gratify one's needs.

Problems may occur in the pursuit of gratifying those needs. They can detach themselves, become independent and determine the person in such a way that they will dictate what the person does in the world. For example, if one lives a life where needs govern all human intercourse and interaction, relationships will be governed by the experience of need. This view will serve an individualistic philosophy of human nature characterized by egotistically motivated human intercourse and the exploitation of others for the gratification of one's own needs.

An active engagement and receptive directedness is not always structured by needs as exemplified by the ethical life phenomena such as compassion and trust. A nurse who has true compassion is not aware that she is compassionate; a trustful nurse does not know that she is trustful. If someone is consciously trying to be compassionate, the attention is directed at oneself, and the focus of attention is one's own situation rather than the situation of the other. Life becomes self-centered, circling around the gratification of one's own needs (Delmar, 2013b).

Needs and Life Phenomena

By pointing out some differences in their characteristics, I hope I have shown some essential differences between needs and life phenomena. This should not be understood as an attempt to explain away that needs exist in human life; they are part of being human. Needs are quite legitimate. Nevertheless, it is important to acknowledge the different human dimensions concerning needs and life phenomena. The nurse's challenge lies in spotting the unnoticed life phenomena so that they are not overlooked or ignored because life phenomena come to the fore in the sick and vulnerable person. Life phenomena have their place in the nursing care model. It is a future challenge for nurses in daily practice to incorporate the thoughts and actions that go beyond the drive to satisfy needs (Thorup, Rundqvist, Roberts, & Delmar, 2012).

Conclusion

Because there is no recipe for good nursing care, development of competence against a sensuous contextual attention is required. Furthermore, it is essential to vocalize a care ethics framework for nurses' actions as a basis for clinical discussions. The framework is a mind-set directed at the patient and family in an attempt to find out what sort of appeal for help the patient expresses. The framework is not a set of rules; however, for nurses to become more conscious and mindful in the concrete practice and more visible in the political context, nurse theorists have to collaborate with clinical nurses with the purpose to make values, philosophies, and theories explicit. To enliven the framework in clinical practice, an entire hospital has to work on the basis of a program that implements the framework in various research projects.

AUTHORS' REFLECTIONS (SEE FIGURE 29-1)

In the asymmetrical nurse-patient relationship, nursing as an ethical demand presents the nurse with the challenge of taking care of the life that has been placed in his or her hand, in trust and with power. This is the essential message of this chapter, but in clinical and practical life, success is not always achievable. A hidden and more or less unconscious restriction of the patient's room for action may result in the excesses of care. The patient's room for action is affected in no lesser degree by the relational ethical and individual existential life phenomena on which the nurse bases her nursing and life philosophy and on her personal demeanor and sensitive attention. The nurse should first and foremost be aware of the power issues that are inherent to the relationship and that every situation is an ethical challenge to be attentive to the patient's appeal for help so that his room for action is expanded. It calls for a systematic development plan focusing on situation-specific sensitive attention skills.

Figure 29–1: Dr. Delmar lecturing to faculty and graduate students on the ethics of nursing in the Danish/Norwegian culture.

Care Ethics Reflections

- Reflect on cases where trust has been shaken in the collaboration with the patient or the family.
- What are your experiences with life-conducive life phenomena?
- What are your experiences with life-constraining life phenomena?
- How do you prefer yourself to have the courage to be and stay together with the patient in his or her existential suffering?
- What is involved in being autonomous and self-managing when one is suffering?
- Is it possible to imagine that the self-managing patient no longer feels that he or she is the master of his own life because the insecurity created by the volatility of the condition is all-pervading or because falling ill has shaken his identity?

References

Delmar, C. (1999). *Tillid og magt—en moralsk udfordring [Trust and power—a moral challenge]*. Copenhagen, Denmark: Munksgaard.

Delmar, C. (2004). Development of ethical expertise: A question of courage. *International Journal for Human Caring, 8*(3), 8–12.

Delmar, C. (2008). No recipe for care as a moral practice. *International Journal for Human Caring, 12*(4), 38–43.

Delmar, C. (2012). The excesses of care: A matter of understanding the asymmetry of power. *Nursing Philosophy, 13*(4), 236–243.

Delmar, C. (2013a). Becoming whole: Kari Martinsen's philosophy of care—selected concepts and the impact on clinical nursing. *International Journal for Human Caring, 17*(3), 20–28.

Delmar, C. (2013b). Beyond the drive to satisfy needs—in the Context of Health Care. *Medicine, Health Care & Philosophy, 16*(2), 141–149.

Delmar, C, Alenius-Karlsson, N., & Mikkelsen, A.H. (2011). The implications of autonomy—viewed in the light of efforts to uphold dignity and integrity. *International Journal of Qualitative Studies on Health and Well-being, 6*(2).

Delmar, C., Bøje, T., Dylmer, D., Forup, L., Jakobsen, C., Møller, M., Sønder, H., & Pedersen, B.D. (2005). Achieving harmony with oneself: Life with a chronic illness. *Scandinavian Journal of Caring Sciences, 19*(3), 204–212.

Delmar, C., Bøje, T., Dylmer, D., Forup, L., Jakobsen, C., Møller, M., Sønder, H., & Pedersen, B.D. (2006). Independence/dependence—a contradictory relationship: life with a chronic illness. *Scandinavian Journal of Caring Sciences, 20*(3), 261–268.

Delmar, C., Rasmussen, B., & Dolmer, I. (2009). Staying in "the stream of life": Rehabilitation of older people in their own homes following total hip replacement. *International Journal of Older People Nursing, 4*, 272–279.

Løgstrup, K.E. (1956/1986). *Den etiske fordring [The Ethical Demand]* (11th ed.). Copenhagen, Denmark: Gyldendal.

Løgstrup, K.E.(1997). *The ethical demand*. Notre Dame, IN: University of Notre Dame Press.

Martinsen, K. (1993). *Fra Marx til Løgstrup. Om etikk og sanselighet i sykepleien [From Marx to Løgstrup. Ethics and sensitivity in nursing]*. Oslo, Norway: Tano A/S.

Martinsen, K. (2006). *Care and vulnerability*. Oslo, Norway: Akribe.

Pahuus, M. (1995). *Livsfilosofi. Lykke og lidelse i eksistens og litteratur [Life philosophy. happiness and suffering in existence and literature]* (2nd ed.). Århus: Philosophia.

Thorup, C.B., Rundqvist, E., Roberts, C., & Delmar, C. (2012). Care ethics as a matter of courage. Vulnerability, suffering and ethical formation in nursing care. *Scandinavian Journal of Caring Sciences, 26*(3), 427–435.

CHAPTER 30

Considerations Within the United Nations for Transcultural Nursing: Global Initiatives for Caring, Peace, and Quality of Life

*T*he call for professional nursing to address the human condition has existed for more than two centuries. The specialty of transcultural nursing has concentrated on cultural understanding and culturally congruent care since its inception over 40 years ago. Rapid changes in science, technology, economics, transportation, demographics, health care, and even innovative interpretations of the meaning of spirituality have challenged us to new paradigm thinking initiated by the sciences of complexity—the authentic meaning of interconnectedness *of all things, the integrality of the human-environment relationship, and attention to communicative caring ethics (Davidson, Ray, & Turkel, 2011; Ray, 2010a, 2010b, 2010c). Discussion ensues of ongoing international cultural conflicts within geopolitical communities, political challenges, global economic analyses, refugee and migrant peoples' crises, the emergence of social media, and communicative action. These lifeworld phenomena present opportunities for transcultural nurses to examine and/or develop new paradigms.*

As our world becomes increasingly connected, it is imperative for nurses to consider the present world order and how human rights and justice, cultural understanding, and culturally congruent care practices, with an emphasis on caring, ethics, context, and spirituality are in need now more than ever (Martin & Ray, in press, 2016; Ray & Turkel, 2014). The purpose of this chapter is to discuss globally relevant development initiatives needed to promote peace and improve the quality of life of world citizens. Ray's (2010a) Transcultural Caring Dynamics in Nursing and Health-Care Theory and Model is discussed as related to goals established as the United Nations Development Program Millennium Development Goals (MDGs) (United Nations Development Program, 2014).

Marilyn and Mary's Stories

On June 4–8, 2012, Dr. Marilyn Ray and Dr. Mary Brigid Martin attended the John C. Whitehead School of Diplomacy and International Relations, United Nations (UN) Intensive Summer Study Program offered by Seton Hall University, South Orange, New Jersey, led by Dr. Courtney Smith.

We were the first and only nurses ever to attend this annual seminar that has been held for years, mostly attended by political science majors, diplomats, and others in leadership positions. The week's presentations were held at the Church Center for the UN across from the UN headquarters in New York City. Topics presented included the structure, processes, and activities of the UN and its components and the roles of nongovernmental organizations, and a comprehensive tour was offered, including a visit with the director of the Institute for Peace. We dialogued with presenters and recorded journal entries about presentations with a focus on health influences.

The UN is charged with the role of guiding nations worldwide in a direction that supports quality of life for humankind. Its main purposes include international peacekeeping; the development of friendly relations among countries; assistance to nations to improve the lives of the poor; fighting hunger, disease, and illiteracy; supporting human rights; and to be a center for harmonized activities among nations (United Nations, 2015a). As globalization impacts practice, it is essential for nurses to understand the work of the UN because these activities are aligned with nursing's interest in the health and well-being of humankind.

The MDGs are development goals agreed on by the UN member states to improve conditions in the world's poorest countries by 2015 and beyond in an attempt to meet the needs of the poorest of humanity (United Nations Development Program, 2014). The establishment of the MDGs represents a concerted attempt to meet these needs and provide direction and accountability toward their achievement. "The UN Department of Economic and Social Affairs (DESA) [in conjunction with the UNDP] is fully engaged in promoting and supporting the emergence of a solid and ambitious post-2015 development agenda with sustainable development at its centre" (Development Agenda Beyond 2015: The United Nations Millennium Development Goals, August, 2015).

There are eight target areas of concern, each of which has specified goals, objectives, and time frames:

1. To eradicate extreme poverty and hunger
2. To achieve universal primary education
3. To promote gender equality and empowering women

4. To reduce child mortality rates
5. To improve maternal health
6. To combat HIV/AIDS, malaria, and other diseases
7. To ensure environmental sustainability
8. To develop a global partnership for development

Promotion of the MDGs supports awareness of all citizens (both professional and nonprofessional) of international common needs and efforts by which these goals may be achieved. In nursing, knowledge of these initiatives is growing in academic circles, and many frontline nurses address these goals and objectives in practice. Greater articulation of and connections to the MDGs must occur so that nurses can refine practice in effective alignment with this work. We envision a day when the MDGs are household words in a world where all people recognize that its citizens are unequivocally interconnected in mutual needs and desires.

Ongoing efforts to accomplish the work of the aforementioned target areas are undertaken by UN programs and affiliated nongovernmental organizations (NGOs). NGOs and multinational corporations play the most significant roles as nonstate entities in the political goings-on of the UN (Smith, 2006). NGOs may embark on an application process to become affiliated with two branches of the UN: (1) the United Nations Department of Public Information (UNDPI) and (2) the Economic and Social Council (ECOSOC). The UNDPI comprises 1300 NGOs, and the ECOSOC comprises 3500 NGOs (United Nations Department of Public Information, 2015).

NGOs create effective mechanisms for social change and improvement of quality of life in cooperation with the UN. They are free to create their own mission, vision, and goals; select and hire qualified staff; and manage their own budgets; most exist to influence social concerns, rather than endorse political alliances. Although they are obliged to follow governmental regulation, their nongovernmental affiliation positions them to be inclusive, rather than divisive (i.e., endorsing political parties) and self-serving (i.e., endorsing national interests), as governmental agencies may be. Resources of NGOs may vary; for example, the United Nations Foundation (UNF) began with a $1 billion donation from Ted Turner. In nursing, the Sigma Theta Tau International Honor Society of Nursing achieved NGO status in 2009 (Sigma Theta Tau International Honor Society of Nursing, 2015) with the intention to support the MDGs. Although this organization has a much smaller budget and resources than, for example, the UNF, its aims are similar in its support for UN initiatives.

An experience at a NGO in Lebanon conveyed the opportunity for one nurse, Mary Brigid Martin, to learn about the needs of a target group at a local level of global proportion. On a trip to the Middle East, Mary visited the Home of Hope Lebanon (Figures 30-1 to 30-4), a nonprofit organization located outside of Beirut, whose mission is to create a safe, nurturing environment for abused, abandoned, and orphaned children in Lebanon. This center also helps children recover from traumatic events that they have endured and aims to educate them to be intellectually, emotionally, and spiritually prepared to face their futures (Home of Hope Lebanon, 2014). Established by the Lebanese Evangelical Society in 1999, in the support of the National Convention of the Rights of the Child, Home of Hope was intended to serve the large number of children at risk residing in Lebanon (Home of Hope Lebanon, 2014). Most of the children at the center come from a background of violence, abuse, and neglect. Most are brought in from the street by police and have been forced, often by family or child labor ringleaders, to steal and beg for money. Other children brought to the center have come from more desperate situations, such as sex trafficking, drug experimentation, and human organ trafficking (Home of Hope Lebanon, 2014). Ages range from 3 to 18 years; many have lost parents in the recent and ongoing Syrian conflict, have parents in prison, and are without documentation of nationality. A tour of the facility and discussion with the director, Maher Taberani, illuminated many basic organizational needs and the lack of a structured health service for the children.

Figure 30–1: Lebanese flag and Home of Hope sign.

Figure 30–2: Home of Hope building.

Figure 30–3: Another view of the Home of Hope building.

Figure 30–4: Sunset view from Home of Hope.

Home of Hope Lebanon has volunteers on intermittent and regular bases, including a more recent visit from an international team of volunteer health providers; however, it lacks its own health clinic/service. As a volunteer activity, Mary spent 2 days conducting an assessment of the facility with a particular focus on health-related needs of the children. Initially, Mary reviewed the admission documentation conducted in Arabic, documented in Arabic and some English, by support staff; often information is scant. On admission, general hygiene is addressed as well as the presence of any contagious/communicable conditions. Because there is no budget for a nurse or health-care provider, the center director, office staff, or supervisor for boys or girls, depending on availability, carry out admission duties.

At the time of the nursing assessment by Mary, approximately 70 children were at the center (Figure 30-5). Records of a recent visit by a volunteer health team were reviewed that revealed mostly episodic evaluations for which medications were provided. Given the age group, health needs of the children include immunizations, growth and development evaluations, screening, adolescent health, and health and hygiene education. The presence of a volunteer nurse on a regular basis, even for a few hours a week, would help establish health maintenance, episodic, and follow-up care. An Arabic-speaking nurse or the presence of an interpreter is essential. An organized location for health care and medical supplies at the center would greatly improve the conditions for providers to care for the children. The center is always in need of basic necessities to accommodate the growing number of children at the facility. Monetary and material donations are always welcome. Further information is available on the Home of Hope Lebanon website (http://www.homeof hopelebanon.org/home.html).

Figure 30–5: Recreation time at Home of Hope.

AUTHORS' REFLECTIONS

Globalization and migration of populations exist worldwide, and nurses may be most effective in addressing these concerns locally in their practice. The evolving role of the transcultural nurse in local, national, and international policy; human rights advocacy; and inclusive interdisciplinary leadership begins at home. Nurses may become involved in nonprofit organizations and NGOs in their communities that address social concerns such as free health clinics, immigration centers, and human rights groups. On an international level, nurses may stay abreast of trends in nursing by maintaining membership in the International Council of Nurses (International Council of Nurses, 2013), whereby membership is included with national nursing associations. Concerns of the ICN include the reduction in nursing representation at the World Health Organization (WHO), from 2.6% in 2000 to 0.7% in 2012, and the need to increase the number of mental health nurse specialists worldwide (World in Brief, 2012). Awareness of global nursing dynamics may affirm the common needs of the profession within and across nations and support knowledge sharing and collaboration. Technology, communication advancements, and travel have enhanced international collaboration through conferences and professional networking, which may only expand in the future.

Application of Ray's Transcultural Caring Dynamics in Nursing and Health-Care Theory and Model

This section explains the evolution of the theory and the model of Transcultural Caring Dynamics in Nursing and Health Care (Ray, 2010a). In 2010, Ray (2010a) published her theoretical model and data related to transcultural caring dynamics in nursing and health care. As a transcultural nursing scholar and a scholar and researcher of the science of caring in complex health-care organizations, Ray has been committed personally and professionally to understanding the meaning of the relationship between human caring and complex health-care systems as small cultures. With initial research in 1981 and over the course of almost 35 years of the study of the meaning of caring in institutional cultures, Ray discovered the Theory of Bureaucratic Caring (1981, 1989a, 1994, 2010b; Ray & Turkel, 2012, 2015), a synthesis of dimensions of human caring (compassion, spiritual, ethical, education) and organizational systems (sociocultural, economic, political, technological, legal). With the investigative assistance of nurse caring scientist, Turkel, Ray furthered the study of the Theory of Bureaucratic Caring by focusing on technology and economics. The Theory of Relational Caring Complexity (Ray & Turkel, 2012, 2014, 2015) emerged as a transtheoretical model of caring, economics, and factors related to complex health-care systems. In terms of this research, a nurse could see and understand that the meaning of caring in health-care institutions not only involved compassion, spirituality, and ethics but also included the context—the political, economic, technological, and legal phenomena of the social and cultural world of an organization. The contextual integration of caring and sociocultural phenomena illuminated the interplay between the organization as a microculture within the macroculture of a nation or the global community-at-large. One significant publication of Ray in 1994, "Transcultural nursing ethics: A framework and model for transcultural ethical analysis" highlighting the interrelationship between caring and the complex context or the human-environment relationship, became the impetus for creating the book and advancing the book with its theoretical model, Transcultural Caring Dynamics in Nursing and Health Care (Ray, 2010a). Not only is the theoretical model a means to put into action professional nursing from a relational perspective, but it also is a framework for understanding human rights and justice, cultural understanding, transcultural nursing and caring, and culturally congruent care practices. (See Section 1, Chapter 1, "Transcultural Caring Dynamics in Nursing and Health Care," p. 4.)

The dimensions of the theory with its model highlighting the Essence of Caring, Transcultural Caring Ethics, Transcultural Context, Universal Sources and Transcultural Caring Awareness, and Understanding and Choice are relational and holographic—that is, one part is in the whole or the whole itself, and the whole is one part or also the whole. The model is archetypal of relatedness, interconnectedness, communicative, patterned, self-organizational, and emergent—many central tenets of the sciences of complexity (Davidson, Ray, & Turkel, 2011). The dimensions of the model relate primarily to a social caring ethic, a social and cultural goal based on respect for human dignity, diverse cultures, caring, ethics, religions, human rights, and social justice. "… [A] social caring ethic is a practice of how we think after identifying through critical reflection, dialogue, reasoned argumentation, beliefs and values of human dignity, human rights, and justice (or fairness) that must be woven into the cultural fabric of daily life" (Ray & Turkel, 2014, p. 132). The social caring ethic highlights the responsibility of nursing toward a commitment to collective ethical action—communitarian ethics (Ray, 2010b), which highlights the need to give full attention to human rights (respect for all) and social justice (cultural fairness) in nursing. In essence, the process in nursing is emancipatory nursing praxis, a manner of transforming relationships and ultimately the world by understanding the meaning of the interrelationship between the individual and community life as a moral enterprise to facilitate action to build local and global civic cultures for peaceful coexistence (Ray, 1989b, 2010a, 2010b, 2010c; Ray & Turkel, 2014). The growing responsibility of our local and global age, not only for nursing but also for the society-at-large, is to appreciate the authentic meaning of community as relational. The action for authentic cultural knowledge today will not only be highlighting the needs of individual cultures but also showing how cultures will recognize and can assimilate the personal and the mutual, the self and the other, the cultural and the transcultural into practice.

A synopsis of Ray's theoretical model (2010a) includes the following dimensions for application in practice for human rights, social justice, cultural understanding, and culturally congruent care (a type of political and economic caring) (Ray, 1989b).

1. APPLICATION OF THE ESSENCE OF CARING DIMENSION

The goal of nursing practice is to be compassionate and to act justly by enhancing the well-being of others through knowledgeable caring actions (Ray, 1989b, 2010a). As caring philosopher Roach (1987/2002) stated, "[h]uman development and human fulfillment are achieved through the unfolding of the human capacity to care, through investment of the self in others; through commitment to something that matters. Caring is the human mode of being. The capacity to care needs to be nurtured and such nurturing is critically dependent on its being called forth by others" (p. 5). In the Essence of Caring dimension, Ray emphasizes caring as love, empathy, authenticity, compassion, co-presence, availability, attendance, and communication. Nurturing caring is a responsibility not only of the nurse himself or herself but also leaders in nursing (educators, administrators) and patients. Plato remarked that nurturing others (statespersonship or leadership) is considered the highest form of art (Ray, 1997). Thus, the Essence of Caring dimension focuses on the nurturing action of compassion/love as the mediating force to guide moral caring behavior and facilitate right action (justice or fairness) within the dynamics of culture. Understanding nurses' ways of being, knowing, and doing from this perspective calls for a willingness to be in relationship and responsive to others, to be in spirit and human existence together (Chinn, 2013). There is a professional obligation to respect divergent caring expressions—ones different from one's own that may be expressions, for example, of folk or traditional caring practices of some patients and family members—as well as the contemporary ways in which nursing science is viewed. The personal and mutual communal life must be captured. At the same time of attention given to the cultural needs of patients and families, there is the mutual professional obligation to preserve the rights of an organization in terms of overall patient safety issues. Values of nursing that promote caring support the patient, staff, and the health-care organization, again a view of the cultural and human rights of all. The scope of practice and competency for transcultural caring in all specialties of nursing highlight social justice, a social caring ethic, which include specialty certifications, standards of excellence, professional affiliations, and the seeking of higher education. All of the eight MDGs are committed to caring—caring for the poor and hungry; the need for education; gender equality and the empowerment of women; the reduction of child mortality; the improvement of maternal health; the combating of HIV/AIDS, malaria, and other diseases; environmental sustainability; and the development of global partnerships for development (United Nations Development Program, 2014).

2. APPLICATION OF TRANSCULTURAL CARING ETHICS DIMENSION

Application of Transcultural Caring Ethics Dimension relates to understanding diverse and universal ethical values of all people. Ethics is concerned with human actions, human character, or virtue (MacIntyre, 1996). The dimension highlights the ethical knowledge that shapes moral caring experience to facilitate transcultural ethical caring (Ray, 2010a). This dimension responds to the challenge stated by Socrates in 390 (BCE) of "how we ought to live" (Rachels, 2003, p. 1). Transcultural caring ethics (social caring ethics) emphasizes the idea of the good (beneficence—doing good or the affirmation of truth) and being responsible for and having respect for others, also a declaration by health-care ethics organizations in many nations. The other truth is doing no harm (nonmalfeasance), a manifestation of human excellence, and exercise in virtue (MacIntyre, 1996). The theoretical dimension illuminates commitment, trust, respect for persons, justice, truth, fidelity, and integrity that emphasizes advocacy of patients' rights, civil and human rights, and social justice to protect against inhumanity to human beings, poor health care, discrimination, racism, cultural and religious misunderstanding, assaults against the environment, bullying, human trafficking, and poverty, to name a few. For example, this dimension includes the American Nurses Association Nursing Code of Ethics with Interpretive Statements (American Nurses Association, 2001), Universal Declaration of Human Rights (United Nations, 2015b), Civil Rights Act of 1964 (1964), the Constitution of Canada (Government of Canada, 2015a) and the Canadian Charter of Rights (Government of Canada, 2015b), and laws in other countries.

3. APPLICATION OF TRANSCULTURAL CONTEXT DIMENSION

Application of Transcultural Context Dimension relates to understanding how the context within which people live and work impacts especially health and well-being and ultimately health care and nursing practice. The Transcultural Context dimension addresses diverse identities and personal, ethnic, cultural, multicultural values, beliefs, and attitudes about relationships, symbols, and rituals that guide transcultural caring experiences in social, communal, health care, and global cultural systems (Ray, 2010a, p. 4). The UN, particularly by outlining the MDGs, recognized that around the world, there is inequality in terms of health care, economics, human rights, and social justice. If we examine the MDGs as well as conferences examining the dire problems that exist in the world, we can see how often the human voices of a nation are silenced to the political voices where issues of power and control prevail. Health, including well-being, is determined by a nation, its political and public goals, its commitment to public health (clean water, sanitation, protection from communicable diseases), general health care for all, and its ability to provide access to adequate health care (Ray, 2010a). Around the Western world, there is a commitment to providing health care for all, and for many nations trying to find the best economic means available is attempted, even though the care may not always be adequate. It used to be said that the last nation to provide universal health care for its citizens in the West was the United States. However, the Patient Protection and Affordable Care Act (The White House, 2013) was instituted to provide health care insurance for all by improving the health insurance system. Its provisions help many low-income citizens, and the law is showing that the cost of health care is decreasing.

Significant local problems persist in many nations that impact on or create global issues, such as terrorist organizations and the Islamic State, which is waging war in Iraq and Syria and threatening nations in the Middle East and others around the world. The global refugee crisis and its fallout are enormous. Displacement of people from their homelands is widespread. Leaders of many nations are trying to exercise compassion and trying to care for them, but the problems do not stop there. Russia has claimed the Crimea for its own nation and is threatening other areas of the Ukraine. Cyber warfare is rearing its head with one nation, North Korea, attacking a corporation, Sony, and threatening the national security of the United States as well as Asian nations. In the United States, racial incidences, such as the killing of an African American man by police officers in Ferguson, Missouri, and New York, have led to retribution against law enforcement officials. All these problems affect local and global community context, either by direct or indirect means, and illuminate the lack of political and economic caring (Ray, 1987, 2004) and fulfillment of responsibilities of the Universal Declaration of Human Rights (United Nations, 2015b).

4. APPLICATION OF UNIVERSAL SOURCES DIMENSION

In Ray's (2010a) model, Universal Sources addresses the universality of spirituality in humankind. Most cultures around the world express a religious, spiritual, or human or traditional preference or belief that influences the way in which decisions are made that shape and guide transcultural experiences—a nation's political values, rules of law, human rights, social justice, health care, suffering, or end-of-life issues. This dimension gives examples of diverse religions and their precepts or spiritual beliefs.

In relation to local and global communities, there is consensus about the nature of religion and spirituality. However, there are many religious misunderstandings, including "religious" wars such as Israel/Palestine and Sunni/Shia, religious fanaticism, religious fundamentalism, and so forth. Each religion must be taken into consideration in terms of evaluating health and well-being and the decision to be made about care and caring. Also within the UN, the fact that many nations have to appreciate each others' fundamental beliefs to make decisions, for example, about the commitments related to the MDGs, is crucial. Universal Sources are complex and require openness to diverse values and viewpoints in decision making by politicians, negotiators, public health officials, physicians, and nurses. Rather than ignore religious or spiritual values, which the world-at-large today will not permit given the number of conflicts, religions need to be respected and values need to be recognized, and phenomena need to be negotiated when health care is at stake.

5. APPLICATION OF TRANSCULTURAL CARING AWARENESS, UNDERSTANDING, AND CHOICE DIMENSION

The center of the theoretical relational model of Ray (2010a) claims that the dimensions of the Essence of Caring, Transcultural Caring Ethics, Transcultural Context, and Universal Sources must be taken into consideration in relation to personal, professional and interprofessional, local, national, and international decision making. The MDGs for the most part relate to health and well-being. It behooves all nurses and other health-care professionals and political figures to be cognizant of what is the full measure of the meaning of human rights (respect for all persons) and social justice (fairness) so that each person is respected and is given the opportunity to be as healthy as possible with the most affordable health care that a nation can provide, and national and international policies are enacted that reflect love and caring for dignity, the right to freedom, equality, and a basic standard of living that includes freedom from hunger and violence and encourages tolerance and solidarity (United Nations Development Program, 2014). Awareness and understanding of cultural caring, transcultural ethics, transcultural context, and universal sources help in understanding of the universality of caring as well as cultural differences to provide the best opportunities for people to make the right choices for lives that achieve the rights put forth by the MDGs.

In this age of complexity, social ethical responsibilities for transcultural emancipatory nursing praxis with respect to Ray's (2010a) theoretical model of Transcultural Caring Dynamics in Nursing and Health Care and the MDGs should include the following (Ray, 2010a, p. 107):

* Awareness of transcultural and intercultural needs and desires
* Openness to the meaning of relatedness as belongingness and interconnectedness
* Openness to the meaning of relatedness as compassion and justice
* Engagement of spiritual reflection (i.e., faith, hope, and love)
* Openness to the other as similar to ourselves
* Recognition of our common humanity with diverse expressions of beliefs, values, and attitudes

- Implementation of the ethics of respect for persons of the personal-mutual sense of community within the mutual human-environment process
- Co-creation of transcultural communicative spiritual-ethical caring action committed to understanding diverse cultural beliefs, values, and attitudes and actions
- Evaluation of democratic ideals of liberty and equality or other ideals that function or should function with good governments and societies
- Enactment of mutual choice making to serve all equitably
- Openness to possibilities (human rights and social justice)
- Emergence of new patterns of caring interaction (e.g., policy contributions and development)

Transcultural Nursing Reflections

- Reflect on your personal expressions of caring for an ill family member and within caring moments. How do you enact caring? Compare and contrast these customs with another cultural group you have encountered in practice, such as Arab, Pakistani, Iranian, African American, Haitian, or Filipino, to name a few.
- Reflect on your religious faith. Identify your beliefs; values; and attitudes about God, (Christ, Muhammad, Buddha), fate, family obligations, doing good, and death and the afterlife. Compare and contrast these with another faith (e.g., Christianity, Buddhism, Islam, Jehovah's Witness, Mormonism).
- Reflect on your residential community and its context. Describe its demographic makeup; political affiliations; and access to education, health care, and recreational facilities. Identify your observations of the values of your neighbors. How are they similar to and different from yours? How do these values affect perceptions of health and well-being? How may these contrast and compare with a community in another country with which you are familiar?
- Reflect on your political views and affiliations. Identify a country with a different political system than yours. Some examples are a member of the European Union, an African nation, a country in the Middle East, Canada, Australia, Japan, and China. How does the political system compare and contrast with yours in its nature—that is, democratic, dictatorship, parliamentarian system, kingdom, socialist government? How do the citizens of nations you have identified access education and health care (private, public, self-pay, free, etc).
- Describe an ethical dilemma you encountered in the workplace or heard of in the media. Describe the dilemma in regard to the principles of autonomy, beneficence, no malfeasance (doing no harm), and respect for persons.
- Discuss how you may enact rights for your patients in the workplace, community, and nation, including patient rights, civil rights, and human rights. Give specific examples and share stories.

Select Bibliography

American Nurses Association. (2001, 2015). Code of ethics for nurses with interpretive statements. Retrieved from http://www.nursingworld.org/MainMenuCategories/EthicsStandards/CodeofEthicsforNurses/Code-of-Ethics-For-Nurses.html

Civil Rights Act of 1964. (1964). Office of the Clerk, U.S. House of Representatives. Retrieved from http://library.clerk.house.gov/reference-files/PPL_CivilRightsAct_1964.pdf

Chinn, P. (2013). *Peace and power: New directions for building community* (8th ed.). Burlington, MA: Jones & Bartlett Learning.

Coffman, S. (2014). Marilyn Anne Ray's Theory of Bureaucratic Caring. In M. Alligood (Ed.). *Nursing theorists and their work* (8th ed.). St. Louis: Mosby.

Davidson, A., Ray, M., & Turkel, M. (2011). *Nursing, caring and complexity science: For human-environment well being*. New York: Springer Publishing Company.

Government of Canada. (2015a). The Canadian Constitution. Retrieved from http://www.justice.gc.ca/eng/csj-sjc/just/05.html

Government of Canada. (2015b). The Canadian Charter of Rights and Freedoms. Retrieved from http://www.pch.gc.ca/eng/1355260548180/1355260638531

Home of Hope Lebanon. (2014). About Home of Hope. Retrieved from http://www.homeofhopelebanon.org/about.html

International Council of Nurses. (2013). Who we are. Retrieved from http://www.icn.ch/who-we-are/who-we-are/

MacIntyre, A. (1996). *A short history of ethics*. New York: Simon & Schuster.

Martin, M.B., & Ray, M. (2016). Enhancing the role of the transcultural nurse in the global environment. In M. McFarland & H. Wehbe-Alamah (Eds.), *Transcultural nursing: Concepts, theories, research and practice* (4th ed.). Boston: McGraw-Hill.

Rachels, J. (2003). *The elements of moral philosophy* (4th ed.). Boston: McGraw-Hill.

Ray, M. (1981). A study of caring within an institutional culture. PhD Dissertation, University of Utah, Salt Lake City, Utah.

Ray, M. (1987). Healthcare economics and human caring: Why the moral conflict must be resolved. *Journal of Family and Community Health, 10*(1), 35–43.

Ray, M. (1989a). The theory of bureaucratic caring for nursing practice in the organizational culture. *Nursing Administration Quarterly, 13*(2), 31–42.

Ray, M. (1989b). Transcultural caring: Political and economic visions. *Journal of Transcultural Nursing, 1*(1), 17–21.

Ray, M. (1994). Transcultural nursing ethics: A framework and model for transcultural ethical analysis. *Journal of Holistic Nursing, 12*(3), 251–264.

Ray, M. (1997). The ethical theory of Existential Authenticity: The lived experience of the art of caring in nursing administration. Canadian Journal of Nursing Research, 22(1), 111–126.

Ray, M. (2004). A process model for policy analysis with the context of political caring. International Journal for Human Caring, 7(3), 17–24.

Ray, M. (2010a). Transcultural caring dynamics in nursing and health care. Philadelphia: F. A. Davis Company.

Ray, M. (2010b). Creating caring organizations and cultures through communitarian ethics. Journal of the World Universities Forum, 3(5), 41–52.

Ray, M. (2010c). A study of caring within an institutional culture: The discovery of the theory of bureaucratic caring. Germany: Lambert Academic Publishers.

Ray, M., & Turkel, M. (2012). A transtheoretical evolution of caring science within complex systems. International Journal for Human Caring, 16(2), 28–49.

Ray, M., & Turkel, M. (2014). Caring as emancipatory nursing praxis: The theory of relational caring complexity. Advances in Nursing Science, 37(2), 132–146.

Ray, M., & Turkel, M. (2015). Marilyn Anne Ray's Theory of Bureaucratic Caring. In M. Parker & M. Smith (Eds.), Nursing theories and nursing practice (4th ed.). Philadelphia: F. A. Davis Company.

Roach, M. (1987/2002). Caring, the human mode of being (2nd rev. ed.). Ottawa, ON: Canadian Hospital Association.

Sigma Theta Tau International Honor Society of Nursing. (2015). STTI and the United Nations. Retrieved from http://www2.nursingsociety.org/GlobalAction/UnitedNations/Pages/STTIandtheUN.aspx

Smith, C. (2006). *Politics and processes at the United Nations: The global dance*. Boulder, CO: Lynne Rienner Publishers.

The White House. (2013). About the Affordable Care Act. Retrieved from http://www.whitehouse.gov/healthreform

United Nations. (2015a). U.N. at a glance. Retrieved from http://www.un.org/en/aboutun/index.shtml

United Nations. (2015b). The Universal Declaration of Human Rights. Retrieved from http://www.un.org/en/documents/udhr/

United Nations Department of Economic and Social Affairs (DESA). Development Agenda Beyond 2015. Retrieved from http: www.un.org/en/development/desa/development-beyond 2015.html

United Nations Department of Public Information. (2015). NGO resources. Retrieved from http://www.un.org/en/hq/dpi/index.shtml

United Nations Development Program. (2014). The Millennium Development Goals. Retrieved from http://www.undp.org/content/undp/en/home/mdgoverview.html

World in Brief. (2012). *Nursing Standard*, 26(43), 10.

CHAPTER 31

Transcultural Caring Among the Indigenous People of the Cordilleras, The Philippines

AUTHORS' REFLECTIONS

I am very gratified with my work with the indigenous peoples in the Cordilleras, The Philippines. I gather my strength from them . . . my feet are on the ground because of them. I am where I am because of them . . . I opted to stay and serve my country (despite the lure of "greener pastures"). My calling was to serve the people . . . and I have no regrets whatsoever.

Building Context

The Cordillera Administrative Region (CAR) of the Philippines, located in the highest and largest mountain range in the country, comprises one-sixth of the Luzon Island and covers the six provinces of Benguet, Ifugao, Mountain Province, Abra, Kalinga, and Apayao. Grand Cordillera boasts colorful ethnic culture and the prime tourist destinations. In contrast to the region's magnificent points of interest, the present plight of the

401

Cordillera people is characterized by widespread poverty, maldevelopment, and inadequate health service.

Cordillera's local development situation is a reflection of the national situation and of a government that regards the region as a natural resource base to be exploited (Cordillera Peoples' Alliance, 2014). The Cordillera region holds 25% of the entire country's gold resources and 39% of its copper reserves. More local and foreign mining companies are poised to exploit the region's mineral wealth with the liberalization of the mining industry. On one hand, present government policy, through the Philippine Mining Act of 1995, considers the mining industry as a profitable sector for foreign direct investments, but it does not account for the costs of chronic environmental degradation and damage to the health of the miners (CRHRDC, 2010, p. 8). On the other hand, the National Economic Development Authority has consistently placed Cordillera among the 15 poorest regions in the country. In 2012, an estimated 65,516 poor families were accounted for in CAR. Apayao recorded a poverty incidence of 54.7%, making it the poorest in the region and the third poorest province in the country (Balaw-ing, 2014). The chronic issue of poverty compels many to migrate to town centers, other regions, or eventually overseas to look for the proverbial "greener pastures." However, the considerable deficiency in human capital limits the opportunities for the people who chose to migrate.

The condition of the region is likewise complicated by government neglect. As Palaganas (2004) articulated, the state's response to the needs of the indigenous people of Cordillera is inadequate with unsubstantial services. Severe deterioration of health service provision as a result of severe cuts in the national budget for social services, especially health, is evident in the region. As elsewhere in the country, the privatization of the delivery of primary health care in Cordillera led to the transformation of health care into a commodity instead of a basic right (CHESTCORE, 2012). This situation impinges further the opportunity for well-being and economic development among the Cordillera people.

The Cordillera health situation is characterized by malnutrition, a high infant mortality rate, poor sanitation, a high incidence of communicable diseases, lack and poor distribution of health personnel and facilities, and the prohibitive cost of health care (Palaganas, 2004; INNABUYOG, 2008). In addition, according to Alcala and Belingon (2005), "double burden of disease, threat from emerging and resurgent diseases, large variation in health status across population groups, income classes, and geographic areas, and the decentralized health delivery system" (p. 5) exacerbate the already dire health-care situation of the region. The situation in most areas in the Cordilleras is proof of how government policies have left poor people with little or no access to health care.

Health Discrimination and Inadequacy for Indigenous People

The indigenous people of the Cordilleras are among the most marginalized groups politically, economically, and socioculturally. As a group of people who have successfully resisted colonial integration and political assimilation, Cordillera people suffer from a deeply entrenched bias, apathy, and neglect (Palaganas, Bagamaspad, Cardenas, Josef, & Tolentino, 2004). "They experience neglect and discrimination in the provision of basic social services by the government" (Carino, 2012, p. 7). The region continues to receive the lowest budget allocation in the national budget. In 2014, CAR got the lowest allocation despite evidence that it needs more support based on its economic performance and continuing poverty (Agreda, 2013; Cordillera Peoples' Alliance, 2014; Quitasol, Sotelo, & Cabreza, 2013). This budget discrimination translates to poor provision of social services, such as health care, for indigenous territories relative to the rest of the country (Asian Development Bank, 2001; Carino, 2012).

The indigenous people of Cordillera live through poverty on a daily basis manifested by poorly maintained farm-to-market roads, poor flow of market-to-farm information, inaccessibility of a just credit system, and inadequacy or inappropriateness of services (Palaganas & Castillo, 2011, p. 15). These facets of poverty as defined and explicated by indigenous people themselves tell tales of experienced government neglect, maldevelopment, and deprivation in the region.

The joint evaluation of development researchers and practitioners in the region points to the pervasiveness of substandard and expensive social services, especially in medical care and education (CRHRDC, 2010, p. 10). For instance, Marco (2013) found that health and nutrition concerns persisting in indigenous communities could be attributed to the continued absence or lack of basic health personnel, facilities, resources, and information in territories of marginalized, indigenous peoples. The same study suggests that "for many indigenous peoples, poor nutrition, especially among children and mothers, is often a direct or indirect cause of their common illnesses and deaths. They have deficient food intake and diet due primarily to the poverty conditions" (Carino, 2012, p. 8).

One of the most neglected aspects of health care in the region is proper and healthy child delivery. A study by Palaganas (2004) found that in Benguet and Kalinga, most cases of maternal deaths are due to postpartum hemorrhage and abortion; in Apayao, pregnancy-induced hypertension and placenta previa are the most common problems. Postpartum hemorrhage, hypertension, and placental retention are most common in Ifugao; eclampsia, bleeding, and uterine prolapse are common causes in Mt. Province; and in Abra, sepsis-induced abortion is common (Palaganas, 2004). In 2009, the Department of Health National Epidemiology Center reported that the region recorded a 0.6 maternal death rate, translating to delivery-related mortality of 19 in every 10,000 live births (p. 13). National statistics also indicate slow progress in reducing maternal and child health concerns in the region. "The Department of Health reported a decline in maternal deaths in 2011, with 19 per 100,000 compared to 22 per 100,000 in 2010. The deaths rose to 23, however [in 2013]" (Quitasol & Cabreza, 2014). The problems in maternal and child care in Cordillera reflect the observation that efforts and activities to improve the health and nutrition status of women and children in indigenous communities are limited (Marco, 2013).

Indigenous Health Knowledge and Practices

The ability of a group of people to survive creatively in harmony with the environment is understood as indigenous knowledge (Olaniyan, 1982). This knowledge becomes a tool with which local people can make a living in their environment, while adapting to the requirements of their conditions. Indigenous knowledge systems are by and large ecological, organized, and dynamic and tested over centuries of use (Palaganas, 2004). According to Grenier (1998), these various forms of knowledge are "stored in people's memories and activities and exposed in stories, songs, folklore, proverbs, dances, myths, cultural values, beliefs, rituals, community laws, local language, and taxonomy, agricultural practices, equipment, materials, plant species and animal breeds" (pp. 1–2).

The people of Cordillera are able to maintain indigenous knowledge and practices related to health. Commonly referred to as traditional medicine, indigenous health knowledge and practices (IHKP) consist of culturally embedded and ecologically sound practices, methods, and procedures used for the prevention or treatment of diseases and the promotion of health and well-being (Landy, 1977; Palaganas et al, 2004; Shiva, 1997).

Amidst the permeating influence of technological advancements and the pressures of cultural change, traditional health and healing systems remain significant aspects of local institutions and culture of Cordillera indigenous people. The people of Cordillera have undeniably adapted to the changing circumstances of daily life. However, in a milieu where mainstream health-care services remain inaccessible for the most marginalized, IHKP still provide the most viable health service option for the region's indigenous people. In the face of inadequate health-care delivery of the Philippine government, the people of Cordillera are able to nurture and propagate medically sound IHKP in maternal and child health (MCH). The focus of this chapter is to highlight and put into proper perspective IHKP in MCH in relation to Ray's model of transcultural caring.

Cordillera Indigenous Health Knowledge and Practices in Maternal and Child Health

IHKP in MCH is among Cordillera's cultural treasures. Indigenous MCH expertise has been documented as among the region's distinct and culturally specific health maintenance as well as disease preventive and curative practices. Four communities and their MCH are highlighted in this chapter: Badeo of Kibungan, Benguet; Amtuagan of Tubo, Abra; Katablangan of Conner, Apayao; and Western Uma, Lubuagan, Kalinga.

BADEO INDIGENOUS HEALTH KNOWLEDGE AND PRACTICES IN MATERNAL AND CHILD CARE

The community of Badeo, Kibungan, Benguet, can be reached only by 6 to 7 hours of difficult trekking up and down rugged mountains. The isolation of Badeo to purveyors of modernity has resulted in its being one of the remaining areas where IHKP are practiced and maintained (Palaganas, 2004). Neglect is reflected in the health condition of the people of Badeo, which includes malnutrition; a high incidence of preventable and communicable diseases; lack of health personnel, services, and facilities; and prohibitive cost and inaccessibility of health care.

Badeo Birthing Practices and Rituals: The Story of Maxilinda Padilla

Maxilinda Padilla, a Badeo woman, has 12 children, each of which sources say she delivered in different positions. An ethnographic study by Palaganas (2001) gleaned that Manang Maxilinda's birthing positions exemplify indigenous creativity and are very different from the birthing positions in the lowlands. The birthing positions Manang Maxilinda has used are designed to facilitate bearing down and delivery of the baby, in contrast to other, more popular positions that cater to the comfort of the woman delivering the child or to the physician assisting the delivery of the baby.

The Badeo women do not lie down while giving birth; instead, they squat or kneel, making full use of gravity to facilitate the delivery of the baby (Palaganas, 2003). When the birth pains or contractions begin, the woman begins to explore various positions until she finds one that is most conducive to her delivery (Figure 31-1). She may squat, kneel (Figure 31-2), half-stand, or sit on her buttocks with her legs folded as she holds on to a pole for support while she bears down or pushes the baby out. To aid these positions, the Badeo also believe that women during prolonged labor should be given a raw egg to eat for additional strength and warmth or sometimes be fed *pinikpikan* (a traditional Cordilleran chicken dish in which an unplucked chicken is repeatedly beaten with a stick without bloodletting) in the belief that the aroma of the chicken can help facilitate the labor process. After a successful traditional delivery the Badeo way, the umbilical cord is cut using a sharpened bamboo tool called an *epal*, the sole purpose of which is to cut umbilical cords. Afterward, the Badeo keep the umbilical cord inside the house with the belief that it will help their children remember their roots, and then they bury the placenta near the house or place it in a basket that they hang in a nearby tree. After childbirth, the mother is given *abusing*, a concoction made with ginger and lentils mixed with pork fat placed in a coconut shell, which the Badeo believe can

Figure 31–1: A woman explores various birthing positions.

help the woman lactate. Finally, the Badeo observe *tanggad*, a rest period ranging from 1 to 3 months (Palaganas et al, 2001, 2004).

AMTUAGAN INDIGENOUS HEALTH KNOWLEDGE AND PRACTICES IN MATERNAL AND CHILD CARE

Barangay Amtuagan is one of the 10 political divisions of Tubo, Abra. The village is located east of the Abra River (Figure 31-3) and is bordered by two mountains overlooking the Damanil River. Amtuagan is located approximately 15 km away from the municipal towns of

Figure 31–2: Kneeling position.

Figure 31–3: The Abra River.

Tubo and may be reached by different routes. One may get to the Barangay by a 5-hour jitney ride from Bangued to the town center of Tubo, followed by a 3-hour hike from Mayabo to Amtua-gan. Another option is 3-hour vehicle travel from Bangued to Luba plus a 2-hour hike setting off from Sabnangan, Luba, to Sitio Likowan. Although there are rough roads connecting Amtuagan with other Tubo and Luba villages, most of these paths are accessible only during the dry season.

Health services remain inaccessible to the people of Amtuagan. Construction of the Barangay health center was stopped because of lack of funds. A Barangay midwife is stationed in the community, and several Barangay health workers serve as frontliners of health care in the area. The nearest health facility available for the Amtuagan people is in Mayabo, which is 3-hour hike away. The rural health unit does not have a physician; thus, people choose to go directly to Bangued to seek medical attention. The people manually transport the patients using impro-vised stretchers made from a blanket tied on a bamboo pole (Figure 31-4).

Learn More: The Maengs' Knowledge and Practices in Pregnancy and Childbirth

Pregnancy

The Maengs, people of Amtuagan, believe that pregnancy and childbirth is a normal part of a woman's life. Pregnancy for this community is indicated by unexplained headache, nausea, vomiting, and strong pulse in the neck. *Manginaw* and *mangangteg* are believed to be experienced by women in the early stage of pregnancy. *Manginaw* is characterized by cravings for specific food types; *mangangteg* is the dislike for certain routines, odor, or food items. The community does not consider pregnancy as an illness; hence, a pregnant woman may continue daily routines. Women elders have ways of foretelling the sex of the conceived child. If the pregnant woman's skin is reddish, it is believed that the child will be male. If the woman's bulge in the abdomen seems sharp, the child will be male. If the bulge is rounded, the child will be female. If the woman always steps the left feet first when starting to walk, the child will be male. If the bulge in the abdomen is large and seems to have a gap, the woman should expect twins.

Childbirth

A traditional birth attendant, who is also a woman, assists the woman while giving birth. Most Amtuagan women seek the help of a traditional birth attendant when giving birth. It has been a practice for the birth attendant to repeat whatever the woman did before

Figure 31–4: Manually transporting patients using improvised stretchers made from a blanket tied on a bamboo pole.

she felt cramps. If the woman was sewing, the birth attendant should do the same. If the woman opened a bottle, the attendant should open and close the bottle again. It is believed that this activity helps in making child delivery easier for the woman. When a woman is about to give birth, the attendant or her companion would prepare the instrument, made of sharpened bamboo, that will be used to cut the umbilical cord and warm water to bathe the baby after birth.

The woman has the freedom to choose the position where she is most comfortable in giving birth. Positions vary per individual and for every child delivered. Some women prefer a sitting position. Some prefer lying down or squatting. After the child has been delivered, the birth attendant waits for the placenta to be delivered before cutting the umbilical cord. The baby is bathed and wrapped in a warm clean cloth. Oil is rubbed in the infant's palms and feet, especially if the infant's hands and feet are cold because this is believed to help keep the baby warm. The infant is then placed beside the mother for the mother to breastfeed her baby.

The *kadkadua ti ubing*, or the placenta, is washed and either is placed in a basket and hung in a tree or is buried under the house, near the house, or near the doorstep. This is done so that the child may always find his way home when he grows. Some Maengs cut a piece of the placenta, roast it, and soak it in water. The roasted placenta is removed, and the water is brought to the mother to drink. It is believed that drinking this water helps in the speedy recovery of the mother. In cases where the infant is not breathing after delivery, the *kadkadua ti ubing* is massaged until the infant starts to breathe.

Postnatal Care

The mother is not allowed to take a bath on the day she gave birth but should bathe the next day. The mother is allowed to do household chores but not work in the *uma* or rice field for 1 month after giving birth. The mother should not carry heavy objects. Certain kinds of food are not allowed for women who just gave birth and for lactating mothers. Vegetables with trichomes are believed to cause skin diseases. It is believed that the trichomes get into the breast milk. Corn and string beans are believed to cause skin diseases that may spread in large areas of the child's body. Dried beans, especially *kardis*, cause the volume of breast milk to decrease, and dried string beans may cause a painful feeling when breastfeeding. Sweet potato when eaten by a woman who just gave birth is believed to cause parasites, such as pinworm, to come out through the anal opening or the vagina of the mother. *Dodiken* or *agodo*, a kind of shell, is also forbidden. It is believed that eating these causes postnatal bleeding.

Abortion

The indigenous people of Amtuagan believe that abortion may occur for many reasons. Abortion is believed to be caused by a spirit when a pregnant woman passes through another village and is met by a spirit. Overwork and extreme heat may cause abortion. Accidents such as falling or slipping may also bring miscarriage. A woman's emotional health is important during pregnancy. Problems and depression are believed to cause abortion. Induced abortion is not culturally accepted among the *Maengs*. However, some pregnant women abort their unborn child through intake of certain drugs or *sumang*, an herb that can be found in the forest. *Dupilan*, a medicinal plant used to cure arthritis, is also believed to induce abortion.

Excerpts from the Terminal Report (2014) of the national research project entitled "Documentation of Philippine Traditional Knowledge and Practices in Health" and "Development of a Digital Library of Philippine Traditional Knowledge and Practices in Health," a collaborative research project led by the Institute of Herbal Medicine, National Institutes of Health, University of the Philippines Manila with the University of the Philippines Baguio (for the three Indigenous Groups in the Cordillera Administration Region [CAR] of Northern Philippines), funded by the Philippine Council for Health Research and Development (PCHRD).

KATABLANGAN INDIGENOUS HEALTH KNOWLEDGE AND PRACTICES IN MATERNAL AND CHILD CARE

Barangay Katablangan is a home for the Isneg tribe in the Municipality of Conner, province of Apayao. This village is found in the uppermost portions of the rich Barren River and in the middle of abundant natural resources in the gentle mountains and rolling hills. The village may be reached via 5 to 7 hours of hike from Manag, Conner, Apayao.

Learn More: The Isnegs' Knowledge and Practices in Pregnancy and Childbirth

Pregnancy

A pregnant Isneg woman is allowed to eat all kinds of food. She is also allowed to travel to other places for as long as she can endure the hike or the trip. The Isnegs believe that when a woman gets pregnant she may experience a condition that they call *ag-inaw*. *Ag-inaw* refers to the condition in which a pregnant woman likes or dislikes a certain food too much or she does not like the smell of certain food. The pregnant woman may also favor a certain person during the time when she is *ag-inaw*. It is expected of the husband to provide the needs of his wife during this stage. Pregnancy outside marriage is shameful for the community. The woman is blamed for not considering the family's reputation. At the present time, teens are the ones who usually get pregnant outside of marriage.

Childbirth

The traditional birth attendants or *partera* assist the woman in giving birth. Being a *partera* is a voluntary job. The woman or her husband sometimes gives money or goods to the *partera*. However, in most cases with families that cannot afford money or goods, the *partera* is invited for a meal usually after childbirth. To make childbirth easier, the *partera* ties a cloth around the body of the woman just above the bulge in the abdomen. This cloth is pushed downward together with the *ubban* (a light blanket used for carrying the baby). The covers of cooking pots are also removed. Oil is very important in childbirth. The mother is asked to drink some of the oil to facilitate childbirth. During a long labor time, the *tapis* (traditional wraparound skirt for women) is hung in the door. It is believed to shorten labor and facilitate childbirth. Saline solution sometimes is given to the mother who is laboring. Another method to hasten childbirth and shorten labor time is to put a ladder upside down. The placenta is buried where the water flows during the rainy season so that the child will be *tolobug* (well traveled or rise above troubles). To ensure that the child is intelligent, paper and pencil are buried with it.

Breastfeeding and Child Rearing

The breast is cleaned using warm water and clean cloth before the first breastfeeding of the child; this is believed to facilitate the flow of breast milk. Women who are believed to have less breast milk are given soup from grated young papaya and coconut milk. In the past when the mother produced less breast milk, the juice of sugarcane was extracted and given to the child. Soup might also be given. However, this practice is no longer followed at the present time. Fried and other dry food should not be given to the mother. She should always be given soup. Bottle feeding is not practiced in Katablangan except when a mother has died after childbirth. The child's name has to be chosen from the names of his or her ancestors. When a grandparent or grand uncle or auntie has died (before, during, or days after a child has been born), the child is named after him or her. To wean the child, chili or extract from bitter food is placed on the tip of the nipple of the breast. A child may be weaned at 1 year of age; however, it is believed that a child should be breastfed until the age of 2.

Postnatal Care

After giving birth, the woman drinks a solution of water and dried bile of snake. This solution is believed to help in cleaning the blood from the woman's womb. The woman is asked to drink warm water after drinking the solution.

Abortion

Abortion is taboo in the community. It is believed that when a woman commits abortion, she may get sick or die.

Excerpts from the Terminal Report (2014) of the national research project entitled "Documentation of Philippine Traditional Knowledge and Practices in Health" and "Development of a Digital Library of Philippine Traditional Knowledge and Practices in Health," a collaborative research project led by the Institute of Herbal Medicine, National Institutes of Health, University of the Philippines Manila with the University of the Philippines Baguio (for the three Indigenous Groups in the Cordillera Administration Region [CAR] of Northern Philippines), funded by the Philippine Council for Health Research and Development (PCHRD).

UMA INDIGENOUS HEALTH KNOWLEDGE AND PRACTICES IN MATERNAL AND CHILD CARE

Western Uma, Lubuagan, Kalinga, is a home of the Uma tribe of Kalinga province; it is one of the barangays within the Municipality of Lubuagan lying 800 m above sea level and found in the eastern part of the CAR. The community is found in the middle of rugged mountains and surrounded by rivers, springs, waterfalls, and creeks. Western Uma according to the elders was once known by the name, *Wowok*, or "water source," because you can find a water source everywhere. From Tabuk City, which is the capital center of Kalinga Province, Western Uma may be reached via a 5- to 7-hour bumpy jitney ride.

Learn More: Uma Beliefs and Rituals on Birthing and Childcare

Ilom

Ilom is a ritual done by the tribe for couples to have a healthy firstborn child. It is conducted when the wife is pregnant and if the couple is having difficulty conceiving. The family of the man is responsible for the *basi* (sugarcane wine), and the family of the woman butchers a pig or chicken to welcome the *basi*; this is called *palanus* of the *basi*. *Palanus* is a ritual for welcoming a person or significant things. During this ritual, the elders in charge of the ritual put a piece of log together with the *gamugam* (combination of various leaves and grass and all the things to be used for the ritual) and a clay pot in front of the couple's house. Sugarcane, rattan, and coconut leaves also are put inside the house. The couple's parents cook *jekot*, which is usually *kilampayay*, and put it in front of the house, after that they call the couple to eat. When the couple are done eating, the people present during the ritual throw *kilampayay* first on the couple, next on their parents, and then on each other. If somebody brings *pilanteyok* (pulverized *jekot* cooked with sugar), the people put it in bowls and pour it on anybody. A merry-making activity starts when everybody runs from the person holding *kilampayay* and *pilanteyok*. However, this activity is done less today because it was realized that food for which the people work hard was being thrown.

Konted

For every newborn baby, parents butcher a native chicken. If the baby is a girl, they butcher a *upa* (hen), and if it is a boy, they butcher a *kawitan* (rooster). This is done to celebrate the birth of the baby. For the Uma tribe, if this ritual is not performed, the baby will grow sickly. Families who can afford to do so complete the ritual of butchering native chickens for a period of 10 days. Poor families must complete the ritual a for a minimum of 3 days. The ritual was patterned to the three rocks in a *jepong* (hearth). If the family performs it for only 1 or 2 days, it is not balanced like the hearth where three rocks are needed to balance a pot. The *konted* should be *lajejepong*, meaning "balanced."

Gabbok

This ritual is not strictly practiced today because it is costly. However, during the time of the tribe's ancestors, it was a requirement. This ritual is done for every firstborn girl and boy in the family. Most of the time, this ritual is performed if the firstborn is sick. The illness is attributed to the spirits of the ancestors, and to appease the spirits, the family has to perform the *gabbok*. A *mandadawak* from the tribe or from the other neighboring tribes facilitates the celebration. The *mandadawak* prays that the couple and the child will be healthy. The parents usually butcher a pig, and the tribe dances to the beat of gongs. The feast also includes a *gamugem* that is composed of *allilison* (a species of fern), *gawed* (a leaf chewed together with the betel nut), *buwa* (betel nut), *iwoy* (rattan), *unas* (sugar cane), *tagaupay* (herb that thrives in upland rivers and in moist soil), coconut leaf, betel nut leaf, *byakka* with the pig's *ogtoy* (liver), and unhusked rice.

Obyen

Obyen is a tradition done usually after the *gabbok*. The parents cook *jekot* and bring the baby to the husband's parents. The *jekot* is distributed to both husband and wife's relatives as a sign that the family already performed the *obyen*. The grandparents welcome the baby by butchering a pig or chicken depending on their social status. All relatives who receive *jekot* help in the ritual. Some important things that they give the family with their firstborn are *fonge* (jade necklace), *piling* (porcelain plate), and the *obyen* (baby carrier cloth), which is also called *kagoy*. When they go back home, the family brings back half of the butchered pig, which they call *liyom*. The *liyom* is an exchange for the *jekot* that they distributed. When the family goes to the house of the wife's parents, the *liyom* is distributed to her relatives. If the wife's parents can afford it, they welcome the baby with butchering another pig.

Excerpts from the Terminal Report (2014) of the national research project entitled "Documentation of Philippine Traditional Knowledge and Practices in Health" and "Development of a Digital Library of Philippine Traditional Knowledge and Practices in Health," a collaborative research project led by the Institute of Herbal Medicine, National Institutes of Health, University of the Philippines Manila with the University of the Philippines Baguio (for the three Indigenous Groups in the Cordillera Administration Region [CAR] of Northern Philippines), funded by the Philippine Council for Health Research and Development (PCHRD).

Western Biomedical Perspective: A Review of Davis-Floyd's Technocratic Model of Birthing and the Technocratic Imperative

The developing world has experienced the massive importation of westernized modes of birth, including adopting Western medical approaches to birth, resulting in devaluing their indigenous practices. Davis-Floyd (2003) writes about the technocratic model of birthing and the role of obstetrics in the resolution of cultural anomaly. This model encompasses the technocratic imperative—if it can be done with technology, it must be done with technology. This imperative has been heavily embraced in the developing world, which has suffered at the hands of Western technologies and now looks to them for progress and equalization.

Davis-Floyd (2003) lays down the standard procedures for normal birth and symbolically analyzes these, constructing a model of birth allowing him to compare the technocratic to the more cultural and natural. He also tackles the ideology of safety, one that is constantly challenged by home remedies when it comes to sensitive processes such as birthing. The contemporary relevance of Davis-Floyd's book is anchored mainly on the dichotomy between the technocratic and holistic paradigms of birth. The technocratic paradigm stresses the distinction—alienation, even—of practitioner from patient, whereas the holistic paradigm stresses the importance of their relationship as well as the emotional content of care. Davis-Floyd (2003) claims that the holistic and more humanistic practice in reality is nearly impossible to achieve, especially in contemporary, public, and highly modernized hospitals.

Most women desire the humanistic practice, yearning for caring, compassion, and respect for their desires, wishes, and choices without the intervening process. Despite the influence of this more emotion-invested paradigm, the technocratic model still remains hegemonic. With increasing evidence of the unnecessary and often harmful nature of obstetrical procedures published by medical, psychological, anthropological, and lay presses, many individuals involved with birth are asking how it is possible that a medical specialty that purports to be scientific can appear to be so irrational (Davis-Floyd, 2003).

Still, most women lean toward hospital delivery; in fact, so few nurses and obstetricians have ever seen truly "natural" childbirth that most have no idea what childbirth can be like when it is left to proceed on its own. Routine obstetrical procedures such as intravenous feeding, electronic monitoring, and episiotomy are believed by the people who perform them to transform the unpredictable and uncontrollable natural process of birth into a relatively predictable and controllable technological phenomenon that reinforces our contemporary society's most fundamental belief about the superiority of technology over nature (Davis-Floyd, 2003).

Davis-Floyd (2003) states that most discussions on the qualitative difference between births with the woman's own rhythm and births on which institutional rhythms are superimposed are almost never heard in medical schools or conferences. Similarly, in the Philippines and most especially in more deprived and remote areas, discussions on the differences of the two paradigms hardly exist, but for a different reason: Because there is only one mode of delivery—the natural one, safe in the confines of the home surrounded by the community. This situation is in stark contrast with the one in more developed countries, with the technocratic imperative hovering above the Western biomedical scene. Traditional midwifery, although still vital, is already a vanishing occupation.

Finally, Davis-Floyd states, "I have a strong commitment to home birth and freestanding birthing centers as safe and viable options deserving the same cultural respect as the choice for hospital birth" (2003), a commitment resulting from the study's result, which demonstrates the safety of planned, midwife-attended home birth. Davis-Floyd is focusing not on eliminating the "overtechnologization" of birth but rather on keeping open the spectrum of choice.

The Truth Behind Ritual Home Birthing

A common tenet of modern thought holds that the transfer of the birthplace from home to hospital that has taken place in U.S. society represents the deritualization of what in other, more "primitive" societies has traditionally been a process laden with superstition and taboo. Originators of this belief, the members of our medical profession, hold that obstetrical procedures are determined by physiological reality. On the contrary, however, I suggest that the removal of birth to the hospital has resulted in a proliferation of rituals surrounding this natural physiological event more elaborate than any heretofore known in the "primitive" world. These rituals, also known as "standard procedures for normal birth," work to effectively convey the core values of American society to birthing women (Davis-Floyd, 2003, pp. 1–2).

It all sounds informed and a good point of interest in the discourse of medical procedures of birth care. Birthing is a very important life event. Not only does it bring about a new life, but it also ushers in a new member of the society. More traditional communities treat it as a rite of passage and proceed to embellish it with cultural items and rituals, such details generally serving to imbue the individual with a sense of cosmic importance within the group.

Various areas of Cordillera are rich with a variety of culture and rituals they apply in all forms of life-changing events, especially when it comes to birthing. Now the question most are probably afraid to ask is: Are their birth delivery practices primarily rituals deeply embedded in their culture, or are these ways for them to cope with the obvious disparity when it comes to primary health care and exposure to technology and health services?

They are first cultural. But more importantly, they are practical choices. Labeling them as "primitive rituals" is a luxury because the reality is these communities are highly deprived of government care and attention. So they make do with what they have—caring community members, indigenous creativity, and a strong belief of their own ideologies.

Most of the women in Cordillera admit to preferring giving birth at home because they are ashamed of showing their bodies to nonfamily members and are afraid of episiotomy or what they call *makartiban*, but mostly because they could not afford hospital bills (Palaganas, 2004). If you can give birth in the comfort of your home surrounded by people you have known since you were a child and who you know truly care for you, it's the best choice for you, naturally. As Davis-Floyd (2003) says, the most important determinants of the outcome of a woman's birth are the attitudes of her primary caregiver.

The Interception of Indigenous Health Knowledge and Practices and Biomedicine

Cultures from all over the world have developed different views of health, healing, and care. "Many of them are rooted in traditional systems of beliefs, which indigenous people use to understand and interpret their biophysical environment" (Laccarino, 2003). Science has become a dominant order often construed not only as foremost but also intolerant toward other systems. Likewise, much of the debate is between science and indigenous knowledge. According to Durie (2004), this debate takes three distinct forms: (1) the opposition to the promotion of science as the only valid body of knowledge, (2) the rejection of science in favor of indigenous knowledge, and (3) the misinterpretation of knowledge by the use of system-bound criteria.

Highlighting the debate on IHKP versus bioscience in MHC, the Department of Health passed an Administrative Order 2008-0029, "Implementing Health Reforms Towards Rapid Reduction in Maternal and Neonatal Mortality," called the "No Home Birthing Policy." This policy discourages home births and home births assisted with traditional birth attendants, including midwives. The goal to provide safe delivery in birthing facilities may be noble, but taking the context of the indigenous peoples of the Cordilleras into consideration, this measure is unrealistic. Instead of recognizing this and providing health services that revolve around IHKP on birthing practices that are widely documented and recognized by medical practitioners (Cunningham, MacDonald, & Gant, 1989; Davis-Floyd, 2003; Johnson, Posner, Biermann, Cordero, Atrash, Parker, 2006; McKay & Mahan, 1984; Oxorn & Foote, 1975), it further widens the gap of transcultural caring in the health-care delivery system. In the case of Cordillera, health knowledge and practices on MHC is at an interface. MCH is informed by both science and indigenous knowledge. Although people do not rely exclusively on bioscience or indigenous knowledge, the inaccessibility of health social services makes IHKP a more viable choice for the prevention and cure of MCH-related concerns.

Concept of Transcultural Caring

In understanding indigenous notions of care, one must relate culture to patterns of learned behavior and values that are interpreted and shared among a group. For this group of people, understanding their beliefs and lifestyle is key to assessing their care system and provision of a culturally congruent health care.

Matay-eo's (2013) paper about the Cordillerans and their philosophy regarding their ancestral domain put in perfect words the Cordilleran concept of care. Care is nurturing indigenous identity. It inculcates an appreciation for cultural processes and not just cultural products. Indigenous knowledge is a temporal awareness of technologies and practices such as farming, health, agriculture, craftsmanship, and artistry explained specifically in contemporary terms. The culture mentality of Cordillera engenders the respect to elders as teachers. There is an intergenerational relationship where children listen to the wisdom of the elders in relation to how life is to be lived. The elders show the primordial importance of community life as something corporate, which must be continual from one generation to another (Matay-eo, 2013, p. 18).

Care, in the most holistic sense for the Cordillerans, is nurturing their indigenous identity. Whether it be in terms of their ancestral domain and dwelling or in terms of individuals as members of a community and of a bigger whole, their concept of care is one that is grounded strongly in their culture and identity—"indigenous ways of knowledge generation, documentation and refinement about listening to wisdom of the elders, dances, chants, real life dramas among others" (Matay-eo, 2013, p. 18). In nurturing their culture and identity is the constant and continuous passing on of their core mentalities as a community. According to Matay-eo, the Cordilleran concept of care took its genesis from the idea of a community's experience of solidarity or empathy. Further, solidarity and acting together is inherent among people in Cordillera. For these indigenous people, reflecting on one's existence in relation to others is a significant aspect of a person's growth as an individual and as a member of a community. Their years of struggle and history of people's movement likewise speak of their spirit of oneness as mountain ethnic tribes.

The people of Cordillera believe that there are stewards for everything on earth (trees, bodies of water, forest, etc). These stewards can be spirits of ancestors or spirits of nature. Whatever activities people are going to conduct in their environment requires rituals to inform and be in accord with the stewards' will. Cordillera indigenous people also deem that all actions of a person toward his or her fellow men or women and to the environment have repercussions to a person's health. Being greedy of hunting and gathering could make the stewards angry and cast illness to the doer of the action. Doing injustice against one's neighbor can make a person suffer ill luck or bad health. Cordillerans' optimum well-being depends on how they respect and care for the environment and their fellows.

Care is more than a dynamic system of beliefs and cultural practices, but rather a long line of indigenous knowledge passed on for the members to take part in the process of healing and wholeness. When one looks at the various cultural embellishments with which the Cordillerans surround their MCH knowledge and practices, one may see a variety of options: (1) a rich and well-preserved cultural bind to their age-old beliefs and rituals, (2) a means of coping with their impoverished situations and insufficient basic health care needs, and (3) the essence of transcultural caring ethics within a community.

Ray's Conceptual Model of Caring

This chapter endeavors to lay out the facts and cases of Cordilleran MCH tradition juxtaposed with the area's obvious lack of primary health care attention. It also aims to apply Ray's (2010) model of transcultural caring to understand better the ways with which Cordillerans cope with their underprivileged situation, while maintaining the long line of indigenous knowledge they hope to preserve by passing on.

DIMENSION 1 OF RAY'S MODEL: THE ESSENCE OF CARING

The Cordilleran concept of caring is one that is rooted in their beliefs and value systems and respect for their ancestral domain. Macli-ing Dulag, a Kalinga elder and leader during the struggles against the construction of Chico Dam in the 1980s, said that *ti daga ket biag* ("land is life") (Carino, Gimenez, Loste, & Verzola, 2009). Ancestral domain, often used interchangeably with ancestral land, covers the biophysical and human environment where indigenous communities live. Land as the central determinant of the lifeways of people was elaborated in accurate terms: In the language of ecology, the organism's right to habitat entails the prior basic rights of the organism to define and set the terms of its relationship with the environment. Land laws or rules of land use and land resource management are inherent expressions of this fundamental relationship (Carino et al, 2009).

Land is the main determinant of the life of the organism, for land is primary environment and habitat. The relationship of the human organism to land, whether in subjugation or in self-determination, constitutes the infrastructure of societal group life. All others—religion, health, laws, all moral and cultural ways, and relationships of the human organisms—are superstructures that reinforce and validate the basal substructure. These bureaucratic structures arise from and are shaped by antecedent orientations by a priori motive forces (CPA, 2009, p. 33).

Cordillera people's IHKP are based on their land and their resources. In their effort to find various ways to survive using the parts of their own homeland, they have developed a holistic concept of care. They use practical knowledge in familiar ways to care for others by focusing on the use of homes, community, and other familiar resources. Health and healing are likewise performed as household or community rituals and activities.

DIMENSION 2 OF RAY'S MODEL: TRANSCULTURAL CARING ETHICS

In the search for ethical understanding, human actions and character or virtue are examined and challenged. Ethics demands serving the good and owning responsibility for others and encourages the virtue of personal fidelity and commitment to a dynamic and dignified system of truths and values (Ray, 2010). The people of Cordillera, in more specific and ethnically sensitive terms, possess a "consistent and highly integrated and ecologically harmonious system of knowledge that involves life cycles, major life events and health issues" (Palaganas, 2004, p. 135).

Life in the Cordilleras is difficult. Despite the rapid technological advancements of the lowlands or the nearby cities, the people of Badeo, Uma, Katablangan, and Amtuagan rely on a way of life that has been passed on to them by their ancestors. They cling to many traditions, not only because they wish to maintain and preserve them but also and more so because they consider their value system important for their survival. The concept of health is one of the most integral in their belief system. Cordilleran health ethics are guided by people's belief in the existence of unseen beings, deities, and spirits that possess mighty power to grant or deprive them of good health. This knowledge shapes their moral caring experience, which facilitates transcultural ethical caring.

One of the basic tenets in the search for ethical understanding is utilitarianism and social contract. These theories underscore right actions and moral rules to gain the benefits of social living. These concepts revolve around the fact that "we must be able to count on each other, so as not to harm each other deliberately, to rely on people to keep their contracts and share their resources," and that "each person's welfare is equally important" (Ray, 2010, p. 67). These concepts, when put in a collage and integrated, build a diverse system of complex and dynamic transcultural ethics as grounded on the community's long line of traditions and beliefs.

The immediate purpose of transcultural ethics is to hear the other and learn from the other with mutual respect. To highlight and to propel forward the Cordilleran communities' cultural health practices as a reflection of poverty is to validate the need to challenge further the lack of support for indigenous health care ethics and knowledge.

DIMENSION 3 OF RAY'S MODEL: TRANSCULTURAL CONTEXT

Tiller wrote: "We are all connected. We are entangled . . . And there is no real separation between us, so that what we do to another, we do to an aspect of our self . . . We can't really turn our backs on it because we are all co-creators somehow or another. And we have to do the right things to try to get the future that is best for all of us" (in Ray, 2010, p. 226).

The experiences of Cordillerans vary widely depending on the social, cultural, economic, and political phenomena of the time. The dimensions of Ray's model (2010) revolve around the person, his or her background and acculturation, and the system of which he or she is a part. A person's diverse identities guide his or her transcultural experience in social, communal health-care, and global cultural systems. Meaning of identity, position, and responsibility of the person in the family, community, society, culture, and world all contribute toward building a transcultural context. This composition changes rapidly and with these changes is the desire to maintain a connection to specific cultural and ethnic identities and traditions (Ray, 2010). The Cordillerans have had quite a past: They have lived and survived generations of struggle to protect their identity, ancestral lands, and cultural traditions (Palaganas, 2004, p. 109). Their concept of care and transcultural ethics is strongly guided by their culture and traditions. Their system of health, illness, healing, and caring is rooted from their past experiences written down in history.

The transcultural context illuminates the interrelationship between the person and the other or a community and one other (Ray, 2010). In this case, it illuminates the interrelationship between the community and their history, the community and their struggles, and the community and the cosmos. According to Thomas (2003, in Ray, 2010, p. 15), "on the one hand, we look outward and attempt to see the world for what it is, and on the other hand, we look inward to grow in understanding of ourselves." We are all linked together, and when it comes to health and caring, it is always just a matter of perspective, of proper context to be successful in the search for understanding and comprehension of a culture's dynamics.

FemPov: Assessing Devlopment: Designing Better Indices of Poverty and Gender Equity

The FemPov (Rural Poverty) Research by Palaganas and Castillo (2011) was developed and tested as an alternative poverty and gender disparity assessment tool. The project engaged participants who are considered poor to illustrate that measures of poverty and gender disparity can be developed by drawing from the points of view of the poor and that there are dimensions other than income that can be considered in deciding whether a person is poor or not. The study was conducted in the Cordilleras, particularly in the Gad-dang indigenous community of Bantay, Paracelis, Mountain Province.

AUTHORS' REFLECTIONS

My work among the indigenous peoples of the Cordilleras as a community health and development researcher exposed me to the various challenges of community and development work in the country. My exposure to the realities of the nursing profession made me a critical thinker and staunch advocate of people's rights, community participation, indigenous knowledge and practice, and genuine community development. It has grounded me to the reality that nurses and health-care practitioners need to espouse a more holistic perspective of caring. We need to be concerned and engaged with transforming the health-care system to address the relationship between poverty and diseases. As such, we need to be aware of the complex array of social, political, economic, and demographic factors that influence human response to health and illness. This means that we should examine the philosophy underlying our practice and be prepared to advocate, lobby, and effect changes that are consistent with the notion of holistic caring that includes social change and empowerment.

Research is a dialogue. My interactions and uninhibited discourses with the indigenous peoples of the Cordilleras opened their world. I recognized and learned from the well-spring of information, wisdom, and knowledge in the stories they shared. I realized that I underwent a journey of understanding and that I should give back. A caring nurse has to respond and use the "data" to improve the lives of the people he or she touches. For this reason among many others, being insightful of indigenous people's context and culture has molded me to be the health activist that I am today. For example, my position as an antimining advocate is rooted in my realization that indigenous health care knowledge is based on the land and resources; hence, advocating for indigenous people's health comes with the inherent recognition of the value of keeping the integrity of their land.

A caring nurse and health professional needs to look at the gamut of community development. A caring nurse engages in a more humanistic relationship by listening to the people and by grounding solutions to health concerns. By listening to people's experiences and aspirations, we are able to advance their interests, and we are able to respond appropriately. This means that we are socially sensitive and value service to the people.

Understanding what has shaped the indigenous people's lives and how they have responded to their context, we must continue exploring their perspectives. Exploring what they think and feel about what we do and how we do things will not only evaluate the relevance and effectiveness of our work but also strengthen the concepts and theories we practice.

Acknowledgments

I thank my colleagues and research teammates, Marian C. Sanchez, Executive Director, Luke Foundation, Inc., and Ruel Caricativo, Instructor, Department of Economics and Political Science, University of the Philippines, Bagio, for their valuable suggestions in the conceptualization, formulation, and critique of this chapter. Research is always a great journey with great people like Marian and Ruel.

For additional information regarding the indigenous people of the Cordillera region of the Philippines, see the following link by Desiree Caluza, a writer, journalist, poet, and painter who covers stories on culture, human rights, rights of indigenous peoples, and traditional healing practices: http://www.positivelyfilipino.com/magazine/?author=53320eabe4b0fba62007d1f6.

References

Agreda, J. (2013). *Cordillera has lowest 2014 budget*. Retrieved from http://www.sunstar.com.ph/baguio/local-news/2013/08/09/cordillera-has-lowest-2014-budget-297007

Alcala, J., & Belingon, E. (2005). Cited in Dacany, E.F. (Ed.). *Regional Health Research Agenda for the Cordillera Administrative Region*. Baguio, Philippines: Saint Louis University College of Medicine.

Asian Development Bank. (2001) Annual report. http://www.adb.org/documents/adb-annual-report-2001

Balaw-ing, S. (2014). *Decrease in poverty seen in Cordillera*. Retrieved January 6, 2015, from http://www.sunstar.com.ph/baguio/local-news/2014/01/02/decrease-poverty-seen-cordillera-321256

Carino, J.K. (2012). *Country Technical Notes on Indigenous Peoples' Issues: Republic of the Philippines*. Retrieved from http://www.ifad.org/english/indigenous/pub/documents/tnotes/philippines.pdf

Carino, J., Gimenez, L.A., Loste, M.A., & Verzola Jr. P. (2009). *Ti Daga ket Biag, Land Is Life*. Baguio City, Philippines: Cordillera Peoples Alliance.

CHESTCORE. (2012). *Annual Program Report*. (Unpublished). Baguio City, Philippines: Community Health Education, Services and Training in the Cordillera Region (CHESTCORE).

CRHRDC, 2010. *Health Research Agenda of the Cordillera Region*. Baguio City, Philippines: PCHRD-DOST.

Cordillera Peoples' Alliance. (2009). Ti Daga Ket Biat (Land is Life): Selected reading from three Cordillera multisectoral land congresses (1983, 1994, adn 2001), Baguio City: Cordillera Peoples' Alliance.

Cordillera Peoples' Alliance. (2014). *Cordillera Day 2014: Central Statement Resist Imperialist Plunder of Our Land and Resources! Assert Our Right to Self Determination!* Retrieved from http://www.katribu.org/content/cordillera-day-2014central-statement-resist-imperialist-plunder-our-land-and-resources-assert

Cordillera Regional Health Research and Development Committee (CRHRDC). (2010). Health Research Agenda of the Cordillera Region. Baguio City, Philippines: PCHRD-DOST.

Cunningham, F.G., MacDonald, P.C., & Gant, N.F. (Eds.). (1989). *Williams obstetrics* (18th ed.). Norwalk, CT: Appleton & Lange.

Davis-Floyd, R.E. (2003). *Birth as an American Rite of Passage*. Oakland, CA: University of California Press.

Department of Health National Epidemiology Center. (2008). The 2008 Philippine heath statistics. Manila: Department of Health.

Durie, M. (2004). Understanding health and illness: Research at the interface between science and indigenous knowledge. *International Journal of Epidemiology, 33*, 1138–1143.

Grenier, L. (1998). *Working with Indigenous Knowledge: A Guide for Researchers*. Ottawa, ON, Canada: International Development Research Centre.

INNABUYOG, Alliance of indigenous women's organizations in the Cordillera, Philippines. (2008). *Statement on the Occasion of World Rural Women's Day and World Foodless Day*. Cordillera, Philippines: Alliance of Peasants in the Cordillera Homeland.

Johnson K, Posner SF, Biermann J, et al. CDC/ATSDR Preconception Care Work Group; Select Panel on Preconception Care. Recommendations to improve preconception health and health care—United States. A report of the CDC/ATSDR Preconception Care Work Group and the Select Panel on Preconception Care. MMWR Recomm Rep. 2006;55(RR-6):1-23. Cited in Kozhimanni, K.B., & Fontaine, P. (2013). Care from family physicians reported by pregnant women in the United States. *Annals of family medicine, 11*(4), 350-354.

Laccarino, M. (2003). Science and culture. *EMBO Reports, 4*, 220–223.

Landy, D. (1977). Medical systems in transcultural perspective. In D. Landy (Ed.), *Culture, disease and healing* (pp. 129–131). New York: Macmillan Publishing.

Marco, J. (2013). *The health and nutrition situation of children and women in indigenous communities: A preliminary review*. Manila, Philippines: DLSU Social Development Research Center.

Matay-eo, F. (April 9, 2013). *Ancestral domain as a philosophy of dwelling among the Cordillera indigenous peoples*. Presented at The Rise of the East and the Decline of the West, Philippine Philosophy at the Crossroads (Philosophical Association of the Philippines, Inc.), Ateneo de Manila University, Quezon City, The Philippines.

McKay, S., & Mahan, C.S. (1984). Routines: Laboring patients need more freedom to move. *Contemporary OB-GYN, 24*, 90–119.

Olaniyan, R. (1982). *African history and culture*. London: Longman Group United Kingdom.

Oxorn, H., & Foote, W. (1975/2013). *Human labor and birth*. New York: McGraw-Hill.

Palaganus, E.C. (2001). Mainstreaming indigenous health Knowledge and Practices. Quezon City: University of the Philippines-Center for Integrative and Development Studies.

Palaganas, E.C. (2003). *Health Care Practice in the Community*. Manila, Philippines: Educational Publishing House.

Palaganas, E.C. (2004). *Health consequences of gender-based knowledge, attitudes and practices*. Baguio, Philippines: UP Baguio Cordillera Studies Center.

Palaganas, E.C., & Castillo, F. (2011). *Terminal report: Assessing development: Designing better indices of poverty and gender equity (Rural poverty)* (FemPov). Canberra, Australian Capital Territory: Australian National University.

Palaganas, E.C., Bagamaspad, A., Cardenas, M, Josef, J., & Tolentino, L. (2004). Science and indigenous health knowledge and practice. In F. Alvarez-Castillo (Ed.). *(Re)framing old issues, bridging divides in Health*. Philippine Health Social Association.

Quitasol, K., & Cabreza, V. (2014). *PH far from hitting dev't target, but RH law may help, say execs*. Retrieved from http://newsinfo.inquirer.net/605814/ph-far-from-hitting-devt-target-but-rh-law-may-help-say-execs.

Quitasol, K., Sotelo, Y., & Cabreza, V. (2013). *Cordillera needs funds most, but gets lowest budget*. Retrieved from http://newsinfo.inquirer.net/462771/cordillera-needs-funds-most-but-gets-lowest-budget#ixzz3QLr8yl7d

Ray, M. (2010). *Transcultural caring dynamics in nursing and health care*. Philadelphia: F. A. Davis Company.

Shiva, V. (1997). *Biopiracy and the plunder of nature and knowledge*. New Delhi: Research Foundation for Science, Technology and Ecology.

Umil, A.M. (2013). *Banning home births to worsen, not improve maternal death rate—health groups*. Retrieved from http://bulatlat.com/main/2013/04/09/banning-home-births-to-worsen-not-improve-maternal-death-rate-health-groups

Coming to Know a Community: A Community Assessment in Rural Haiti

*R*esponding to a call for nursing, we, a team of nurses and clergy, arrived in Haiti midmorning, anxious to help a country so recently devastated by a 7.0 magnitude earthquake. From our taxi windows we could see partially crumbled buildings, piles of debris, and a tent city sheltering thousands of families who lost their homes, livelihoods, and, in many cases, family members and friends in the earthquake. Yet the streets in downtown Port-au-Prince were bustling with vendors selling wares and buyers bargaining for a good price. As outsiders, we seemed to be in the midst of a population struggling with loss while picking up the pieces and living life to the fullest.

The drive through the capital to our destination in rural Haiti was hot, bumpy, and spellbinding. The road along the coast revealed the beautiful hues of the Caribbean Sea, while the streams of children walking to school dressed in distinct colorful uniforms added to the uniqueness of the towns and villagesalong the way. We finally reached our destination and found the village marked for the first time with a public road sign. We all thought this is progress toward becoming a name and place on a map.

The parochial school community was waiting for us. The children emerged from class-rooms. The girls were dressed in the school uniform, green gingham shirts, matching hair ribbons, and khaki colored jumpers. The boys were dressed in green gingham shirts and khaki shorts. The students, teachers, and pastor greeted us warmly. A hot lunch had been pre-pared for us, and after a tour of the grounds, a group of leaders and elders was gathered for an inquiry group focused on coming to know the hopes and dreams for health and wellness in this community.

Coming to Know a Community: History

The story of Haiti and the Haitian people is a complex picture of exploration, beauty, natural resources, and wealth as well as poverty, exploitation, oppression, and colonization. The Arawak/Taino Indians inhabited the land and referred to their home as "Hayti" for the mountainous land of palm trees and colorful flowers. Christopher Columbus arrived in 1492 and called the island Hispaniola. Because of its location in the Caribbean and its natural resources, the land was sought after by many nations. In the 17th century, France and Spain fought over the land and finally in 1697 divided the land into two countries, Haiti and the Dominican Republic (World Health Organization, 2010).

During the next 100 years, the Haitian people were enslaved and suffered infamous brutality and inhumane treatment. The French elite became rich through the slave trade and the export of cotton, sugarcane, tobacco, and coffee. In the last decade of the 18th century, Toussaint L'Ouverture, a self-educated former slave, led a revolution in Haiti to abolish slavery. This revolution is known as the only successful slave revolution in human history. In 1804, Haiti became the first independent black republic in the world. Over the course of the next 100 years, the country was ravaged by wars and disputes. The Americans invaded in 1915 and left in 1934. The infrastructure and economy improved under the U.S. occupation; however, most profits were realized by investors and bankers in the United States.

The transition to democracy and prosperity has been tumultuous for this country steeped in a history of strength and independence. Government instability and ineffectiveness has been a barrier to progress. Decimation of natural resources, natural disasters, and weak infrastructure have led to a dominant structure of nongovernmental organizations (NGOs). The deep poverty and lack of capacity of the Haitian state have been exacerbated by a political economy of NGOs within the country, which focuses on providing services to populations rather than state building (Zanotti, 2010). Haiti is currently a republic with a president elected by popular vote and a prime minister appointed by the president.

Coming to Know a Community: Culture

The culture of Haiti is steeped in African, French, and Spanish heritage. Haiti's ethnicity is 95% black and 5% white and mulatto. French and Creole are the two official languages of Haiti with Creole being the first language spoken by almost 90% of the population. Haiti has the largest Creole-speaking population in the world. The primary religions practiced in Haiti are Roman Catholic (80%) and Protestant (16%), and approximately one-half of the population practice voodoo along with Christianity (Embassy of the Republic of Haiti, 2015).

Most of the population lives in rural areas organized around clusters of extended family units forming an interdependent community sharing a common courtyard (World Health Organization, 2010). Gender roles tend to be well-defined, with women responsible for managing the family budget, caring for the children, and handling market transactions and men responsible for providing for the family, agricultural work, and repair of the home (Miller, 2000; World Health Organization, 2010). Traditionally, older parents and grandparents are highly respected and are often cared for by their children or relatives. Children also are highly valued, with boys often accorded more privilege than girls (World Health Organization, 2010).

Haiti's literacy rate of 53% is low compared with other Caribbean countries, where the literacy rate is 90% (The Haitian Alliance, 2015). Most children attend primary schools operated by religious groups, nongovernmental agencies, or for-profit organizations for an average of 4.9 years; only 29% attend secondary school (United Nations Development Programme, 2014).

Haiti is considered one of the poorest countries in the Western hemisphere. Unemployment rates in the country are high; approximately 59% of the population live below the national poverty level of $2.44 per day, and 24% live below the extreme poverty level of $1.24 per day (The World Bank, 2015). One-half of the population experiences "multidimensional poverty," which is determined by income, health, education, and standard of living (United Nations Development Programme, 2015). The index of income equality for Haiti is ranked one of the lowest in the Western hemisphere (United Nations Development Programme, 2014). Challenged with high poverty rates, low educational levels, and repeated natural disasters, the economy remains fragile. Haiti is characterized by a powerful class hierarchy based on language, culture, education, and economic background, which stems from its colonial history.

Coming to Know a Community: Health

Health is a major challenge in Haiti because only 40% of its estimated population of 10.2 million have access to health care. The World Health Organization ranking of 190 worldwide health systems places Haiti at 138. In comparison, the United States is ranked at 38, Slovenia at 39, and Uganda at 149 (World Health Organization, 2000). The average life expectancy is 62.51 years of age with the overall population being relatively young; in 2012, only 4% were 65 years old and older (Embassy of the Republic of Haiti, 2015).

Haiti's maternal and infant mortality rates, two critical indices of a country's health, are among the worst in the region and the world. Haiti is ranked 31st for maternal mortality (number of female deaths/100,000 live births) (World Health Organization, 2013), with 380,000 deaths/100,000 live births, and 40th for infant mortality, with 56.5 infant deaths per 1,000 live births (World Health Organization, 2012). Additionally, Haiti has the largest population of persons living with HIV/AIDS in the Caribbean (Pan American Health Organization, 2006). The country continues to experience the largest cholera epidemic in the Western hemisphere, claiming thousands of lives and remaining a major public health threat (United Nations, 2014). Haiti ranks as a country with one of the highest exposures and vulnerability to multiple disasters including earthquakes and flooding, which is compounded by large-scale urbanization, poverty, and migration.

Community Assessment: Introduction

In 2013, the authors were invited to collaborate with a community in rural Haiti to assess the health of their community. This chapter describes a specific approach to a community assessment grounded in the community nursing practice model (CNPM) (Parker, Barry, & King, 2015) (Figure 32-1) and a type of community-based participatory research (CBPR), the inquiry group method (Parker, Barry, & King, 2000).

Based in the values of respect, wholeness, and caring, the CNPM promotes community participation and intersectoral collaboration. Within the context of this model, the focus of the community assessment is to identify the strengths, challenges, and hopes and dreams of the community. The CNPM is grounded in the following beliefs: respect for person, persons are caring, and persons are whole and connected to the community and environment. In addition, services and activities are intentionally guided by the concepts of community participation/partnership, empowerment, access, essentiality, and intersectoral collaboration (World Health Organization, 1978).

**The Community Nursing Practice Model:
Concentric Circles of Empathetic Concern**

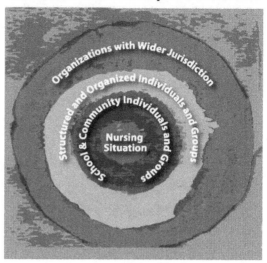

Figure 32–1: Community nursing practice
model. (Printed with permission from the
Florida Atlantic University.)

Community-Based Participatory Research

The community-based participatory research (CBPR) approach is an ideal method for working with communities and underserved populations. CBPR focuses on "social structural, and physical environmental inequities through active involvement of community members, organizational representatives, and researchers in all aspects of the research process" (Israel, Schulz, Parker, & Becker, 2001, p. 182). According to Israel et al (2001), "key principles of CBPR are: (1) recognizes community as a unit of identity; (2) builds on strengths and resources within the community; (3) facilitates collaborative, equitable involvement of all partners in all phases of the research; (4) integrates knowledge and action for mutual benefit of all partners; (5) promotes a co-learning and empowering process that attends to social inequities; (6) involves a cyclical and iterative process; (7) addresses health from both positive and ecological perspectives; (8) disseminates findings and knowledge gained to all partners; and (9) involves a long-term commitment by all partners" (p. 184).

Through partnership with communities, nurses support empowerment of community leaders and members to advocate for solutions to their health-care challenges as well as to address social issues, which may negatively affect the quality of their lives individually and collectively. In contrast to more traditional methods of research, where participants are observed and the relationships are not measured equally, CBPR allows the researchers to learn from the community as equal partners. Instead of research being conducted on the participants, it is conducted with the participants (Lindsey, Sheilds, & Stajduhar, 1999). The community is respected as being the expert and guardian of collectively shared beliefs, values, traditions, and health-care practices. The goal of community-based participatory action research is to discover the strengths and challenges of the community with the purpose of combining resources to build on the common strengths and, through shared reflection, empower the researchers and community to address the challenges. The voice of the community becomes incorporated into the process and the outcome.

Inquiry Group Method

The inquiry group method (Parker et al, 2000), grounded in the values of the CNPM and the principles of CBPR, is an ideal approach to assess the health of a community. The values of respect and humility guide and direct the inquiry group methodology, as the community members are considered experts in their own health as well as community strengths and challenges, and the nurse facilitator is expert in the method and nursing care.

The inquiry group method requires a facilitator to develop an environment conducive to sharing information and a recorder to document information shared, such as impressions of the process. Groups are gathered together, and the facilitator introduces him or herself, other participants, and the purpose of the group. Focused questions guide the discussion: (1) What do you care most about for yourself (family or community)? (2) What do you do on a day-to-day basis to care for yourself (family or community)? (3) What are your hopes and dreams for yourself (family or community)? (4) What are ways nurses can be helpful to you (family or community)?

Application of Model and Method of Community Assessment to a Rural Community in Haiti

Narrative From an Inquiry Group

We left the guest house early to prepare for a second inquiry group with women in the village. The meeting was to be held in the church, and as we approached, we saw the sanctuary crowded with approximately 80 women and children in their "Sunday best" clothes waiting to meet us. We began with a greeting in French, "Bonjour," and through the voices of our language facilitators, we thanked them for coming to meet with us. The purpose of the meeting was explained as wanting to know more about their expert care of themselves, their families, and their community. We were described as experts in nursing care and wanted to find out from them how we could be helpful to them. Immediately after the explanation of the inquiry group format, the group format unfolded into individual consultations about the women's health concerns. We intently and respectfully listened to each woman, and through two language facilitators, we heard their stories of "tired backs and feet, sore eyes, stomachaches, headaches, and skin rashes." One woman, with a very distended abdomen, waited to be heard last. She explained she had terrible abdominal pain and needed help.

The meeting was scheduled for 1 hour and lasted 31/2 hours. At the end, we thanked the women for coming; sharing with us how they cared for themselves, families, and community; and their acceptance of us. We affirmed their care for themselves, their children, and their community. We told them we were in the process of assessing the health resources in the country and would work with them to advocate for more resources in their village. Table 32-1 depicts the translation and application of the CNPM values during the community assessment and inquiry group process.

TABLE 32-1 Translation and Application of the Community Nurse Practice Model

TRANSCENDENT VALUES: PRESENT IN ALL NURSING SITUATIONS	DEFINITION/DESCRIPTION	EXPRESSION OF VALUE THROUGH INQUIRY GROUP METHOD
Respect for person	Refers to honoring the inherent dignity and uniqueness of each individual	The question "How can we be helpful to you?" recognizes the person and communities are experts of their own care and community. Humility and being open to learn from the other allows for

TABLE 32-1 Translation and Application of the Community Nurse Practice Model—cont'd

TRANSCENDENT VALUES: PRESENT IN ALL NURSING SITUATIONS	DEFINITION/DESCRIPTION	EXPRESSION OF VALUE THROUGH INQUIRY GROUP METHOD
		coparticipation. This inquiry group followed our initial meeting with community leaders and elders, mostly men and a few women. Wanting to hear the voice of all participants, we requested a second inquiry group for women only. During this meeting, the women voiced their health concerns for themselves and their families. In this situation, women wanted to meet with us individually to tell us their story. Wanting to respect each one, we altered our format and individually met with each person.
Caring	Understand that to be human is to be caring and that caring is the essence of nursing	The question "How do you care for yourself, your family, and your community?" was evidenced by the number of women that attended the meeting. It seemed as though every woman within a 2-mile radius was there to meet with us. They wanted us to hear their call for care and for their children to be healthy and educated.
Wholeness	Views persons as whole in the moment and always connected with others in families and communities and environment	Participation by persons and their community is vital to the community assessment process. The inquiry group method allows for a way to come to know and understand the needs of the community. Each community member is a coparticipant and an expert with his or her own experience. The four questions that guided the inquiry method facilitated the understanding of persons as a whole and the hopes and dreams of the community. The connection to the environment was most evident by view of the beautiful blue ocean

Continued

TABLE 32–1 Translation and Application of the Community Nurse Practice Model—cont'd

TRANSCENDENT VALUES: PRESENT IN ALL NURSING SITUATIONS	DEFINITION/DESCRIPTION	EXPRESSION OF VALUE THROUGH INQUIRY GROUP METHOD
		and also in the immediate by the lack of safe drinking water and sanitation.
ACTUALIZING VALUES: GUIDES PRACTICES IN SPECIFIC NURSING SITUATIONS	**DEFINITION/DESCRIPTION**	**EXPRESSION OF VALUE THROUGH INQUIRY GROUP METHOD**
Access	Views as ongoing and constant availability of health care that is competent, culturally acceptable, respectful, and cost-effective	Access to health care was a call heard throughout the inquiry groups. When we asked "How can we help you?" the response we heard was "We need a hospital." The closest hospital is 2 hours away. Others described walking miles into town seeking medicines. The school had a health room at one time, but it was not used today. Yearly medical missions had come to the community, but access to ongoing care was unavailable.
Essentiality	Described from the client's view as what is necessary for well-being	The community identified the need for a hospital for access to care.
Community participation	Described as the active engagement with members of a community fostered by openness to listen to calls for nursing and to create nursing responses	Partnerships are essential for the success of community assessments. In this situation, the church and local minister as well as community leaders were our main partners in the beginning. As we came to understand the call for health, we reached out to the broader community. We met with the Dean from a College of Nursing, met with others providing care in Haiti, and participated in the first Best Health Practices for Haiti Conference. Stateside, we reported back to local churches and developed relationships with Haitian Nurses Associations.

TABLE 32–1 Translation and Application of the Community Nurse Practice Model—cont'd

ACTUALIZING VALUES: GUIDES PRACTICES IN SPECIFIC NURSING SITUATIONS	DEFINITION/DESCRIPTION	EXPRESSION OF VALUE THROUGH INQUIRY GROUP METHOD
Empowerment	Understood as the client's awareness of making individual choices that influence health and well-being	Central to the community nursing practice model is empowerment of the community and individual persons.
Intersectoral collaboration	Refers to the openness to seek and honor the expertise of providers and agencies to potentiate the outcomes of services essential to well being	Knowing the value of partnerships, we committed to working within the community to develop partnerships for health care, met with church leaders within the community to seek funding for health care, and met with the dean of a nursing program to discuss the possibility of students participating in health care in the community. Also, doctors at the hospital were consulted about caring for the woman with severe abdominal pain, and plans were made for transportation and payment. Funding was sought from local organizations and churches.

Summary of the Community Nursing Practice Model

The values of the CNPM guide practice and offer an ethical framework for community assessment, the inquiry group method. The inquiry group method is conducted with respect for all participants and acknowledges the expertise of the other. The facilitators' intentional approach is grounded in cultural humility and compassion: To lay aside assumptions, to be open to know the other, and to put oneself in the other's shoes so that calls for nursing are heard and nursing responses are developed from the community's hopes and dreams for well-being. The inquiry group method facilitated knowing the community directly from its members.

The exploration of Haiti's history, cultural patterns, and health-care system were viewed through the lens of Leininger's Theory of Culture Care Diversity and Universality (Wehbe-Alamah, 2015). The Sunrise Enabler Model (Leininger & McFarland, 2006) illuminates the major factors influencing health-care beliefs and practices: Technological, religion/philosophy, kinship/social, political/legal, economic, and educational. Leininger's enabler model guided knowing the background of Haiti.

The exploration of self-knowing for the authors was guided by the values embedded in the CNPM. In particular, the definition of community as a synthesis of several understandings is ignited with the idea that members of a community share values, share a willingness to risk, and tolerate a certain lack of structure (Parker & Barry, 2010, p. 454). This understanding grounded the authors in the sacredness of community work: The shared values between the authors and participants, the shared risk of being with each other, and the shared expertise of participants' self care and the authors' expertise in nursing care.

The actualizing values of the CNPM—access, essentiality, empowerment, community participation, and intersectional collaboration—were developed from the World Health Organization Declaration of Primary Health Care formulated at Alma Ata in 1978 (World Health Organization, 1978). The declaration invited a spirit of cooperation among all countries to ensure that the populations of all countries have equal access to health care that is practical, cost-effective, scientific, and culturally sensitive. It is the first point of care with a local provider and the entry point into the country's health-care system. The ideals of the primary health care declaration are yet to be realized in Haiti. However, the spirit of the CNPM and inquiry group method for nursing are useful in moving closer to the goal of health for all.

Transcultural Caring–Based Learning Approach

The theoretical approach to transcultural care/caring is grounded in an intentional respectful engagement with others to discover health beliefs and practices and to provide nursing care that responds to the others' hopes and dreams for health and well-being. In your group, identify a nursing situation in which the caring between the nurse and the one nursed nurtures wholeness and well-being within the context of transcultural caring. Use the dimensions of the transcultural caring dynamics and health-care model (Ray, 2010); Leininger's theory of Culture Care Diversity and Universality (Wehbe-Alamah, 2015) or the work of Parker, Barry, and King (2015) to describe your approach to transcultural caring. The Reflections with Questions section is a guide to assist in identifying essential knowing of the health of the population, identifying calls for nursing, and developing nursing responses that nurture wholeness and well-being within the context of transcultural caring.

Reflections with Questions

Compare and contrast the health of Haiti with the (1) Pan American Health Organization goal of "Health: A right for all" (Pan American Health Organization, 2006), (2) the World Health Organization's social determinants of health (World Health Organization, 2015), and (3) the United Nations millennium development and health goals (United Nations Development Programme, 2015).

Transcultural Nursing Reflections

- To understand this rural community in Haiti, contemplate what has occurred in Haiti throughout its history. What are the population, economic, and geopolitical structures of Haiti? What is the political structure of Haiti, the military and peacekeeping presence in Haiti?
- How do the elements of poverty, literacy, health-care access, education, and crime in Haiti compare with other Caribbean countries, the United States, and Canada?
- What are the differences in immigration policies between Haiti, the United States, Canada, and other Caribbean countries?
- What is the nature of poverty, health, health care, and education in Haiti? What are the health beliefs and practices in Haiti? What is the nature of maternal-child care and what is the health of children and life expectancy of the Haitian people? What is the nutritional status of the people of Haiti?
- What are the spiritual beliefs and religions of Haiti and their impact on health-care beliefs and practice? What is the influence on family planning, health promotion and prevention, use of folk healing practices, and death and dying rituals?

- What is the literacy level and health literacy in Haiti? How does this affect the population of this community?
- How do the elements of health, public health, health-care access, and human safety of Haiti compare with the standards of the World Health Organization and Pan American Health Organization?
- How are missionary groups contributing to the population of Haiti? How do NGOs contribute to the health of Haiti?
- What is the meaning of the role of a nurse researcher in a transcultural nursing situation within a global community?
- How would you provide care for this population in a village in rural Haiti?
- What resources would be available through the public health system or private health systems to care for families in Haiti?
- What organizations and resources inside the country or outside the country are available from the global community to support health care in this community?
- Overall, what may be the short-term and long-term prospects for health care in this community?

References

Embassy of the Republic of Haiti. (2015). *Haiti at a glance.* Retrieved from http://www.haiti.org/index.php/economic-xm-affairs-xm/26-the-embassy/content/121-haiti-at-a-glance

Israel, B.A., Schulz, A.J., Parker, E.A., & Becker, A.B. (2001). Community-based participatory research: Policy recommendations for promoting a partnership approach in health research. *Education for Health*, 14(2), 182–197.

Leininger, M.M., & McFarland, M.R. (Eds.). (2006). *Cultural care diversity and universality: A worldwide nursing theory* (2nd ed.). Sudbury, MA: Jones & Bartlett.

Lindsey, E., Sheilds, L., & Stajduhar, K. (1999). Creating effective nursing partnerships: Relating community development to participatory action research. *Journal of Advanced Nursing*, 29(5), 1238–1245.

Miller, N.L. (2000). Haitian ethnomedical systems and biomedical practitioners: Directions for clinicians. *Journal of Transcultural Nursing*, 11(3), 204–211.

Pan American Health Organization. (2006). *The challenge of Haiti: Health a right for all.* Retrieved from http://iris.paho.org/xmlui/handle/123456789/3662

Parker, M.E., & Barry, C.D. (2010). The community nursing practice model. In M. Parker and M. Smith (Eds.), *Nursing theories and nursing practice* (3rd ed., pp. 451–459). Philadelphia: F. A. Davis Company.

Parker, M.E., Barry, C.D., & King, B.M. (2015). The development of a community nursing practice model. In M. Smith and M. Parker (Eds.), *Nursing theories and nursing practice* (4th ed., pp. 435–447). Philadelphia: F. A. Davis Company.

Parker, M., Barry, C., & King, B. (2000). Use of inquiry group method for assessment and evaluation in a school-based community nursing project. *Journal of Family and Community Health*, 23(2), 51–61.

Ray, M.A. (2010). *Transcultural caring dynamics in nursing and health care.* Philadelphia, PA: F. A. Davis Company.

The Haitian Alliance. (2015). *Haiti literate.* Retrieved from http://transformhaiti.com/?page_id=789

The World Bank. (2015). *Haiti overview.* Retrieved from http://www.worldbank.org/en/country/haiti/overview

United Nations. (2014). *UN fact sheet: Combating cholera in Haiti.* Retrieved from http://www.un.org/News/dh/infocus/haiti/Cholera_UN_Factsheet_24%20Feb_2014.pdf

United Nations. (2015). *Millennium development goals and beyond 2015*. Retrieved from http://www.un.org/millenniumgoals/

United Nations Development Programme. (2014). *Human development reports Haiti*. Retrieved from http://hdr.undp.org/en/countries/profiles/HTI

United Nations Development Programme. (2015). *Multidimensional poverty index*. Retrieved from http://hdr.undp.org/en/content/multidimensional-poverty-index-mpi

Wehbe-Alamah, H. (2015). Madeleine Leininger's theory of culture care diversity and universality. In M. Smith & M. Parker (Eds.), *Nursing theories and nursing practice* (4th ed., pp. 303–319). Philadelphia, PA: F. A. Davis Company.

World Health Organization. (1978). *Declaration of Alma-Ata. Primary health care*. Geneva, Switzerland: World Health Organization.

World Health Organization. (2000). *The world health report 2000*. Retrieved from http://www.who.int/whr/2000/en/

World Health Organization. (2010). *Mental health in Haiti: A literature review*. Retrieved from http://www.who.int/mental_health/emergencies/culture_mental_health_haiti_eng.pdf

World Health Organization. (2012). *Haiti Neonatal and child health profile*. Retrieved from www.who.int/maternal_child_adolescent/epidemiology/profiles/neonatal_child/hti.pdf

World Health Organization. (2013). *Maternal mortality in 1990-2013*. Retrieved from http://www.who.int/reproductivehealth/publications/monitoring/maternal-mortality-2013/en/

World Health Organization. (2015). Social determinants of health. Retrieved from http://www.who.int/social_determinants/en/

Zanotti, L. (2010). Cacophonies of aid, failed state building and NGOs in Haiti: Setting the stage for disaster, envisioning the future. *Third World Quarterly, 31*(5), 755–771.

CHAPTER 33

Reflections on the Universality of Caring

AUTHORS' REFLECTIONS

My professional journey reflects the universality of caring. I started courses for my Masters of Science in Nursing (Administration track) in 1989, and this was a special time within the College of Nursing at Florida Atlantic University. Nursing theorists Dr. Madeline Leininger, Sister Simone Roach, and Dr. Jean Watson came to the college to dialogue and interact with students. Dr. Boykin and Dr. Schoenhofer were beginning their own scholarship related to Nursing as Caring. I was privileged, humbled, and honored to meet Dr. Marilyn Ray while I was a graduate student, as we had a shared research interest related to caring within complex systems, caring and economics, and caring leadership. I also became involved with the International Association for Human Caring (IAHC) and served in leadership roles as treasurer, president-elect, and president for more than 12 years. I am currently immediate past president. I reconnected with Dr. Jean Watson in 2007 and became faculty in the Watson Caring Science Institute (WCSI). Through my work with IAHC and WCSI, I have the opportunity to participate in international conferences and mentor nurses from around the world on caring. The epistemology of the universality of caring is the scholarship of knowing related to caring from nurses around the world, the ontology is the meaning and expression of caring within different cultures, and the praxis is how nurses from around the world cocreate caring into their practice of nursing. Examples presented are from a review over the past few years of conference abstracts from the IAHC, International Caritas Consortium, and the Middle Eastern Nurses United in Peace and Caring.

The Lived Experience of the Universality of Caring

Dr. Ray and I attended the first Caring and Peace Conference in Hiroshima, Japan, in 2012. Before the conference, we shared the rich history of caring with nursing students to help them understand caring as a substantive area of study within the discipline of nursing and as a way to advance and transform nursing practice. During the conference, we shared the scholarship of caring through multiple ways of knowing. The presentation was didactic and experiential as nurse participants engaged in expressions of caring. We presented an overview of the multiple ways of knowing (empirical, aesthetic, personal, ethical) and creatively provided specific examples of how they inform the practice of nursing and allowed participants to experience the multiple ways of knowing through experiential interactive activities. We had nurses from the United States, Japan, China, New Zealand, and Thailand in our session participating in caring-healing modalities of dance, storytelling, music, authentic listening, centering, art, and aromatherapy.

This exchange illustrated personal knowing, coming to know self and others as caring, and was a reflection of understanding our humanity and our interconnectedness with others, what informs us as human beings, and valuing caring practices from "the heart." A memory of that session was nurses from all over the world engaged in singing and dancing to the music of the British rock group Coldplay. Although we could not speak each other's languages, music and dance united us. It was at that conference that Dr. Marilyn Ray and Dr. Naohiro Hohashi from Tokyo and Kobe, Japan, began the dialogue to host the 35th International Association for Human Caring Conference in Kyoto, Japan (Figures 33-1 to 33-5).

Drs. Madeline Leininger and Jean Watson and a group of doctoral students including Marilyn Ray (now Dr. Marilyn Ray) gathered for the first conference 36 years ago to present research and philosophical reflections related to caring and nursing. This group continued to meet every year to reflect, dialogue, and share research and philosophical assumptions about caring. In 1988, the group formalized and became known as the International Association for Human Caring. The 35th International Association for Human Caring Conference, held in Kyoto, Japan, May 2014, with a theme of the universality of caring, represented the largest conference in the history of the IAHC and the largest gathering of caring scholars from

Figure 33-1: The 35th International Association for Human Caring Conference in Kyoto, Japan.

Figure 33-2: Left to right: Marian Turkel, Patrick Dean, and Marilyn Ray.

Figure 33-3: Left to right: Junko Honda, Marian Turkel, Naohiro Hohashi, and Marilyn Ray.

around the world being together and creating sacred space that was caring, healing, and welcoming. Members of the IAHC, the Special Interest Group on Transcultural Nursing and Caring, and the Society of Cultural Nursing Studies were present. Dr. Jean Watson (Figs. 33-6 and 33-7) opened the conference with "Universality of Human Caring in Our World," and Dr. Rozzano Locsin presented the closing keynote "Affirming the Universality of Caring in Nursing."

At the conference, 500 podium and poster sessions with more than 600 colleagues in attendance representing Canada, Australia, New Zealand, Thailand, Hong Kong, Macao, China, Taiwan, The Philippines, United Kingdom, Finland, Norway, Kenya, India, Portugal, Columbia, Indonesia, Saudi Arabia, Mongolia, Vietnam, Singapore, Turkey, Japan, and the United States shared their research and ideas. The common values of authentic presence,

Figure 33-4: Left to right: Marian Turkel, Naohiro Hohashi, Marilyn Ray, Junko Honda, Patrice McCarthy, and Nancey France.

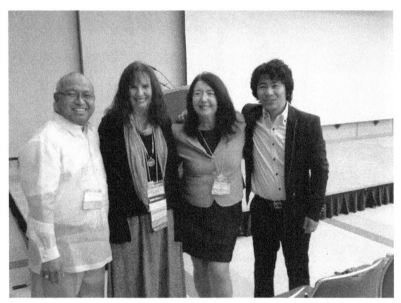

Figure 33-5: Left to right: Danny Bolima, Marian Turkel, Diane Breckenridge, and Naohiro Hohashi.

belonging, caring, connection, compassion, commitment, creativity, dedication, healing, hope, gratitude, kindness, love, peace, and sensitivity to others were illuminated (see Figure 33-8 for more conference attendees).

I was privileged to be part of the review of the abstracts for this 35th anniversary conference. We received close to 500 abstracts. Dr. Ide from Japan and I became e-mail buddies, keeping track of the abstracts, sending them out for reviews, receiving them, receiving the edits, and moving them forward to Dr. Zane Wolf for publication in the *International Journal of Human Caring*. Dr. Ide and I worked many long hours on the computer. When it was morning for her, it was evening for me, and when it was evening for me, it was morning for

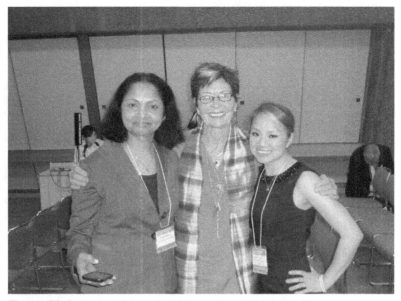

Figure 33-6: Left to right: Lalitha Mathew, Jean Watson, Nga Nguyen.

Figure 33-7: Jean Watson with conference attendees.

her. We became caring colleagues over the computer. We developed mutual respect for each other and practiced transcultural caring by treating each other with caring and reminding each other to take time to practice self-care.

The epistemology of the universality of caring was reflected in the scholarly presentations at the conference and the emerging themes of the conference abstracts. Emerging overarching themes on the initial metasynthesis of the conference abstracts included the following: Being open to unfolding possibilities; caring is a way of being; cocreating caring moments; practicing from the heart; serving those who need us most; and transforming self, others, and systems through intentional caring.

Figure 33-8: Left to right: Marie-Pierre Avoine, Susan Knibbs, Meagan Miyagishima, Paula Clark, Meredith Porter, Colleen Maykut, Leanne Topola, Melissa Meunier, Marlienne Goldin, and Rosemary Hoffman.

As I was reading the abstracts alone in my office, many a night the tears just came. I read the story of a nurse in Thailand caring for patients in the emergency department committed and dedicated to practicing caring and doing her best when at times the resources (staffing and supplies) were limited. It reminded me of the emergency departments in the United States. Nurses have experiences of not having enough staff; the environment can be complex, hectic, and stressful. Similar to our colleagues in Thailand, nurses in the United States create caring moments, including buying a birthday card and a cake for an 80-year-old man who has no family and allowing the parents of a child with pediatric trauma to stay in the room with their child. I read the story of nurses from Japan who were caring compassionately for elders and who were still suffering and hurting from being involved in the earthquake; the nurses were practicing caring—they were healing. I read the stories of nurses who care for elders in many different countries. Elderly patients sometimes are vulnerable, they are frail, and they are scared, and the person who is providing care with intentionality and authenticity and meeting basic human needs with respect and dignity is the nurse.

The abstracts from Thailand and Indonesia related to caring in the neonatal intensive care unit and highlighted being with the father and mother when their child is stillborn or when their child does not survive after a few days in the neonatal intensive care unit. These practices and care patterns were almost identical to caring practices in the United States, focusing on understanding the experience and being present for the parents.

I read stories from nurses caring for people who had open heart surgery. I started to cry when I read those because when I practiced at the bedside, that was my area of specialty. I was privileged to care for patients who had just had their hearts touched by the human hands of the physician. I remembered one special time when a patient was waking up from surgery and I was talking to him and letting him know that he was in the intensive care unit, and tears started coming down his face. I just held his hand and told him my name and said, "I'm here for you, I'm your nurse, I'll be with you." When the patient woke up, he told me the reason that he started crying was because he thought he had died and was in heaven. He thought that the voice he heard was that of an angel. When I touched him and told him I was his nurse and that he would be okay, that's when the tears came. They were not tears of fear or sadness; they were tears of joy for he was happy to know that he was alive.

I read stories of nurses caring for ill pediatric patients and taking care of them and their family members. How important that is for us as nurses to have the families at the center of the care. We are committed to patient-centered and family-centered care. At the same time I was reading the stories, I became very sad because I remembered a time when I was a nurse caring for a little boy who had open heart surgery. He was sleeping and stable; then he bolted up and screamed, "Mommy!" and we went over to his bedside. His mother was not with him; she had stepped out just for a few minutes to go to the cafeteria to get something to eat. One nurse ran down to the cafeteria to find her and bring her back while the rest of us stayed in the unit with the child. He never woke up. The doctor said with the type of surgery he had, one of the rare complications was that you could go into ventricular fibrillation. That is what happened, and we could not save him. I was glad that I did not tell the mother that she could not stay at the bedside with her child. I was also glad that I did not tell her she should stay either.

Relevance to Ray's Theory and Model of Transcultural Caring Dynamics in Nursing and Health Care

Ray's theory and model of transcultural caring dynamics in nursing and health care is congruent with the epistemology, ontology, and praxis of the universality of caring. The first dimension of the model, the essence of caring, is illustrated when nurses from around the world share values of love, empathy, and compassion and integrate authentic presence and authentic listening when in communication with colleagues, patients, and families. Examples include staying at the bedside with a critically ill patient so the family can have some respite time, buying clothes and food for patients who have none, giving a bath to a patient covered in feces and lice, focusing on what is most important to the family and patients, centering oneself before going into a patient's room, and practicing self-care to have the energy to be loving and compassionate with others. An emergency department nurse from the United States shared the following: Nurses open their hearts and love the ones that others will not look in the face. A nurse from Japan noted how nurses washed and bathed the elderly who were displaced in shelters after the recent earthquake.

Transcultural caring ethics, the second dimension of the model, is a shared experience for nurses when caring for patients from different cultures or religions, especially when practicing nursing and caring in countries at war or caring for patients who exhibit violent behavior. Personal safety and security is at risk, yet there is a sense of duty to provide the best care. Nurses working in emergency departments in the United States are seeing more and more patients coming in with guns and threatening health-care workers. Also, there is an increase in patients with mental health disorders. Nurses from the Middle East tell of how they practice under the threat of terrorist attacks at all times. For both groups under threat, there is a sense of fear and feeling vulnerable, while knowing that they need to care for those who need them the most. Nursing is a calling, not just a job. Nurse leaders experience ethical choice making. The changing physical practice environments to ensure safety require decisions in the reallocation of economic and material resources, including the provision of more staffing to provide the needed quality of care.

The third dimension related to the transcultural context are congruent with Ray's theory of bureaucratic caring. Professional nursing practice involves the understanding of personal, family, economic, educational, and cultural needs of the patient. Practicing within complex systems means nurses also need to understand the influence of the complex health-care context—the political, legal, technological, and economic systems. Themes include working without enough staff, making do with limited supplies, intense focus on regulatory requirements, overwhelming paperwork, computers taking time away from rather than freeing up time for patients, and families who are living with hunger and poverty. Abstracts representing such difficulties were dominant at the 35th International Caring Conference. One of the most profound abstracts was from a hospital manager in East Jerusalem where nurses worked for almost 4 months at a very modest salary while the hospital was experiencing financial crisis. The manager and nurses worked in collaboration with hospital leaders to provide care, continued to treat refugees, and maintained a working labor and delivery room.

Universal sources is the fourth dimension of the model and involves religion, spirituality, energy, creativity, and healing. The cover of the issue of the *International Journal for Human Caring* in which the abstracts from the conference were published has words that represent care and caring in 16 different languages. God, Christ, Buddha, and a Divine Force all represent love and compassion—the essence of caring.

Throughout Ray's book, stories of nurses from many distinct cultures emphasize the creation of caring-healing environments for self, patients, families, and complex systems. In many of the shared transcultural caring experiences (case studies, stories), indigenous modalities of diverse culture groups for healing are underscored. Rituals including healing ceremonies are part of nursing practice in many countries. An example of this took place at the A-Bomb Museum in Hiroshima, Japan, at the time of the 2012 Caring and Peace Conference. Nurses from several different countries gathered in a circle in the rain in front of the Eternal Flame and began to sing "give peace a chance" (from the John Lennon song originally recorded May 31, 1969) (Fig. 33-9). The circle grew larger as the nurses opened their hands to anyone who wanted to join the group. For many, this ritual created a sense of healing and peace knowing the pain, suffering, and destruction that the A-bomb brought to Hiroshima.

In closing, remember, "Never believe that a few caring people can't change the world for indeed, that's all who ever have" (Margaret Mead; retrieved from www.goodreads.com)

Transcultural Caring Reflections

- How can caring be made more explicit in nursing education, practice, and research within your culture or cultural setting?
- What does the universality of caring mean to you?
- When attending national or international nursing conferences, look for stories and experiences of being open to unfolding possibilities. Reflect on caring as a way of being by cocreating caring moments; practicing from the heart; serving those who need us most; and transforming self, others, and systems through intentional caring.

Figure 33-9: Left to right: Gayle Casterline, Marlienne Goldin, Lynne Wagner, Marian Turkel, Michael Brooks Turkel, and Marilyn Ray.

- Identify a self-care practice so as to have the energy to care compassionately for others.
- Reflect on an ethical caring experience. What was that like for you? How did you resolve the ethical dilemmas, conflicts, issues, and concerns?
- How can you, as a nurse, create a caring-healing environment within your practice setting?
- Is caring for patients exhibiting violence a concern in your practice environment? How can you be an advocate for change?
- Language is universal, and the language of caring reflects the universality of caring. Within your practice, use positive words such as "acceptance," "compassion," "healing," and "relationship" in place of negative words such as "anger," "fear," or "hate" when you are in dialogue with patients, families, or colleagues. What is an experience of using caring words like? Do you as a nurse change the energy pattern?

Index

Note: Page numbers followed by "b," "f," and "t" indicate boxes, figures, and tables, respectively.

Aboriginal/native religions, 140–141
  spiritual belongingness and, 145
Abortion
  Amtuagan people and, 408
  Isneg people and, 410
Accountability, in transcultural caring
  competency, 208–209
Acculturation (cultural assimilation), 110,
  113–114, 172–173
Advocacy, in transcultural communicative
  spiritual-ethical caring, 119
African-American community,
  transcultural caring experiences of,
  223–229
Agape. See Love
Allah, 137
Alternative therapies. *See*
  Complementary/alternative
  therapies
American Mexican transcultural caring
  experience, 216–222
Ancient Greek ethics, 70
Anthropology, caring and, 41–42
Aquinas, Thomas, 70
Aristotle, 70, 72
Art, caring and, 47–48
Asian Indian widow, transcultural caring
  experiences of, 235–238
Assimilation, 15
Augustine, Saint, 45, 70
Autonomy, 44, 74
Avoine, Marie-Pierre, 436f
Awareness, in transcultural caring inquiry,
  168

Baha'i faith, 142
Beatitudes, 71, 145
Belonging/belongingness, 10, 14, 134,
  173, 179. *See also* Spiritual
  belongingness
Beneficence, 73–74
Bentham, Jeremy, 72
Bible, 42, 69, 70, 137, 145–146
Biomedical ethics, 73–74
Birthing/childbirth practices
  among Amtuagan people,
  407–408
  among Isneg people, 409
  Davis-Floyd's technocratic model of,
  411–412
  indigenous, in Cordilleras, the
  Philippines, 405f, 406f
Bolima, Danny, 434f
Bonhoeffer, Dietrich, 79
Breckenridge, Diane, 434f
Buber, Martin, 45

Buddhism, 139
  caring and, 42
Buddhists, in Thailand, transcultural
  caring experiences, 342–351

Canada
  ethnic/immigrant populations in, 6
  preservation of native cultures in, 16
  transcultural caring experiences of
  multiculturalism/interculturality in,
  320–327
Cardiovascular intensive care unit,
  transcultural caring experiences of
  nurse manager in, 260–266
Caring. *See also* Transcultural caring
  basis of, in contemporary nursing, 39
  classification system of, 50f
  components of, 10
  concept of, 8–9
  contemporary perceptions of, in
  nursing, 49–52
  definitions of, 41
  perspectives on, in non-nursing
  disciplines, 41–48
  philosophical/empirical categories of,
  39–41
  reflections on universality of, 431–439
  spiritual-ethical
    meaning of, 50f
    process of, 50f
  through self-reflection, 9
Casterline, Gayle, 438f
Categorical Imperative (Kant), 71
CBPR. *See* Community-based
  participatory research
Charity, as pillar of Islam,
  137, 146
Childbirth practices. *See*
  Birthing/childbirth practices
China, American Chinese family in,
  transcultural caring experiences of,
  290–295
Choice, in transcultural caring inquiry,
  168–169
Christian ethics, 70–71
Christianity, 69, 136–137
  caring and, 42
  spiritual belongingness and,
  145–146
Clark, Paula, 436f
CNPM. *See* Community nursing practice
  model
Commitment, in transcultural
  communicative spiritual-ethical
  caring, 119
Communal theologies, 142–144

Communication
  ethic of, 188, 188f
  language and, 182–183
  symbols and, 181
  in transcultural communicative
  spiritual-ethical caring, 119
Communication ethics, 89
Community
  culture as, 101
  identity and, 109, 113–114
  meaning of membership in, 106
Community-based participatory research
  (CBPR), 423
Community nursing practice model
  (CNPM), 422, 423f, 427–428
  translation/application of, 424t–427t
Compassion, 83
  caring and, 10
  in concept of caring, 41
  spiritual suffering/healing and, 152
  in transcultural caring, 52
  in transcultural communicative
  spiritual-ethical caring, 119
Competence, in transcultural
  communicative spiritual-ethical
  caring, 119
Complementary/alternative therapies, 8
Complexity sciences, 12–15, 46
  spiritual belongingness and, 146–148
  transcultural context and, 102–104
Confidentiality, 74
Conflict, 108, 115, 118. *See also*
  Culture-value conflict
  assessment tool
  cultural, 12, 15
  ethical, 78–83
  intergenerational/multigenerational,
  184–185
  in transcultural caring inquiry,
  172–174
Confucianism, 139–140
Conscience, 70
  caring and, 86
  Christianity and, 145
  ethics and, 76–77, 79, 80, 83
  in Roach's six Cs of caring, 44, 49
  reflective practice and, 205
  in transcultural communicative
  spiritual-ethical caring, 119
Consequentialism, 72
Copresence, in transcultural
  communicative spiritual-ethical
  caring, 119
Cordilleras (the Philippines), transcultural
  caring experiences of indigenous
  people of, 401–419

Correctional facilities, adolescent, transcultural caring experiences of nurse practitioner in, 277–281
Creed, as pillar of Islam, 137, 146
Critical caring inquiry, 203
  reflective practice in transcultural communicative spiritual-ethical caring action, 205
  in TCCBL (Transcultural Caring-Based Learning), 204, 209
Cuba/Cuban culture, 250–251
Cuban American transcultural caring experience, 250–255
Cultural competency
  definition of, 208
  Ray's Transcultural Communicative Spiritual-Ethical CARING tool for, 51f
Cultural dynamics, caring and, 10
Cultural incompetence, 208–209
Cultural practices, dynamic cultural context and, 106–107
Cultural relativism, 84–85
Cultural transformation, in transcultural caring inquiry, 172–174
Culture
  concept of, 10
  historical meanings, 11–12
  meaning of health and, 18–19
  multiculturalism and, 15–16
  in transcultural caring inquiry, 172–173
  transcultural context and, 101
  transglobalization and, 12–15
Culture-value conflict assessment tool, 178–180, 180f
  different cultural histories and, 181
  different cultural rituals and, 182–183
  different symbols/meanings of reality and health and, 181
  dimensions of, 180–181
  diversity of health-care models, 185–186
  ethnocentrism, 183
  fear, 185
  gender, 184
  intergeneration interactions, 184–185
  language/communication and, 181–182
  legislation, 186–188
  marginal status/marginality, 184
  prejudice, 185
  social class, 183–184
  stereotyping, 183
  time, 185

Dalai Lama, 78
Danish/Norwegian culture nursing care model, transcultural caring experiences in, 374–387
Davis-Floyd's technocratic model of birthing/technocratic imperative, 411–412

Dean, Patrick, 433f
Demographics, racial/ethnic in North America, 6
Deontology, 71
Descartes, René, 38
Diversity
  in American culture, 15
  creation of multicultural self and, 16
Diversity fatigue, 15–16
Divine Command Theory, 69
Dynamic complexity, cultural transglobalization and, 12–15

Ebola, in sub-Saharan Africa, transcultural caring experiences relating to, 352–357
Ecuador, shamanism in, transcultural caring experiences of, 307–312
Education, caring and, 47
Empathy, caring and, 10
Essence of Caring model, 36f, 50
Ethics. See also Transcultural caring ethics
  ancient Greek, 70
  biomedical, 73–74
  of care/caring, 75
  caring and, 44–45
  Christian, 70–71
  Medieval/Renaissance, 70
  nursing and theories of, 77–78
Ethics committees, transcultural nurses participating in, 88–89
Ethics of care/caring, 75
Ethnicity, racialized, 111
Ethnocentrism, culture-value conflict assessment tool and, 183
Evidence, of transcultural caring, 207
  elements of, 167f, 168–169
  nature of, 169–170
Evil, 69, 71
  ethical conflict and, 78
  ethics and, 68
  idea of, 45, 80–81
Expanded consciousness, 18

Fairness, 74, 90, 107. See also Justice
Fear, culture-value conflict assessment tool and, 185
Feminist ethics, 75
Fidelity, 74
Filipino nurse, transcultural caring experiences of, 239–243
France, Nancey, 434f
Frankl, Viktor, 79

Gabbok (Uma ritual), 410
Gender, culture-value conflict assessment tool and, 184
Generational names, 185b
Globalization
  health issues and, 8
  in nursing, 7–8

God
  approaches to, 144
  in monotheistic religions, 136–138
Golden Rule, 70–71, 78
Goldin, Marlienne, 436f, 438f
the Good, 78
  idea of, 79–80
Guatemalan Mayan farmworker, transcultural caring experiences of, 230–234

Haiti, rural, transcultural caring experiences in, 420–430
Haitian family in U.S., transcultural caring experiences of, 267–270
Haitian girl and nurse practitioner in adolescent correctional facility, transcultural caring experiences of, 277–281
Health
  cultural complexity and meanings of, 18–19
  globalization and, 8
Health-care models, diversity of, culture-value conflict assessment tool and, 185–186
Heidegger, Martin, 43, 106
Hinduism, 138–139
Hobbes, Thomas, 72
Hoffman, Rosemary, 436f
Hohashi, Naohiro, 433f, 434f
Holism, 133, 149, 152
Home of Hope (Lebanon), 391f, 392f, 393f
Honda, Junko, 433f, 434f
Human-environment totality paradigm, 17

Identity, derivation of, 109–110
Identity politics, 112
Ilom (Uma ritual), 410
Immigration, 109, 113, 220, 221
  conflict and, 173
  North American population growth and, 6
Integrative spirituality. See New Age/integrative spirituality
Interculturality (transculturality), 16
Intergeneration interactions, culture-value conflict assessment tool and, 184–185
Islam, 69, 137–138
  caring and, 42
  spiritual belongingness and, 145
Isneg people, pregnancy/childbirth practices of, 409–410

Jamaican transcultural caring experiences, 244–249
Japanese graduate nursing students, transcultural caring experiences of, 328–341

Jesus, 70–71, 137
Jewish spiritual culture, transcultural
    caring experiences in, 282–289
Judaism, 136
    caring and, 42
    spiritual belongingness and, 145
Jung, Carl, 80
Justice, 52, 74, 83
    caring and, 10
    in transcultural communicative
        spiritual-ethical caring, 119

Kabala, 136
Kant, Immanuel, 44, 71
Kingdom of Ends (Kant), 71
Kinship structure, 101
    race/lineage in, 110–111
Knibbs, Susan, 436f
Konted (Uma ritual), 410

Language
    culture-value conflict assessment tool
        and, 181–182
    in transcultural communicative
        spiritual-ethical caring, 119
Legislation, culture-value conflict
    assessment tool and, 186–188
Leininger, Madeleine, 7, 20, 38, 39, 42,
    105–106
Love (agape), 42, 143
    caring and, 10
    in transcultural caring, 52

Maeng people, pregnancy/childbirth
    practices of, 407–408
Maleficence, in nursing, 81–83
Mance, Jeanne, 38
Marginal status/marginality, culture-value
    conflict assessment tool and, 184
Maslow's hierarchy of needs, 18
Mathew, Lalitha, 435f
Maykut, Colleen, 436f
McCarthy, Patrice, 434f
Medieval ethics, 70
Meunier, Melissa, 436f
Mill, John Stuart, 72
Miyagishima, Meagan, 436f
Mohammed (the Prophet), 69
Moral concepts, changes in, 68–69
Moses, 69
Multicultural self, 16
Multiculturalism, 10, 111–112
    culture and, 15–16
    transcultural context and,
        112–114
Muslims
    in Thailand, transcultural caring
        experiences, 342–351
    in U.S., transcultural caring experiences
        of, 296–306
Myth spirituality, 141

Native American spirituality, 42. See also
    Aboriginal/native religions
Natural Law, 69
Navajo elder in nursing home,
    transcultural caring experiences of,
    271–276
Needs, hierarchy of (Maslow), 18
New Age/integrative spirituality, 141–142
Nguyen, Nga, 435f
Nightingale, Florence, 37–39, 45
    caring philosophy of, 44
    on mystical experience, 148–149
    spiritual calling of, 132
    virtue ethics and, 73
Nonmaleficence, 74
Nursing
    basis of caring in, 39
    contemporary perceptions of caring in,
        49–52
    globalization in, 7–8
    maleficence in, 81–83
    spiritual belongingness and, 148–149
    spiritual caring in, 149–150
    spiritual healing and, 152
    spirituality and, 132–133
    transcultural, in practice, 19–20
    transcultural caring ethics in, 85–90
    transcultural caring
        evidence/competency in, 206–209

Obama, Barack, 15, 250
Obyen (Uma ritual), 410
Old Testament, 69, 136

Panethnic choice, 113–114
Panethnicity, 10, 111–112
Paradigm(s)
    definition of, 16
    of nursing, 17, 21
    ways of knowing and, 17–18
Patient Protection and Affordable Care
    Act (PPACA, 2010), 19, 45, 52
Philippines, transcultural caring
    experiences of indigenous
    people of Cordilleras region,
    401–419
Philosophy, caring and, 43–44
Pilgrimage, as pillar of Islam, 138
Plato, 70
Political science, caring and, 47–48
Political theologies, 142–144
Population(s), North American,
    racial/ethnic demographics in, 6
Porter, Meredith, 436f
Postnatal care, among Amtuagan
    people, 408
PPACA. See Patient Protection and
    Affordable Care Act
Pregnancy
    Isneg practices, 409
    Maeng practices, 407

Prejudice, culture-value conflict
    assessment tool and, 185
Principle-based universalism, 84
Puerto Rican community, Western
    New York, transcultural caring
    experiences of, 256–259

Qur'an, 42, 69, 138, 146

Race
    controversy over concept of, 10
    in kinship structure, 110–111
Racialized ethnicity, 111
Ramadan, 137–138, 146
Ray, Marilyn, 433f, 434f, 438f
Religion, 144
    caring and, 42
    idea of the good and, 79
Religious, definition of, 135
Religious women, 38
Renaissance ethics, 70
Respect, in transcultural communicative
    spiritual-ethical caring, 119
Responsibility, in transcultural caring
    competency, 208–209
Rights, individual/collective,
    multiculturalism and, 112
Rituals, cultural
    birthing/childcare
        of Badeo community, 404–405
        of Isneg people, 409–410
        of Uma people, 410–411
    culture-value conflict assessment tool
        and, 182–183

Salat (prayer), as pillar of Islam,
    137, 146
Science, caring and, 45–47
The Self, multicultural, 16
Self-reflection, caring through, 9
Sermon on the Mount, 71, 145–146
Sex worker, abused HIV-infected, healed
    through education/love, 313–319
Shamanism, in Ecuador, transcultural
    caring experiences of, 307–312
Shi'a Islam, 138
Shintoism, 140
Simultaneity paradigm, 17
Social categories, 101
Social class, culture-value conflict
    assessment tool and, 183–184
Social contract theory, 72
Sociocultural behavior, dynamic cultural
    context and, 107
Socrates, 70
Spiritual belongingness, 145–146
    complexity sciences and, 146–148
    nursing and, 148–149
    world community and, 148
Spiritual-ethical caring, 170–172
Spiritual healing, 151–153

Spiritual/spirituality
  caring and, 42–43
  definition of, 135
  myth, 141
Spiritual suffering, 151
Stereotyping, culture-value conflict
  assessment tool and, 183
Sufism, 138
Summa Theologiae (Aquinas), 70
Sunni Islam, 138
Symbols/symbolism
  in Christianity, 137
  cultural practices and, 106–107
  in culture-value conflict assessment
    tool, 181
  in Hinduism, 138–139
  in indigenous religious culture, 146
  in Islam, 138
  in myth spirituality, 141
  in Shintoism, 140

TCCBL. *See* Transcultural caring-based
    learning
Ten Commandments, 69, 146
Thailand, Buddhists/Muslims in,
    transcultural caring experiences,
    342–351
Theological, definition of, 134–135
Theory of Bureaucratic Caring, 41
35th International Association for Human
    Caring Conference (Kyoto, Japan),
    432–439, 432f
Time, culture-value conflict assessment
    tool and, 185
Topola, Leanne, 436f
Transactional relationship, nursing as, 39
Transcultural caring, 9–10, 19–20
  concepts in ensuring, 22b
  dynamics of, 50–52
  fundamentals of, 5
Transcultural caring-based learning
    (TCCBL), 4, 203–206
  learning group formation, 211–212
  pattern identification process in,
    209–211
  transcultural caring experiences
    and, 212
Transcultural Caring Dynamics in
    Nursing and Health-Care
    Theoretical Model, 4f, 20–21, 50
  center of, 168f
  dimensions of, 5
Transcultural caring dynamics tool,
    176–178
  universal environment, 176f

Transcultural caring ethics, 67–99
  dimension of model, 68f
  ethical theories, 69–78
  good/evil, as ethical conflict, 78–83
  in nursing, 85–90
  search for understanding through,
    83–85
Transcultural caring experiences
  of abused HIV-infected sex worker
    healed through education/love,
    313–319
  of African-American community,
    223–229
  of American Chinese family in China,
    290–295
  American Mexican, 216–222
  of Asian Indian widow, 235–238
  in awareness/understanding/choice,
    190–192
  of Buddhists/Muslims in Thailand,
    342–351
  Cuban American, 250–255
  in Danish/Norwegian culture nursing
    care model, 374–387
  in essence of caring, 53–58
  of Filipino nurse, 239–243
  of Guatemalan Mayan farmworker,
    230–234
  of Haitian family in U.S., 267–270
  of Haitian girl and nurse practitioner in
    adolescent correctional facility,
    277–281
  of indigenous people of Cordilleras, the
    Philippines, 401–419
  Jamaican, 244–249
  of Japanese graduate nursing students,
    328–341
  in Jewish spiritual culture, 282–289
  of multiculturalism/interculturality in
    Canada, 320–327
  of Muslims in U.S., 296–306
  of Navajo elder in nursing home,
    271–276
  of nurse manager in cardiovascular
    ICU, 260–266
  of Puerto Rican community in Western
    New York, 256–259
  relating to Ebola in sub-Saharan Africa,
    352–357
  relating to UN global initiatives for
    caring/peace/quality of life, 388–400
  in rural Haiti, 420–430
  of shamanism in Ecuador, 307–312
  transcultural caring-based learning
    process and, 212

in transcultural caring dynamics, 24–26
  in transcultural caring ethics, 91–94
  in transcultural context for transcultural
    nursing, 121–123
  in universal sources, 155–159
Transcultural caring negotiation tool, 189,
    189f
Transcultural caring tool for choice,
    188–189, 188f
Transcultural Communicative
    Spiritual-Ethical CARING tool
    for Cultural Competency, 51f,
    178, 179f
Transcultural consciousness, 20
Transcultural context, 100–130
  model of, 101f
Transcultural ethics, 75–77
Transcultural spiritual ethical caring
    action of nursing, 175f
Transcultural worldview, paradigms/ways
    of knowing in, 16–18
Turkel, Marian, 433f, 434f, 438f
Turkel, Michael Brooks, 438f

Uma people, pregnancy/childbirth
    practices of, 410–411
Understanding, in transcultural caring
    inquiry, 168
Unitary-transformative (UT) paradigm, 17
United Nations' global initiatives for
    caring/peace/quality of life,
    transcultural caring experiences
    relating to, 388–400
United States, immigration and population
    growth in, 6
Universal Sources, 131–165
  dimension of model, 132f
  dynamics of, 133–136
  major religions/philosophies,
    136–144
  the religious person, 144–145
  spiritual belongingness and,
    145–153
Utilitarianism, 72, 73

Vedas, 138
Veracity, 74
Virtue ethics, 72–73

Wagner, Lynne, 438f
Wahhabism, 138
Watson, Jean, 435f
Ways of knowing (epistemology),
    47, 48
  in transcultural worldview, 17–18